AUTOIMMUNE DISEASES – CONTRIBUTING FACTORS, SPECIFIC CASES OF AUTOIMMUNE DISEASES, AND STEM CELL AND OTHER THERAPIES

Edited by **James Chan**

Autoimmune Diseases – Contributing Factors, Specific Cases of Autoimmune Diseases, and Stem Cell and Other Therapies
http://dx.doi.org/10.5772/2896
Edited by James Chan

Contributors

Marcus Muller, Rachael Terry, Stephen D. Miller, Daniel R. Getts, Ahmad Massoud, Amir Hossein Massoud, Nicola Gagliani, Samuel Huber, Dan Li, Miranda Piccioni, Zhimei Gao, Chen Chen, Zuojia Chen, Jia Nie, Zhao Shan, Yangyang Li, Andy Tsun, Bin Li, Reginald Halaby, Alla Arefieva, Marina Krasilshchikova, Olga Zatsepina, Anna Pituch-Noworolska, Katarzyna Zwonarz, J.P.S. Peron, D. Oliveira, W. N. Brandão, A. Fickinger, A. P. Ligeiro de Oliveira, L. V. Rizzo, N.O.S. Câmara, Reuben Mari Valenzuela, Paayal Patel, Jorge C. Kattah, Marco Wiltgen, Gernot P. Tilz, Eun Wha Choi, Jesus Ciriza, Jennifer O. Manilay, Rizwanul Haque, Fengyang Lei, Xiaofang Xiong, Jianxun Song, Katerina Chatzidionysiou, A.A. Baranov, E.I. Alexeeva, L.S. Namazova-Baranova, T.M. Bzarova, S.I. Valiyeva, R.V. Denisova, K.B. Isayeva, A.M. Chomakhidze, E.G. Chistyakova, T.V. Sleptsova, E.V. Mitenko, E.I. Zelikovich, G.V. Kurilenko, E.L. Semikina, A.V. Anikin, A.M. Stepanchenko, N.I. Taybulatov, A.V. Starikova, I.V. Dvoryakovskiy, M.V. Ryazanov

Published by InTech

Janeza Trdine 9, 51000 Rijeka, Croatia

Publishing Process Manager Marijan Polić
Technical Editor InTech Prepress, Novi Sad
Cover InTech Design team

Additional hard copies can be obtained from orders@intechopen.com

Autoimmune Diseases – Contributing Factors, Specific Cases of
Autoimmune Diseases, and Stem Cell and Other Therapies, Edited by James Chan
p. cm.
ISBN 978-953-51-0693-7

For EU product safety concerns:
IN TECH d.o.o., Prolaz Marije Krucifikse Kozulić 3, 51000 Rijeka, Croatia,
info@intechopen.com or visit our website at intechopen.com.

Meet the editor

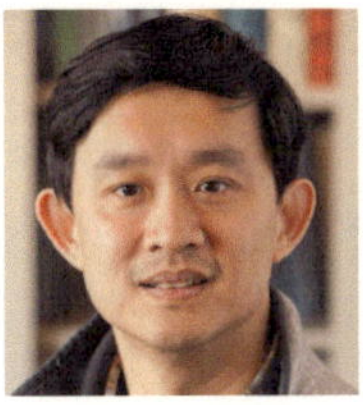

Dr James Chan's main research interests focus on tolerance induction, autoimmune diseases, gene therapy and stem cell therapy. It is the aim of combining these areas of research that one day the fruits of this research can benefit patients at the clinic. He conducts his research using two autoimmune disease models, namely diabetes and experimental autoimmune encephalomyelitis (EAE), a model for the human disease multiple sclerosis. There are 2 main areas in his research namely 1) using gene therapy technique to genetically modify haematopoietic stem cells to induce immune tolerance for the treatment of autoimmune disease and 2) the use of stem cells from various tissues such as placental stem cells and bone marrow mesenchymal stem cells for the treatment of autoimmune diseases.

Contents

Preface XI

Section 1 Pathogenesis of Autoimmune Disease 1

Chapter 1 **Current Theories for Multiple Sclerosis Pathogenesis and Treatment 3**
Marcus Muller, Rachael Terry, Stephen D. Miller and Daniel R. Getts

Chapter 2 **Immunologic and Genetic Factors in Type 1 Diabetes Mellitus 25**
Ahmad Massoud and Amir Hossein Massoud

Chapter 3 **Balancing Pro- and Anti-Inflammatory CD4+ T Helper Cells in the Intestine 51**
Nicola Gagliani and Samuel Huber

Chapter 4 **T Cell Metabolism in Autoimmune Diseases 77**
Dan Li, Miranda Piccioni, Zhimei Gao, Chen Chen, Zuojia Chen, Jia Nie, Zhao Shan, Yangyang Li, Andy Tsun and Bin Li

Chapter 5 **Apoptosis and Autoimmune Disorders 99**
Reginald Halaby

Section 2 Specific Autoimmune Diseases 117

Chapter 6 **Immune Complex Deposits as a Characteristic Feature of Mercury-Induced SLE-Like Autoimmune Process in Inbred and Outbred Mice 119**
Alla Arefieva, Marina Krasilshchikova and Olga Zatsepina

Chapter 7 **Celiac and Inflammatory Bowel Diseases in Children with Primary Humoral Immunodeficiency 151**
Anna Pituch-Noworolska and Katarzyna Zwonarz

Chapter 8 **Central Nervous System Resident Cells in Neuroinflammation: A Brave New World 173**
J.P.S. Peron, D. Oliveira, W. N. Brandão, A. Fickinger, A. P. Ligeiro de Oliveira, L. V. Rizzo and N.O.S. Câmara

Chapter 9 **Autoimmune Encephalitis in Rural Central Illinois 193**
Reuben Mari Valenzuela, Paayal Patel and Jorge C. Kattah

Chapter 10 **The Role of the Antigen GAD 65 in Diabetes Mellitus Type 1: A Molecular Analysis 207**
Marco Wiltgen and Gernot P. Tilz

Section 3 Stem Cell and Other Therapies for Autoimmune Disease 251

Chapter 11 **New Therapeutic Challenges in Autoimmune Diseases 253**
Eun Wha Choi

Chapter 12 **Stem Cell Therapies for Type I Diabetes 281**
Jesus Ciriza and Jennifer O. Manilay

Chapter 13 **Stem Cell-Based Cellular Therapy in Rheumatoid Arthritis 319**
Rizwanul Haque, Fengyang Lei, Xiaofang Xiong and Jianxun Song

Chapter 14 **Biologic Treatment in Rheumatoid Arthritis 343**
Katerina Chatzidionysiou

Chapter 15 **Biologic Therapy in Patients with Juvenile Idiopathic Arthritis – A Unique Single Centre Experience at the Scientific-Research Pediatric Centre in the Russian Federation 357**
A.A. Baranov, E.I. Alexeeva, L.S. Namazova-Baranova, T.M. Bzarova, S.I. Valiyeva, R.V. Denisova, K.B. Isayeva, A.M. Chomakhidze, E.G. Chistyakova, T.V. Sleptsova, E.V. Mitenko, E.I. Zelikovich, G.V. Kurilenko, E.L. Semikina, A.V. Anikin, A.M. Stepanchenko, N.I. Taybulatov, A.V. Starikova, I.V. Dvoryakovskiy and M.V. Ryazanov

Preface

Autoimmune disease represents a group of more than 60 different chronic autoimmune diseases that affect approximately 6% of the population. It is the third major category of illness in the United States and many industrialized countries, following heart disease and cancer. Autoimmune diseases arise when one's immune system actively targets and destroys self tissue resulting in clinical disease. Common examples include Systemic Lupus Erythematosus, Type 1 Diabetes, Rheumatoid Arthritis and Multiple Sclerosis. While different in clinical features and may involve different organs, the underlying mechanism is the failure of immune tolerance of the adaptive immune system.

The immune system is designed to protect us from foreign pathogens such as viruses and bacteria, and in particular the adaptive immune system mounts antigen specific attack on targets. The underlying mechanism that enables recognition and responses to unknown targets is the generation of antigen receptors on lymphocytes through the process of random gene recombination. A negative consequence of this process is the generation of self-reactive receptors capable of responding to self-antigens and causing pathology. Although a number of mechanisms such as clonal deletion and other immune regulations are in place to eliminate or counter the action of these self-reactive clones, a number of known factors can interfere and breakdown these regulatory mechanisms.

This book entitled "Autoimmune Diseases - Contributing Factors, Specific Cases of Autoimmune Diseases, and Stem Cell and Other Therapies" aims to present the latest knowledge and insights regarding the different contributing factors and their interplay, discussions on several autoimmune diseases and their case studies, and therapeutic treatments, including stem cell, for autoimmune diseases. The quest in this field of research is to better understand the underlying factors and pathways leading to autoimmune diseases and derive proper treatment for each disease.

I believe this book will provide an invaluable resource for researchers and students in the field of autoimmunity/immune tolerance, and also for a general readership to better understanding autoimmune diseases.

James Chan Ph.D.
Department of Medicine, Monash University,
Australia

Section 1

Pathogenesis of Autoimmune Disease

Chapter 1

Current Theories for Multiple Sclerosis Pathogenesis and Treatment

Marcus Muller, Rachael Terry, Stephen D. Miller and Daniel R. Getts

Additional information is available at the end of the chapter

http://dx.doi.org/10.5772/50005

1. Introduction

Multiple Sclerosis (MS) is a chronic, progressive, immune mediated central nervous system (CNS) disorder that affects both adults and children. MS is characterized by the formation of multiple lesions along the nerve fibers in the brain, spinal cord and optic nerves (Bradl and Lassmann, 2009; Bruck, 2005; Bruck and Stadelmann, 2005; Chitnis *et al.*, 2009; Hafler, 2004; Holland, 2009; Mah and Thannhauser, 2010; Pohl *et al.*, 2007). The precise triggers of autoreactive T cell development remain to be fully understood, however, it is clear that myelin antigens are the major target (Grau-Lopez *et al.*, 2009). T cell activation results in cytokine release and recruitment of other immune cells that results in tissue damage not only to the myelin sheath but, over time and with repeated attacks, to the underlying axons as well. Demyelination and axonal damage impairs or interrupts nerve transmission, giving rise to clinical signs and symptoms.

Clinically, neurological symptoms in patients with MS vary from mild to severe and typically include one or more of the following: sensory symptoms (numbness, tingling, other abnormal sensations, visual disturbances, dizziness), motor symptoms (weakness, difficulty walking, tremor, bowel/bladder problems, poor coordination, and stiffness), and other symptoms such as heat sensitivity, fatigue, emotional changes, cognitive changes and sexual symptoms (Bronner *et al.*, 2010). While some persons have a limited number of "attacks" or "relapses" and remain fairly healthy for decades, others may deteriorate rapidly from the time of diagnosis, with poor quality of life and shortened lifespan. There is no way of knowing at the clinical onset what course the disease will take (Andersen, 2010; Bradl and Lassmann, 2009; Bruck, 2005).

In this chapter how the autoimmune process is triggered as well as current clinical options to try and reduce disease symptoms are addressed. While the induction of long-term durable antigen-specific T cell tolerance is the desired treatment option, such a therapy remains to be clinically developed. Instead, once a diagnosis of MS is made, immune based treatment is generally begun, with numerous therapies aimed primarily at inactivating T cells and other immune functions.

2. Multiple Sclerosis triggers and animal models

The ability for the immune system to differentiate between self and non-self is critical for host preservation. Deficits in self-non-self discrimination can result in opportunistic infections or immunological over-reactivity resulting in immunopathology and autoimmunity. It is therefore, not surprising that multiple genetic factors that influence the sensitivity of the immune system are known to trigger autoimmune mediated diseases. However it is hypothesized that clinical symptom development may only manifest after exposure to certain environmental factors, including viral infection. The interplay of genetics and the environment in regards to the development of MS, and other autoimmune diseases, has not been completely elucidated. No matter what the potential switch that causes MS initiation the activation, proliferation and effector functions of auto-reactive $CD4^+$ T cells appears to be critical for disease development and progression (Goverman, 2009; Miller and Eagar, 2001; Miller et al., 2001).

i. Predisposing genetic factors

The significantly higher concordance rates of MS in monozygotic twins compared to dizygotic twins (Hansen *et al.*, 2005; Islam *et al.*, 2006; Willer *et al.*, 2003), the 2-fold increased risk of disease development in siblings of affected individuals (Ebers *et al.*, 2004) as well as the observed increased susceptibility in offspring from two affected parents, compared to those with only one affected parent (Ebers *et al.*, 2000; Robertson *et al.*, 1997) all point to a strong genetic component in the pathogenesis of MS. However, like many other complex autoimmune diseases, MS is not transferred from parent to offspring via classic Mendelian genetics and the disease trait involves a large number of genes (Hoffjan and Akkad, 2010). Until recently, most gene variations associated with increased or decreased susceptibility were thought to be within the human leukocyte antigen (HLA) loci (Ramagopalan *et al.*, 2009). However, recent studies have also identified risk-conferring alleles within several non-HLA genes (Nischwitz *et al.*, 2011). Importantly, most of these genes are known to play important roles in T cell activation and function, which further supports the concept that a dysfunctional immune process is involved in the initiation and progression of MS (Nischwitz *et al.*, 2011).

ii. HLA genes

Allelic variations within the major histocompatibility complex (MHC) exert the greatest individual effect on the risk of MS (Ramagopalan *et al.*, 2009). Initial studies published in 1972 identified the HLA Class I antigens *HLA-A*03* and *HLA-B*07* as risk-conferring alleles (Jersild *et al.*, 1972; Naito *et al.*, 1972). Between 1973 and 1976, several studies reported a significant link between the HLA Class II gene HLA-DR2 and MS (Jersild *et al.*, 1973; Terasaki *et al.*, 1976; Winchester *et al.*, 1975). This has been further subtyped into a strong and consistent association between the *HLA-DRB5*0101*, *HLA-DRB1*1501*, *HLA-DQA1*0102* and *HLA-DQB1*0602* extended haplotype and disease (Fogdell *et al.*, 1995). As these genes are tightly linked, early genetic studies failed to identify which of these alleles confers the greatest risk for MS (Hoppenbrouwers and Hintzen, 2011). However, statistically-powered studies conducted in the past decade, including several international genome-wide association studies (GWAS), have identified *HLA-DRB1*1501* as the major risk conferring gene for the development of MS (2007; 2009; Hafler *et al.*, 2007; Lincoln *et al.*, 2005; Oksenberg *et al.*, 2004; Sawcer *et al.*, 2011).

Other HLA-DR2 alleles that confer susceptibility in some populations include *HLA-DRB1*17* and *HLA-DRB1*08*, however the effects of these alleles are modest compared to *HLA-DRB1*1501* (Dyment *et al.*, 2005; Modin *et al.*, 2004). Some variants are also reported to confer protection from the development of MS, including *HLA-DRB1*14*, *HLA-DRB1*01*, *HLA-DRB1*10* and *HLA-DRB1*11* (Brynedal *et al.*, 2007; Dyment *et al.*, 2005; Ramagopalan *et al.*, 2007).

iii. Non-HLA genes

Early gene linkage studies failed to validate associations between non-HLA genes and the development of MS, potentially due to the small individual contribution of each gene to disease (Nischwitz *et al.*, 2011). However, in recent years, several GWAS have identified polymorphisms within a number of non-HLA genes that play an important role in the development of MS (Pravica *et al.*, 2012). These include genes that are involved in cytokine pathways, such as those encoding the IL-2, IL-7, IL-12 and TNF receptors, which are important for T cell development, homeostasis, proliferation and differentiation (2009; Baranzini *et al.*, 2009; Sawcer *et al.*, 2011).

Also, variations within genes coding for co-stimulatory molecules, such as CD40, CD58, CD80 and CD86, which promote the activation of T cells, were also implicated in susceptibility to MS (2009; Baranzini *et al.*, 2009; Sawcer *et al.*, 2011). Polymorphisms within genes encoding for molecules such as STAT3 and TYK2, which are involved in several signal transduction pathways including those that mediate T cell activation and Th17 differentiation, were also linked with the development of MS (2009; Baranzini *et al.*, 2009; Sawcer *et al.*, 2011).

Variations within other genes that can affect T cell functioning, including CD6, CLEC16A, and the vitamin D alpha hydroxylase gene CYP27B1 are also implicated in the pathogenesis of MS (2009; Baranzini *et al.*, 2009; Sawcer *et al.*, 2011). Although the individual contribution of each gene to the development of MS is modest, the identification of such genes is critical, as they will provide novel targets or approaches for therapeutic intervention in MS (Nischwitz *et al.*, 2011).

There is clearly further research to be performed to better understand the role of genetics and MS development. However the data clearly show that genes associated with T cell activation and other immune functions certainly highlight the importance of targeting immune factors when treating disease.

3. Environmental factors

Although it is clear that genetics play a key role in determining susceptibility to MS, concordance rates between monozygotic twins (*i.e.* with identical genomes) varies between 6 and 30 percent (Dyment *et al.*, 2004). This suggests that other non-inheritable factors play an important role in the initiation of the auto-reactive immune response. A number of infectious and non-infectious stimuli have been identified as key factors that increase the risk of MS development.

i. Infectious factors

For many years, underlying infections have been implicated in the induction of the autoreactive $CD4^+$ T cell response that leads to MS (Kakalacheva and Lunemann, 2011). Roles for several pathogens, including Epstein Barr Virus (EBV), Human Herpes Virus-6 (HHV-6) and Varicella Zoster Virus (VZV) have been investigated. There is considerable evidence that links EBV with the initiation and progression of MS (Ascherio and Munger, 2007a, b; Dyment *et al.*, 2004). EBV infects over 90% of the world population and causes infectious mononucleosis (IM) in a large proportion of individuals, which is characterized by glandular fever and the massive expansion of virus-specific T cells (Vetsika and Callan, 2004). Pooled data from 18 clinical studies revealed a significant link between IM and an elevated risk of MS (Kakalacheva *et al.*, 2011).

Furthermore, in individuals that concurrently tested positive for IM and the HLA allele *HLA-DRB1*1501*, the risk of developing MS was increased by 7-fold (Kakalacheva and Lunemann, 2011). Also, an increased proportion of MS patients are seropositive for EBV, however, it is important to note that not all patients are seropositive which suggests that EBV infection is not critical for the development of disease (Kakalacheva and Lunemann, 2011; Kakalacheva *et al.*, 2011). Nevertheless, taken together these studies support the concept that EBV infection may at least increase the risk of MS development in genetically susceptible individuals. The mechanisms by which EBV infection trigger the autoreactive immune response are unclear, but some data suggest that $CD4^+$ T cells in MS patients are specific for an increased range of EBV nuclear antigens, which frequently recognize myelin peptides (Lang *et al.*, 2002; Olson *et al.*, 2001). Further investigations into the role of infection in the development of disease are needed to show definitively the role of virus infection in the pathogenesis of MS.

ii. Non-infectious factors

Smoking and Vitamin D have been identified as the two primary non-infectious environmental factors that can contribute to MS susceptibility. Although the elevated risk of MS development in individuals who smoke was originally identified in a study in the 1960's (reviewed in (Wingerchuk, 2012)), it has become more prominent in recent years. Smoking is argued to increase the chance of MS development by a factor of 1.5 (Wingerchuk, 2012). In addition, patients that smoke increase the potential for rapid MS development. In a recent Belgium study, patients that smoked were more likely to develop a score of 6 on the Extended Disability Status Scale. This represents an increased potential to develop intermittent or unilateral constant assistance (cane, crutch or brace) required to walk 100 meters without resting (D'Hooghe M *et al.*, 2012). The amount or timing of cigarette exposure to enhance MS risk remains to be defined, with linkage between smoking and MS remaining a predominately epidemiological observation. Further research is required to better define the role and process of smoking exposure in MS development and progression.

Vitamin D is a potent immunomodulatory molecule that has been shown to affect numbers and activity of regulatory T cells. Several epidemiological studies have identified a significant link between the incidence of MS and distance from the equator (Kurtzke *et al.*, 1979; Miller *et al.*, 1990; Vukusic *et al.*, 2007). Although MS occurred more frequently at high latitudes, this effect was negated in populations that consumed a vitamin D-rich diet (Agranoff and Goldberg, 1974; Swank *et al.*, 1952; Westlund, 1970). These findings are supported by a large study in which high serum levels of the vitamin D metabolite 25(OH)D were shown to correspond with a significantly decreased risk of MS (Munger *et al.*, 2006). In a separate study, low serum levels of 25(OH)D were associated with relapse and the degree of disability in MS patients (Smolders *et al.*, 2008a).

A possible explanation for these findings is the indirect immunomodulatory functions of vitamin D on T cells (Bartels *et al.*, 2010; Smolders *et al.*, 2008b). Also, T cells express vitamin D receptors (VDR), suggesting a direct vitamin D- T cell interaction resulting in T cell regulation (Cantorna, 2011). Indeed, a recent study using the EAE mouse model demonstrated that vitamin D could inhibit auto-reactive T cells, which express high levels of VDR, but did not affect numbers of regulatory T cells, which express low levels of VDR (Mayne *et al.*, 2011). An earlier study also showed that survival of EAE-induced mice could be prolonged with vitamin D injection (Hayes, 2000).

4. Epitope spreading and disease progression

Multiple sclerosis is initiated by the activation of auto-reactive $CD4^+$ T cells specific for a single or few myelin epitopes in the CNS (Vanderlugt and Miller, 2002). Inflammation caused by this initial response recruits and activates other $CD4^+$ T cell clones specific for a range of other self-epitopes, a process which is referred to as "epitope spreading" (Lehmann *et al.*, 1992). This process occurs, within experimental settings, in a hierarchical fashion, likely the result of differential antigen liberation, processing and presentation by various antigen-presenting cell (APC) populations. In addition the availability of self-reactive $CD4^+$ T cell clones throughout the course of disease is also important. Epitope spreading was originally described and characterized in the Experimental Autoimmune Encephalomyelitis (EAE) model of MS, but also occurs in Theiler's murine encephalomyelitis virus induced demeylinating disease (TMEV-IDD) (Lehmann *et al.*, 1992; Miller *et al.*, 2001; Miller *et al.*, 1997b; Vanderlugt *et al.*, 2000). Evidence has also accumulated supporting the existence of epitope spreading within the human context.

1. Epitope spreading in EAE

Experimental autoimmune encephalomyelitis is induced in susceptible murine strains by immunization with myelin peptides in conjunction with adjuvant (Miller *et al.*, 2010). This disease initiation method, with a single and defined myelin peptide allows for the observation and measurement of changing T cell specificities over time (Vanderlugt and Miller, 2002). Using this model epitope spreading has been described as a hierarchical event, with a defined path through which T cells specific for certain epitopes emerge. Epitope spreading is a critical phenomenon in the SJL model of EAE, as it is responsible for the relapsing remitting pattern of disease (Vanderlugt and Miller, 2002).

The first study to demonstrate epitope spreading was reported in 1992 by Lehmann and colleagues (Lehmann *et al.*, 1992), in which susceptible (SJLxB10.PL)F_1 mice were immunized with guinea-pig MBP. T cell responses in the draining lymph node and spleen were measured 9 days after immunization. At this time point, T cells only responded to MBP_{Ac1-11}, and not MBP_{35-47}, MBP_{81-100} or $MBP_{121-140}$. In comparison, T cells isolated from the spleen 40 days after immunization responded to all of these peptides. These findings demonstrate that epitopes that are initially hidden or sequestered during the initial phase of disease can become liberated as disease progresses (Lehmann *et al.*, 1992).

Studies in our laboratory have also characterized epitope spreading in EAE induced by immunization of SJL mice with the immunodominant PLP epitope $PLP_{139-151}$(Vanderlugt *et al.*, 2000). In this model, T cell responses are initially specific for $PLP_{139-151}$. However, the first relapse, which occurs within 30-40 days after immunization, coincides with T cell responses against $PLP_{178-191}$. During the second relapse, which occurs between 50-70 days after immunization, T cells are also shown to respond to MBP_{84-104}. Understanding of the epitope spreading hierarchy has allowed for epitope specific therapeutic targeting in EAE. The induction of tolerance against relapse-associated peptides blocks the progression of disease, even though $PLP_{139-151}$ responses remain intact (Vanderlugt *et al.*, 2000). These observations highlight the role of changing T cell specificities in mediating chronic disease as well as the need for therapeutic strategies that address these specific T cells populations (Vanderlugt and Miller, 2002).

2. Epitope spreading in TMEV-IDD

Theiler's murine encephalomyelitis virus- induced demyelinating disease is induced by intracranial inoculation of SJL/J mice with TMEV, resulting in low-level chronic CNS infection that progresses into myelin-specific autoimmune disease (Getts *et al.*, 2010). The initial $CD4^+$ T cell-mediated immune response against chronic TMEV infection of the CNS causes significant damage to myelin, which in turn results in the activation of myelin-specific T cell clones (Karpus *et al.*, 1995; Miller *et al.*, 1997a). Similar to EAE, this occurs in a hierarchical order, beginning with the immunodominant $PLP_{139-151}$ epitope (Miller *et al.*, 1997b). Subsequent T cell reactivity against other peptides, including $PLP_{178-191}$, PLP_{56-70} and MOG_{92-106} has been demonstrated as disease progresses (Miller *et al.*, 2001).

These findings correspond with antigen presentation by CNS APC. These cells present viral peptides but not myelin peptides up to day 40 post-immunization, at which time point there are still no clinical signs of disease and no evidence of myelin destruction (Katz-Levy *et al.*, 1999; Katz-Levy *et al.*, 2000). However, by day 90 post-infection, microglia and macrophages isolated from the CNS present both viral and myelin antigens to T cells *in vitro* (Katz-Levy *et al.*, 1999; Katz-Levy *et al.*, 2000).

In further support of epitope spreading after TMEV inoculation, tolerance induction to multiple myelin epitopes using MP-4 during ongoing TMEV-IDD in SJL mice was shown to significantly attenuate disease progression, reduce demyelination and decrease CNS leukocyte infiltration (Neville *et al.*, 2002).

3. Epitope spreading in MS

Evidence of epitope spreading in human MS patients is growing, with a number of small studies at least supporting a potential for epitope spreading in human disease. A study by Tuohy and colleagues conducted over several years followed peripheral T cell responses to myelin epitopes in three patients with isolated monosymptomatic demyelinating syndrome (IMDS) (Tuohy *et al.*, 1997; Tuohy *et al.*, 1999a; Tuohy *et al.*, 1999b). T cell autoreactivity to several myelin epitopes was initially shown to be strong, waning with time. However, when two of these three patients progressed to clinically-defined MS, peripheral T cells isolated from these patients showed expanded reactivity to different myelin peptides than originally observed during the patients IMDS stage (Tuohy *et al.*, 1997; Tuohy *et al.*, 1999a; Tuohy *et al.*, 1999b). A separate study by Goebels and colleagues investigated MBP-specific responses of five MS patients over 6-7 years (Goebels *et al.*, 2000). Two of these patients showed a focused T cell response that broadened over the course of 6 years, thus providing evidence of epitope spreading in human disease. The pattern was non-consistent, however, with two patients showing a broad epitope response that fluctuated over time, with the other patient exhibiting a very focused response to a cluster of MBP epitopes. Together the data suggest that unlike the EAE model, patient T cell epitopes exhibit strong heterogeneity with the precise epitope spreading hierarchy likely to be variable between patients. Not withstanding, the liberation of antigens and activation of novel T cell clones over time in MS patients supports the role of epitope spreading in human MS patients (Goebels *et al.*, 2000).

5. Current clinical strategies in Multiple Sclerosis to modify the course of disease

The pathologic role of T cells in driving MS has resulted in numerous therapies aimed at inactivating T cells and/or the induction of T cell tolerance. Tolerance induction in autoimmune disease refers to a reinstatement of sustained, specific non-responsiveness of the native immune system to self-antigen. Manipulation of T cell activation and differentiation pathways has been at the center of current tolerance induction theory, and the basis of tolerance induction utilizing current immunosuppressive agents. Over recent years, experimental models have shown that it is possible to exploit the mechanisms that normally maintain immune homeostasis and tolerance to self-antigens, as well as to reintroduce tolerance to self-antigen in an autoimmune setting (Getts *et al.*, 2011; Kohm *et al.*, 2005; Podojil *et al.*, 2008; Turley and Miller, 2007). However, in the clinical setting the utilization of co-stimulatory blockade, soluble peptide, altered peptide ligands among others have yielded disappointing results. As such while the induction of tolerance remains the optimal future treatment for MS current therapies are focused on agents that are disease modifying.

Over the last three decades a number of broad acting immune modifying therapeutic options have been developed and introduced to treat MS patients. None of these therapeutic options is a cure, currently available therapies aim instead to prevent or at least reduce the frequency of relapsing inflammatory events, with the idea of reducing impact of disease on overall quality of life over time (Miller and Rhoades, 2012; Rio *et al.*, 2011). In addition to the clear efficacy requirement long-term safety is also paramount for any MS therapy, with typical MS patients requiring treatment for many decades. The available MS therapies may be divided based on function into "immune modulatory" or "disease modifying" drugs (DMFs) as well as classic immune suppressive substances. In addition, a third group has recently emerged, which includes monoclonal antibodies (biologics). These drugs act by direct interference with specific immune system functions or by broad immune subset depletion. DMFs are typically used early in the course of the disease, whereas immune suppressive drugs and biologics are mostly viewed as treatment options in those patients with abnormally high disease activity, a high risk of sustained disability and/or show poor response to the front line therapeutics (Table 1).

The most widely used disease modifying drugs are Interferon-β (IFNβ) and glatiramer acetate (GLAT) (Johnson, 2012). Both drugs were approved after large phase III studies, which were conducted in the 1990s. These studies proved the efficacy of these drugs in relapsing remitting MS. IFN-β and GLAT reduce the relapse rate in relapsing remitting MS patients by up to 50% (Boster *et al.*, 2011; Johnson, 2012; Limmroth *et al.*, 2011). Furthermore, both agents significantly slowed the progression of disease and have an excellent safety profile allowing for long-term utilization. However, there remain a number of administration and efficacy issues with these drugs. Administration is required weekly at a minimum via subcutaneous or intramuscular injection, resulting in significant discomfort to patients. In addition, while IFN-β and GLAT have relatively comparable efficacy, there is some patient to patient variability. For example a patient that is not responsive to IFN-β may be responsive to GLAT and vice versa. Unfortunately no marker exists that may predict those populations that should be prescribed IFN-β over GLAT or GLAT over IFN-β. Currently trial and error serve as the best strategy for physicians to use when determining the optimal treatment regimen.

The exact mechanism(s) through which GLAT or IFN-β modify disease progression in MS patients are not completely defined, with multiple mechanisms likely to be involved. There is evidence suggesting IFN-β can inhibit T-cell co-stimulation and activation (Chen *et al.*, 2012). In an experimental setting, IFN-β inhibits immune-cell migration by increasing soluble Intercellular Adhesion Molecule 1 (ICAM-1) and Vascular Cell Adhesion Molecule-1 (VCAM-1), as well as by decreasing very late antigen-4 (VL4-4) on the cell surface of T cells. It has also been shown that IFN-β can stabilize the blood brain barrier by reducing matrix metalloproteinase-9, an important tissue degradation enzyme.

GLAT is a randomized mixture of synthetic polypeptides consisting of the amino acids l-alanine, l-lysine, l-glutamic acid and l-tyrosine. GLAT was originally designed to induce CNS inflammation in animals by stimulating the myelin auto-antigen MBP, however, subsequent studies showed that the product appeared to be a protective immunomodulator. The ability for this drug to prevent relapses and disease progression is supported by large clinical studies. Mechanistically, GLAT may compete with myelin peptides for access to peptide binding cleft in MHC complex (Racke and Lovett-Racke, 2011). In addition to MHC binding, GLAT may stimulate a TH2 environment through its ability to modulate APC such as dendritic cells and monocytes (Miller *et al.*, 1998). Evidence for the ability of GLAT to induce a TH2 biased immune response includes the finding that GLAT promotes the expression of anti-inflammatory cytokines such as IL-10 and TGF-β in the CNS of MS patients (Neuhaus *et al.*, 2001). More recent studies revealed that GLAT elevates the levels of T-regulatory (Tregs) cells and reduces the levels of potentially harmful Th-17 cells (Lalive *et al.*, 2011).

It is difficult to establish the long-term efficacy of drugs in MS because the disease can be highly variable and unpredictable. Still, the available long-term observational data point toward a significant prevention and delay of disability in most MS patients treated with either GLAT or IFN-β over a long time. Furthermore, there is sparse evidence that the early treatment reduces the long-term mortality of MS patients (Goodin *et al.*, 2012).

More recently, new disease-modifying drugs have become or are expected to soon be available (Buck and Hemmer, 2011; Fox and Rhoades, 2012) (Table 1). These drugs include more convenient agents that can be applied orally and may have enhanced efficacy in regards to reducing patient disease activity relative to GLAT or IFN-β (Killestein *et al.*, 2011) (Hartung and Aktas, 2011). However, the long-term safety profiles of these substances remains questionable, with more time needed to adequately address the safety profile of these agents.

If front line disease modifying therapies fail to provide sufficient relief, therapeutic escalation to include more effective therapies has to be considered (Repovic and Lublin, 2011). The most effective currently available therapy for escalation is the monoclonal antibody Natalizumab (Tysabri®). Natalizumab acts via the blockade of the VLA-4 receptor, which plays a significant role in leukocyte migration into the brain parenchyma (Rudick and Sandrock, 2004). Clinical studies with Natalizumab have shown this drug to have high efficacy in terms of its ability to prevent disease relapses and progression (Chaudhuri and Behan, 2003; O'Connor *et al.*, 2004). However, this efficacy comes at the cost of some significant safety issues. For example severe JC-Virus mediated encephalitis called "progressive multifocal leukencephalopathy" (PML) has been recorded in numerous patients receiving Natalizumab. This severe complication occurs in approximately 1:1000 patients. PML is severe, not only because it can potentiate MS symptoms, but because it can cause death (Berger and Koralnik, 2005; Langer-Gould *et al.*, 2005; Ransohoff, 2005). As a result of this treatment related risk, Natalizumab utilization is usually reserved for patients with highly active MS, who do not respond sufficiently to standard disease modifying therapies and subsequently likely to suffer rapid disease progression (Kappos *et al.*, 2011a; Keegan, 2011). Finally, Natalizumab must be given chronically for it to maximize its clinical effect. Patients that stop taking Natalizumab usually relapse, with patients developing symptoms similar to those experienced before Natalizumab therapy was initiated

Substance	Indication	Side-Effects	Comments
Interferon-β	**Scheme 1.** RR-MS, CIS	**Scheme 2.** Flu-like symptoms	**Scheme 3.** good safety profile, inconvenient administr., moderate efficacy (Sanford and Lyseng-Williamson, 2011)
Scheme 4. Glatirameracetate	**Scheme 5.** RR-MS, CIS	**Scheme 6.** Local irritation,	**Scheme 7.** good safety profile, inconvenient administr., moderate efficacy (Lalive *et al.*, 2011)
Scheme 8. Fingolimod	**Scheme 9.** RR-MS or escalation in RR-MS[1]	**Scheme 10.** Lymphopenia, arrhythmia, macular edema	**Scheme 11.** Increased relapse reduction compared to IFN-β (Singh *et al.*, 2011) (Jeffery *et al.*, 2011)
Scheme 12. Natalizumab	**Scheme 13.** Escalation in RR-MS	**Scheme 14.** Infections, hepatopathy, allergic response, PML	**Scheme 15.** Excellent efficacy, severe viral encephalitis as a dangerous side-effect (Keegan, 2011; Pucci *et al.*, 2011)
Scheme 16. Mitoxantrone	**Scheme 17.** Escalation in RR-MS, PP-MS, SP-MS, with fast progression	**Scheme 18.** Leukopenia, infections, cardiomyopathy, leukemia	**Scheme 19.** Immunosupressive escalation option. Option in progressive MS courses (Rizvi *et al.*, 2004; Stuve *et al.*, 2004)
Scheme 20. Cyclophosphamide	**Scheme 21.** Escalation in RR-MS, PP-MS, SP-MS, with fast progression	**Scheme 22.** Leukopenia, infections	**Scheme 23.** Therapeutic option if other escalation therapies including mitoxantrone fail (Rinaldi *et al.*, 2009; Weiner *et al.*, 1984)
Scheme 24. Teriflunomide	**Scheme 25.** RR-MS? (phase-III trial ongoing)	**Scheme 26.** lymphopenia, hepathopathy	**Scheme 27.** (Warnke *et al.*, 2009; Wood, 2011)
Scheme 28. BG-12 (fumaric acid)	**Scheme 29.** RR-MS? (phase-III trial ongoing)	**Scheme 30.** gastrointestinal complaints	**Scheme 31.** (Kappos *et al.*, 2008; Papadopoulou *et al.*, 2010)
Scheme 32. Laquinimode	**Scheme 33.** RR-MS? (phase-III trial ongoing)	**Scheme 34.** Hepatopathy, thrombosis?	**Scheme 35.** (Thone and Gold, 2011)
Scheme 36. Ocrelizumab	**Scheme 37.** Escalation therapy? (trials ongoing)	**Scheme 38.** Severe infections and sepsis possible, allergic response	**Scheme 39.** (Chaudhuri, 2012; Kappos *et al.*, 2011b)

Scheme 40. **Daclizumab**	**Scheme 41.** RR-MS, escalatation? (trials ongoing)	**Scheme 42.** Cutaneous rash, infections	**Scheme 43.** Increased relapse reduction compared to IFN-β likely (Stuve and Greenberg, 2010)
Scheme 44. **Alemtuzumab**	**Scheme 45.** Escalation therapy? (trials ongoing)	**Scheme 46.** Induction of autoimmune diseases, infections (Cossburn *et al.*, 2011)	**Scheme 47.** Increased relapse reduction compared to IFN-β (Coles *et al.*, 2012; Klotz *et al.*, 2012)

RR-MS: relapsing remitting Multiple sclerosis, CIS: clinical isolated syndrome, PP-MS: primary progressive Multiple Sclerosis, SP-MS: secondary progressive Multiple Sclerosis, [1]: Fingolimod is recommended as a first-line treamtent in the US but as an escalation therapy in the EU

Table 1.

(O'Connor *et al.*, 2011). The chronic treatment requirement increases patient risk and highlights the ongoing conundrum for all MS therapies, which is how to balance immune modulation efficacy with safety. The emergence of PML with Natalizumab is one striking example, however, more recent cardiac issues have been associated with the recently approved oral DMF, ingolomid (Gilyena), highlighting the point that all therapies focused on immune intervention require diligent safety studies.

The need for safer therapies, combined with animal data showing the ability for short course immune induction therapy (SCIIT) to induce long term disease remission, has supported a new approach to treating MS. SCIIT is a therapeutic strategy employing rapid, specific, short-term modulation of the immune system usually using a biologic therapeutic to induce long term T cell non-responsiveness. Alemtuzumab clinical studies are leading the way in employing this therapeutic concept. In this example, a one week dosing regimen with Alemtuzumab has been in phase 2 and 3 studies shown to have a long term dramatic impact on disease, reducing disease relapses for over a year (Coles *et al.*, 2008; Hauser, 2008; Moreau *et al.*, 1996). The ability for long lasting relapse prevention even after the treatment is discontinued is the primary objective of SCIIT. Unfortunately, from an immunological perspective, tolerance is the result of a number of T cell reprogramming pathways, not induced by Alemtuzumab. Alemtuzumab functions through long term whole scale immune cell depletion. While this drug may have great efficacy it come has added consequences including the potential for JC-virus infection, cancer and up to 20% of patients may develop other autoimmune diseases (notably Thyroiditis). As such newer therapies are required that focus on immune reprogramming and less on immune depletion. Some potential candidates in development may include Daclizumab (Wynn *et al.*, 2010), Ocrelizumab (Chaudhuri, 2012; Kappos *et al.*, 2011b) or the anti-alpha beta T cell receptor antibody, TOL101 (Table 1).

In situations where all other avenues have been exhausted and disease continues to progress at an unusually rapid rate, physicians may prescribe the chemotherapy drugs mitoxantrone or cyclophosphamide (Neuhaus *et al.*, 2006; Perini *et al.*, 2006; Rinaldi *et al.*, 2009; Stuve *et al.*, 2004; Theys *et al.*, 1981). These drugs are often considered as final options due to their potent immunosuppressive and other serious effects. These drugs can suppress both cell-mediated and humoral immunity and often result in lymphopenia, increasing malignancy and infection risk. Results from smaller clinical studies suggest, that treating with these immunosuppressive drugs at the very beginning of the disease and in addition to immune modulating drugs might have a beneficial impact on the course of the disease. However, the harmful side effects associated with these drugs means their use is usually restricted to patients that have failed other treatment options, such as Natalizumab.

6. Summary

Multiple Sclerosis (MS) is a chronic, progressive, immune mediated central nervous system disorder that affects both adults and children. The precise triggers of autoreactive T cell development remain to be fully understood, however, it appears that a host of genetic and environmental factors contribute to disease development. Disease initiation may be the result of a single myelin specific T cell clone being activated, however, animal models and preliminary human data suggest that epitope spreading which results in the activation of numerous myelin specific T cells is important for disease progression. Therapies capable of inducing T cell tolerance, thereby rendering these myelin specific T cells inactive remain to be developed for human use. Instead a number of disease modifying agents are available, with GLAT and IFN-β being the primary front line MS treatments. In those patients refractory to these therapies or who show a rapid disease progression, escalation to more broad acting therapies, such as Natalizumab may be considered. Unfortunately, while escalating therapies may have enhanced efficacy this comes with increases in safety concerns. In progressive MS patients whereby all other therapies have failed or no longer show efficacy more toxic chemotherapeutic agents are usually the last resort.

Currently within the field of MS treatment, reduction of relapse rates by around 50% is considered to be a success. As such even patients who are considered treatment successes suffer relapses. During these relapses CNS damage and epitope spreading continue to occur with further neurological impairment the result. Future therapies need to have a higher objective and bring the relapse rate down by 75-100%. This goal may not be out of reach with short course Alemtuzumab therapy shown to induce disease remission for an extended period of time. While the safety profile of this drug remains highly questionable, the observed efficacy certainly generates promise that safer more efficacious therapeutic options for MS treatment may soon be available.

Author details

Rachael Terry, Stephen D Miller and Daniel R. Getts
Microbiology-Immunology Department, Feinberg School of Medicine, Northwestern University, Chicago IL, USA

Marcus Muller
Department of Neurology, University of Bonn, Germany

Daniel R. Getts
Tolera Therapeutics, Inc, Kalamazoo, MI, USA

7. References

(2007) Genome-wide association study of 14,000 cases of seven common diseases and 3,000 shared controls. *Nature* 447, 661-678.

(2009) Genome-wide association study identifies new multiple sclerosis susceptibility loci on chromosomes 12 and 20. *Nat Genet* 41, 824-828.

Agranoff, B. W. and Goldberg, D. (1974) Diet and the geographical distribution of multiple sclerosis. *Lancet* 2, 1061-1066.

Andersen, O. (2010) Predicting a window of therapeutic opportunity in multiple sclerosis. *Brain* 133, 1863-1865.

Ascherio, A. and Munger, K. L. (2007a) Environmental risk factors for multiple sclerosis. Part I: the role of infection. *Ann Neurol* 61, 288-299.

Ascherio, A. and Munger, K. L. (2007b) Environmental risk factors for multiple sclerosis. Part II: Noninfectious factors. *Ann Neurol* 61, 504-513.

Baranzini, S. E., Wang, J., Gibson, R. A., Galwey, N., Naegelin, Y., Barkhof, F., Radue, E. W., Lindberg, R. L., Uitdehaag, B. M., Johnson, M. R., Angelakopoulou, A., Hall, L., Richardson, J. C., Prinjha, R. K., Gass, A., Geurts, J. J., Kragt, J., Sombekke, M., Vrenken, H., Qualley, P., Lincoln, R. R., Gomez, R., Caillier, S. J., George, M. F., Mousavi, H., Guerrero, R., Okuda, D. T., Cree, B. A., Green, A. J., Waubant, E., Goodin, D. S., Pelletier, D., Matthews, P. M., Hauser, S. L., Kappos, L., Polman, C. H. and Oksenberg, J. R. (2009) Genome-wide association analysis of susceptibility and clinical phenotype in multiple sclerosis. *Hum Mol Genet* 18, 767-778.

Bartels, L. E., Hvas, C. L., Agnholt, J., Dahlerup, J. F. and Agger, R. (2010) Human dendritic cell antigen presentation and chemotaxis are inhibited by intrinsic 25-hydroxy vitamin D activation. *Int Immunopharmacol* 10, 922-928.

Berger, J. R. and Koralnik, I. J. (2005) Progressive multifocal leukoencephalopathy and natalizumab--unforeseen consequences. *N Engl J Med* 353, 414-416.

Boster, A., Bartoszek, M. P., O'Connell, C., Pitt, D. and Racke, M. (2011) Efficacy, safety, and cost-effectiveness of glatiramer acetate in the treatment of relapsing-remitting multiple sclerosis. *Ther Adv Neurol Disord* 4, 319-332.

Bradl, M. and Lassmann, H. (2009) Progressive multiple sclerosis. *Semin Immunopathol.*

Bronner, G., Elran, E., Golomb, J. and Korczyn, A. D. (2010) Female sexuality in multiple sclerosis: the multidimensional nature of the problem and the intervention. *Acta Neurol Scand* 121, 289-301.

Bruck, W. (2005) The pathology of multiple sclerosis is the result of focal inflammatory demyelination with axonal damage. *J Neurol* 252 Suppl 5, v3-9.

Bruck, W. and Stadelmann, C. (2005) The spectrum of multiple sclerosis: new lessons from pathology. *Curr Opin Neurol* 18, 221-224.

Brynedal, B., Duvefelt, K., Jonasdottir, G., Roos, I. M., Akesson, E., Palmgren, J. and Hillert, J. (2007) HLA-A confers an HLA-DRB1 independent influence on the risk of multiple sclerosis. *PLoS One* 2, e664.

Buck, D. and Hemmer, B. (2011) Treatment of multiple sclerosis: current concepts and future perspectives. *J Neurol* 258, 1747-1762.

Cantorna, M. T. (2011) Why do T cells express the vitamin D receptor? *Ann N Y Acad Sci* 1217, 77-82.

Chaudhuri, A. (2012) Ocrelizumab in multiple sclerosis: risks and benefits. *Lancet* 379, 1196-1197; author reply 1197.

Chaudhuri, A. and Behan, P. O. (2003) Natalizumab for relapsing multiple sclerosis. *N Engl J Med* 348, 1598-1599; author reply 1598-1599.

Chen, M., Chen, G., Deng, S., Liu, X., Hutton, G. J. and Hong, J. (2012) IFN-beta induces the proliferation of CD4+CD25+Foxp3+ regulatory T cells through upregulation of GITRL on dendritic cells in the treatment of multiple sclerosis. *J Neuroimmunol* 242, 39-46.

Chitnis, T., Glanz, B., Jaffin, S. and Healy, B. (2009) Demographics of pediatric-onset multiple sclerosis in an MS center population from the Northeastern United States. *Mult Scler* 15, 627-631.

Coles, A. J., Compston, D. A., Selmaj, K. W., Lake, S. L., Moran, S., Margolin, D. H., Norris, K. and Tandon, P. K. (2008) Alemtuzumab vs. interferon beta-1a in early multiple sclerosis. *N Engl J Med* 359, 1786-1801.

Coles, A. J., Fox, E., Vladic, A., Gazda, S. K., Brinar, V., Selmaj, K. W., Skoromets, A., Stolyarov, I., Bass, A., Sullivan, H., Margolin, D. H., Lake, S. L., Moran, S., Palmer, J., Smith, M. S. and Compston, D. A. (2012) Alemtuzumab more effective than interferon beta-1a at 5-year follow-up of CAMMS223 Clinical Trial. *Neurology* 78, 1069-1078.

Cossburn, M., Pace, A. A., Jones, J., Ali, R., Ingram, G., Baker, K., Hirst, C., Zajicek, J., Scolding, N., Boggild, M., Pickersgill, T., Ben-Shlomo, Y., Coles, A. and Robertson, N. P. (2011) Autoimmune disease after alemtuzumab treatment for multiple sclerosis in a multicenter cohort. *Neurology* 77, 573-579.

D'Hooghe M, B., Haentjens, P., Nagels, G. and De Keyser, J. (2012) Alcohol, coffee, fish, smoking and disease progression in multiple sclerosis. *Eur J Neurol* 19, 616-624.

Dyment, D. A., Ebers, G. C. and Sadovnick, A. D. (2004) Genetics of multiple sclerosis. *Lancet Neurol* 3, 104-110.

Dyment, D. A., Herrera, B. M., Cader, M. Z., Willer, C. J., Lincoln, M. R., Sadovnick, A. D., Risch, N. and Ebers, G. C. (2005) Complex interactions among MHC haplotypes in multiple sclerosis: susceptibility and resistance. *Hum Mol Genet* 14, 2019-2026.

Ebers, G. C., Sadovnick, A. D., Dyment, D. A., Yee, I. M., Willer, C. J. and Risch, N. (2004) Parent-of-origin effect in multiple sclerosis: observations in half-siblings. *Lancet* 363, 1773-1774.

Ebers, G. C., Yee, I. M., Sadovnick, A. D. and Duquette, P. (2000) Conjugal multiple sclerosis: population-based prevalence and recurrence risks in offspring. Canadian Collaborative Study Group. *Ann Neurol* 48, 927-931.

Fogdell, A., Hillert, J., Sachs, C. and Olerup, O. (1995) The multiple sclerosis- and narcolepsy-associated HLA class II haplotype includes the DRB5*0101 allele. *Tissue Antigens* 46, 333-336.

Fox, E. J. and Rhoades, R. W. (2012) New treatments and treatment goals for patients with relapsing-remitting multiple sclerosis. *Curr Opin Neurol* 25 Suppl, S11-19.

Getts, D. R., Turley, D. M., Smith, C. E., Harp, C. T., McCarthy, D., Feeney, E. M., Getts, M. T., Martin, A. J., Luo, X., Terry, R. L., King, N. J. and Miller, S. D. (2011) Tolerance induced by apoptotic antigen-coupled leukocytes is induced by PD-L1+ and IL-10-producing splenic macrophages and maintained by T regulatory cells. *J Immunol* 187, 2405-2417.

Getts, M. T., Richards, M. H. and Miller, S. D. (2010) A critical role for virus-specific CD8(+) CTLs in protection from Theiler's virus-induced demyelination in disease-susceptible SJL mice. *Virology* 402, 102-111.

Goebels, N., Hofstetter, H., Schmidt, S., Brunner, C., Wekerle, H. and Hohlfeld, R. (2000) Repertoire dynamics of autoreactive T cells in multiple sclerosis patients and healthy subjects: epitope spreading versus clonal persistence. *Brain* 123 Pt 3, 508-518.

Goodin, D. S., Traboulsee, A., Knappertz, V., Reder, A. T., Li, D., Langdon, D., Wolf, C., Beckmann, K., Konieczny, A., Ebers, G. C. and Year Long Term Follow-up Study, I. (2012) Relationship between early clinical characteristics and long term disability outcomes: 16 year cohort study (follow-up) of the pivotal interferon beta-1b trial in multiple sclerosis. *J Neurol Neurosurg Psychiatry* 83, 282-287.

Goverman, J. (2009) Autoimmune T cell responses in the central nervous system. *Nat Rev Immunol* 9, 393-407.

Grau-Lopez, L., Raich, D., Ramo-Tello, C., Naranjo-Gomez, M., Davalos, A., Pujol-Borrell, R., Borras, F. E. and Martinez-Caceres, E. (2009) Myelin peptides in multiple sclerosis. *Autoimmun Rev* 8, 650-653.

Hafler, D. A. (2004) Multiple sclerosis. *J Clin Invest* 113, 788-794.

Hafler, D. A., Compston, A., Sawcer, S., Lander, E. S., Daly, M. J., De Jager, P. L., de Bakker, P. I., Gabriel, S. B., Mirel, D. B., Ivinson, A. J., Pericak-Vance, M. A., Gregory, S. G., Rioux, J. D., McCauley, J. L., Haines, J. L., Barcellos, L. F., Cree, B., Oksenberg, J. R. and Hauser, S. L. (2007) Risk alleles for multiple sclerosis identified by a genomewide study. *N Engl J Med* 357, 851-862.

Hansen, T., Skytthe, A., Stenager, E., Petersen, H. C., Bronnum-Hansen, H. and Kyvik, K. O. (2005) Concordance for multiple sclerosis in Danish twins: an update of a nationwide study. *Mult Scler* 11, 504-510.

Hartung, H. P. and Aktas, O. (2011) Evolution of multiple sclerosis treatment: next generation therapies meet next generation efficacy criteria. *Lancet Neurol* 10, 293-295.

Hauser, S. L. (2008) Multiple lessons for multiple sclerosis. *N Engl J Med* 359, 1838-1841.

Hayes, C. E. (2000) Vitamin D: a natural inhibitor of multiple sclerosis. *Proc Nutr Soc* 59, 531-535.

Hoffjan, S. and Akkad, D. A. (2010) The genetics of multiple sclerosis: an update 2010. *Mol Cell Probes* 24, 237-243.

Holland, N. J. (2009) Overview of Multiple Sclerosis. *Clinical Bulletin, Information for health professionals. National Multiple Sclerosis Soceity.*

Hoppenbrouwers, I. A. and Hintzen, R. Q. (2011) Genetics of multiple sclerosis. *Biochim Biophys Acta* 1812, 194-201.

Islam, T., Gauderman, W. J., Cozen, W., Hamilton, A. S., Burnett, M. E. and Mack, T. M. (2006) Differential twin concordance for multiple sclerosis by latitude of birthplace. *Ann Neurol* 60, 56-64.

Jeffery, D. R., Markowitz, C. E., Reder, A. T., Weinstock-Guttman, B. and Tobias, K. (2011) Fingolimod for the treatment of relapsing multiple sclerosis. *Expert Rev Neurother* 11, 165-183.

Jersild, C., Fog, T., Hansen, G. S., Thomsen, M., Svejgaard, A. and Dupont, B. (1973) Histocompatibility determinants in multiple sclerosis, with special reference to clinical course. *Lancet* 2, 1221-1225.

Jersild, C., Svejgaard, A. and Fog, T. (1972) HL-A antigens and multiple sclerosis. *Lancet* 1, 1240-1241.

Johnson, K. P. (2012) Glatiramer acetate for treatment of relapsing-remitting multiple sclerosis. *Expert Rev Neurother* 12, 371-384.

Kakalacheva, K. and Lunemann, J. D. (2011) Environmental triggers of multiple sclerosis. *FEBS Lett* 585, 3724-3729.

Kakalacheva, K., Munz, C. and Lunemann, J. D. (2011) Viral triggers of multiple sclerosis. *Biochim Biophys Acta* 1812, 132-140.

Kappos, L., Bates, D., Edan, G., Eraksoy, M., Garcia-Merino, A., Grigoriadis, N., Hartung, H. P., Havrdova, E., Hillert, J., Hohlfeld, R., Kremenchutzky, M., Lyon-Caen, O., Miller, A., Pozzilli, C., Ravnborg, M., Saida, T., Sindic, C., Vass, K., Clifford, D. B., Hauser, S., Major, E. O., O'Connor, P. W., Weiner, H. L., Clanet, M., Gold, R., Hirsch, H. H., Radu, E. W., Sorensen, P. S. and King, J. (2011a) Natalizumab treatment for multiple sclerosis: updated recommendations for patient selection and monitoring. *Lancet Neurol* 10, 745-758.

Kappos, L., Gold, R., Miller, D. H., Macmanus, D. G., Havrdova, E., Limmroth, V., Polman, C. H., Schmierer, K., Yousry, T. A., Yang, M., Eraksoy, M., Meluzinova, E., Rektor, I., Dawson, K. T., Sandrock, A. W., O'Neill, G. N. and Investigators, B. G. P. I. S. (2008) Efficacy and safety of oral fumarate in patients with relapsing-remitting multiple sclerosis: a multicentre, randomised, double-blind, placebo-controlled phase IIb study. *Lancet* 372, 1463-1472.

Kappos, L., Li, D., Calabresi, P. A., O'Connor, P., Bar-Or, A., Barkhof, F., Yin, M., Leppert, D., Glanzman, R., Tinbergen, J. and Hauser, S. L. (2011b) Ocrelizumab in relapsing-remitting multiple sclerosis: a phase 2, randomised, placebo-controlled, multicentre trial. *Lancet* 378, 1779-1787.

Karpus, W. J., Pope, J. G., Peterson, J. D., Dal Canto, M. C. and Miller, S. D. (1995) Inhibition of Theiler's virus-mediated demyelination by peripheral immune tolerance induction. *J Immunol* 155, 947-957.

Katz-Levy, Y., Neville, K. L., Girvin, A. M., Vanderlugt, C. L., Pope, J. G., Tan, L. J. and Miller, S. D. (1999) Endogenous presentation of self myelin epitopes by CNS-resident APCs in Theiler's virus-infected mice. *J Clin Invest* 104, 599-610.

Katz-Levy, Y., Neville, K. L., Padilla, J., Rahbe, S., Begolka, W. S., Girvin, A. M., Olson, J. K., Vanderlugt, C. L. and Miller, S. D. (2000) Temporal development of autoreactive Th1 responses and endogenous presentation of self myelin epitopes by central nervous system-resident APCs in Theiler's virus-infected mice. *J Immunol* 165, 5304-5314.

Keegan, B. M. (2011) Natalizumab for multiple sclerosis: a complicated treatment. *Lancet Neurol* 10, 677-678.

Killestein, J., Rudick, R. A. and Polman, C. H. (2011) Oral treatment for multiple sclerosis. *Lancet Neurol* 10, 1026-1034.

Klotz, L., Meuth, S. G. and Wiendl, H. (2012) Immune mechanisms of new therapeutic strategies in multiple sclerosis-A focus on alemtuzumab. *Clin Immunol* 142, 25-30.

Kohm, A. P., Turley, D. M. and Miller, S. D. (2005) Targeting the TCR: T-cell receptor and peptide-specific tolerance-based strategies for restoring self-tolerance in CNS autoimmune disease. *Int Rev Immunol* 24, 361-392.

Kurtzke, J. F., Beebe, G. W. and Norman, J. E., Jr. (1979) Epidemiology of multiple sclerosis in U.S. veterans: 1. Race, sex, and geographic distribution. *Neurology* 29, 1228-1235.

Lalive, P. H., Neuhaus, O., Benkhoucha, M., Burger, D., Hohlfeld, R., Zamvil, S. S. and Weber, M. S. (2011) Glatiramer acetate in the treatment of multiple sclerosis: emerging concepts regarding its mechanism of action. *CNS Drugs* 25, 401-414.

Lang, H. L., Jacobsen, H., Ikemizu, S., Andersson, C., Harlos, K., Madsen, L., Hjorth, P., Sondergaard, L., Svejgaard, A., Wucherpfennig, K., Stuart, D. I., Bell, J. I., Jones, E. Y. and Fugger, L. (2002) A functional and structural basis for TCR cross-reactivity in multiple sclerosis. *Nat Immunol* 3, 940-943.

Langer-Gould, A., Atlas, S. W., Green, A. J., Bollen, A. W. and Pelletier, D. (2005) Progressive multifocal leukoencephalopathy in a patient treated with natalizumab. *N Engl J Med* 353, 375-381.

Lehmann, P. V., Forsthuber, T., Miller, A. and Sercarz, E. E. (1992) Spreading of T-cell autoimmunity to cryptic determinants of an autoantigen. *Nature* 358, 155-157.

Limmroth, V., Putzki, N. and Kachuck, N. J. (2011) The interferon beta therapies for treatment of relapsing-remitting multiple sclerosis: are they equally efficacious? A comparative review of open-label studies evaluating the efficacy, safety, or dosing of different interferon beta formulations alone or in combination. *Ther Adv Neurol Disord* 4, 281-296.

Lincoln, M. R., Montpetit, A., Cader, M. Z., Saarela, J., Dyment, D. A., Tiislar, M., Ferretti, V., Tienari, P. J., Sadovnick, A. D., Peltonen, L., Ebers, G. C. and Hudson, T. J. (2005) A predominant role for the HLA class II region in the association of the MHC region with multiple sclerosis. *Nat Genet* 37, 1108-1112.

Mah, J. K. and Thannhauser, J. E. (2010) Management of multiple sclerosis in adolescents-current treatment options related adherence issues. *Adolescent Health, Medicine and Therapeutics* 1, 31-43.

Mayne, C. G., Spanier, J. A., Relland, L. M., Williams, C. B. and Hayes, C. E. (2011) 1,25-Dihydroxyvitamin D3 acts directly on the T lymphocyte vitamin D receptor to inhibit experimental autoimmune encephalomyelitis. *Eur J Immunol* 41, 822-832.

Miller, A., Shapiro, S., Gershtein, R., Kinarty, A., Rawashdeh, H., Honigman, S. and Lahat, N. (1998) Treatment of multiple sclerosis with copolymer-1 (Copaxone): implicating mechanisms of Th1 to Th2/Th3 immune-deviation. *J Neuroimmunol* 92, 113-121.

Miller, A. E. and Rhoades, R. W. (2012) Treatment of relapsing-remitting multiple sclerosis: current approaches and unmet needs. *Curr Opin Neurol* 25 Suppl, S4-10.

Miller, D. H., Hammond, S. R., McLeod, J. G., Purdie, G. and Skegg, D. C. (1990) Multiple sclerosis in Australia and New Zealand: are the determinants genetic or environmental? *J Neurol Neurosurg Psychiatry* 53, 903-905.

Miller, S. D. and Eagar, T. N. (2001) Functional role of epitope spreading in the chronic pathogenesis of autoimmune and virus-induced demyelinating diseases. *Adv Exp Med Biol* 490, 99-107.

Miller, S. D., Karpus, W. J. and Davidson, T. S. (2010) Experimental autoimmune encephalomyelitis in the mouse. *Curr Protoc Immunol* Chapter 15, Unit 15 11.

Miller, S. D., Katz-Levy, Y., Neville, K. L. and Vanderlugt, C. L. (2001) Virus-induced autoimmunity: epitope spreading to myelin autoepitopes in Theiler's virus infection of the central nervous system. *Adv Virus Res* 56, 199-217.

Miller, S. D., Vanderlugt, C. L., Begolka, W. S., Pao, W., Neville, K. L., Yauch, R. L. and Kim, B. S. (1997a) Epitope spreading leads to myelin-specific autoimmune responses in SJL mice chronically infected with Theiler's virus. *J Neurovirol* 3 Suppl 1, S62-65.

Miller, S. D., Vanderlugt, C. L., Begolka, W. S., Pao, W., Yauch, R. L., Neville, K. L., Katz-Levy, Y., Carrizosa, A. and Kim, B. S. (1997b) Persistent infection with Theiler's virus leads to CNS autoimmunity via epitope spreading. *Nat Med* 3, 1133-1136.

Modin, H., Olsson, W., Hillert, J. and Masterman, T. (2004) Modes of action of HLA-DR susceptibility specificities in multiple sclerosis. *Am J Hum Genet* 74, 1321-1322.

Moreau, T., Coles, A., Wing, M., Thorpe, J., Miller, D., Moseley, I., Issacs, J., Hale, G., Clayton, D., Scolding, N., Waldmann, H. and Compston, A. (1996) CAMPATH-IH in multiple sclerosis. *Mult Scler* 1, 357-365.

Munger, K. L., Levin, L. I., Hollis, B. W., Howard, N. S. and Ascherio, A. (2006) Serum 25-hydroxyvitamin D levels and risk of multiple sclerosis. *JAMA* 296, 2832-2838.

Naito, S., Namerow, N., Mickey, M. R. and Terasaki, P. I. (1972) Multiple sclerosis: association with HL-A3. *Tissue Antigens* 2, 1-4.

Neuhaus, O., Farina, C., Wekerle, H. and Hohlfeld, R. (2001) Mechanisms of action of glatiramer acetate in multiple sclerosis. *Neurology* 56, 702-708.

Neuhaus, O., Kieseier, B. C. and Hartung, H. P. (2006) Therapeutic role of mitoxantrone in multiple sclerosis. *Pharmacol Ther* 109, 198-209.

Neville, K. L., Padilla, J. and Miller, S. D. (2002) Myelin-specific tolerance attenuates the progression of a virus-induced demyelinating disease: implications for the treatment of MS. *J Neuroimmunol* 123, 18-29.

Nischwitz, S., Muller-Myhsok, B. and Weber, F. (2011) Risk conferring genes in multiple sclerosis. *FEBS Lett* 585, 3789-3797.

O'Connor, P. W., Goodman, A., Kappos, L., Lublin, F. D., Miller, D. H., Polman, C., Rudick, R. A., Aschenbach, W. and Lucas, N. (2011) Disease activity return during natalizumab treatment interruption in patients with multiple sclerosis. *Neurology* 76, 1858-1865.

O'Connor, P. W., Goodman, A., Willmer-Hulme, A. J., Libonati, M. A., Metz, L., Murray, R. S., Sheremata, W. A., Vollmer, T. L., Stone, L. A. and Natalizumab Multiple Sclerosis Trial, G. (2004) Randomized multicenter trial of natalizumab in acute MS relapses: clinical and MRI effects. *Neurology* 62, 2038-2043.

Oksenberg, J. R., Barcellos, L. F., Cree, B. A., Baranzini, S. E., Bugawan, T. L., Khan, O., Lincoln, R. R., Swerdlin, A., Mignot, E., Lin, L., Goodin, D., Erlich, H. A., Schmidt, S., Thomson, G., Reich, D. E., Pericak-Vance, M. A., Haines, J. L. and Hauser, S. L. (2004) Mapping multiple sclerosis susceptibility to the HLA-DR locus in African Americans. *Am J Hum Genet* 74, 160-167.

Olson, J. K., Croxford, J. L., Calenoff, M. A., Dal Canto, M. C. and Miller, S. D. (2001) A virus-induced molecular mimicry model of multiple sclerosis. *J Clin Invest* 108, 311-318.

Papadopoulou, A., D'Souza, M., Kappos, L. and Yaldizli, O. (2010) Dimethyl fumarate for multiple sclerosis. *Expert Opin Investig Drugs* 19, 1603-1612.

Perini, P., Calabrese, M., Tiberio, M., Ranzato, F., Battistin, L. and Gallo, P. (2006) Mitoxantrone versus cyclophosphamide in secondary-progressive multiple sclerosis: a comparative study. *J Neurol* 253, 1034-1040.

Podojil, J. R., Turley, D. M. and Miller, S. D. (2008) Therapeutic blockade of T-cell antigen receptor signal transduction and costimulation in autoimmune disease. *Adv Exp Med Biol* 640, 234-251.

Pohl, D., Waubant, E., Banwell, B., Chabas, D., Chitnis, T., Weinstock-Guttman, B. and Tenembaum, S. (2007) Treatment of pediatric multiple sclerosis and variants. *Neurology* 68, S54-65.

Pravica, V., Popadic, D., Savic, E., Markovic, M., Drulovic, J. and Mostarica-Stojkovic, M. (2012) Single nucleotide polymorphisms in multiple sclerosis: disease susceptibility and treatment response biomarkers. *Immunol Res.*

Pucci, E., Giuliani, G., Solari, A., Simi, S., Minozzi, S., Di Pietrantonj, C. and Galea, I. (2011) Natalizumab for relapsing remitting multiple sclerosis. *Cochrane Database Syst Rev*, CD007621.

Racke, M. K. and Lovett-Racke, A. E. (2011) Glatiramer acetate treatment of multiple sclerosis: an immunological perspective. *J Immunol* 186, 1887-1890.

Ramagopalan, S. V., Knight, J. C. and Ebers, G. C. (2009) Multiple sclerosis and the major histocompatibility complex. *Curr Opin Neurol* 22, 219-225.

Ramagopalan, S. V., Morris, A. P., Dyment, D. A., Herrera, B. M., DeLuca, G. C., Lincoln, M. R., Orton, S. M., Chao, M. J., Sadovnick, A. D. and Ebers, G. C. (2007) The inheritance of resistance alleles in multiple sclerosis. *PLoS Genet* 3, 1607-1613.

Ransohoff, R. M. (2005) Natalizumab and PML. *Nat Neurosci* 8, 1275.

Repovic, P. and Lublin, F. D. (2011) Treatment of multiple sclerosis exacerbations. *Neurol Clin* 29, 389-400.

Rinaldi, L., Perini, P., Calabrese, M. and Gallo, P. (2009) Cyclophosphamide as second-line therapy in multiple sclerosis: benefits and risks. *Neurol Sci* 30 Suppl 2, S171-173.

Rio, J., Comabella, M. and Montalban, X. (2011) Multiple sclerosis: current treatment algorithms. *Curr Opin Neurol* 24, 230-237.

Rizvi, S. A., Zwibel, H. and Fox, E. J. (2004) Mitoxantrone for multiple sclerosis in clinical practice. *Neurology* 63, S25-27.

Robertson, N. P., O'Riordan, J. I., Chataway, J., Kingsley, D. P., Miller, D. H., Clayton, D. and Compston, D. A. (1997) Offspring recurrence rates and clinical characteristics of conjugal multiple sclerosis. *Lancet* 349, 1587-1590.

Rudick, R. A. and Sandrock, A. (2004) Natalizumab: alpha 4-integrin antagonist selective adhesion molecule inhibitors for MS. *Expert Rev Neurother* 4, 571-580.

Sanford, M. and Lyseng-Williamson, K. A. (2011) Subcutaneous recombinant interferon-beta-1a (Rebif(R)): a review of its use in the treatment of relapsing multiple sclerosis. *Drugs* 71, 1865-1891.

Sawcer, S., Hellenthal, G., Pirinen, M., Spencer, C. C., Patsopoulos, N. A., Moutsianas, L., Dilthey, A., Su, Z., Freeman, C., Hunt, S. E., Edkins, S., Gray, E., Booth, D. R., Potter, S. C., Goris, A., Band, G., Oturai, A. B., Strange, A., Saarela, J., Bellenguez, C., Fontaine, B., Gillman, M., Hemmer, B., Gwilliam, R., Zipp, F., Jayakumar, A., Martin, R., Leslie, S., Hawkins, S., Giannoulatou, E., D'Alfonso, S., Blackburn, H., Martinelli Boneschi, F., Liddle, J., Harbo, H. F., Perez, M. L., Spurkland, A., Waller, M. J., Mycko, M. P., Ricketts, M., Comabella, M., Hammond, N., Kockum, I., McCann, O. T., Ban, M., Whittaker, P., Kemppinen, A., Weston, P., Hawkins, C., Widaa, S., Zajicek, J., Dronov, S., Robertson, N., Bumpstead, S. J., Barcellos, L. F., Ravindrarajah, R., Abraham, R., Alfredsson, L., Ardlie, K., Aubin, C., Baker, A., Baker, K., Baranzini, S. E., Bergamaschi, L., Bergamaschi, R., Bernstein, A., Berthele, A., Boggild, M., Bradfield, J. P., Brassat, D., Broadley, S. A., Buck, D., Butzkueven, H., Capra, R., Carroll, W. M., Cavalla, P., Celius, E. G., Cepok, S., Chiavacci, R., Clerget-Darpoux, F., Clysters, K., Comi, G., Cossburn, M., Cournu-Rebeix, I., Cox, M. B., Cozen, W., Cree, B. A., Cross, A. H., Cusi, D., Daly, M. J., Davis, E., de Bakker, P. I., Debouverie, M., D'Hooghe M, B., Dixon, K., Dobosi, R., Dubois, B., Ellinghaus, D., Elovaara, I., Esposito, F., Fontenille, C., Foote, S., Franke, A., Galimberti, D., Ghezzi, A., Glessner, J., Gomez, R., Gout, O., Graham, C., Grant, S. F., Guerini, F. R., Hakonarson, H., Hall, P., Hamsten, A., Hartung, H. P., Heard, R. N., Heath, S., Hobart, J., Hoshi, M., Infante-Duarte, C., Ingram, G., Ingram, W., Islam, T., Jagodic, M., Kabesch, M., Kermode, A. G., Kilpatrick, T. J., Kim, C., Klopp, N., Koivisto, K., Larsson, M., Lathrop, M., Lechner-Scott, J. S., Leone, M. A., Leppa, V., Liljedahl, U., Bomfim, I. L., Lincoln, R. R., Link, J., Liu, J., Lorentzen, A. R., Lupoli, S., Macciardi, F., Mack, T., Marriott, M., Martinelli, V., Mason, D., McCauley, J. L., Mentch, F., Mero, I. L., Mihalova, T., Montalban, X., Mottershead, J., Myhr, K. M., Naldi, P., Ollier, W., Page, A., Palotie, A., Pelletier, J., Piccio, L., Pickersgill, T., Piehl, F., Pobywajlo, S., Quach, H. L., Ramsay, P. P., Reunanen, M., Reynolds, R., Rioux, J. D., Rodegher, M., Roesner, S., Rubio, J. P., Ruckert, I. M., Salvetti, M., Salvi, E., Santaniello, A., Schaefer, C. A., Schreiber, S., Schulze, C., Scott, R. J., Sellebjerg, F., Selmaj, K. W., Sexton, D., Shen, L., Simms-Acuna, B., Skidmore, S., Sleiman, P. M., Smestad, C., Sorensen, P. S., Sondergaard, H. B., Stankovich, J., Strange, R. C., Sulonen, A. M., Sundqvist, E., Syvanen, A. C., Taddeo, F., Taylor, B., Blackwell, J. M., Tienari, P., Bramon, E., Tourbah, A., Brown, M. A., Tronczynska, E., Casas, J. P., Tubridy, N., Corvin, A., Vickery, J., Jankowski, J., Villoslada, P., Markus, H. S., Wang, K., Mathew, C. G., Wason, J., Palmer, C. N., Wichmann, H. E., Plomin, R., Willoughby, E., Rautanen, A., Winkelmann, J., Wittig, M., Trembath, R. C., Yaouanq, J., Viswanathan, A. C., Zhang, H., Wood, N. W., Zuvich, R., Deloukas, P., Langford, C., Duncanson, A., Oksenberg, J. R., Pericak-Vance, M. A., Haines, J. L., Olsson, T., Hillert, J., Ivinson, A. J., De Jager, P. L., Peltonen, L., Stewart, G. J., Hafler, D. A., Hauser, S. L., McVean, G., Donnelly, P. and Compston, A.

(2011) Genetic risk and a primary role for cell-mediated immune mechanisms in multiple sclerosis. *Nature* 476, 214-219.

Singh, M., Cugati, G., Singh, P. and Singh, A. K. (2011) Fingolimod: The first oral drug approved by food and drug administration; A breakthrough in treatment of multiple sclerosis. *J Pharm Bioallied Sci* 3, 460-461.

Smolders, J., Damoiseaux, J., Menheere, P. and Hupperts, R. (2008a) Vitamin D as an immune modulator in multiple sclerosis, a review. *J Neuroimmunol* 194, 7-17.

Smolders, J., Menheere, P., Kessels, A., Damoiseaux, J. and Hupperts, R. (2008b) Association of vitamin D metabolite levels with relapse rate and disability in multiple sclerosis. *Mult Scler* 14, 1220-1224.

Stuve, O. and Greenberg, B. M. (2010) Anticipated benefits and surprising effects of daclizumab in multiple sclerosis. *Lancet Neurol* 9, 337-338.

Stuve, O., Kita, M., Pelletier, D., Fox, R. J., Stone, J., Goodkin, D. E. and Zamvil, S. S. (2004) Mitoxantrone as a potential therapy for primary progressive multiple sclerosis. *Mult Scler* 10 Suppl 1, S58-61.

Swank, R. L., Lerstad, O., Strom, A. and Backer, J. (1952) Multiple sclerosis in rural Norway its geographic and occupational incidence in relation to nutrition. *N Engl J Med* 246, 722-728.

Terasaki, P. I., Park, M. S., Opelz, G. and Ting, A. (1976) Multiple sclerosis and high incidence of a B lymphocyte antigen. *Science* 193, 1245-1247.

Theys, P., Gosseye-Lissoir, F., Ketelaer, P. and Carton, H. (1981) Short-term intensive cyclophosphamide treatment in multiple sclerosis. A retrospective controlled study. *J Neurol* 225, 119-133.

Thone, J. and Gold, R. (2011) Laquinimod: a promising oral medication for the treatment of relapsing-remitting multiple sclerosis. *Expert Opin Drug Metab Toxicol* 7, 365-370.

Tuohy, V. K., Yu, M., Weinstock-Guttman, B. and Kinkel, R. P. (1997) Diversity and plasticity of self recognition during the development of multiple sclerosis. *J Clin Invest* 99, 1682-1690.

Tuohy, V. K., Yu, M., Yin, L., Kawczak, J. A. and Kinkel, P. R. (1999a) Regression and spreading of self-recognition during the development of autoimmune demyelinating disease. *J Autoimmun* 13, 11-20.

Tuohy, V. K., Yu, M., Yin, L., Kawczak, J. A. and Kinkel, R. P. (1999b) Spontaneous regression of primary autoreactivity during chronic progression of experimental autoimmune encephalomyelitis and multiple sclerosis. *J Exp Med* 189, 1033-1042.

Turley, D. M. and Miller, S. D. (2007) Peripheral tolerance induction using ethylenecarbodiimide-fixed APCs uses both direct and indirect mechanisms of antigen presentation for prevention of experimental autoimmune encephalomyelitis. *J Immunol* 178, 2212-2220.

Vanderlugt, C. L. and Miller, S. D. (2002) Epitope spreading in immune-mediated diseases: implications for immunotherapy. *Nat Rev Immunol* 2, 85-95.

Vanderlugt, C. L., Neville, K. L., Nikcevich, K. M., Eagar, T. N., Bluestone, J. A. and Miller, S. D. (2000) Pathologic role and temporal appearance of newly emerging autoepitopes in relapsing experimental autoimmune encephalomyelitis. *J Immunol* 164, 670-678.

Vetsika, E. K. and Callan, M. (2004) Infectious mononucleosis and Epstein-Barr virus. *Expert Rev Mol Med* 6, 1-16.

Vukusic, S., Van Bockstael, V., Gosselin, S. and Confavreux, C. (2007) Regional variations in the prevalence of multiple sclerosis in French farmers. *J Neurol Neurosurg Psychiatry* 78, 707-709.

Warnke, C., Meyer zu Horste, G., Hartung, H. P., Stuve, O. and Kieseier, B. C. (2009) Review of teriflunomide and its potential in the treatment of multiple sclerosis. *Neuropsychiatr Dis Treat* 5, 333-340.

Weiner, H. L., Hauser, S. L., Hafler, D. A., Fallis, R. J., Lehrich, J. R. and Dawson, D. M. (1984) The use of cyclophosphamide in the treatment of multiple sclerosis. *Ann N Y Acad Sci* 436, 373-381.

Westlund, K. (1970) Distribution and mortality time trend of multiple sclerosis and some other diseases in Norway. *Acta Neurol Scand* 46, 455-483.

Willer, C. J., Dyment, D. A., Risch, N. J., Sadovnick, A. D. and Ebers, G. C. (2003) Twin concordance and sibling recurrence rates in multiple sclerosis. *Proc Natl Acad Sci U S A* 100, 12877-12882.

Winchester, R., Ebers, G., Fu, S. M., Espinosa, L., Zabriskie, J. and Kunkel, H. G. (1975) B-cell alloantigen Ag 7a in multiple sclerosis. *Lancet* 2, 814.

Wingerchuk, D. M. (2012) Smoking: effects on multiple sclerosis susceptibility and disease progression. *Ther Adv Neurol Disord* 5, 13-22.

Wood, H. (2011) Multiple sclerosis: Teriflunomide shows promise for MS treatment in phase III trial. *Nat Rev Neurol* 7, 657.

Wynn, D., Kaufman, M., Montalban, X., Vollmer, T., Simon, J., Elkins, J., O'Neill, G., Neyer, L., Sheridan, J., Wang, C., Fong, A., Rose, J. W. and investigators, C. (2010) Daclizumab in active relapsing multiple sclerosis (CHOICE study): a phase 2, randomised, double-blind, placebo-controlled, add-on trial with interferon beta. *Lancet Neurol* 9, 381-390.

Chapter 2

Immunologic and Genetic Factors in Type 1 Diabetes Mellitus

Ahmad Massoud and Amir Hossein Massoud

Additional information is available at the end of the chapter

http://dx.doi.org/10.5772/48141

1. Introduction

Diabetes mellitus (DM) is a metabolic disorder resulting from a defect in insulin secretion, insulin action, or both (Kumar et al., 2002). In type 1 diabetes, the body does not produce insulin. Insulin is a hormone that is needed to convert sugar, starches and other food into energy needed for daily life. Insulin deficiency in turn leads to chronic hyperglycaemia with disturbances of carbohydrate, fat and protein metabolism (Kumar et al., 2002). As the disease progresses tissue or vascular damage ensues leading to severe diabetic complications such as retinopathy, neuropathy, nephropathy, cardiovascular complications and ulceration (Huang, Kim et al. 2002; Wallace, Reiber et al. 2002; Bearse, Han et al. 2004; Seki, Tanaka et al. 2004; Svensson, Eriksson et al. 2004). Thus, diabetes covers a wide range of heterogeneous diseases. Diabetes is the most common endocrine disorder and by the year 2015, it is estimated that more than 200 million people worldwide will have DM and 300 million will subsequently have the disease by 2025. Type 1 diabetes is usually diagnosed in children and young adults, and was previously known as juvenile diabetes.

The diagnostic criteria and the classification of diabetes was first put forward by the World Health Organization (WHO) in 1965 then by the National Diabetes Data Group (NDDG) in 1979, and the latest recommendations have been published by the American Diabetes Association (ADA) in 1997 and by the WHO in 1999(Genuth, Alberti et al. 2003). According to the ADA recommendation, the fasting glucose concentration should be used in routine screening for diabetes as well as epidemiological studies; the threshold for fasting glucose is fasting glucose = 7.0 mmol/L (126 mg/dl) and /or a 2-h glucose = 11.1 mmol/L (200 mg/dL). For the diagnosis of diabetes, at least one criteria must also apply:

- Symptoms of diabetes (polyurea, polydipsia, unexplained weight loss, etc) as well as casual plasma glucose concentration = 11.1 mmol/L (200mg/dL).
- Fasting plasma glucose = 7.0 mmol/L (126mg/dL), with no caloric intake for at least 8 h.

Diabetes Mellitus may be categorized into several types but the two major types are type 1 and type 2. The term type 1 and type 2 were widely used to describe Insulin-Dependent Diabetes Mellitus (IDDM) and Noninsulin-Dependent Diabetes Mellitus (NIDDM), respectively. On the basis of etiology, Type 1 (DM) is present in patients who have little or no endogenous insulin secretory capacity and who therefore require insulin therapy. The two main forms of clinical type 1 diabetes are type 1a (about 90% of type 1 cases) which is thought to be due to immunological destruction of pancreatic beta-cells resulting in insulin deficiency, and type 1b (idiopathic, about 10% of type 1 diabetes), in which there is no evidence of autoimmunity. Type 1a is characterized by the presence of islet cell antibody (ICA), anti-glutamic acid decarboxylate (anti-GAD), IA-2 or insulin antibodies that identify the autoimmune process with beta-cell destruction. Autoimmune diseases such as Grave's disease, Hashimoto's thyroiditis and Addison's disease may be associated with Type 1 (DM) (Betterle, Zanette et al. 1984; Atkinson and Maclaren 1994). There is no known etiological basis for type 1b diabetes mellitus. Some of Type1b patients have permanent insulinopaenia and are prone to ketoacidosis, but have no evidence of autoimmunity. This form is more prevalent among individuals of African and Asian origins.

Type 2 diabetes is the commonest form of DM and is characterized by disorders of insulin secretion and insulin resistance.

Type 1 (DM) is a multifactorial disease characterized by the autoimmune destruction of insulin-secreting pancreatic beta-cells causing tissue damage. The peak age of onset is about 12 years, and from then onwards daily injections of insulin are required by affected individuals. With a frequency of about 0.4% in Caucasians of European descent, Type 1 (DM) is second to asthma as the most serious chronic childhood disease in the Western world (Wan, Yang et al. 2010). There is a marked geographic variation of Type 1 (DM), with a higher incidence in the European and North American than the Asian and south American countries. The current global increase in incidence of 3% per year is well reported. This rapid rise strongly suggests that the action of the environment on susceptibility genes contributes to the evolving epidemiology of this disease(Wan, Yang et al. 2010).

Type 1 (DM) shows a complex mode of inheritance, with disease susceptibility caused both by genetic and by environmental components. The penetrance of disease genes being determined by unknown environmental factors. Identical twins of affected individuals have a risk of developing the disease of only 36% (Owerbach and Gabbay 1996), demonstrating the importance of the environmental factors. Nevertheless, genetic factors are essential, as measured by the quantity (i.e. the ratio of the risk to siblings of patients compared with the population prevalence). The disease is polygenic in humans and in mice, with a number of different susceptibility genes each accounting for a portion of the familial clustering of the disease (Pharoah, Dunning et al. 2004). Around the time of clinical presentation, insulitis, a chronic inflammatory infiltrate of the islets affecting primarily insulin containing islets, is present in the majority of cases. The mononuclear cell infiltrates in the islet, which results in the development of insulitis (a prerequisite step for the development of diabetes) are primarily composed of T cells. It is now well accepted that these T cells play important roles in initiating and propagating an autoimmune process, which in turn destroys insulin-producing islet beta-cells in the pancreas (Toyoda and Formby 1998). Understanding insights of the mechanism of immune-mediated islet cell destruction and the interaction between the immune system and pancreatic islets provide new therapeutic means of preventing this chronic debilitating disease.

Before safe and rational therapies can be offered in a clinical setting, a detailed understanding of the immune-mediated process that results in Type 1 (DM) is required, as is the accurate identification of those at risk of the disease. The immunogenetics of type 1 diabetes has become the model upon which other complex disorders are studied, and in this chapter we focus on the importance of recent insights into the pathogenesis and natural history of Type 1 (DM) with consideration to current therapeutic strategies, and future perspective for the efficient treatment.

2. Diabetes mellitus clinical manifestation and diagnosis

The symptoms of diabetes are more readily recognizable in children than in adults, so it is surprising that the diagnosis may sometimes be missed or delayed. Those families with a strong family history of diabetes should suspect diabetes, especially if there is one child in the family with diabetes. Main manifestations are: polyuria, polydipsia, polyphagia, progressive cachexia, glucosuria, hyperglycemia, increasing of specific gravity of urine, blurred vision, fatigue, cramps and candidiasis. Diabetic retinopathy is a major complication of diabetes (Bakker, Tushuizen et al. 2012). Diabetes causes high blood sugar levels, which can damage blood vessels. The damaged vessels around the retina can leak protein and fats, forming deposits that can interfere with vision. The damaged blood vessels are also not as effective at carrying oxygen to the retina, which can also cause damage (Bakker, Tushuizen et al. 2012).

When blood glucose concentrations increase, more glucose is filtered by the glomeruli of the kidneys than can be reabsorbed by the kidney tubules, resulting in glucose excretion in the urine. High glucose concentrations in the urine create an osmotic effect that reduces the reabsorption of water by the kidneys, causing polyuria (excretion of large volumes of urine) (Katavetin 2009). The loss of water from the circulation stimulates thirst. Therefore, patients with moderate or severe hyperglycemia typically have polyuria and polydipsia (excessive thirst). The loss of glucose in the urine results in weakness, fatigue, weight loss, and increased appetite (polyphagia). Patients with hyperglycemia are prone to infections, particularly vaginal and urinary tract infections and an infection may be the presenting manifestation of diabetes (Katavetin 2009).

There are two acute life-threatening complications of diabetes: hyperglycemia and acidosis (increased acidity of the blood), either of which may be the presenting manifestation of diabetes. In patients with Type 1 (DM), insulin deficiency, if not recognized and treated properly, leads to severe hyperglycemia and to a marked increase in lipolysis (the breakdown of lipids), with a greatly increased rate of release of fatty acids from adipose tissue (Wajchenberg 2007). In the liver, much of the excess fatty acid is converted to the keto acids beta-hydroxybutyric acid and acetoacetic acid. The increased release of fatty acids and keto acids from adipose, liver, and muscle tissues raises the acid content of the blood, thereby lowering the pH of the blood. The combination of hyperglycemia and acidosis is called diabetic ketoacidosis and leads to hyperventilation and to impaired central nervous system function, culminating in coma and death.

Many studies have also shown that hyperglycemia causes oxidative stress in tissues that are susceptible to complications of diabetes mellitus, including peripheral nerves (Ziegler, Sohr et al. 2004). The autonomic nervous system modulates the electrical and contractile activity of the myocardium via the interplay of sympathetic and parasympathetic activity (Lahiri, Kannankeril et al. 2008). An imbalance of autonomic control is implicated in the pathophysiology of Type 1 (DM). Cardiovascular autonomic neuropathy, a common form of autonomic dysfunction found in patients with diabetes mellitus (Maser and Lenhard 2005), as well, and causes abnormalities in heart rate control, as well as defects in central and peripheral vascular dynamics.

Symptoms are similar in both types of diabetes but they vary in their intensity. Longstanding Type 1 (DM) patients are susceptible to microvascular complications; and macrovascular disease (coronary artery, heart, and peripheral vascular diseases) (Saely, Aczel et al. 2004; Svensson, Eriksson et al. 2004)and end stage renal disease. Ketoacidosis is usually not a problem in patients with type II diabetes because they secrete enough insulin to restrain lipolysis.

Symptoms in type 2 DM are similar but usually milder and insidious in onset. Geographical differences exist in both the magnitude of these problems and their relative contributions to overall morbidity and mortality.

3. Composition of the islet infiltrates and the mechanism of beta-cell destruction

The histopathology of type 1 diabetes is defined by a decreased beta-cell mass in association with insulitis, a characteristic lymphocytic infiltration limited to the islets of Langerhans and prominent in early stage disease in children. It is considered to be pathognomonic for recent onset disease. The infiltrate consists predominantly of T cells, in which CD8+ lymphocytes dominate, but may also contain CD4+ lymphocytes, B-lymphocytes and macrophages (Willcox, Richardson et al. 2009).

The cellular response is accompanied by a humoral response that includes autoantibodies against a wide array of beta-cell antigens (which will be discussed later). However, the precipitating (auto)antigen against which the inflammatory response is directed has not been identified, nor has it been established whether the humoral response that is considered to be part of our current diagnostic criteria is a cause or a consequence of the disease. Although animal models for the disease exist, like the spontaneously non-obese diabetic (NOD) mouse, they are found to differ from the human disease in many key aspects and it is an open question whether data derived from such models will be applicable to patients. In fact, even after a century of research we know very little about the etiology and histopathology of the human disease.

The pancreas is a difficult organ to biopsy and most of the material is therefore post-mortem. The islets are scattered in a matrix of exocrine tissue and thus form only 1–2% of the parenchymal tissue. In addition the beta-cells are not homogeneously distributed throughout the gland and are often located within a few lobes. In a diabetic condition, the lesions are mainly found in islets in which beta-cells are still present and the lesions will largely disappear together with the beta-cells against which the reaction appears to be directed. In addition, the few cases that were brought to autopsy often died in ketoacidosis, they may thus represent a more fulminant version of the disease that is not necessarily characteristic for the disease process in the rest of the population. Lastly, and perhaps most importantly, the histopathological lesions that we observe in cases with recent onset disease will only show the final stages of a process that has been going on for a long period of time, and until recently, we had no material available of earlier stages of the disease. Identifying patients with pre-clinical disease and studying the immunological processes occurring at this stage may prove to be indispensable for a breakthrough in our quest for the etiology of the disease.

3.1. A Brief history of insulitis

Inflammatory infiltrates in the islets of Langerhans were first described in 1902 by the German pathologist Schmidt (Nagler and Taylor 1963), who found foci of small-cell infiltration in the periphery of islets of Langerhans from a 10 year old diabetic child with an unknown duration of disease. This islet-specific inflammation, later termed "insulitis" by the Swiss pathologist von Meyenburg, was long considered to be a rare event. Cecil (Cecil 1909) described leucocytic infiltration associated with islets in 9 out of 90 patients with diabetes, but often under conditions in which a more generalized pancreatitis was present; he observed islet-specific inflammation in only a single case, involving a young adult patient with recent onset disease. In 1928 Stansfield and Warren were the first to draw attention to the association between insulitis and the age of the patient; they described insulitis in a six year old girl who died in a diabetic coma two months after onset of the disease, and in an 11 year old girl who died in a diabetic coma within four weeks after the initiation of symptoms. In their view, the striking lymphocytic infiltration in the islets of both cases suggested a causal relationship between the inflammation and the diabetic condition in these two young patients with recent onset fulminant disease. On the other hand, it was clear from their studies in larger groups of children that insulitis was not always observed. These observations were revisited in 1958 by LeCompte (Lecompte 1958) who collected four cases with insulitis, all involving acute onset disease and short duration in children. He proposed four possible explanations for the presence of the cellular infiltrate: a direct invasion of the islets by an infectious agent, a manifestation of functional overstimulation or strain, a reaction to damage by some unknown nonbacterial agent and lastly an antigen-antibody reaction.

Fifty years later one could still make the same list, as none of these possibilities has been excluded. In a 1965 landmark study, Willy Gepts (Gepts 1965) reported the presence of the lesion in 15/22 (68%) recent onset cases below the age of 40 and noted that it was not present in patients with a disease duration of more than a year. He also noted that beta-cell mass appeared to be reduced to approximately 10% of that in non-diabetic controls. Other authors supported the findings as well. Foulis et al (Foulis, Liddle et al. 1986) using a 25-year computerized survey of deaths in the UK to identify 119 young patients who died in ketoacidosis before the age of 20, in combination with immunohistochemistry to identify islets and infiltrating leucocytes, confirmed that insulitis was present in 47 out of 60 (78%) of young patients with recent onset disease (<1 year). These investigators, however, also pointed out that certain heterogeneity seemed to exist in their patient population, as it is observed that young-adult patients with a short duration of the disease showed no evidence of insulitis and in which all islets contained insulin. Together it appears that insulitis exist predominantly in (pre) diabetic patients in which it is limited to islets that were still insulin-containing.

3.2. Pathogenic autoantigen in type 1 diabetes

The major autoantigens in Type 1 (DM), identified by circulating autoantibodies, are glutamic acid decarboxylase (GAD), tyrosine phosphatase-like insulinoma antigen and (pro) insulin. It is not clear, however, which if any drive pathogenic T cells. So far, no antigen has emerged as dominant, although both glutamic acid decarboxylase and insulin have been postulated to be principal autoantigens (Pugliese, Brown et al. 2001).

With the possible exception of rare self-antigen-expressing cells in lymphoid tissue (Pugliese, Brown et al. 2001), proinsulin is expressed uniquely in beta-cells. Investigation on humans (Kent, Chen et al. 2005), and murine model (Nakayama, Abiru et al. 2005), highlight the pancreatic beta-cell hormone insulin as a major target for T cell attack. If insulin, or peptides of the β chain of insulin, is given orally (Bergerot, Fabien et al. 1994) intranasally (Harrison, Dempsey-Collier et al. 1996) or subcutaneously(Hutchings and Cooke 1998), diabetes is suppressed. In addition, when proinsulin is expressed in the NOD mice under the control of a MHC class II promoter, such that it is expressed on antigen-presenting cells and in the thymus, the incidence of diabetes is decreased (French, Allison et al. 1997). There are some reports demonstrating that insulin gene polymorphism is associated with predisposition to Type 1 (DM) (which will be discussed later). In some studies specificity of the T cell response was confirmed by isolation of $CD4^+$ and $CD8^+$ T cell clones specific for the insulin epitopes. The most convincing evidence of a pathogenic role of insulin specific $CD4^+$ T cells came from a study in which the insulin A1–15 specific T cells were expanded from pancreatic lymph nodes of deceased patients affected by Type 1 (DM) (Kent, Chen et al. 2005).

Moreover, Multiple T-cell epitopes against GAD65 (glutamate decarboxylase 65) have been associated with Type 1 (DM). GAD65 is expressed in the endocrine cells of the islets of Langerhans and in the central nervous system (Karlsen, Hagopian et al. 1991). The major autoantigens, in which there are evidence that are associated to the pathogenesis of Type 1 (DM) are listed below.

3.3. Phenotyping insulitis

Immunophenotyping of the infiltrate showed that most cells corresponded to T cells, with T cytotoxic/suppressor cells being most abundant, although helper $CD4^+$ T cells and NK cells were also present (In't Veld 2011). CD8+ T lymphocytes (T cytotoxic/suppressor) were the main infiltrating cell type. In addition to lymphocytes, macrophages were a prominent feature of the infiltrate; although it is controversial and in some studies macrophages were not found in insulitic lesions. The composition of the cellular infiltrate is stratified according to the percent beta-cells present in islets collected across patients (In't Veld 2011). The percent beta-cells would be a surrogate marker for the stages of advent of the insulitic lesion, with 50–69% insulin-positive area taken as starting point and 0% insulin-positive area as end-stage (In't Veld 2011). In all stages, CD8+ T cells are predominant, increasing in number with decreasing insulin-positive area, but disappearing when insulin-positivity is completely lost. CD20+ B-cells were found to be the second most prominent cell type, following the dynamics of CD8+ cells, while macrophages were present at relatively constant levels becoming the most prominent infiltrating cell type in insulin-deficient islets.

autoantigen	Expression	Subcellular location	Involvement in the NOD mouse	Human T1D		
				autoantibodies	$CD4^+$ T cells	$CD8^+$ T cells
Insulin	β-cell, thymus	secretory granule	+	+	+	+
GAD 65	neuroendocrine	synaptic-like microvesicles	+	+	+	+
GAD 67	neuroendocrine	cytosol	+	+	+	+
IA-2 (ICA512)	neuroendocrine	secretory granule		+	+	+
IA-2 β/phogrin	neuroendocrine	secretory granule		+	+	+
IGRP	β-cell	endoplasmic reticulum	+	?	+	+
Chromogranin	neuroendocrine	Secretory granule	+	?	?	?
ZnT8	β-cell	secretory granule	?	+	?	?
HSP-60 HSP-70	Ubiquitous	mitochondria	+	+	+	?
Glima-38		secretory granule	?	+	?	?
Amylin/IAPP		secretory granule	?	?	?	+
CD38	Ubiquitous	?	?	±	?	?

Table 1. Autoantigens defined as recognized by T cells in human and NOD mice type 1 (DM).

Phenotyping the infiltrating cells in insulitic lesions is only a first step in a process to identify the antigen against which the infiltrate is directed. The key step will be to analyze their specificity. Direct analysis of insulitic T cell specificity has been reported to date is limited, although some studies suggest that CD4+ T cells isolated from pancreases of Type 1 (DM) patients are specific to some parts of the insulin molecule (Kent, Chen et al. 2005). Although the predominantly CD3+CD8+ phenotype of the infiltrating cells is compatible with a cytotoxic T cell mediated beta-cell destruction, it has not yet been proven that the cells in the insulitic lesion are the cells that are actually responsible for the destruction of the beta-cell component. However many studies suggest that a cytotoxic T cell mediated destruction of insulin-producing beta-cells is initiated by an unknown (auto)antigen, leading to the destruction of beta-cell mass.

It is equally well possible that a large part of such infiltrates are the consequence of beta-cell destruction rather than its cause, at least at this relatively late time point in the progression of the disease. What we observe at clinical presentation is the final stage of a process that may have been going on for a long period of time. If the presence of circulating autoantibodies against islet cell antigens is considered as a surrogate marker for beta-cell destruction, then the process may take years before the clinical threshold is reached. Determining the incidence and time course of insulitis prior to diagnosis and correlating it to the presence, and persistence of circulating immune markers, will be crucial for our understanding of the disease and for the development of immune intervention strategies. It is important to correlate such information to the regenerative capacity of the beta-cell mass. Not all individuals who are autoantibody-positive progress to overt disease and the process may well involve episodes of fulminant destruction followed by episodes of repair and regeneration.

Islets with insulitis contain replicating beta-cells, indicating that beta-cells retain a substantial capacity for growth that appears to be activated under conditions of inflammation. It cannot be excluded that such newly formed cells attract recurrent autoimmune attack and that islets with a low insulin-positive area represent islets with regeneration rather than islets in the last stages of beta-cell destruction.

3.4. Mechanisms of beta-cell destruction and initiation of pathogenesis

Although the pathogenesis of Type 1 (DM) has been extensively studied, the precise mechanisms involved in the initiation and progression of beta-cell destruction remain unclear. Animal models used in the study of Type 1 (DM), such as the (BB) rat and (NOD) mouse, have greatly enhanced our understanding of the pathogenic mechanisms involved in this disease. In these animals, macrophages and/or dendritic cells are the first cell types to infiltrate the pancreatic islets (Yoon and Jun 2005). Macrophages must be involved in the pathogenesis of Type 1 (DM) early on, since inactivation of macrophages results in the near-complete prevention of insulitis and diabetes in both NOD mice and BB rats (Yoon and Jun 2005). The activated macrophages secrete IL-12, which stimulates Th1 type CD4+ T cells. The

CD4+ T cells secrete IFN-γ and IL-2. IFN-γ activates other resting macrophages, which, in turn, release cytokines, such as IL-1β, TNF-α, and free radicals, which are toxic to beta-cells. During this process, IL-2 and other cytokines induce the migration of $CD8^+$ peripheral T cells to the inflamed islets, perhaps by inducing the expression of a specific homing receptor. The precytotoxic $CD8^+$ T cells that bear beta-cell-specific autoantigen receptors differentiate into cytotoxic effector T cells upon recognition of the beta-cell-specific peptide bound to MHC class I molecules in the presence of beta-cell-specific $CD4^+$ T helper cells. The cytotoxic $CD8^+$ T cells then affect beta-cell damage by releasing perforin and granzyme, and by Fas-mediated apoptosis. In this way, macrophages, CD4+ T cells, and CD8+ T cells synergistically destroy beta-cells, resulting in the onset of autoimmune Type 1 (DM).

Both direct and indirect killing of beta-cells, mediated by $CD8^+$cytotoxic T cells and $CD4^+$helper T cells respectively, are thought to occur by apoptosis following activation of caspases, but necrosis also might play some role (Rasche, Busick et al. 2009). Based upon animal models, it is now generally believed that multiple effector molecules and pathways are involved in beta cell killing. In addition to apoptosis being the main mechanism by which beta-cells are destroyed, beta-cell apoptosis has been implicated in the initiation of Type 1 (DM) through antigen cross-presentation mechanisms that lead to beta-cell-specific T cell activation (The term cross-presentation denotes the ability of certain antigen-presenting cells to take up, process and present extracellular antigens with MHC class I molecules to CD8+cytotoxic T cells). In mammals, there are 14 caspases, of which many participate in the apoptotic pathways. Caspase-3 is the major effector caspase involved in apoptotic pathways. Caspase-3 knockout mice were protected from developing diabetes in autoimmune diabetes model.

As explained before, autoantibodies have turned out to be excellent diagnostic and predictive markers for Type 1 (DM). However, it is generally thought that they play only a minor role, if any, in the actual pathogenesis of the disease. Instead, the cell-mediated immune response is believed to be responsible for beta-cell killing as explained above. Inflammatory cells are found in and around the pancreatic islets. However, human studies show that in some individuals these inflammatory cells are present for years without clinical symptoms. In fact, some individuals with autoantibodies and insulitis do not go on to develop clinical disease. The outcome appears to be related to the amount of beta-cell destruction. It is estimated from animal studies that between 80 and 90% of the beta-cells must be destroyed before the diabetes becomes clinically apparent. In humans, however, the temporal and quantitative relationships between inflammatory cells, beta-cell damage, and clinical diabetes have been difficult to determine because pancreatic biopsies are not easy to be performed. Finally, much of our information about cell-mediated immune pathogenesis and beta-cell killing comes from animal models. These animals spontaneously develop an autoimmune disease similar, although not identical, to human autoimmune Type 1 (DM).

The possible dysregulation of Regulatory T cells (Treg) suppressor activity is shown to association to Type 1 (DM) as well.

3.5. Immunoregulatory problems underlie loss to beta-cell tolerance

Regulatory CD4+ T-cells (Treg), whose development and function is dictated by the Foxp3 gene in mice and humans have the primary function of pouring a cold shower on inflammatory responses. They suppress and regulate the function of various immune responses to microbes, tumors, allergens and transplants (Sakaguchi, Setoguchi et al. 2006). It is suspected that defects in Treg number and activity are causally related to the development of Type 1 (DM). It is likely, that certain genetic predispositions, coupled with the possible contribution of external environmental factors or infections, could potentially alter regulatory T-cell function in susceptible individuals and trigger a full-scale diabetic autoimmune reaction in the pancreas.

Many studies have implicated Treg cells in the control of diabetes onset and progression, and that reduced Foxp3+ Treg cell frequencies or functions in NOD mice, represent a primary predisposing factor to diabetes. Whether thymic development of Treg cells is normal in NOD mice has been a contentious issue. Recent studies show that thymic development of Treg cells seems to be normal, as thymectomy in NOD mice up to 3 weeks of age results in exacerbated Type 1 (DM) due to a marked reduction in Treg cells (Dardenne, Lepault et al. 1989). Surprisingly, the NOD background proved superior in generating Treg cells in the thymus relative to non-autoimmune prone strain C57/BL6, suggesting that central tolerance mechanisms are intact. Furthermore, the frequency and function of single-positive Foxp3+ Treg cells in the thymus of NOD was comparable to diabetes-resistant C57/BL6 mice (Tritt, Sgouroudis et al. 2008).

It is believed that regulatory T cells may represent a kind of master switch, and by understanding how they are made, how they function and how they survive, we may be able to stop disease from occurring. The use of beta-cell specific Tregs is also leading to a tissue specific immunotolerance without perturbing the general immunocompetence. If subsequent studies show that Tregs represent a safe and efficient source for therapy, they could become an important weapon in the fight against immune mediated pathology.

4. Triggers of autoimmune cascade

A critical question, independent of the mechanism by which the immune response kills beta-cells, is what actually triggers the autoimmune cascade. Immunologic, genetic, and environmental factors have been implicated. Normally an individual's T lymphocytes are immunologically anergic or tolerant to self-antigens. T lymphocyte education and selection takes place in the thymus. T cells that do not receive a signal from an HLA-autoantigen complex die by neglect. T cells that receive a signal from an HLA-autoantigen complex that is too strong die by apoptosis. However, T cells that receive a weak, low affinity signal from an HLA-autoantigen complex are positively selected. These positively selected autoantigen-specific T cells, generally present in very low numbers, escape from the thymus and migrate to peripheral organs throughout the body including the pancreas. Under ordinary circumstances they remain dormant and are kept under strict regulatory control by still poorly defined regulatory mechanisms (*e.g.* CD4+CD25+Foxp3+ Regulatory T cells or other regulatory pathway). If, however, these antigen-specific T cells come in contact with cognate autoantigens presented by beta-cells or APCs, through MHC-I and MHC-II respectively, in the pancreas and if the regulatory controls fail, these dormant, antigen-specific T cells will be activated and the autoimmune cascade of beta-cell killing will be initiated. Thus, immune dysregulation may serve as one of the triggers for autoimmunity. Genetic and environmental factors have been implicated as possible initiating triggers. The fact that in identical twins the concordance rate for Type 1 (DM) is less than 50% argues for genetic predisposition upon which an environmental insult is superimposed. More than 20 putative diabetes predisposing genes have been identified, but most of them have only a weak association, and in many cases the association has been difficult to confirm. The one exception is the HLA genes, which are thought to contribute as much as 50% of the genetic risk for Type 1 (DM) (Noble, Valdes et al. 2010). Although HLA genes may be necessary, by themselves they seem not to be sufficient to produce the disease. From a genetic point of view, all the evidence points to Type 1 (DM) as a complex disease involving a combination of several different genes. However, it may be that there is no specific "diabetes" gene(s). Instead, there may be the "wrong combination" of perfectly normal genes (*i.e.* alleles, haplotypes) that regulate, at the level of the beta-cell, processes such as apoptosis or antigen processing and presentation which, in turn, may trigger an autoimmune response.Various environmental triggers, e.g. certain viruses and dietary factors, are also thought to initiate the autoimmune process, leading to the destruction of pancreatic beta-cells and consequent Type 1 (DM). The major focus of the following parts is on genetic and environmental factors that predispose and triggers the autoimmune cascade.

4.1 Genetic etiology of Type 1 (DM)

To date, twelve separate chromosome regions have been implicated in the development of human Type 1 (DM). The major disease locus, *IDDM1* in the major histocompatibility complex (MHC) on chromosome 6p21, accounts for about 35% of the observed familial clustering and its contribution to disease susceptibility is likely to involve polymorphic residues of class II molecules in T-cell-mediated autoimmunity (Huber, Menconi et al. 2008). *IDDM2* is encoded by a minisatellite locus embedded in the regulatory region of the insulin gene. Familial clustering of disease can be explained by the sharing of alleles of at least 10 loci. *IDDM1* and *IDDM2* interact epistatically. For a multifactorial disease, such as Type 1 (DM), important information concerning the pathways and mechanisms involved can be gained from examining such interactions between loci, using methods that simultaneously take account of the joint effects of the various underlying genetic components.

The task of identifying susceptibility genes for complex human traits can be facilitated by first mapping susceptibility genes in an experimental species, such as the mouse or rat, and then performing mapping studies in humans by examining regions of disease in an animal model. However the animal models might not be same as the human susceptibility genes, in terms of the number of genes involved, interactions between loci and the physiological disease processes. For *IDDM*, the (NOD) mouse spontaneously develops Type1 (DM) with remarkable similarities to the human disorder. Moreover, *IDDM1*, the major genetic locus contributing to human *IDDM* in the MHC has been shown to be conserved between the two species of human and murine. A second locus, *IDDM7* on chromosome 2q31, is homologous to a region containing the *NOD* locus, *Idd5,* on chromosome 1 (Copeman, Cucca et al. 1995). Thirdly, there is evidence that the gene region encoding the human interleukin 1 (IL-1) on chromosome 2q12-q21 is associated and linked to Type 1 (DM). This region would correspond to mouse chromosome 2, in which the region encoding IL-1 has also been linked to NOD diabetes (Serreze, Prochazka et al. 1994).

A key issue in the identification of disease susceptibility genes is that of testing association versus testing linkage. Only through demonstrating association between specific alleles at a disease locus and the disease can the causal role of particular polymorphisms in the physiological disease processes be investigated. For mapping of disease loci, however, demonstration of linkage and estimation of the recombination fraction between a disease locus and known marker loci is required. Having mapped a disease locus to a particular chromosome region, the position of the disease locus can be further localized using tests of linkage disequilibrium between particular marker alleles and the disease, which assumes a founder effect for the ancestral mutation or selection of the mutation in the study population.

The strongest genetic association for Type 1 (DM) is with the HLA class I and II genes, with a 30–50% of the genetic risk for progression of the disease. Therefor in the next section the contribution of HLA genes predisposing to Type 1 (DM) will be addressed more extensively.

4.1.1. HLA genes predisposing to Type 1 (DM)

From a genetic point of view, combinations of several different genes are involved in predisposition to Type1 (DM), and there is no specific diabetes gene(s). Human Leukocyte Antigen (HLA) genes are thought to contribute the massive part of the genetic risk for Type1 (DM). In humans, the MHC is known as the HLA complex and contains over 200 genes. It is located on chromosome 6 and encodes HLA class I and class II molecules. The main function of these molecules is to present antigens that have been processed into peptides to antigen-specific receptors on CD4 and $CD8^{+}$T lymphocytes. Class I molecules, expressed on most nucleated cells, are encoded by genes within the HLA-A, -B, and -C loci, whereas class II molecules, expressed primarily on antigen-presenting cells (*e.g.* macrophages and dendritic cells), are encoded by genes within the HLA-DP, -DQ, and -DR loci.

HLA class I and II genes are highly polymorphic and consist of many different alleles. In type 1 diabetes, certain HLA class II alleles or combinations of alleles (haplotypes) show a strong association with the development of diabetes, whereas other haplotypes show a weak or even protective association. It is well established that the HLA-DR3 and HLA-DR4 genes at the HLA-DR locus on chromosome 6 are strongly associated with increased susceptibility to insulin-dependent diabetes (Field and McArthur 1987), and that the predisposition is greatest among individuals who possess both of these genes (HLA-DR3/4 heterozygotes). Furthermore, individuals with the HLA haplotype DRB1*0302- DQA1*0301, especially when combined with DRB1*0201- DQA1*0501, are highly susceptible (10–20-fold increase) to Type1 (DM) (Pociot and McDermott 2002). In contrast, individuals with the haplotype DRB1*0602-DQA1*0102 rarely develop type 1 diabetes. Many other high and low risk haplotypes have been identified, and the frequency of specific haplotypes differs among ethnic groups (Pociot and McDermott 2002). Other genes within the HLA complex, particularly class I genes, also have been linked to type 1 diabetes, but the strongest linkage by far is with the DQ and DR class II genes.

Experimental support for the importance of class II genes in the development of diabetes comes from a variety of sources including the deletion of specific MHC loci in mice and their replacement with human HLA homologs. Although the linkage of HLA class II molecules with Type1 (DM) is now well established and the binding of peptides to pockets within the groove of the HLA class II molecule understood, why the binding of peptides to certain HLA class II molecules, and not to others, is associated with autoimmune Type 1 (DM) remains unresolved (concerning the fact that CD8+ T cell have the largest contribution in the pathogenesis of Type 1 (DM)). Regardless of mechanism, HLA typing has proved useful in population screening for identification and follow-up of individuals at high risk for disease.

4.1.2. Non-HLA genes contributing to Type 1 (DM)

Multiple studies have recently linked Type 1 (DM) to 50 non-HLA gene polymorphisms (Pociot and McDermott 2002). Major efforts have therefore been made to identify non-HLA genetic risk factors for Type 1 (DM). Interestingly enough, many of the genetic factors are important to the function of the immune system. For instance *PTPN22* is a regulator of T-cell function and a genetic polymorphism results in a phosphatase variant that is increasing the risk not only for Type 1 (DM) but also for rheumatoid arthritis, juvenile rheumatoid arthritis, systemic lupus erythematosus, Graves' disease, generalized vitiligo, and other human autoimmune diseases (Herr, Dudbridge et al. 2000). The *PTPN22* polymorphism seems in particular to affect progression from pre-diabetes to clinical disease (Herr, Dudbridge et al. 2000) also in individuals with lower risk HLA genotypes. The variable nucleotide tandem repeat in the promoter region of the insulin gene *INS VNTR* seems to contribute to Type 1(DM) by the mechanisms of central tolerance (Takase, Yu et al. 2005). In newly diagnosed Type 1 (DM) patients the presence of insulin autoantibodies is associated with the *INS VNTR* polymorphism (Takase, Yu et al. 2005).

The majority of the non-HLA genetic factors seem to be associated with the immune system. We have also demonstrated the association of the polymorphism of Th1 type cytokines (IL-12, IL-18) as well as TGF-β in human patients with Type 1 (DM). It is therefore attractive to speculate that their contribution is related to the ability of the immune system to mount an autoimmune reaction specifically directed toward the islet beta-cells.

The existence of genes predisposing to Type 1 (DM) in the region of the insulin (INS) gene now also established. Association analysis has demonstrated an increased frequency of class 1 alleles of the 5' INS polymorphism in diabetics compared with controls. Interestingly, the effect of INS region susceptibility on Type 1 (DM) cannot be detected by linkage analysis, suggesting that if a genetic marker locus is close to a disease susceptibility locus, association analysis may be a more sensitive method than linkage analysis for detecting the susceptibility locus.

4.2. Potential environmental triggers of beta-cell autoimmunity in Type 1 (DM)

The clinical presentation of type 1 diabetes is preceded by an asymptomatic period of highly variable duration. Aggressive beta-cell destruction may lead to disease manifestation within a few months in infants and young children, whereas in other individuals, the process may continue for years (in some cases, even for >10 years) before the eventual presentation of overt disease.

Several lines of evidence support a critical role of exogenous factors in the pathogenesis of Type 1 (DM). Studies in monozygotic twins indicate that only 13–33% are pairwise concordant for Type 1 (DM) (Barnett, Eff et al. 1981), suggesting that there is either acquired postconceptional genetic discordance or differential exposure to the putative environmental factor(s). The geographic variation in the incidence of Type 1 (DM) in children is conspicuous. This difference in incidence can hardly be explained by genetic factors. A substantial increase in the incidence of Type 1 (DM) among children has been documented over the last decades, particularly in Europe—for example, in Finland, the incidence has increased 4.5-fold from the early 1950s (Gale 2002). Such an increase cannot be the consequence only of enhanced genetic disease susceptibility in the population but must mostly be due to changes in lifestyle and environment. As well, available data indicate that the incidence of Type 1 (DM) has increased in population groups who have moved from a low-incidence region to a high-incidence area, emphasizing the influence of environmental conditions (Akerblom and Knip 1998). Accumulating evidence suggests that the proportion of subjects with high-risk HLA genotypes has decreased over the last decades among patients with newly diagnosed type 1 diabetes, whereas the proportion of people with low-risk or even protective HLA genotypes has increased (Resic-Lindehammer, Larsson et al. 2008). These data are compatible with an increased environmental pressure resulting in progression to clinical diabetes with less genetic susceptibility.

As mentioned earlier, the first signs of beta-cell autoimmunity and the autoantibodies may appear very early in life. Many studies have revealed that there is an unequivocal temporal variation in the appearance of the diabetes-associated autoantibodies reflecting the initiation of the disease process and paralleling the seasonal variation. Most initial autoantibodies appear during the cold period in the fall and winter but rarely in the spring or in the summer. There also seems to be some variation from one year to another in the timing and height of the autoantibody peaks.

The pattern of the autoantibody appearance strongly points to the role of infectious agents with conspicuous seasonal variation as triggers of beta-cell autoimmunity. Such variations are typical for viral infections, and the pattern of laboratory-confirmed enterovirus infections. In addition to viral infections, one should also consider other environmental variables with seasonal variation. There is definitely seasonal variation in the amount of daylight and sunshine hours, especially in Northern Europe, which has the highest incidence of Type 1 (DM) in the world (Moltchanova, Penttinen et al. 2005). Without oral substitution, the sunlight-dependent synthesis of vitamin D in the skin is the most important source of this immunologically active hormone. Some studies have indicated that the lack of oral vitamin D substitution in infancy increases the subsequent risk of type 1 diabetes. Also improved insulin sensitivity in the spring and summer because of more physical exercise can be taken into account as well. Improved insulin sensitivity diminishes beta-cell stress, as the workload on the beta-cells decreases. However, it is unlikely that there should be substantial seasonal variation in physical exercise in very young children, the target group in whom the seasonal variation in the appearance of the first diabetes-associated autoantibodies has been observed.

Accordingly, we are left with viral infections as the most likely explanation for the seasonal variation in the emergence of the first signs of beta-cell autoimmunity. Taken into account the timing and profiles of the autoantibody peaks, such as enterovirus infections, appear to be the most probable trigger of beta-cell autoimmunity. The frequency of enterovirus infections has decreased over the last decades in the background population in developed countries, e.g., in Finland and Sweden (Viskari, Ludvigsson et al. 2005). Despite that, these countries have a high and increasing incidence of Type 1 (DM) among children. This appears to be paradoxical. The paradox can, however, be explained by the so-called "polio hypothesis" introduced by Viskari et al (Viskari, Koskela et al. 2000). The polioviruses comprise three serotypes among >60 enterovirus serotypes. When the frequency of acute poliovirus infections started to decrease at the beginning of the last century among the general population in countries with an increasing standard of hygiene, the incidence of paralytic polio being a complication of the acute infection began to increase. This was obviously the consequence of decreased levels of protective maternal poliovirus antibodies transferred transplacentally and through breast milk to the infant, leading to a situation where the risk increased that the infant would get his or her first poliovirus infection at the time of no maternal protection. Similarly, the decreasing frequency of enterovirus infections in the background population would increase the susceptibility of young children to the diabetogenic effect of enteroviruses. The same phenomenon may also contribute to the marked international variation in Type 1 (DM) incidence, because enterovirus infections seem to be rare in countries where the rate of type 1 diabetes is high.

The tropism phenomenon (the characteristic of a virus to infect a particular tissue or cell type), in which the attachment of the virus to the viral receptors on the cell surface together with other interactions with cellular proteins is a central feature, is thought to explain why some variants of enteroviruses may be diabetogenic and others not. It has been proposed that pancreatic beta-cell tropic variants of the coxsackie B virus are present in the general population and that they are able to induce beta-cell damage in susceptible individuals. In vitro studies have shown that enteroviruses infect beta-cells easily and induce functional impairment and cell death (Roivainen, Rasilainen et al. 2000).

Taken together, accumulated data support the hypothesis that a diabetogenic enterovirus infection is the likely trigger of beta-cell autoimmunity. This is supported by the observed temporal variation in the appearance of the first diabetes-associated autoantibodies in young children, the profile of which resembles the temporal profile of enterovirus infections in the background population.

Some other viruses, such as encephalomyocarditis virus, act directly by replicating in and destroying pancreatic beta-cells. A single amino acid substitution in the virus, presumably by altering its binding to beta-cells, determines whether or not diabetes develops. The Kilham rat virus, on the other hand, produces diabetes not by infecting beta-cells but by altering the immunoregulatory network of the host (Herr, Dudbridge et al. 2000). Still other viruses are thought to initiate or accelerate the autoimmune response through molecular mimicry (Copeman, Cucca et al. 1995) or by releasing sequestrated autoantigens from damaged beta-cells. In a transgenic autoimmune model (Serreze, Prochazka et al. 1994), the administration of infectious lymphocytic choriomeningitis virus (LCM) to transgenic animals expressing LCM viral proteins in their beta-cells results in diabetes, but the same LCM virus does not produce diabetes in non-transgenic animals.

A recent study has also found evidence of Coxsackie virus infection in beta-cells in three out of six pancreases of patients with recent-onset Type 1 (DM). Coxsackie viruses are known to induce interferon alpha secretion by beta-cells and this could initiate the sequence of events that culminates in their autoimmune destruction.

In summary of this part, Type 1 (DM) may be triggered by an environmental culprit at any age, although a majority of the processes appear to start early in childhood. Viruses have been the leading candidates. In animal experiments viruses have been shown to produce diabetes as well. In humans, case reports and sero-epidemiologic studies (Herr, Dudbridge et al. 2000) suggest that viruses, particularly enteroviruses, may play a role, but most likely as a cofactor, in individuals who already have suffered some autoimmune beta-cell loss. However, for the vast majority of the cases of Type 1 (DM) in humans, a viral cause has not been established.

The identification of exogenous factors triggering and driving beta-cell destruction offers potential means for intervention aimed at the prevention of Type 1 (DM). Therefore, it is important to pursue studies on the role of environmental factors in the pathogenesis of this disease. Environmental modification is likely to offer the most powerful strategy for effective prevention of Type 1 (DM), since such an approach can target the whole population or at least that proportion of the population carrying increased genetic disease susceptibility and would therefore prevent both sporadic and familial type 1 diabetes if successful.

5. Therapeutic interventions

Before the isolation of insulin in the 1920s, most patients died within a short time after onset of Type 1 (DM). Untreated diabetes leads to ketoacidosis, the accumulation of ketones (products of fat breakdown) and acid in the blood. Continued buildup of these products of disordered carbohydrate and fat metabolism result in nausea and vomiting, and eventually the patient goes into a diabetic coma.

Treatment for diabetes mellitus is aimed at reducing blood glucose concentrations to normal levels. Achieving this is important in promoting well-being and in minimizing the development and progression of the long-term complications of diabetes. Despite the widespread use of exogenous insulin, morbidity and mortality caused by Type 1 (DM) continue to place a significant burden on society, both in terms of human suffering and cost. The care of diabetes on self-management is based on the patient's clinical status and his/her ability to participate in self-care. Insulin replacement therapy is the mainstay for patients with Type 1 (DM) while diet and lifestyle modifications are also crucial for the treatment and management of this disease.

Diabetics who are unable to produce insulin in their bodies receive regular injections of the insulin, which are often customized according to their individual and variable requirements. Beef or pork insulin, made from the pancreatic extracts of cattle or pigs, can be used to treat humans with diabetes. However, in the United States, beef and pork forms of insulin are no longer manufactured, having been discontinued in favor of human insulin production. Modern human insulin treatments are based on recombinant DNA technology. Human insulin may be given as a form that is identical to the natural form found in the body, which acts quickly but transiently, or as a form that has been biochemically modified so as to prolong its action for up to 24 hours. The optimal regimen of insulin administration is one that most closely mimics the normal pattern of insulin secretion, which is a constant low level of insulin secretion plus a pulse of secretion after each meal. This can be achieved by administration of a long-acting insulin preparation once daily plus administration of a rapid-acting insulin preparation with or just before each meal. Patients also have the option of using an insulin pump, which allows them to control variations in the rate of insulin administration. A satisfactory compromise for some patients is twice-daily administration of mixtures of intermediate-acting and short-acting insulin. Patients taking insulin also may need to vary food intake from meal to meal, according to their level of activity; as exercise frequency and intensity increase, less insulin and more food intake may be necessary.

There are also several classes of oral drugs used to control blood glucose levels, including sulfonylureas, biguanides, and thiazolidinediones. Sulfonylureas, such as glipizide and glimepiride, are considered hypoglycemic agents because they stimulate the release of insulin from beta-cells in the pancreas, thus reducing blood glucose levels (Pernet, Trimble et al. 1985). The most common side effect associated with sulfonylureas is hypoglycemia (abnormally low blood glucose levels), which occurs most often in elderly patients who have impaired liver or kidney function.

Biguanides, of which metformin is the primary member, are considered antihyperglycemic agents because they work by decreasing the production of glucose in the liver and by increasing the action of insulin on muscle and adipose tissues (Spaans, Kleefstra et al. 2011). A potentially fatal side effect of metformin is the accumulation of lactic acid in blood and tissues, often causing vague symptoms such as nausea and weakness.

Thiazolidinediones, such as rosiglitazone and pioglitazone, act by reducing insulin resistance of muscle and adipose cells and by increasing glucose transport into these tissues

(Garg 2011). These agents can cause edema (fluid accumulation in tissues), liver toxicity, and adverse cardiovascular events in certain patients. Furthermore, oral hypoglycemic agents lower mean blood glucose concentrations by only about 50–80 mg per 100 ml (2.8–4.4 mmol/l), and sensitivity to these drugs tends to decrease with time(Garg 2011).

There are several other agents that can be highly effective in the treatment of diabetes. Pramlintide is an injectable synthetic hormone (based on the human hormone amylin) that regulates blood glucose levels by slowing the absorption of food in the stomach and by inhibiting glucagon, which normally stimulates liver glucose production(Riddle and Drucker 2006). Exenatide is an injectable antihyperglycemic drug that works similarly to incretins, or gastrointestinal hormones, such as gastric inhibitory polypeptide, that stimulate insulin release from the pancreas. Exenatide has a longer duration of action than incretins produced by the body because it is less susceptible to degradation by an enzyme called dipeptidyl peptidase-4 (DPP-4)(Sena, Nunes et al. 2008). A drug called sitagliptin specifically inhibits DPP-4, thereby increasing levels of naturally produced incretins. Side effects associated with these drugs are often mild, although pramlintide can cause profound hypoglycemia in patients with Type 1 (DM).

All patients with diabetes mellitus, particularly those taking insulin, should measure blood glucose concentrations periodically at home, especially when they have symptoms of hypoglycemia. Diet and lifestyle strategies also are required to reduce weight, improve glycaemic control and reduce the risk of cardiovascular complications, which account for 70% to 80% of deaths among those with diabetes.

Research into other areas of insulin therapy includes pancreas transplantation, beta-cell transplantation, and generation of beta-cells from existing exocrine cells in the pancreas. Patients with Type I (DM) have been treated by transplantation of the pancreas or of the islets of Langerhans. However, limited quantities of pancreatic tissue are available for transplantation, prolonged immunosuppressive therapy is needed, and there is a high likelihood that the transplanted tissue be rejected even when the patient is receiving immunosuppressive therapy. Attempts to improve the outcome of transplantation and to develop mechanical islets are ongoing.

Whole pancreas or islet transplantation is another treatment continues to develop and reduced the need for insulin, achieve better glucose stability, and reduce problems with hypoglycemia. The transplantation of vascularized pancreas, from a deceased donor, developed in the 1960s and usually performed concurrently with renal transplantation, can cure Type 1 (DM), as shown by results in more than 15,000 such transplants over about 30 years. Transplantation of isolated pancreatic islets, instead of the whole organ, however, offers an attractive alternative that minimizes surgery and its complications. Although islet transplantation initially met with only modest success, recent changes in patient selection criteria, number and treatment of islets transplanted, and better immunosuppressive regimens dramatically improved the results. The development of clinical islet transplantation was driven by an unmet medical need within the diabetes mellitus patient population and was preceded by the introduction of transplantation of whole, vascularized pancreas. Despite this promise, organ/islet availability remains an important limitation to this technology. A solution to the problem of limited materials for transplantation may be in the use of stem/progenitor cells.

The presence of beta-cells in patients with long-standing Type 1 (DM), despite ongoing autoimmunity, implies that new formation of beta-cells may be occurring. Although an ambitious aim currently targeted regeneration of such beta-cells offers another strategy to prevent Type 1 (DM). Regeneration of beta-cells is therefore an area of major active investigation, with recent studies reporting differentiation of pancreatic and nonpancreatic progenitors as well as replication of existing islet beta-cells. In this regard some studies have shown that pre-existing beta-cells, rather than pluripotent stem cells, are the main source of new beta-cells during adult life and after pancreatectomy in mice.

6. Cellular and molecular strategy for inhibition of the initiation and progression of beta-cell destruction

Mononuclear cell infiltration into the islets of the pancreas (insulitis) is characteristic of autoimmune diabetes. T lymphocytes are the predominant subpopulation seen in insulitis, and are involved in the autoimmune process. Insulin-producing beta-cells are thought to be destroyed by cytotoxic T cells, cytokines or nitric oxide, and beta-cell death occurs, at least partly, via apoptosis. Beta-cell death induced by inflammatory cytokines can be inhibited by forced expression of Bcl-2 (*B-cell lymphoma 2,* thought to implicate in cell growth and survival) in those cells, suggesting its potential as a tool for gene therapy (Iwahashi, Itoh et al. 1998). The Fas/Fas-ligand system plays a critical role in inducing insulitis and overt diabetes in (NOD) mice as well. Beta-cells are destroyed by apoptosis through Fas-Fas ligand and TNF-TNF receptor interactions and by granzymes and perforin released from cytotoxic effector T cells. Therefore, the activated macrophages and T cells, and cytokines secreted from these immunocytes, act synergistically to destroy beta-cells, resulting in the development of Type 1 (DM). Preventive strategies might be developed by focusing on these molecules involved in beta-cell destruction.

The feasibility of gene therapy in NOD mice by *ex vivo* genetic manipulation of normal hematopoietic stem cells (HSCs) with proinsulin II followed by transfer to recipient mice has been examined as an approach to treat T1D recently (10). The incidence and degree of insulitis was significantly reduced in recipient, and thus this molecular chimerism can potentially protect from destructive insulitis in an antigen-specific manner (10).

In some studies the anti–T cell strategies were also examined to inhibit insulitis. Early studies of cyclosporin in the 1980s provided a proof of principal for the usefulness of immunomodulators in the treatment of Type 1 (DM); the adverse effects of cyclosporin, however, were incompatible with their widespread use. More sophisticated anti–T-cell strategies have been developed more recently. In the hOKT3γ1(Ala-Ala) trial, a humanized, modified anti-CD3 monoclonal antibody, analysis of peripheral blood samples demonstrated an increase in the CD8/CD4 ratio and in particular an increase in CD4+CD25+

regulatory T cells (36). Most studies of regulatory T cells have focused on a subset of naturally occurring CD4+ cells that have the capacity to control self-reactive T cells, and their depletion results in autoimmunity. Strategies that target the action of regulatory T cells *in vivo* offer one of the most attractive options for therapy in Type 1 (DM). The establishment of screening techniques for detecting prediabetic patients is also necessary to allow successful intervention.

Immunosuppressive drugs and anti-T cell antibodies have shown varying degrees of success in suppression of beta-cell autoimmunity in NOD mice. However, these strategies require repeated drug administration and may cause nonspecific harmful effects such as interference with normal immune system functions. A new therapeutic approach for type 1 diabetes is based on prevention of beta-cell loss through vaccine restoration of normal immune system function. Traditionally, vaccination refers to prevention of an infectious disease by exposing the immune system to a weakened or dead infectious agent. Alternatively, "inverse vaccination" (the inhibition of an immune response) arrests autoimmunity through manipulation of the innate and adaptive arms of the immune system (Steinman 2010). In type 1 diabetes, vaccination with β-cell autoantigens was shown to induce a partial state of immunological tolerance in NOD mice (Peakman and von Herrath 2010). Beta-cell self-antigens can induce tolerance through three possible mechanisms: (1) induction of T cell deletion/anergy, (2) induction of anti-inflammatory T helper 2 (Th2) cells, and (3) stimulation of regulatory T cell proliferation (Maldonado and von Andrian 2010). Insulin, GAD and some heat shock proteins are considered to be the first pancreatic autoantigens detected early during diabetes onset in both humans and NOD mice. However, the primary beta-cell antigen responsible for triggering autoimmunity in Type 1 (DM) remains under dispute. Thus, several pancreatic autoantigens have been selected for development into type 1 diabetes vaccines. These results suggest that multi-component vaccine strategies are promising for prevention and reversal of diabetes autoimmunity in humans, although some antigens determined to be most immunogenic, and not successful in trials.

We are still some way from developing a pill to prevent Type 1 (DM), but all the divergent strands of ongoing research, from epidemiology to molecular biology, immunology to clinical trials, appear to be converging to provide clear perspectives on the therapeutic interventions that are most likely to be successful. Two strategies are open to physicians who have patients with Type 1 (DM): the first is to prevent initiation of autoimmunity; the second is to reverse the effects of ongoing autoimmunity coupled with beta-cell regeneration. Although highly ambitious, the prevention of Type 1 (DM) could be possible by identifying and eliminating environmental risk factors. The next line of defense would be to re-educate the immune system through exposure to beta-cell antigens with the use of oral or nasal tolerance strategies. The observation that insulin may be the primary autoantigen provides support for therapies using insulin to induce tolerance. The potential to re-educate the immune system, or to divert it using regulatory T cells, and the rapidly expanding field of islet beta-cell differentiation give hope that improved strategies to manage this chronic disease are on the horizon.

7. Concluding remarks

Type 1 (DM), formerly known as juvenile diabetes is a complex disease caused by multiple environmental and genetic risk factors. It is a T cell-mediated disease characterized by the destruction of the endocrine insulin-producing beta-cells of the pancreatic islets, resulting in plasma glucose dysregulation, persistent hyperglycemia and long-term complications. Evidence for a constant global increase of incidents is worrisome. There is a major international challenge for optimal intervention and prevention strategies. Thus, a better understanding of the events going on in the autoimmune processes and understanding the relative contribution of genetics and environmental factors is necessary for the ultimate prevention/treatment.

Research is ongoing to discover the exact cause of Type 1 (DM), which remains unknown. Eepidemiological studies support the notion that viral infections play a causative role in Type 1 (DM). Indeed, there is a strong association between certain HLA and non-HLA alleles or combinations of alleles that predispose to development of Type 1 (DM). HLA typing is one means in screening to identify individuals at high risk as well.

Based on experimental results from studies using NOD mice and BB rats over the past 3 decades, the possible interactions between beta-cell autoantigens and immunocytes such as macrophages, dendritic cells, T cells, and their secretory products in connection with MHC class I and II molecules has shown in this autoimmune disease. The animal models may not encompass all aspects of the pathogenic mechanisms involved in autoimmune diabetes in humans; nevertheless, it may provide helpful information with respect to the synergistic destruction of beta-cells by immunocytes and their cytokines and a basis for the formation of new hypotheses for further investigation.

Although rarer than type 2, Type 1 (DM) is more severe, and constitutes the fourth or fifth leading cause of death worldwide. There is currently no cure or preventative measure for Type 1 (DM). Patients are dependent for the rest of their lives on regular injections of insulin to control their blood sugar levels. Combined with some conservative lifestyle choices, insulin lets people manage their diabetes, but the control of blood sugar is never perfect. In the long term, tolerogenic, antigen-specific and beta-cell-specific regenerative agents could provide a promising platform for the development of disease-modifying therapies. Thus, combination therapies could be most effective in delivering the long-sought cure.

Author details

Ahmad Massoud
Tehran University of Medical Science, Iran

Amir Hossein Massoud
McGill University, Canada

8. References

Akerblom, H. K. and M. Knip (1998). "Putative environmental factors in Type 1 diabetes." *Diabetes/metabolism reviews* 14(1): 31-67.

Atkinson, M. A. and N. K. Maclaren (1994). "The pathogenesis of insulin-dependent diabetes mellitus." *The New England journal of medicine* 331(21): 1428-1436.

Bakker, S. F., M. E. Tushuizen, et al. (2012). "Type 1 diabetes and celiac disease in adults: glycemic control and diabetic complications." *Acta diabetologica.*

Barnett, A. H., C. Eff, et al. (1981). "Diabetes in identical twins. A study of 200 pairs." *Diabetologia* 20(2): 87-93.

Bearse, M. A., Jr., Y. Han, et al. (2004). "Local multifocal oscillatory potential abnormalities in diabetes and early diabetic retinopathy." *Investigative ophthalmology & visual science* 45(9): 3259-3265.

Bergerot, I., N. Fabien, et al. (1994). "Oral administration of human insulin to NOD mice generates CD4+ T cells that suppress adoptive transfer of diabetes." *Journal of autoimmunity* 7(5): 655-663.

Betterle, C., F. Zanette, et al. (1984). "Clinical and subclinical organ-specific autoimmune manifestations in type 1 (insulin-dependent) diabetic patients and their first-degree relatives." *Diabetologia* 26(6): 431-436.

Cecil, R. L. (1909). "A Study of the Pathological Anatomy of the Pancreas in Ninety Cases of Diabetes Mellitus." *The Journal of experimental medicine* 11(2): 266-290.

Copeman, J. B., F. Cucca, et al. (1995). "Linkage disequilibrium mapping of a type 1 diabetes susceptibility gene (IDDM7) to chromosome 2q31-q33." *Nature genetics* 9(1): 80-85.

Dardenne, M., F. Lepault, et al. (1989). "Acceleration of the onset of diabetes in NOD mice by thymectomy at weaning." *European journal of immunology* 19(5): 889-895.

Field, L. L. and R. G. McArthur (1987). "The genetics of susceptibility to insulin-dependent diabetes mellitus--possible new markers." *Clinical and investigative medicine. Medecine clinique et experimentale* 10(5): 437-443.

Foulis, A. K., C. N. Liddle, et al. (1986). "The histopathology of the pancreas in type 1 (insulin-dependent) diabetes mellitus: a 25-year review of deaths in patients under 20 years of age in the United Kingdom." *Diabetologia* 29(5): 267-274.

French, M. B., J. Allison, et al. (1997). "Transgenic expression of mouse proinsulin II prevents diabetes in nonobese diabetic mice." *Diabetes* 46(1): 34-39.

Gale, E. A. (2002). "The rise of childhood type 1 diabetes in the 20th century." *Diabetes* 51(12): 3353-3361.

Garg, V. (2011). "Noninsulin pharmacological management of type 1 diabetes mellitus." *Indian journal of endocrinology and metabolism* 15(Suppl 1): S5-S11.

Genuth, S., K. G. Alberti, et al. (2003). "Follow-up report on the diagnosis of diabetes mellitus." *Diabetes care* 26(11): 3160-3167.

Gepts, W. (1965). "Pathologic anatomy of the pancreas in juvenile diabetes mellitus." *Diabetes* 14(10): 619-633.

Harrison, L. C., M. Dempsey-Collier, et al. (1996). "Aerosol insulin induces regulatory CD8 gamma delta T cells that prevent murine insulin-dependent diabetes." *The Journal of experimental medicine* 184(6): 2167-2174.

Herr, M., F. Dudbridge, et al. (2000). "Evaluation of fine mapping strategies for a multifactorial disease locus: systematic linkage and association analysis of IDDM1 in the HLA region on chromosome 6p21." *Human molecular genetics* 9(9): 1291-1301.

Huang, C., Y. Kim, et al. (2002). "Cellular basis of diabetic nephropathy: II. The transforming growth factor-beta system and diabetic nephropathy lesions in type 1 diabetes." *Diabetes* 51(12): 3577-3581.

Huber, A., F. Menconi, et al. (2008). "Joint genetic susceptibility to type 1 diabetes and autoimmune thyroiditis: from epidemiology to mechanisms." *Endocrine reviews* 29(6): 697-725.

Hutchings, P. and A. Cooke (1998). "Protection from insulin dependent diabetes mellitus afforded by insulin antigens in incomplete Freund's adjuvant depends on route of administration." *Journal of autoimmunity* 11(2): 127-130.

In't Veld, P. (2011). "Insulitis in human type 1 diabetes: The quest for an elusive lesion." *Islets* 3(4): 131-138.

Iwahashi, H., N. Itoh, et al. (1998). "Molecular mechanisms of pancreatic beta-cell destruction in autoimmune diabetes: potential targets for preventive therapy." *Cytokines, cellular & molecular therapy* 4(1): 45-51.

Karlsen, A. E., W. A. Hagopian, et al. (1991). "Cloning and primary structure of a human islet isoform of glutamic acid decarboxylase from chromosome 10." *Proceedings of the National Academy of Sciences of the United States of America* 88(19): 8337-8341.

Katavetin, P. (2009). "Renal and retinal effects of enalapril and losartan in type 1 diabetes." *The New England journal of medicine* 361(14): 1410-1411; author reply 1411.

Kent, S. C., Y. Chen, et al. (2005). "Expanded T cells from pancreatic lymph nodes of type 1 diabetic subjects recognize an insulin epitope." *Nature* 435(7039): 224-228.

Lahiri, M. K., P. J. Kannankeril, et al. (2008). "Assessment of autonomic function in cardiovascular disease: physiological basis and prognostic implications." *Journal of the American College of Cardiology* 51(18): 1725-1733.

Lecompte, P. M. (1958). "Insulitis in early juvenile diabetes." *A.M.A. archives of pathology* 66(4): 450-457.

Maldonado, R. A. and U. H. von Andrian (2010). "How tolerogenic dendritic cells induce regulatory T cells." *Advances in immunology* 108: 111-165.

Maser, R. E. and M. J. Lenhard (2005). "Cardiovascular autonomic neuropathy due to diabetes mellitus: clinical manifestations, consequences, and treatment." *The Journal of clinical endocrinology and metabolism* 90(10): 5896-5903.

Moltchanova, E., A. Penttinen, et al. (2005). "A hierarchical Bayesian birth cohort analysis from incomplete registry data: evaluating the trends in the age of onset of insulin-dependent diabetes mellitus (T1DM)." *Statistics in medicine* 24(19): 2989-3004.

Nagler, W. and H. Taylor (1963). "Diabetic coma with acute inflammation of Islets of Langerhans." *JAMA : the journal of the American Medical Association* 184: 723-725.

Nakayama, M., N. Abiru, et al. (2005). "Prime role for an insulin epitope in the development of type 1 diabetes in NOD mice." *Nature* 435(7039): 220-223.

Noble, J. A., A. M. Valdes, et al. (2010). "HLA class I and genetic susceptibility to type 1 diabetes: results from the Type 1 Diabetes Genetics Consortium." *Diabetes* 59(11): 2972-2979.

Owerbach, D. and K. H. Gabbay (1996). "The search for IDDM susceptibility genes: the next generation." *Diabetes* 45(5): 544-551.

Peakman, M. and M. von Herrath (2010). "Antigen-specific immunotherapy for type 1 diabetes: maximizing the potential." *Diabetes* 59(9): 2087-2093.

Pernet, A., E. R. Trimble, et al. (1985). "Sulfonylureas in insulin-dependent (type I) diabetes: evidence for an extrapancreatic effect in vivo." *The Journal of clinical endocrinology and metabolism* 61(2): 247-251.

Pharoah, P. D., A. M. Dunning, et al. (2004). "Association studies for finding cancer-susceptibility genetic variants." *Nature reviews. Cancer* 4(11): 850-860.

Pociot, F. and M. F. McDermott (2002). "Genetics of type 1 diabetes mellitus." *Genes and immunity* 3(5): 235-249.

Pugliese, A., D. Brown, et al. (2001). "Self-antigen-presenting cells expressing diabetes-associated autoantigens exist in both thymus and peripheral lymphoid organs." *The Journal of clinical investigation* 107(5): 555-564.

Rasche, S., R. Y. Busick, et al. (2009). "GAD65-Specific Cytotoxic T Lymphocytes Mediate Beta-Cell Death and Loss of Function." *The review of diabetic studies : RDS* 6(1): 43-53.

Resic-Lindehammer, S., K. Larsson, et al. (2008). "Temporal trends of HLA genotype frequencies of type 1 diabetes patients in Sweden from 1986 to 2005 suggest altered risk." *Acta diabetologica* 45(4): 231-235.

Riddle, M. C. and D. J. Drucker (2006). "Emerging therapies mimicking the effects of amylin and glucagon-like peptide 1." *Diabetes care* 29(2): 435-449.

Roivainen, M., S. Rasilainen, et al. (2000). "Mechanisms of coxsackievirus-induced damage to human pancreatic beta-cells." *The Journal of clinical endocrinology and metabolism* 85(1): 432-440.

Saely, C. H., S. Aczel, et al. (2004). "Cardiovascular complications in Type 2 diabetes mellitus depend on the coronary angiographic state rather than on the diabetic state." *Diabetologia* 47(1): 145-146.

Sakaguchi, S., R. Setoguchi, et al. (2006). "Naturally arising Foxp3-expressing CD25+CD4+ regulatory T cells in self-tolerance and autoimmune disease." *Current topics in microbiology and immunology* 305: 51-66.

Seki, M., T. Tanaka, et al. (2004). "Involvement of brain-derived neurotrophic factor in early retinal neuropathy of streptozotocin-induced diabetes in rats: therapeutic potential of brain-derived neurotrophic factor for dopaminergic amacrine cells." *Diabetes* 53(9): 2412-2419.

Sena, C. M., E. Nunes, et al. (2008). "Supplementation of coenzyme Q10 and alpha-tocopherol lowers glycated hemoglobin level and lipid peroxidation in pancreas of diabetic rats." *Nutrition research* 28(2): 113-121.

Serreze, D. V., M. Prochazka, et al. (1994). "Use of recombinant congenic and congenic strains of NOD mice to identify a new insulin-dependent diabetes resistance gene." *The Journal of experimental medicine* 180(4): 1553-1558.

Spaans, E. A., N. Kleefstra, et al. (2011). "[Metformin in adolescents and adults with type 1 diabetes mellitus: not evidence-based]." *Nederlands tijdschrift voor geneeskunde* 155(39): A3166.

Steinman, L. (2010). "Inverse vaccination, the opposite of Jenner's concept, for therapy of autoimmunity." *Journal of internal medicine* 267(5): 441-451.

Svensson, M., J. W. Eriksson, et al. (2004). "Early glycemic control, age at onset, and development of microvascular complications in childhood-onset type 1 diabetes: a population-based study in northern Sweden." *Diabetes care* 27(4): 955-962.

Takase, H., C. R. Yu, et al. (2005). "Thymic expression of peripheral tissue antigens in humans: a remarkable variability among individuals." *International immunology* 17(8): 1131-1140.

Toyoda, H. and B. Formby (1998). "Contribution of T cells to the development of autoimmune diabetes in the NOD mouse model." *BioEssays : news and reviews in molecular, cellular and developmental biology* 20(9): 750-757.

Tritt, M., E. Sgouroudis, et al. (2008). "Functional waning of naturally occurring CD4+ regulatory T-cells contributes to the onset of autoimmune diabetes." *Diabetes* 57(1): 113-123.

Viskari, H., J. Ludvigsson, et al. (2005). "Relationship between the incidence of type 1 diabetes and maternal enterovirus antibodies: time trends and geographical variation." *Diabetologia* 48(7): 1280-1287.

Viskari, H. R., P. Koskela, et al. (2000). "Can enterovirus infections explain the increasing incidence of type 1 diabetes?" *Diabetes care* 23(3): 414-416.

Wajchenberg, B. L. (2007). "beta-cell failure in diabetes and preservation by clinical treatment." *Endocrine reviews* 28(2): 187-218.

Wallace, C., G. E. Reiber, et al. (2002). "Incidence of falls, risk factors for falls, and fall-related fractures in individuals with diabetes and a prior foot ulcer." *Diabetes care* 25(11): 1983-1986.

Wan, X., C. Yang, et al. (2010). "BOOST: A fast approach to detecting gene-gene interactions in genome-wide case-control studies." *American journal of human genetics* 87(3): 325-340.

Willcox, A., S. J. Richardson, et al. (2009). "Analysis of islet inflammation in human type 1 diabetes." *Clinical and experimental immunology* 155(2): 173-181.

Yoon, J. W. and H. S. Jun (2005). "Autoimmune destruction of pancreatic beta cells." *American journal of therapeutics* 12(6): 580-591.

Ziegler, D., C. G. Sohr, et al. (2004). "Oxidative stress and antioxidant defense in relation to the severity of diabetic polyneuropathy and cardiovascular autonomic neuropathy." *Diabetes care* 27(9): 2178-2183.

Chapter 3

Balancing Pro- and Anti-Inflammatory CD4+ T Helper Cells in the Intestine

Nicola Gagliani and Samuel Huber

Additional information is available at the end of the chapter

http://dx.doi.org/10.5772/48183

1. Introduction

The intestinal mucosal surface represents a huge border where different pathogenic particles, such as bacteria, fungi, viruses or parasites can potentially invade and harm the body. One crucial task of the immune system in the intestine is to maintain this epithelial barrier, in order to prohibit or defeat a microbial invasion. Pro-inflammatory effector $CD4^{+}$ T helper cells play a crucial role during this task. These effector T helper cells can be subdivided into different subsets (Figure 1), which are characterized by a master transcriptional regulator and a unique cytokine profile: Th17 cells express RORγt that in turn promotes the transcription of *Il17a, Il17f, Il21* and *Il22*. Th1 cells express T-bet and produce IFN-γ, IL-2 and TNF-α. Th2 cells express GATA-3 and secrete IL-4, IL-5 and IL-13 [1-5]. The intestine also contains numerous non-pathogenic bacteria (commensal bacteria), which are beneficial to the host, as well as food antigens. This vast collection of non-self antigens can also promote the activation of T helper cells, and in turn cause immune-pathology. Therefore it is important for the immune system to control effector T helper cells. Indeed different types of regulatory T cells with anti-inflammatory properties team up in order to control effector T cells. The two most studied regulatory T cell subtypes are Foxp3+ regulatory T cells, which can be generated either in the thymus (nTreg) or induced in peripheral lymphoid organs (iTregs) and type 1 regulatory T cells (Tr1), which are induced in the periphery (Figure 1).

2. Differentiation of naïve CD4+ T cells into effector T helper cells

Naïve T cells, which are functionally immature, can be differentiated into different subsets of effector T cells upon activation. The fate of naïve T cell is directed by cytokines. These cytokines signal via different members of the STAT family, which induce master transcriptional regulators. Most of these transcriptional factors bind then to the effector cytokine gene thereby inducing gene activation, repression or epigenetic modification [6] (Figure 1). It should be noted that there is a certain amount of T helper cell heterogeneity and plasticity regarding cytokine production and expression of the master transcriptional factor of each T helper cell subset. This fact is currently also one of the most intriguing aspect of the ongoing research in Immunobiology. However, the model of different T helper cell lineages as first proposed by Mosmann and Coffman [7] is still the most useful one in order to understand the function and differentiation of T helper cells.

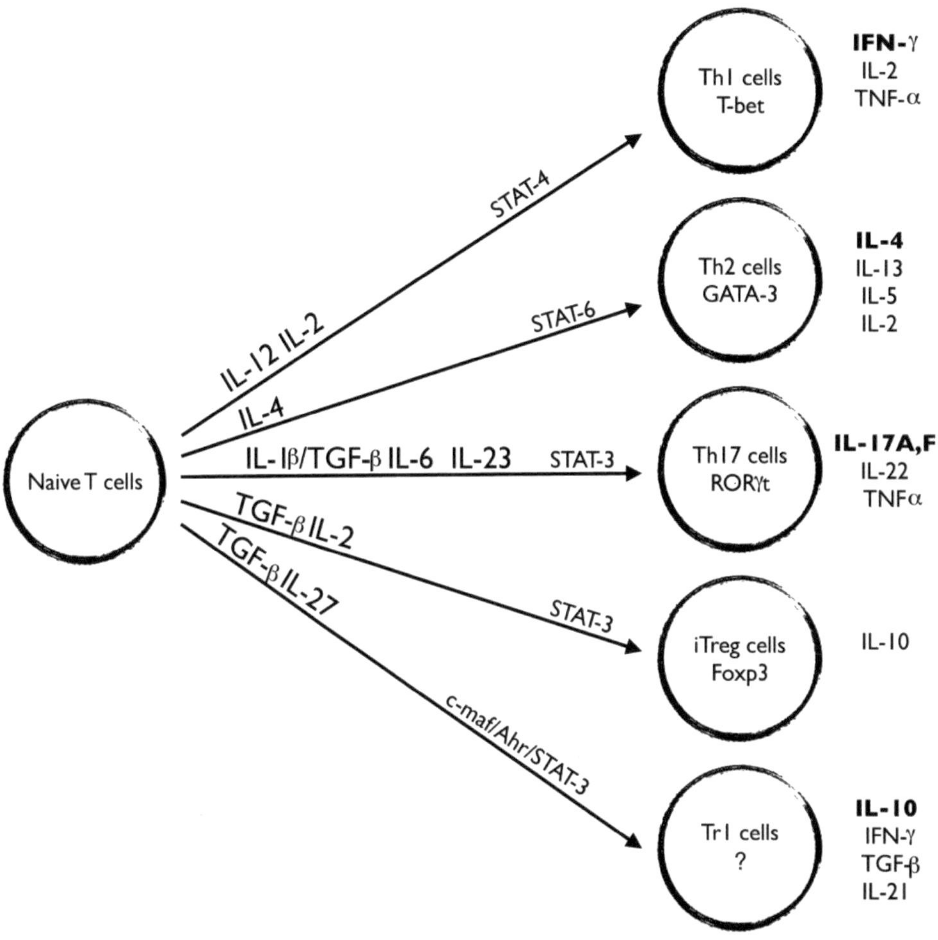

Figure 1. Differentiation of naïve T cells into different effector and regulatory T cells. A specific combination of cytokine signals leads to the differentiation of naïve T cells into different T helper cell subsets. Each T helper cell subset is characterized by the production of a combination of cytokines and exerts specific functions.

2.1. Differentiation and function of Th1 cells

Th1 cells produce IFN-γ as their signature cytokine. Th1 cells secrete also IL-2 and/ or TNF-α. Naive T cells upon TCR stimulation in the presence of IL-12 differentiate in Th1 cells [8].

IL-12 signals via STAT4 promoting the expression of T-bet, which transcribes the *Ifng* gene [9, 10]. T-bet is the master transcriptional regulator of Th1 cells, which is essential for the IFN-γ production [5]. Accordingly T-bet deficient mice have a defective Th1 differentiation [11]. One other important function of T-bet is the inhibition of GATA-3 expression, the master transcriptional regulator of Th2 cells [9].

Th1 cells are particularly important for the defense against intra-cellular bacteria. Some microorganisms such as mycobacteria, like *Mycobacterium tuberculosis* or *Mycobacterium lepromatosis*, are examples for these intracellular pathogens. These bacteria grow primarily in phagolysosomes of macrophages. Because of this feature these microorganisms are protected from the effects of antibodies and cytotoxic T cells. These bacteria can inhibit the fusion of lysosomes to the phagosomes, in which they grow and prevent the activation of the lysosomal proteases. The defense against these microorganisms is the important task of Th1 effector cells because they can activate macrophages, which are then able to kill ingested pathogens. Accordingly, deficiency in Th1 cells increases the susceptibility to infections with intracellular pathogens in humans [12]. These patients suffer from infections with mycobacteria, particularly *Mycobacterium tuberculosis,* but also with *Salmonella.* Of note both of these bacteria strains can typically infect the gastrointestinal system.

2.2 Differentiation and function of Th2 cells

The signature cytokines of Th2 cells are IL-4, IL-5, and IL-13. Some Th2 cells also produce TNF-α and/ or IL-9. Additionally, some Th2 cells can secrete small amounts of IL-2. The cytokines leading to Th2 differentiation are IL-2 and IL-4. Therefore the signature cytokine of Th2 cells, IL-4 also promotes the differentiation of Th2 cells [13-15]. STAT6 is the major signaling pathway of IL-4 mediated Th2 differentiation, and induces GATA-3 expression [16-20]. GATA-3 is the master transcriptional regulator of Th2 cells [3, 21] and the differentiation of these cells is indeed dependent on the induction of this master transcriptional regulator [22]. GATA-3 binds to the promoters of *Il5* and *Il13,* and the enhancer of *Il4* thereby promoting their transcription [6]. Additionally STAT5, which can be activated by IL-2, is important for Th2 differentiation and for the maintenance of GATA-3 expression [23].

Th2 cells and their effector cytokines IL-4, IL-5, and IL-13 are essential to control helminth infections in the intestine. In line with this, mice deficient in IL-4 receptor a-chain (IL-4Rα), STAT6 or GATA-3 show highly compromised anti-helminth immunity [24]. One of the most unique tasks of Th2 cells is the induction of B-cell immunoglobulin class switching. Through CD40-CD40L interaction, Th2 cells promote B cells to secret IgG1, IgE and (in humans) IgG4 isotype antibodies. These antibodies are again important for mediating protection against helminth infections. The Th2-immune response involves also eosinophils, basophils and mast cells, which all together mount the immune response controlling helminth infection. The release of IL-4 and IL-13 is key for eliciting the alternative activation of macrophage, which is crucial in order to trap the intestinal parasite [25, 26]. Th2-cytokines, in particular

IL-4 and IL-13, promote the goblet cell differentiation, the enhancement of mucus secretion and the production of resistin-like molecule-β (RELMβ), an innate protein with direct anti-helminth activity [27-29]. Moreover IL-4 stimulates intestinal muscle hyper-contractility and accelerates epithelial turnover to promote the 'epithelial escalator', which functions together with epithelial secretions to dislodge resident parasites [30, 31]. Another Th2 associated cytokine, namely IL-9, promotes the release of mast cell protease that can depredate tight junctions and in turn increase the fluid flow in the intestine. All together these mechanisms are part of the "weep and sweep" response, which is key for the control of a helminth invasion.

2.3. Differentiation and function of Th17 cells

The signature cytokines of Th17 cells are Il-17A and IL-17F. Th17 cells produce also, IL-22 and TNF-α. TGF-β, IL-1β, IL-6, and IL-23 are the cytokines, which are important for Th17 cell differentiation. IL-6 can activate STAT3, which induces IL-23R and RORγt [32-34], the master transcriptional regulator of Th17 cells. This master transcriptional regulator leads to the production of IL-17A and IL-17F [1, 4, 35, 36]. IL-6 also promotes the release of IL-21 [33], which synergizes with TGF-β, IL-6, and IL-1β, for the induction of IL-23 receptor expression [37]. In the presence of IL-23, $CD4^+$ $ROR\gamma t^+$ $IL\text{-}17A^+$ T cells can expand and fully mature in Th17 cells [38, 39].

Human and mouse Th17 cells are rare in a non-pathological state [2, 40]. A specific member of commensal microbiota, known as segmented filamentous bacteria (SFB), attracts Th17 cells in the terminal ileum of mice [41]. Therefore in steady state condition most of the few Th17 cells accumulate mainly in the intestine. The commensal microbiota promotes the release of serum amyloid A [41] and adenosine 5′-triphosphate (ATP), which activates lamima propria mononuclear phagocytes. These phagocytes in turn promote Th17 cell differentiation [42]. Among all cytokines known to induce the differentiation of Th17 cells, the presence of IL-1β rather than IL-6 is essential in the intestine [43]. TGF- β 1 is also not essential for the differentiation of Th17 cells in the intestine, but may influence the phenotype of Th17 cells together with IL-1β [44]. Th17 cells, which have been differentiated in the presence of TGF-β1 are less pathogenic and produce more IL-10 compared to Th17 cell differentiated in the presence of IL-1β [45, 46].

Th17 cells also produce several other cytokines besides IL-17A and IL-17F. Cytokine production by Th17 cells is also modulated by environmental factors in the intestine. For example, the activation of the environmental chemical receptor and transcription factor aryl hydrocarbon receptor in Th17 cells is important for the production of IL-22 [47-49]. IL-22 is a critical cytokine for antimicrobial immunity exerted by Th17 cells [50]. On the other hand, the induction of c-maf upon stimulation with IL-27, promotes the release of IL-10 from Th17 cells [51], and these IL-10 producing Th17 cells are also particularly induced in the intestine [40]. Therefore Th17 cells can have different cytokine profiles depending on environment factors.

In the absence of pathology, Th17 cells are very rare. However pathogenic infections, such as fungi infection with *Candida albicans*, or bacterial infection with gram positive or gram negative extracellular bacteria, such as *Citrobacter rodentium* or *Klebsiella pneumoniae* lead to a dramatic increase of the number of Th17 cells [52-56]. Viral infection also promotes a Th17-cell mediated immune response [40]. In line with this, Th17 cells and their effector cytokines IL-17A, IL-17F, and IL-22 are critical for proper host defense against various infections, especially against extracellular bacteria and fungi. The receptors for IL-17A, IL-17F and IL-22 are broadly expressed throughout the intestinal epithelial tissue. Therefore Th17 cells can provide crosstalk between immune system and tissues [2, 57].

IL-17A and IL-17F strongly induce the recruitment of neutrophils to the inflammatory site. The subsequent induction of the chemokine CCL20 attracts even more Th17 cells via CCR6, the chemokine receptor of CCL20, which is highly expressed by Th17 cells [58]. Additionally, both IL-17A and IL-17F promote β-defensin production [56, 59, 60]. β-defensins play an important role in the immune responses against bacterial infections. Interestingly, IL-17A and IL-17F can compensate each other during the host defense against *S. aureus* [56]. However during other infections, such as *Citrobacter rodentium*, IL-17A and IL-17F are both required in order to control the bacterial dissemination [56].

At the mucosal surface IL-22 has a crucial function for host defence and tissue homeostasis. IL-22 induces the expression of antimicrobial peptides from epithelial cells and limits bacterial replication and dissemination during *Citrobacter rodentium* infection [57, 61]. Furthermore IL-22 can promote epithelial cell proliferation, survival, and tissue repair in the intestine [62-64].

However it should be noted that several other immune cells besides Th17 cells can produce IL-17A and IL-22, thereby also contributing to the defense against pathogens (for review see [50]).

2.4. Differentiation and function of Foxp3$^+$ Treg cells

In 1995 Sakaguchi et al. first described a subpopulation of regulatory T cells characterized by the constitutive expression of the IL-2 receptor α-chain (CD25). These regulatory T cells were called CD4$^+$CD25$^+$ Treg [65]. Foxp3 was identified later on as the master transcriptional regulator of CD4$^+$CD25$^+$ Treg cells, which have been called Foxp3$^+$ Treg cells thereafter [66, 67]. Foxp3$^+$ Treg cells can be generated within the thymus (tTreg) [65]. However, Foxp3$^+$ Treg cell numbers are also regulated in peripheral lymphoid organs both by expansion of pre-existing Foxp3$^+$ Treg and by de novo generation of induced regulatory T cells (iTreg). The combination of the cytokines IL-2 and TGF-β1 are key for the differentiation of naïve T cells into Foxp3$^+$ iTreg cells [68-73]. Foxp3$^+$ Treg cells are essential to control auto-reactive T cells, which can react to self-antigens and cause damage to the host. The key role of Foxp3$^+$ Treg cells in the peripheral immune response is evident in murine models [74] and in humans [75]: scurfy mice [74] and IPEX (immunodysregulation polyendocrinopathy enteropathy X-linked syndrome) patients [75] lacking the master transcriptional factor of regulatory T cells - Foxp3 - consequently develop strong autoimmune disorders. Importantly, a severe form of autoimmune enteropathy is characteristic for scurfy mice and IPEX patients [75]. This underlines the importance of Foxp3$^+$ Treg cells for controlling the immune response in the intestine. Foxp3$^+$ Treg cells have different mechanism to suppress effector T cells. Some of these are mediated via soluble factors (i.e. IL-10, TGF-β1 [76, 77]) and others are cell contact dependent (i.e. CTLA-4, cAMP [78, 79]). Recent studies have demonstrated that Foxp3$^+$ Treg cells can acquire some features of effector T helper cells in order to better control them (see paragraph 4.3).

2.5. Differentiation and function of Tr1 cells

In 1994, T regulatory type 1 (Tr1) cells were isolated from severe combined immuno deficiency (SCID) patients transplanted with allogeneic haematopoietic stem cells (HSCT). Subsequently it was possible to test the regulatory capacity of this new type of T cells directly in murine IBD models. To date Tr1 cells lack a defined cell surface signature, and their identification relays therefore on their unique cytokine profile. Tr1 cells secrete high levels of IL-10 as compared to IL-4 and IL-17A, the hallmark cytokines of Th2 and Th17 cells respectively. Depending on the milieu Tr1 cells can produce variable levels of IFN-γ, the key cytokine produced by Th1 cells [80]. However, Tr1 cells posses the capacity to suppress inflammatory T cell responses and, therefore are distinct from bona fide Th1, Th2 and Th17 cells that largely promote rather than suppress the inflammatory responses.

Tr1 cells are induced in the periphery, and they respond selectively to persistent foreign and self-antigens under steady-state conditions [81].

After the discovery of Foxp3 as the master transcriptional regulator of Foxp3$^+$ Treg cells, it became a key point, if also Tr1 cells express a master regulator. The double reporter mouse model for IL-10 and Foxp3 was instrumental in order to demonstrate that these two types of regulatory T cells are distinct. Indeed, Tr1 cells do not constitutively express Foxp3 [82, 83] and can be induced from IPEX patients who lack Foxp3 [84]. However the master transcriptional regulator for Tr1 cells has not been identified so far.

IL-10 has been considered to be the driving force for Tr1-cell generation on the basis of experiments in which antigen-specific Tr1 cells are induced *in vitro* by repeated TCR stimulation in the presence of high doses of IL-10 [85, 86]. However, the frequency of Tr1 cells in IL-10 deficient mice is not altered. Several recent publications have demonstrated a key role of IL-27, which can even synergize with TGF-β, in the induction of Tr1 cells. During the induction of Tr1 cells by IL-27, the ligand-activated transcription factor hydrocarbon receptor (AhR) physically associates with c-avian musculoaponeurotic fibrosarcoma (c-Maf) and transactivates the *Il10* and *Il21* promoters. The secretion of IL-21 acts as an autocrine growth factor for Tr1 cells (Reviewed in [87]).

Tr1 cells can control Th1, Th2 and Th17 cell, and regulate immune responses mainly through the secretion of the immunosuppressive cytokines IL-10 and TGF-β1 [88]. The antigen-specific activation of Tr1 cells is important to potentiate their regulatory function [86]. IL-10 acts by limiting the magnitude of immune responses, as proved by mice that lack IL-10 and that exhibit spontaneous enterocolitis. IL-10 down-regulates the expression of co-stimulatory molecules, such as CD80, CD86, and MHC Class II, and pro-inflammatory cytokine production by APCs and inhibits the secretion of IL-2, TNF-α and IL-17 by effector T cells [89]. In particular, Tr1-cell supernatant diminishes the capacity of monocytes to stimulate Th1-cell responses and blocks the differentiation and maturation of DCs *via* IL-10 [90]. TGF-β down-regulates the functions of APCs [91] and inhibits the proliferation and cytokine production by T cells [92]. Therefore, the suppressive effects of Tr1 cells are reversed by the addition of anti-IL10 and anti-TGF-β neutralizing antibodies [85, 93, 94], but additional mechanisms may also contribute. Human Tr1 cells generated *in vitro* by crosslinking CD3 with CD46 can kill target cells through a granzyme B/ perforin dependent mechanism [95] [96]. Accordingly human Tr1 cells selectively kill myeloid cells (i.e., DC and monocytes) through granzyme B/ perforin [97]. This selective cell-killing is mediated by CD226, which is expressed on Tr1 cells. Only myeloid cells express the CD226-ligand (CD155). Thus, this type of regulatory mechanism by Tr1 cells requires a cell-cell contact with APCs.

3. The immune homeostasis in the intestine

The immune system has to respond selectively to harmful non-self pathogens and at the same time needs to minimize reactions against self and not-harmful antigens. This highly fine-tuned mechanism is possible due to a strict selection process, which happens in the thymus. Potentially auto-reactive $CD4^+$ T cell progenitors, which recognize self-antigens with their T cell receptor (TCR), are either deleted or converted into thymic-derived $CD4^+$ regulatory T cells (tTreg) with anti-inflammatory properties. This process, called central tolerance, is essential for the education of $CD4^+$ T cells to respond selectively against foreign antigens. However this thymic control appears still to be insufficient. Therefore the immune system developed several other mechanisms to control potentially auto-reactive T cells, which take places in the periphery (peripheral tolerance). Among these mechanisms, the action of $CD4^+$ regulatory T cells, which can be either selected in the thymus, (tTreg) or induced in the periphery (iTreg)[98], is one of the most studied. Treg cells are essential to control auto-reactive T cells, which can react to self-antigens and cause damage to the host.

The intestine is not only a source of self-antigens, but also contains a vast collection of non-self antigens, such as commensal bacteria. These antigens can promote the activation of naïve T cells causing immune-pathology such as inflammatory bowel disease (IBD). Therefore the immune system has established a second checkpoint in the intestine where naïve T cells, which are potentially able to respond to non self-antigens, are educated to be tolerant. There are important differences between thymus and intestine in tolerance induction. The driving force for the selection in the thymus is the affinity of TCRs to

MHC, while the flora and cytokines are crucial to determine the fate of naïve T cells in the intestine. Accordingly different commensal bacteria can selectively drive a tolerogenic or pro-infammatory response. In line with this, the bacterial composition of the intestine has a substantial impact on the balance between pro-inflammatory and regulatory T cells in the intestine, and can also affect other organ specific diseases [41, 99-101]: For example mice lacking an innate sensor, which controls the intestinal micro-flora, are more susceptible to develop colitis [100]. Another interaction between the gut flora and an autoimmune disease was found in EAE (experimental autoimmune encephalomyelitis, a mouse model for multiple sclerosis). Multiple sclerosis is caused by an attack by auto-reactive T cells against brain white matter. Interestingly it was shown that the commensal gut flora can trigger these auto-reactive T cells, which then drive the disease. Finally it is known that the bacterial colonization between neonates born vaginally or by cesarean delivery differs, and interestingly these differences have been linked to an increased risk for atopic diseases such as allergic rhinitis and asthma in children born by cesarean delivery [102].

Considering the amount of self- and none self-antigens present in this organ and with it the potential to generate an unwanted immune response, different players are required to control the immune homeostasis in the intestine. The first one is a specialized subset of DC, which through the release of TGF-β and retinoic acid, is able to induce iTreg cells [103]. These iTreg cells represent then the second players. It is also known that naïve T cells migrate to the intestine in order to acquire an iTreg cell phenotype [104, 105]. Interestingly, these iTreg cells have a TCR repertoire, which is specific to an individuals microflora. Based on these results, one could hypothesize that iTreg cells have an advantage over tTreg cells (3th player), which are also present in the intestine, but are obviously non-bacteria specific. However, it was shown that specific commensal bacteria can directly activate tTreg cells bypassing the antigen specificity [106]. Both tTreg and iTreg are able to suppress effector T cells in the intestine, thereby curing or preventing colitis development [68, 98, 107-110]. It seems that tTregs and iTreg can also supplement the function of each other partially by expanding the TCR diversity [111]. Tr1 cells (4th players) are expanded in the absence of iTregs, and can at least partially compensate the absence of iTregs [112, 113]. Consistent with this, Tr1 cells and Treg cells can compensate each other to suppress effector T cells in the intestine [114].

In conclusion, commensal antigens in the intestine play an essential role in the regulation of the immune homeostasis. Naïve T cells, which could be potentially auto reactive, are converted into different types of regulatory T cells, which in turn control other effector T helper cells. The regulatory T cells originated in the thymus (nTregs) also participate in this regulatory environment by expanding the antigen specificity of the immune response.

4. Breakdown of the immune homeostasis in the intestine

Imbalance between pro- and anti-inflammatory T helper cells can cause intestinal pathology, such as IBD in humans. Crohn's disease (CD) and ulcerative colitis (UC) are the two main forms of IBD. CD can attack any part of the digestive tract. It typically manifests in the ileum, although it can also selectively affect the large intestine. Histological Crohn's disease shows a transmural inflammation. This inflammation is characterized by focal infiltration of neutrophils into the epithelium. These neutrophils, along with mononuclear cells, can infiltrate the crypts, leading to inflammation or abscess. Granulomas, aggregates of macrophage derivatives, known as giant cells, are found in CD and are specific for the disease. Ulceration can also be seen in highly active CD. On the other hand, UC is a disease mainly of the colon that includes ulcerations. UC normally begins in the rectum, and can continuously affect the whole colon and also the terminal ileum. The pathology in ulcerative colitis involves distortion of crypt architecture, inflammation of crypts and hemorrhage. The inflammation is more superficial compared to CD and affects the mucosa and submucosa.

The aetiology of IBD is still unknown, but it seems that genetic and environmental factors contribute to disease development. Initial studies suggested that CD and UC are mediated by Th1 and Th2 cells respectively. This was based on the cytokine profile seen in CD (IL-12 and IFN-γ) and UC (IL-5, IL-13) [115]. However more recent work has shown that Th17 cells also infiltrate the intestine in CD and UC patients as well [116-118]. Accordingly the signature cytokines of Th17 cells (IL-17A, IL-17F, IL-22) are produced in the intestine of CD and UC patients [116, 118-120]. Additionally, genome wide association studies have linked polymorphism in Th17-related genes, such as *IL-23R* and *STAT3* with IBD [121-124]. In line with these associations murine studies have also shown that Th17 cells are involved in numerous autoimmune and chronic inflammatory diseases [2], and IBD is one of these diseases [125]: RORγt deficient mice, which lack Th17 cells, exhibit attenuated experimentally induced autoimmune disease [4]. Adoptive transfer of *in vitro* or *in vivo* differentiated Th17 cells into lymphopenic hosts leads to the development of colitis [114, 126-128]. IL-23, which is important for the maintenance, expansion and pathogenicity of Th17 cells [38, 39], is essential for the induction of colitis in mouse models. All together, these data argue for an important role of Th17 cells in IBD. However, Th17 cells produce several factors. And it is currently not completely understood, which of these is/are responsible for the pathogenicity of Th17 cells in the intestine [129-132].

One key feature of Th17 cells is their plasticity, which might also contribute to the pathogenic potential of Th17 cells. Epigenetic studies have shown that Th17 cells are more plastic compared to Th1 and Th2 cells [56, 133-135]. Th17 cells have bivalent domains of histone modifications in the *Tbx21* locus, which encodes for T-bet, the key transcriptional factor for Th1 cells. On the contrary, Th1 cells have only repressive markers in both *Rorc* and *Il17a* loci. These differences might account for the higher plasticity of Th17 cells relative to Th1 cells [133]. In line with these data, $CD4^+$ T cells, which express both the key transcriptional factors and cytokines of Th17 and Th1 cells, have been found in the colon of mouse colitis models and moreover in colon of human IBD patients. They are also suggested to play an important role for the development of chronic disease [39, 114, 118].

Human IBD is characterized by a mixture of effector T cells. Therefore it is difficult to assess the relative contribution of a specific T helper cell subset in patients. However there are mouse IBD models, which are dominated by one specific T helper cells subset: Selective deficiency in iTreg cells causes Th2 dominated intestinal pathology, which is characterized by gastritis and plasmacytic enteritis with increased frequencies of plasma cells in the intestinal lamina propria [113]. Another mouse model of colitis, which is induced by the transfer of naïve T cells into a lymphopenic host, is dominated by Th1 cells. This colitis model is characterized by IFN-γ dependent mucosal ulceration in the colon [136, 137]. Th17 cell-dominated intestinal pathology is characterized by mucosal hyperplasia but not ulceration [76, 136, 138]. IL-22, a signature cytokine of Th17 cells, can promote epithelial cell survival and proliferation. It is also important for the repair of the intestinal mucosa [63, 136, 139]. Accordingly, IL-22 induces the hyperplasia in the Th17 dominated colitis models [136]. On the contrary IL-22 is beneficial in Th1 dominated colitis models, which are characterized by ulceration [62]. Of note, the histomorphology in these Th1, Th2, or Th17 cell dominated mouse IBD models features only some characteristics of human IBD. But still these models are useful to evaluate the function of specific T helper cell subsets.

5. Control of pro-inflammatory T helper cells in the intestine

There are three ways to control effector T cells. First, inhibition of the differentiation of naïve T cells into effector T cells. Second, endogenous mechanism limiting the pathogenic potential of effector T cells. Third, control of effector T cells through regulatory T cells.

5.1. Inhibition of the *de novo* differentiation of effector T cells

One possibility is to inhibit the *de novo* differentiation of naïve T cells into effector T cells and generate regulatory T cells in stead. Such a reciprocal development pathway has been described for Th17 cells: High concentrations of TGF-β and/or retinoic acid up-regulate Foxp3 [140, 141], which in turn inhibits the induction of RORγt [37], thereby preventing the differentiation of Th17 cells. Moreover, IL-2 together with TGF-β1 promotes the induction of $Foxp3^+$ regulatory T cells (iTregs) instead of Th17 cells [142]. Interestingly, IL-2 blocks Th17 cell differentiation by directly inhibiting *Il17a* transcription. This second mechanism is largely independent of Foxp3 or RORγt expression, but dependent on the induction of STAT5, which competes with STAT3 for the common sites across the locus encoding IL-17A [143]. Finally, IL-27 through the activation and interaction of AhR and c-maf promotes the induction of type 1 regulatory T cells (Tr1) and efficiently counteracts the effects of TGF-β and IL-6 on $CD4^+$ T cells, resulting in the inhibition of Th17 development in a STAT1-dependent manner (Reviewed in [144]).

5.2. Endogenous control of effector T cells

All effector T cell subsets (Th1, Th2, Th17) have the ability to acquire IL-10 production, thereby limiting their own pathogenicity [145]. This mechanism of self control has been very well described for Th17 cells (Figure 2): During particular bacterial and viral infection, naïve T cells maturate in effector Th17 cells and contribute to the eradication of infections. However, if the Th17 response is too strong and potentially life threatening, Th17 cells are redirected to the small intestine in order to be controlled [40]. The reason why mature Th17 cells migrate mainly to the small intestine is because of the high expression of the chemokine receptor CCR6 [146]. The highest concentration of CCL20, the ligand of CCR6, is indeed in the small intestine [40]. Interestingly, IL-17A and IL-17F promote the release of CCL20 from epithelial cells in the duodenum. The recruited Th17 cells also produce CCL20, furthermore amplifying CCL20 production. This suggests that Th17 cells implement through a positive feedback loop the recruitment of other Th17 cells to the small intestine. Once effector Th17 cells migrated to the intestine, two complementary mechanisms occur in order to control them. First, effector Th17 cells are washed out and eliminated via the intestinal lumen due to the strong tissue destruction and diarrhoea. Secondly, Th17 cells are reprogrammed in regulatory Th17 (rTh17) cells. This last mechanism relays on the plasticity of these cells. In the intestine, effector Th17 cells acquire the capacity to produce IL-10 [40] and in parallel express IL-10Rα. If Th17 cells cannot respond to IL-10, they acquire a "promiscuous" phenotype co-expressing IFN-γ and promote the inflammation in the small intestine [114].

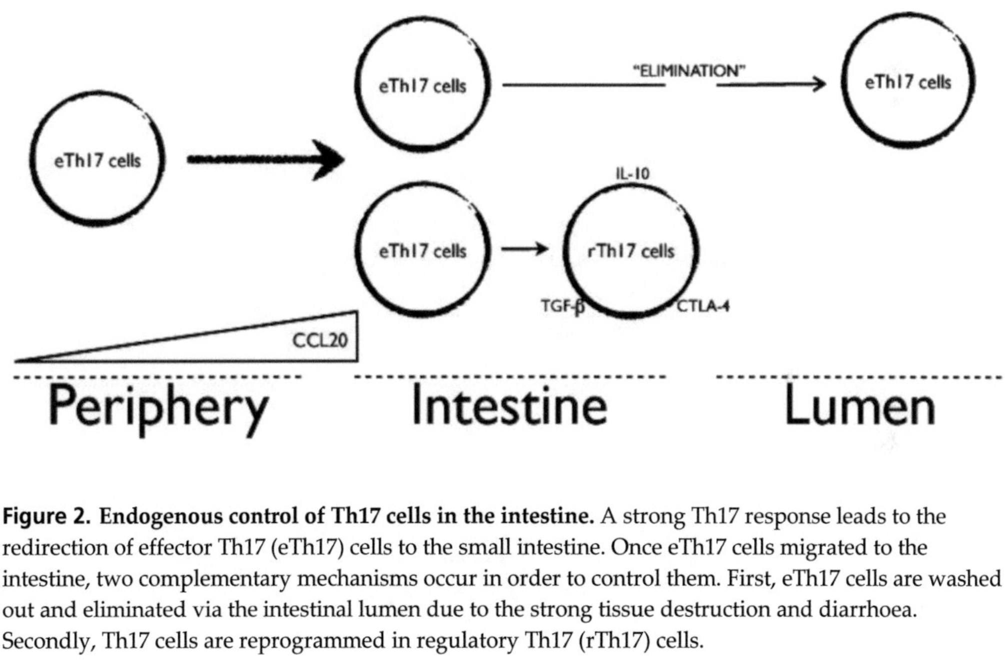

Figure 2. Endogenous control of Th17 cells in the intestine. A strong Th17 response leads to the redirection of effector Th17 (eTh17) cells to the small intestine. Once eTh17 cells migrated to the intestine, two complementary mechanisms occur in order to control them. First, eTh17 cells are washed out and eliminated via the intestinal lumen due to the strong tissue destruction and diarrhoea. Secondly, Th17 cells are reprogrammed in regulatory Th17 (rTh17) cells.

5.3. Exogenous control of effector T cells via regulatory T cells

Importantly, other control mechanisms, which do not rely on the "sense of responsibility" of effector T helper cells, are also present (Figure 3). Regulatory T cells play an essential role for controlling T helper cells. The two most studied regulatory T cell subsets are Foxp3$^+$ Treg and Tr1 cells. Foxp3$^+$ Tregs can be induced in the periphery (Foxp3$^+$ iTregs) or in the thymus (Foxp3$^+$ tTregs). Interestingly, Foxp3$^+$ iTregs are induced in the intestine by TCR recognition of commensal antigens [101, 104, 105, 147]. Foxp3$^+$ tTregs cells are obviously non-bacteria specific, but nevertheless can be activated by some bacterial species in the intestine [106]. It is also important that Foxp3+ iTregs and Foxp3+ tTregs perform complementary functions, in part by expanding the TCR diversity [111].

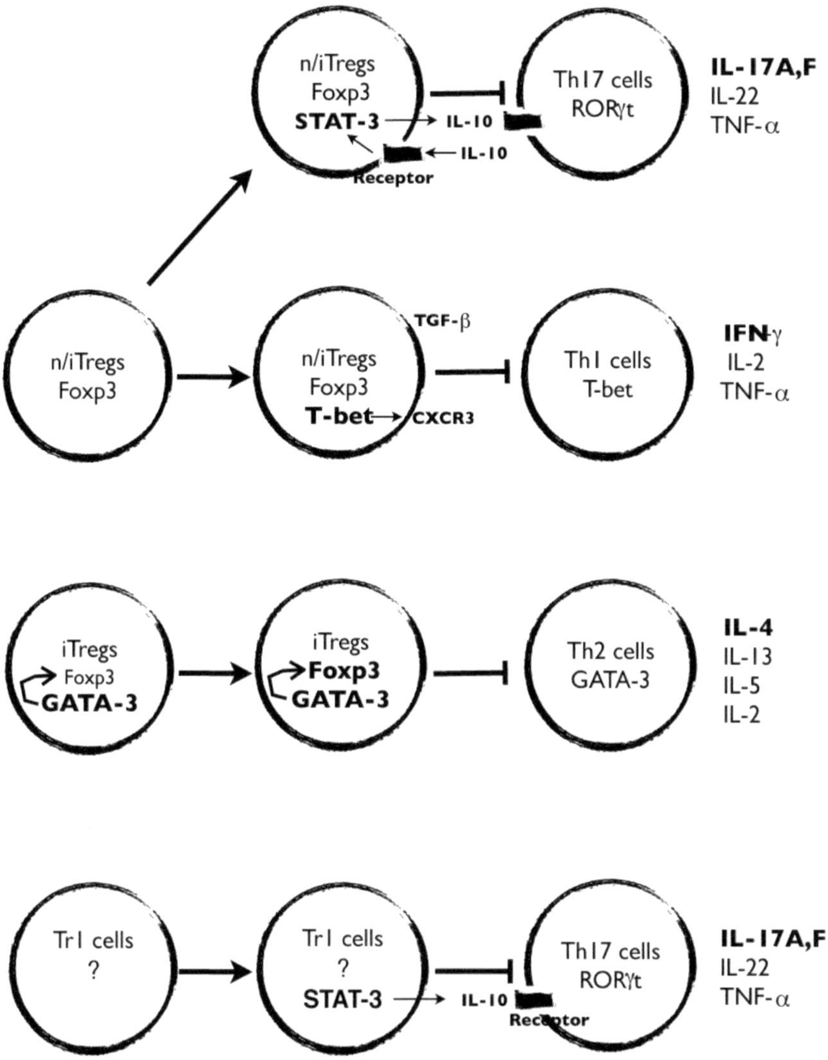

Figure 3. Control of effector T helper cells in the intestine. Different regulatory T cells can efficiently suppress specific T helper cell subsets in the intestine.

Although different types of regulatory T cells can partially compensate each other, it seems that regulatory T cells can also have a more specialized function, and suppress specific types of effector T cells more potent then others: mice with a selective deficiency in iTreg cells develop spontaneous intestinal inflammation, which is characterized by an expansion of Th2 cells [113], indicating that iTregs play an important role in controlling Th2 cells in the intestine. Moreover expression of GATA-3 and IRF-4, master regulators of Th2 cells, by Foxp3+ Treg cells is important for the control of Th2 cells [148, 149]. Additionally, some

$Foxp3^+$ Treg cells can express T-bet the master transcriptional regulator of Th1 cells. These T-bet^+Foxp3^+ Tregs express CXCR3, which is also highly expressed by Th1 cells. Thanks to the expression of the same chemokine receptor T-bet^+Foxp3^+ Treg cells can better "follow" and in turn suppress Th1 cells [150]. Finally, it was shown that IL-10 can induce IL-10 production by $Foxp3^+$ Treg via STAT3 activation, and $Foxp3^+IL\text{-}10^+$ Tregs are particularly important to control Th17 cells [76, 138, 151]. In addition to $Foxp3^+$ Treg the immune system uses an alternative type of regulatory T cell, which can compensate a possible paucity of $Foxp3^+$ Treg in order to avoid immune pathology in the intestine [112]. These cells, Tr1 cells, which are characterized by an abundant production of IL-10 and by the absence of Foxp3 expression, exert an efficient regulation of Th17 cells in the intestine [114]. Interestingly, IL-10 seems to play a non-redundant role in controlling Th17 cells: acting on both Th17 cells and regulatory T cells. Th17 cells are suppressed directly via IL-10, which is produced by Tr1 and $Foxp3^+$Treg cells [114, 136]. Additionally, IL-10 acts on $Foxp3^+$Treg. It activates STAT3 in $Foxp3^+$Tregs, which is crucial to enable them to suppress Th17 cells [138, 151]. Moreover IL-10 signalling in $Foxp3^+$Treg cells is required to promote IL-10 production [138] (Figure 3).

In conclusion $Foxp3^+$ Treg cells can have different phenotypes. This feature allows $Foxp3^+$ Tregs to suppress specific effector T cells more efficiently. Additionally $Foxp3^+$ Tregs can team up with Tr1 cells to maintain the immune homeostasis in the intestine.

However, regulatory T cells do not only suppress effector T cells but can also promote effector T cell function in some settings [152, 153], indicating that the immune system aims to maintain a proper balance between regulatory and effector T cells rather then uncontrolled suppression of effector T cells.

6. Conclusions

$CD4^+$ T helper cells have important physiological functions at the large intestinal mucosal surface: they secrete cytokines thereby attracting other immune cells, inducing anti-microbial peptides, and promoting tissue repair. Therefore effector $CD4^+$ T helper cells play an important 'border patrol' function, and protect the body against infections. Thymic derived naïve $CD4^+$ T cells express bacterial antigen specific TCRs. Encounter with these bacterial derived foreign antigens in the colon can drive the differentiation of regulatory T cells or pro-inflammatory effector T cells dependent on the bacteria and the environmental milieu. If effector $CD4^+$ T helper cells are uncontrolled, they can elicit tissue damage and induce disease such as IBD. Therefore the immune system has established several mechanisms in order to control pro-inflammatory T helper cells. These mechanisms are primarily important to avoid immune pathology and in turn to maintain tolerance in the intestine. However a growing body of evidence suggests that these mechanisms can also be used to suppress other organ specific diseases. One example for this interaction between the intestine and another organ is that the commensal gut flora can trigger a T-cell mediated immune response, which leads to autoimmune disease in the brain [99]. Therefore one possible strategy for the treatment of autoimmune diseases in future would be to specifically target the gut flora. Although the mechanisms controlling effector T cells in the intestine work well in most humans, the frequency of autoimmune and chronic inflammatory disease is steadily increasing. Unfortunately, there are currently no curative treatments for these diseases available. Therefore the patients suffer from the side effects of the drugs and from the relapses of their disease. The the challenge will be to better understand the mechanisms controlling effector T cells in order to establish new and potentially curative treatments for autoimmune and chronic inflammatory diseases. The intestine has the potential to serve as the key target organ of these therapies.

Author details

Nicola Gagliani
Department of Immunobiology, School of Medicine,
Yale University, New Haven, USA

Samuel Huber*
I. Medical Department, University Hospital
Hamburg-Eppendorf, Hamburg, Germany

7. References

[1] Bettelli E, Carrier Y, Gao W, Korn T, Strom TB, Oukka M, Weiner HL, Kuchroo VK (2006) Reciprocal developmental pathways for the generation of pathogenic effector TH17 and regulatory T cells. Nature. 7090: 235-8.

[2] Korn T, Bettelli E, Oukka M, Kuchroo VK (2009) IL-17 and Th17 Cells. Annu Rev Immunol. 485-517.

[3] Zheng W, Flavell RA (1997) The transcription factor GATA-3 is necessary and sufficient for Th2 cytokine gene expression in CD4 T cells. Cell. 4: 587-96.

[4] Ivanov, II, McKenzie BS, Zhou L, Tadokoro CE, Lepelley A, Lafaille JJ, Cua DJ, Littman DR (2006) The orphan nuclear receptor RORgammat directs the differentiation program of proinflammatory IL-17+ T helper cells. Cell. 6: 1121-33.

[5] Szabo SJ, Kim ST, Costa GL, Zhang X, Fathman CG, Glimcher LH (2000) A novel transcription factor, T-bet, directs Th1 lineage commitment. Cell. 6: 655-69.

[6] Zhu J, Yamane H, Paul WE (2010) Differentiation of effector CD4 T cell populations (*). Annu Rev Immunol. 445-89.

[7] Mosmann TR, Cherwinski H, Bond MW, Giedlin MA, Coffman RL (1986) Two types of murine helper T cell clone. I. Definition according to profiles of lymphokine activities and secreted proteins. J Immunol. 7: 2348-57.

[8] Hsieh CS, Macatonia SE, Tripp CS, Wolf SF, O'Garra A, Murphy KM (1993) Development of TH1 CD4+ T cells through IL-12 produced by Listeria-induced macrophages. Science. 5107: 547-9.

* Corresponding Author

[9] Usui T, Preiss JC, Kanno Y, Yao ZJ, Bream JH, O'Shea JJ, Strober W (2006) T-bet regulates Th1 responses through essential effects on GATA-3 function rather than on IFNG gene acetylation and transcription. J Exp Med. 3: 755-66.

[10] Usui T, Nishikomori R, Kitani A, Strober W (2003) GATA-3 suppresses Th1 development by downregulation of Stat4 and not through effects on IL-12Rbeta2 chain or T-bet. Immunity. 3: 415-28.

[11] Szabo SJ, Sullivan BM, Stemmann C, Satoskar AR, Sleckman BP, Glimcher LH (2002) Distinct effects of T-bet in TH1 lineage commitment and IFN-gamma production in CD4 and CD8 T cells. Science. 5553: 338-42.

[12] Filipe-Santos O, Bustamante J, Chapgier A, Vogt G, de Beaucoudrey L, Feinberg J, Jouanguy E, Boisson-Dupuis S, Fieschi C, Picard C, Casanova JL (2006) Inborn errors of IL-12/23- and IFN-gamma-mediated immunity: molecular, cellular, and clinical features. Semin Immunol. 6: 347-61.

[13] Le Gros G, Ben-Sasson SZ, Seder R, Finkelman FD, Paul WE (1990) Generation of interleukin 4 (IL-4)-producing cells in vivo and in vitro: IL-2 and IL-4 are required for in vitro generation of IL-4-producing cells. J Exp Med. 3: 921-9.

[14] Seder RA, Boulay JL, Finkelman F, Barbier S, Ben-Sasson SZ, Le Gros G, Paul WE (1992) CD8+ T cells can be primed in vitro to produce IL-4. J Immunol. 6: 1652-6.

[15] Swain SL, Weinberg AD, English M, Huston G (1990) IL-4 directs the development of Th2-like helper effectors. J Immunol. 11: 3796-806.

[16] Kaplan MH, Schindler U, Smiley ST, Grusby MJ (1996) Stat6 is required for mediating responses to IL-4 and for development of Th2 cells. Immunity. 3: 313-9.

[17] Shimoda K, van Deursen J, Sangster MY, Sarawar SR, Carson RT, Tripp RA, Chu C, Quelle FW, Nosaka T, Vignali DA, Doherty PC, Grosveld G, Paul WE, Ihle JN (1996) Lack of IL-4-induced Th2 response and IgE class switching in mice with disrupted Stat6 gene. Nature. 6575: 630-3.

[18] Takeda K, Tanaka T, Shi W, Matsumoto M, Minami M, Kashiwamura S, Nakanishi K, Yoshida N, Kishimoto T, Akira S (1996) Essential role of Stat6 in IL-4 signalling. Nature. 6575: 627-30.

[19] Kurata H, Lee HJ, O'Garra A, Arai N (1999) Ectopic expression of activated Stat6 induces the expression of Th2-specific cytokines and transcription factors in developing Th1 cells. Immunity. 6: 677-88.

[20] Zhu J, Guo L, Watson CJ, Hu-Li J, Paul WE (2001) Stat6 is necessary and sufficient for IL-4's role in Th2 differentiation and cell expansion. J Immunol. 12: 7276-81.

[21] Zhang DH, Cohn L, Ray P, Bottomly K, Ray A (1997) Transcription factor GATA-3 is differentially expressed in murine Th1 and Th2 cells and controls Th2-specific expression of the interleukin-5 gene. J Biol Chem. 34: 21597-603.

[22] Zhu J, Min B, Hu-Li J, Watson CJ, Grinberg A, Wang Q, Killeen N, Urban JF, Jr., Guo L, Paul WE (2004) Conditional deletion of Gata3 shows its essential function in T(H)1-T(H)2 responses. Nat Immunol. 11: 1157-65.

[23] Zhu J, Cote-Sierra J, Guo L, Paul WE (2003) Stat5 activation plays a critical role in Th2 differentiation. Immunity. 5: 739-48.

[24] Urban JF, Jr., Noben-Trauth N, Donaldson DD, Madden KB, Morris SC, Collins M, Finkelman FD (1998) IL-13, IL-4Ralpha, and Stat6 are required for the expulsion of the gastrointestinal nematode parasite Nippostrongylus brasiliensis. Immunity. 2: 255-64.

[25] Anthony RM, Rutitzky LI, Urban JF, Jr., Stadecker MJ, Gause WC (2007) Protective immune mechanisms in helminth infection. Nat Rev Immunol. 12: 975-87.

[26] Anthony RM, Urban JF, Jr., Alem F, Hamed HA, Rozo CT, Boucher JL, Van Rooijen N, Gause WC (2006) Memory T(H)2 cells induce alternatively activated macrophages to mediate protection against nematode parasites. Nat Med. 8: 955-60.

[27] Hasnain SZ, Evans CM, Roy M, Gallagher AL, Kindrachuk KN, Barron L, Dickey BF, Wilson MS, Wynn TA, Grencis RK, Thornton DJ (2011) Muc5ac: a critical component mediating the rejection of enteric nematodes. J Exp Med. 5: 893-900.

[28] Herbert DR, Yang JQ, Hogan SP, Groschwitz K, Khodoun M, Munitz A, Orekov T, Perkins C, Wang Q, Brombacher F, Urban JF, Jr., Rothenberg ME, Finkelman FD (2009) Intestinal epithelial cell secretion of RELM-beta protects against gastrointestinal worm infection. J Exp Med. 13: 2947-57.

[29] Artis D, Wang ML, Keilbaugh SA, He W, Brenes M, Swain GP, Knight PA, Donaldson DD, Lazar MA, Miller HR, Schad GA, Scott P, Wu GD (2004) RELMbeta/FIZZ2 is a goblet cell-specific immune-effector molecule in the gastrointestinal tract. Proc Natl Acad Sci U S A. 37: 13596-600.

[30] Akiho H, Blennerhassett P, Deng Y, Collins SM (2002) Role of IL-4, IL-13, and STAT6 in inflammation-induced hypercontractility of murine smooth muscle cells. Am J Physiol Gastrointest Liver Physiol. 2: G226-32.

[31] Cliffe LJ, Humphreys NE, Lane TE, Potten CS, Booth C, Grencis RK (2005) Accelerated intestinal epithelial cell turnover: a new mechanism of parasite expulsion. Science. 5727: 1463-5.

[32] Zhou L, Ivanov, II, Spolski R, Min R, Shenderov K, Egawa T, Levy DE, Leonard WJ, Littman DR (2007) IL-6 programs T(H)-17 cell differentiation by promoting sequential engagement of the IL-21 and IL-23 pathways. Nat Immunol. 9: 967-74.

[33] Nurieva R, Yang XO, Martinez G, Zhang Y, Panopoulos AD, Ma L, Schluns K, Tian Q, Watowich SS, Jetten AM, Dong C (2007) Essential autocrine regulation by IL-21 in the generation of inflammatory T cells. Nature. 7152: 480-3.

[34] Yang XO, Panopoulos AD, Nurieva R, Chang SH, Wang D, Watowich SS, Dong C (2007) STAT3 regulates cytokine-mediated generation of inflammatory helper T cells. J Biol Chem. 13: 9358-63.

[35] Veldhoen M, Hocking RJ, Atkins CJ, Locksley RM, Stockinger B (2006) TGFbeta in the context of an inflammatory cytokine milieu supports de novo differentiation of IL-17-producing T cells. Immunity. 2: 179-89.

[36] Mangan PR, Harrington LE, O'Quinn DB, Helms WS, Bullard DC, Elson CO, Hatton RD, Wahl SM, Schoeb TR, Weaver CT (2006) Transforming growth factor-beta induces development of the T(H)17 lineage. Nature. 7090: 231-4.

[37] Zhou L, Lopes JE, Chong MM, Ivanov, II, Min R, Victora GD, Shen Y, Du J, Rubtsov YP, Rudensky AY, Ziegler SF, Littman DR (2008) TGF-beta-induced Foxp3 inhibits T(H)17 cell differentiation by antagonizing RORgammat function. Nature. 7192: 236-40.

[38] McGeachy MJ, Chen Y, Tato CM, Laurence A, Joyce-Shaikh B, Blumenschein WM, McClanahan TK, O'Shea JJ, Cua DJ (2009) The interleukin 23 receptor is essential for the terminal differentiation of interleukin 17-producing effector T helper cells in vivo. Nat Immunol. 3: 314-24.

[39] Ahern PP, Schiering C, Buonocore S, McGeachy MJ, Cua DJ, Maloy KJ, Powrie F (2010) Interleukin-23 drives intestinal inflammation through direct activity on T cells. Immunity. 2: 279-88.

[40] Esplugues E, Huber S, Gagliani N, Hauser AE, Town T, Wan YY, O'Connor W, Jr., Rongvaux A, Van Rooijen N, Haberman AM, Iwakura Y, Kuchroo VK, Kolls JK, Bluestone JA, Herold KC, Flavell RA (2011) Control of TH17 cells occurs in the small intestine. Nature. 7357: 514-8.

[41] Ivanov, II, Atarashi K, Manel N, Brodie EL, Shima T, Karaoz U, Wei D, Goldfarb KC, Santee CA, Lynch SV, Tanoue T, Imaoka A, Itoh K, Takeda K, Umesaki Y, Honda K, Littman DR (2009) Induction of intestinal Th17 cells by segmented filamentous bacteria. Cell. 3: 485-98.

[42] Atarashi K, Nishimura J, Shima T, Umesaki Y, Yamamoto M, Onoue M, Yagita H, Ishii N, Evans R, Honda K, Takeda K (2008) ATP drives lamina propria T(H)17 cell differentiation. Nature. 7214: 808-12.

[43] Shaw MH, Kamada N, Kim YG, Nunez G (2012) Microbiota-induced IL-1beta, but not IL-6, is critical for the development of steady-state TH17 cells in the intestine. J Exp Med. 2: 251-8.

[44] Zielinski CE, Mele F, Aschenbrenner D, Jarrossay D, Ronchi F, Gattorno M, Monticelli S, Lanzavecchia A, Sallusto F (2012) Pathogen-induced human T(H)17 cells produce IFN-gamma or IL-10 and are regulated by IL-1beta. Nature.

[45] Ghoreschi K, Laurence A, Yang XP, Tato CM, McGeachy MJ, Konkel JE, Ramos HL, Wei L, Davidson TS, Bouladoux N, Grainger JR, Chen Q, Kanno Y, Watford WT, Sun HW, Eberl G, Shevach EM, Belkaid Y, Cua DJ, Chen W, O'Shea JJ (2010) Generation of pathogenic T(H)17 cells in the absence of TGF-beta signalling. Nature. 7318: 967-71.

[46] McGeachy MJ, Bak-Jensen KS, Chen Y, Tato CM, Blumenschein W, McClanahan T, Cua DJ (2007) TGF-beta and IL-6 drive the production of IL-17 and IL-10 by T cells and restrain T(H)-17 cell-mediated pathology. Nat Immunol. 12: 1390-7.

[47] Veldhoen M, Hirota K, Christensen J, O'Garra A, Stockinger B (2009) Natural agonists for aryl hydrocarbon receptor in culture medium are essential for optimal differentiation of Th17 T cells. J Exp Med. 1: 43-9.

[48] Veldhoen M, Hirota K, Westendorf AM, Buer J, Dumoutier L, Renauld JC, Stockinger B (2008) The aryl hydrocarbon receptor links TH17-cell-mediated autoimmunity to environmental toxins. Nature. 7191: 106-9.

[49] Quintana FJ, Basso AS, Iglesias AH, Korn T, Farez MF, Bettelli E, Caccamo M, Oukka M, Weiner HL (2008) Control of T(reg) and T(H)17 cell differentiation by the aryl hydrocarbon receptor. Nature. 7191: 65-71.

[50] O'Connor W, Jr., Zenewicz LA, Flavell RA (2010) The dual nature of T(H)17 cells: shifting the focus to function. Nat Immunol. 6: 471-6.

[51] Apetoh L, Quintana FJ, Pot C, Joller N, Xiao S, Kumar D, Burns EJ, Sherr DH, Weiner HL, Kuchroo VK (2010) The aryl hydrocarbon receptor interacts with c-Maf to promote the differentiation of type 1 regulatory T cells induced by IL-27. Nat Immunol. 9: 854-61.
[52] Conti HR, Shen F, Nayyar N, Stocum E, Sun JN, Lindemann MJ, Ho AW, Hai JH, Yu JJ, Jung JW, Filler SG, Masso-Welch P, Edgerton M, Gaffen SL (2009) Th17 cells and IL-17 receptor signaling are essential for mucosal host defense against oral candidiasis. J Exp Med. 2: 299-311.
[53] Huang W, Na L, Fidel PL, Schwarzenberger P (2004) Requirement of interleukin-17A for systemic anti-Candida albicans host defense in mice. J Infect Dis. 3: 624-31.
[54] Ye P, Garvey PB, Zhang P, Nelson S, Bagby G, Summer WR, Schwarzenberger P, Shellito JE, Kolls JK (2001) Interleukin-17 and lung host defense against Klebsiella pneumoniae infection. Am J Respir Cell Mol Biol. 3: 335-40.
[55] Iwakura Y, Nakae S, Saijo S, Ishigame H (2008) The roles of IL-17A in inflammatory immune responses and host defense against pathogens. Immunol Rev. 57-79.
[56] Ishigame H, Kakuta S, Nagai T, Kadoki M, Nambu A, Komiyama Y, Fujikado N, Tanahashi Y, Akitsu A, Kotaki H, Sudo K, Nakae S, Sasakawa C, Iwakura Y (2009) Differential roles of interleukin-17A and -17F in host defense against mucoepithelial bacterial infection and allergic responses. Immunity. 1: 108-19.
[57] Ouyang W, Kolls JK, Zheng Y (2008) The biological functions of T helper 17 cell effector cytokines in inflammation. Immunity. 4: 454-67.
[58] Pelletier M, Maggi L, Micheletti A, Lazzeri E, Tamassia N, Costantini C, Cosmi L, Lunardi C, Annunziato F, Romagnani S, Cassatella MA (2010) Evidence for a cross-talk between human neutrophils and Th17 cells. Blood. 2: 335-43.
[59] Kao CY, Chen Y, Thai P, Wachi S, Huang F, Kim C, Harper RW, Wu R (2004) IL-17 markedly up-regulates beta-defensin-2 expression in human airway epithelium via JAK and NF-kappaB signaling pathways. J Immunol. 5: 3482-91.
[60] Liang SC, Tan XY, Luxenberg DP, Karim R, Dunussi-Joannopoulos K, Collins M, Fouser LA (2006) Interleukin (IL)-22 and IL-17 are coexpressed by Th17 cells and cooperatively enhance expression of antimicrobial peptides. J Exp Med. 10: 2271-9.
[61] Zheng Y, Valdez PA, Danilenko DM, Hu Y, Sa SM, Gong Q, Abbas AR, Modrusan Z, Ghilardi N, de Sauvage FJ, Ouyang W (2008) Interleukin-22 mediates early host defense against attaching and effacing bacterial pathogens. Nat Med. 3: 282-9.
[62] Zenewicz LA, Yancopoulos GD, Valenzuela DM, Murphy AJ, Stevens S, Flavell RA (2008) Innate and adaptive interleukin-22 protects mice from inflammatory bowel disease. Immunity. 6: 947-57.
[63] Pickert G, Neufert C, Leppkes M, Zheng Y, Wittkopf N, Warntjen M, Lehr HA, Hirth S, Weigmann B, Wirtz S, Ouyang W, Neurath MF, Becker C (2009) STAT3 links IL-22 signaling in intestinal epithelial cells to mucosal wound healing. J Exp Med. 7: 1465-72.
[64] Sugimoto K, Ogawa A, Mizoguchi E, Shimomura Y, Andoh A, Bhan AK, Blumberg RS, Xavier RJ, Mizoguchi A (2008) IL-22 ameliorates intestinal inflammation in a mouse model of ulcerative colitis. J Clin Invest. 2: 534-44.
[65] Sakaguchi S, Sakaguchi N, Asano M, Itoh M, Toda M (1995) Immunologic self-tolerance maintained by activated T cells expressing IL-2 receptor alpha-chains (CD25).

Breakdown of a single mechanism of self-tolerance causes various autoimmune diseases. J Immunol. 3: 1151-64.

[66] Fontenot JD, Gavin MA, Rudensky AY (2003) Foxp3 programs the development and function of CD4+CD25+ regulatory T cells. Nat Immunol. 4: 330-6.

[67] Hori S, Nomura T, Sakaguchi S (2003) Control of regulatory T cell development by the transcription factor Foxp3. Science. 5609: 1057-61.

[68] Huber S, Schramm C, Lehr HA, Mann A, Schmitt S, Becker C, Protschka M, Galle PR, Neurath MF, Blessing M (2004) Cutting edge: TGF-beta signaling is required for the in vivo expansion and immunosuppressive capacity of regulatory CD4+CD25+ T cells. J Immunol. 11: 6526-31.

[69] Schramm C, Huber S, Protschka M, Czochra P, Burg J, Schmitt E, Lohse AW, Galle PR, Blessing M (2004) TGFbeta regulates the CD4+CD25+ T-cell pool and the expression of Foxp3 in vivo. Int Immunol. 9: 1241-9.

[70] Fantini MC, Becker C, Monteleone G, Pallone F, Galle PR, Neurath MF (2004) Cutting edge: TGF-beta induces a regulatory phenotype in CD4+CD25- T cells through Foxp3 induction and down-regulation of Smad7. J Immunol. 9: 5149-53.

[71] Chen W, Jin W, Hardegen N, Lei KJ, Li L, Marinos N, McGrady G, Wahl SM (2003) Conversion of peripheral CD4+CD25- naive T cells to CD4+CD25+ regulatory T cells by TGF-beta induction of transcription factor Foxp3. J Exp Med. 12: 1875-86.

[72] Kretschmer K, Apostolou I, Hawiger D, Khazaie K, Nussenzweig MC, von Boehmer H (2005) Inducing and expanding regulatory T cell populations by foreign antigen. Nat Immunol. 12: 1219-27.

[73] Marie JC, Letterio JJ, Gavin M, Rudensky AY (2005) TGF-beta1 maintains suppressor function and Foxp3 expression in CD4+CD25+ regulatory T cells. J Exp Med. 7: 1061-7.

[74] Bennett CL, Christie J, Ramsdell F, Brunkow ME, Ferguson PJ, Whitesell L, Kelly TE, Saulsbury FT, Chance PF, Ochs HD (2001) The immune dysregulation, polyendocrinopathy, enteropathy, X-linked syndrome (IPEX) is caused by mutations of FOXP3. Nat Genet. 1: 20-1.

[75] Brunkow ME, Jeffery EW, Hjerrild KA, Paeper B, Clark LB, Yasayko SA, Wilkinson JE, Galas D, Ziegler SF, Ramsdell F (2001) Disruption of a new forkhead/winged-helix protein, scurfin, results in the fatal lymphoproliferative disorder of the scurfy mouse. Nat Genet. 1: 68-73.

[76] Huber S, Gagliani N, Esplugues E, O'Connor W, Jr., Huber FJ, Chaudhry A, Kamanaka M, Kobayashi Y, Booth CJ, Rudensky AY, Roncarolo MG, Battaglia M, Flavell RA (2011) Th17 cells express interleukin-10 receptor and are controlled by Foxp3- and Foxp3+ regulatory CD4+ T cells in an interleukin-10-dependent manner. Immunity. 4: 554-65.

[77] Fahlen L, Read S, Gorelik L, Hurst SD, Coffman RL, Flavell RA, Powrie F (2005) T cells that cannot respond to TGF-{beta} escape control by CD4+CD25+ regulatory T cells. J Exp Med. 5: 737-46.

[78] Annunziato F, Cosmi L, Liotta F, Lazzeri E, Manetti R, Vanini V, Romagnani P, Maggi E, Romagnani S (2002) Phenotype, localization, and mechanism of suppression of CD4(+)CD25(+) human thymocytes. J Exp Med. 3: 379-87.

[79] Bopp T, Becker C, Klein M, Klein-Hessling S, Palmetshofer A, Serfling E, Heib V, Becker M, Kubach J, Schmitt S, Stoll S, Schild H, Staege MS, Stassen M, Jonuleit H, Schmitt E (2007) Cyclic adenosine monophosphate is a key component of regulatory T cell-mediated suppression. J Exp Med. 6: 1303-10.

[80] Roncarolo MG, Gregori S, Battaglia M, Bacchetta R, Fleischhauer K, Levings MK (2006) Interleukin-10-secreting type 1 regulatory T cells in rodents and humans. Immunol Rev. 28-50.

[81] Haringer B, Lozza L, Steckel B, Geginat J (2009) Identification and characterization of IL-10/IFN-gamma-producing effector-like T cells with regulatory function in human blood. J Exp Med. 5: 1009-17.

[82] Vieira PL, Christensen JR, Minaee S, O'Neill EJ, Barrat FJ, Boonstra A, Barthlott T, Stockinger B, Wraith DC, O'Garra A (2004) IL-10-secreting regulatory T cells do not express Foxp3 but have comparable regulatory function to naturally occurring CD4+CD25+ regulatory T cells. J Immunol. 10: 5986-93.

[83] Maynard CL, Harrington LE, Janowski KM, Oliver JR, Zindl CL, Rudensky AY, Weaver CT (2007) Regulatory T cells expressing interleukin 10 develop from Foxp3+ and Foxp3- precursor cells in the absence of interleukin 10. Nat Immunol. 9: 931-41.

[84] Passerini L, Di Nunzio S, Gregori S, Gambineri E, Cecconi M, Seidel MG, Cazzola G, Perroni L, Tommasini A, Vignola S, Guidi L, Roncarolo MG, Bacchetta R (2011) Functional type 1 regulatory T cells develop regardless of FOXP3 mutations in patients with IPEX syndrome. Eur J Immunol. 4: 1120-31.

[85] Groux H, O'Garra A, Bigler M, Rouleau M, Antonenko S, de Vries JE, Roncarolo MG (1997) A CD4+ T-cell subset inhibits antigen-specific T-cell responses and prevents colitis. Nature. 6652: 737-42.

[86] Gagliani N, Jofra T, Stabilini A, Valle A, Atkinson M, Roncarolo MG, Battaglia M (2010) Antigen-specific dependence of Tr1-cell therapy in preclinical models of islet transplant. Diabetes. 2: 433-9.

[87] Pot C, Apetoh L, Awasthi A, Kuchroo VK (2010) Molecular pathways in the induction of interleukin-27-driven regulatory type 1 cells. J Interferon Cytokine Res. 6: 381-8.

[88] Cobbold SP, Nolan KF, Graca L, Castejon R, Le Moine A, Frewin M, Humm S, Adams E, Thompson S, Zelenika D, Paterson A, Yates S, Fairchild PJ, Waldmann H (2003) Regulatory T cells and dendritic cells in transplantation tolerance: molecular markers and mechanisms. Immunol Rev. 109-24.

[89] Pestka S, Krause CD, Sarkar D, Walter MR, Shi Y, Fisher PB (2004) Interleukin-10 and related cytokines and receptors. Annu Rev Immunol. 929-79.

[90] Cavani A, Nasorri F, Prezzi C, Sebastiani S, Albanesi C, Girolomoni G (2000) Human CD4+ T lymphocytes with remarkable regulatory functions on dendritic cells and nickel-specific Th1 immune responses. J Invest Dermatol. 2: 295-302.

[91] Strobl H, Emshoff R, Rothler G (1999) Conservative treatment of unilateral condylar fractures in children: a long-term clinical and radiologic follow-up of 55 patients. Int J Oral Maxillofac Surg. 2: 95-8.

[92] Cerwenka A, Swain SL (1999) TGF-beta1: immunosuppressant and viability factor for T lymphocytes. Microbes Infect. 15: 1291-6.

[93] Levings MK, Gregori S, Tresoldi E, Cazzaniga S, Bonini C, Roncarolo MG (2005) Differentiation of Tr1 cells by immature dendritic cells requires IL-10 but not CD25+CD4+ Tr cells. Blood. 3: 1162-9.

[94] Gregori S, Tomasoni D, Pacciani V, Scirpoli M, Battaglia M, Magnani CF, Hauben E, Roncarolo MG (2010) Differentiation of type 1 T regulatory cells (Tr1) by tolerogenic DC-10 requires the IL-10-dependent ILT4/HLA-G pathway. Blood. 6: 935-44.

[95] Grossman WJ, Verbsky JW, Tollefsen BL, Kemper C, Atkinson JP, Ley TJ (2004) Differential expression of granzymes A and B in human cytotoxic lymphocyte subsets and T regulatory cells. Blood. 9: 2840-8.

[96] Grossman WJ, Verbsky JW, Barchet W, Colonna M, Atkinson JP, Ley TJ (2004) Human T regulatory cells can use the perforin pathway to cause autologous target cell death. Immunity. 4: 589-601.

[97] Magnani CF, Alberigo G, Bacchetta R, Serafini G, Andreani M, Roncarolo MG, Gregori S (2011) Killing of myeloid APCs via HLA class I, CD2 and CD226 defines a novel mechanism of suppression by human Tr1 cells. Eur J Immunol. 6: 1652-62.

[98] Huber S, Schramm C (2006) TGF-beta and CD4+CD25+ regulatory T cells. Front Biosci. 1014-23.

[99] Berer K, Mues M, Koutrolos M, Rasbi ZA, Boziki M, Johner C, Wekerle H, Krishnamoorthy G (2011) Commensal microbiota and myelin autoantigen cooperate to trigger autoimmune demyelination. Nature. 7374: 538-41.

[100] Elinav E, Strowig T, Kau AL, Henao-Mejia J, Thaiss CA, Booth CJ, Peaper DR, Bertin J, Eisenbarth SC, Gordon JI, Flavell RA (2011) NLRP6 inflammasome regulates colonic microbial ecology and risk for colitis. Cell. 5: 745-57.

[101] Lathrop SK, Bloom SM, Rao SM, Nutsch K, Lio CW, Santacruz N, Peterson DA, Stappenbeck TS, Hsieh CS (2011) Peripheral education of the immune system by colonic commensal microbiota. Nature. 7368: 250-4.

[102] Decker E, Hornef M, Stockinger S (2011) Cesarean delivery is associated with celiac disease but not inflammatory bowel disease in children. Gut Microbes. 2: 91-8.

[103] Benson MJ, Pino-Lagos K, Rosemblatt M, Noelle RJ (2007) All-trans retinoic acid mediates enhanced T reg cell growth, differentiation, and gut homing in the face of high levels of co-stimulation. J Exp Med. 8: 1765-74.

[104] Hadis U, Wahl B, Schulz O, Hardtke-Wolenski M, Schippers A, Wagner N, Muller W, Sparwasser T, Forster R, Pabst O (2011) Intestinal tolerance requires gut homing and expansion of FoxP3+ regulatory T cells in the lamina propria. Immunity. 2: 237-46.

[105] Cassani B, Villablanca EJ, Quintana FJ, Love PE, Lacy-Hulbert A, Blaner WS, Sparwasser T, Snapper SB, Weiner HL, Mora JR (2011) Gut-Tropic T Cells That Express Integrin alpha4beta7 and CCR9 Are Required for Induction of Oral Immune Tolerance in Mice. Gastroenterology.

[106] Geuking MB, Cahenzli J, Lawson MA, Ng DC, Slack E, Hapfelmeier S, McCoy KD, Macpherson AJ (2011) Intestinal bacterial colonization induces mutualistic regulatory T cell responses. Immunity. 5: 794-806.

[107] Huber S, Schramm C (2011) Role of activin A in the induction of Foxp3+ and Foxp3- CD4+ regulatory T cells. Crit Rev Immunol. 1: 53-60.

[108] Huber S, Stahl FR, Schrader J, Luth S, Presser K, Carambia A, Flavell RA, Werner S, Blessing M, Herkel J, Schramm C (2009) Activin a promotes the TGF-beta-induced conversion of CD4+CD25- T cells into Foxp3+ induced regulatory T cells. J Immunol. 8: 4633-40.

[109] Fantini MC, Becker C, Tubbe I, Nikolaev A, Lehr HA, Galle P, Neurath MF (2006) Transforming growth factor beta induced FoxP3+ regulatory T cells suppress Th1 mediated experimental colitis. Gut. 5: 671-80.

[110] Mottet C, Uhlig HH, Powrie F (2003) Cutting edge: cure of colitis by CD4+CD25+ regulatory T cells. J Immunol. 8: 3939-43.

[111] Haribhai D, Williams JB, Jia S, Nickerson D, Schmitt EG, Edwards B, Ziegelbauer J, Yassai M, Li SH, Relland LM, Wise PM, Chen A, Zheng YQ, Simpson PM, Gorski J, Salzman NH, Hessner MJ, Chatila TA, Williams CB (2011) A requisite role for induced regulatory T cells in tolerance based on expanding antigen receptor diversity. Immunity. 1: 109-22.

[112] Zheng Y, Josefowicz S, Chaudhry A, Peng XP, Forbush K, Rudensky AY (2010) Role of conserved non-coding DNA elements in the Foxp3 gene in regulatory T-cell fate. Nature. 7282: 808-12.

[113] Josefowicz SZ, Niec RE, Kim HY, Treuting P, Chinen T, Zheng Y, Umetsu DT, Rudensky AY (2012) Extrathymically generated regulatory T cells control mucosal TH2 inflammation. Nature. 7385: 395-9.

[114] Huber S, Gagliani N, Esplugues E, O'Connor W, Jr., Huber FJ, Chaudhry A, Kamanaka M, Kobayashi Y, Booth CJ, Rudensky AY, Roncarolo MG, Battaglia M, Flavell RA (2011) Th17 cells express interleukin-10 receptor and are controlled by Foxp3 and Foxp3+ regulatory CD4+ T cells in an interleukin-10-dependent manner. Immunity. 4: 554-65.

[115] Fuss IJ, Neurath M, Boirivant M, Klein JS, de la Motte C, Strong SA, Fiocchi C, Strober W (1996) Disparate CD4+ lamina propria (LP) lymphokine secretion profiles in inflammatory bowel disease. Crohn's disease LP cells manifest increased secretion of IFN-gamma, whereas ulcerative colitis LP cells manifest increased secretion of IL-5. J Immunol. 3: 1261-70.

[116] Fujino S, Andoh A, Bamba S, Ogawa A, Hata K, Araki Y, Bamba T, Fujiyama Y (2003) Increased expression of interleukin 17 in inflammatory bowel disease. Gut. 1: 65-70.

[117] Rovedatti L, Kudo T, Biancheri P, Sarra M, Knowles CH, Rampton DS, Corazza GR, Monteleone G, Di Sabatino A, Macdonald TT (2009) Differential regulation of interleukin 17 and interferon gamma production in inflammatory bowel disease. Gut. 12: 1629-36.

[118] Annunziato F, Cosmi L, Santarlasci V, Maggi L, Liotta F, Mazzinghi B, Parente E, Fili L, Ferri S, Frosali F, Giudici F, Romagnani P, Parronchi P, Tonelli F, Maggi E, Romagnani S (2007) Phenotypic and functional features of human Th17 cells. J Exp Med. 8: 1849-61.

[119] Brand S, Beigel F, Olszak T, Zitzmann K, Eichhorst ST, Otte JM, Diepolder H, Marquardt A, Jagla W, Popp A, Leclair S, Herrmann K, Seiderer J, Ochsenkuhn T, Goke B, Auernhammer CJ, Dambacher J (2006) IL-22 is increased in active Crohn's disease

and promotes proinflammatory gene expression and intestinal epithelial cell migration. Am J Physiol Gastrointest Liver Physiol. 4: G827-38.

[120] Seiderer J, Elben I, Diegelmann J, Glas J, Stallhofer J, Tillack C, Pfennig S, Jurgens M, Schmechel S, Konrad A, Goke B, Ochsenkuhn T, Muller-Myhsok B, Lohse P, Brand S (2008) Role of the novel Th17 cytokine IL-17F in inflammatory bowel disease (IBD): upregulated colonic IL-17F expression in active Crohn's disease and analysis of the IL17F p.His161Arg polymorphism in IBD. Inflamm Bowel Dis. 4: 437-45.

[121] Duerr RH, Taylor KD, Brant SR, Rioux JD, Silverberg MS, Daly MJ, Steinhart AH, Abraham C, Regueiro M, Griffiths A, Dassopoulos T, Bitton A, Yang H, Targan S, Datta LW, Kistner EO, Schumm LP, Lee AT, Gregersen PK, Barmada MM, Rotter JI, Nicolae DL, Cho JH (2006) A genome-wide association study identifies IL23R as an inflammatory bowel disease gene. Science. 5804: 1461-3.

[122] Franke A, McGovern DP, Barrett JC, Wang K, Radford-Smith GL, Ahmad T, Lees CW, Balschun T, Lee J, Roberts R, Anderson CA, Bis JC, Bumpstead S, Ellinghaus D, Festen EM, Georges M, Green T, Haritunians T, Jostins L, Latiano A, Mathew CG, Montgomery GW, Prescott NJ, Raychaudhuri S, Rotter JI, Schumm P, Sharma Y, Simms LA, Taylor KD, Whiteman D, Wijmenga C, Baldassano RN, Barclay M, Bayless TM, Brand S, Buning C, Cohen A, Colombel JF, Cottone M, Stronati L, Denson T, De Vos M, D'Inca R, Dubinsky M, Edwards C, Florin T, Franchimont D, Gearry R, Glas J, Van Gossum A, Guthery SL, Halfvarson J, Verspaget HW, Hugot JP, Karban A, Laukens D, Lawrance I, Lemann M, Levine A, Libioulle C, Louis E, Mowat C, Newman W, Panes J, Phillips A, Proctor DD, Regueiro M, Russell R, Rutgeerts P, Sanderson J, Sans M, Seibold F, Steinhart AH, Stokkers PC, Torkvist L, Kullak-Ublick G, Wilson D, Walters T, Targan SR, Brant SR, Rioux JD, D'Amato M, Weersma RK, Kugathasan S, Griffiths AM, Mansfield JC, Vermeire S, Duerr RH, Silverberg MS, Satsangi J, Schreiber S, Cho JH, Annese V, Hakonarson H, Daly MJ, Parkes M (2010) Genome-wide meta-analysis increases to 71 the number of confirmed Crohn's disease susceptibility loci. Nat Genet. 12: 1118-25.

[123] Anderson CA, Boucher G, Lees CW, Franke A, D'Amato M, Taylor KD, Lee JC, Goyette P, Imielinski M, Latiano A, Lagace C, Scott R, Amininejad L, Bumpstead S, Baidoo L, Baldassano RN, Barclay M, Bayless TM, Brand S, Buning C, Colombel JF, Denson LA, De Vos M, Dubinsky M, Edwards C, Ellinghaus D, Fehrmann RS, Floyd JA, Florin T, Franchimont D, Franke L, Georges M, Glas J, Glazer NL, Guthery SL, Haritunians T, Hayward NK, Hugot JP, Jobin G, Laukens D, Lawrance I, Lemann M, Levine A, Libioulle C, Louis E, McGovern DP, Milla M, Montgomery GW, Morley KI, Mowat C, Ng A, Newman W, Ophoff RA, Papi L, Palmieri O, Peyrin-Biroulet L, Panes J, Phillips A, Prescott NJ, Proctor DD, Roberts R, Russell R, Rutgeerts P, Sanderson J, Sans M, Schumm P, Seibold F, Sharma Y, Simms LA, Seielstad M, Steinhart AH, Targan SR, van den Berg LH, Vatn M, Verspaget H, Walters T, Wijmenga C, Wilson DC, Westra HJ, Xavier RJ, Zhao ZZ, Ponsioen CY, Andersen V, Torkvist L, Gazouli M, Anagnou NP, Karlsen TH, Kupcinskas L, Sventoraityte J, Mansfield JC, Kugathasan S, Silverberg MS, Halfvarson J, Rotter JI, Mathew CG, Griffiths AM, Gearry R, Ahmad T, Brant SR, Chamaillard M, Satsangi J, Cho JH, Schreiber S, Daly MJ, Barrett JC, Parkes M, Annese

V, Hakonarson H, Radford-Smith G, Duerr RH, Vermeire S, Weersma RK, Rioux JD (2011) Meta-analysis identifies 29 additional ulcerative colitis risk loci, increasing the number of confirmed associations to 47. Nat Genet. 3: 246-52.

[124] Glas J, Stallhofer J, Ripke S, Wetzke M, Pfennig S, Klein W, Epplen JT, Griga T, Schiemann U, Lacher M, Koletzko S, Folwaczny M, Lohse P, Goke B, Ochsenkuhn T, Muller-Myhsok B, Brand S (2009) Novel genetic risk markers for ulcerative colitis in the IL2/IL21 region are in epistasis with IL23R and suggest a common genetic background for ulcerative colitis and celiac disease. Am J Gastroenterol. 7: 1737-44.

[125] Miossec P, Korn T, Kuchroo VK (2009) Interleukin-17 and type 17 helper T cells. N Engl J Med. 9: 888-98.

[126] Lee YK, Turner H, Maynard CL, Oliver JR, Chen D, Elson CO, Weaver CT (2009) Late developmental plasticity in the T helper 17 lineage. Immunity. 1: 92-107.

[127] Wang C, Kang SG, Lee J, Sun Z, Kim CH (2009) The roles of CCR6 in migration of Th17 cells and regulation of effector T-cell balance in the gut. Mucosal Immunol. 2: 173-83.

[128] Elson CO, Cong Y, Weaver CT, Schoeb TR, McClanahan TK, Fick RB, Kastelein RA (2007) Monoclonal anti-interleukin 23 reverses active colitis in a T cell-mediated model in mice. Gastroenterology. 7: 2359-70.

[129] Zhang Z, Zheng M, Bindas J, Schwarzenberger P, Kolls JK (2006) Critical role of IL-17 receptor signaling in acute TNBS-induced colitis. Inflamm Bowel Dis. 5: 382-8.

[130] Ogawa A, Andoh A, Araki Y, Bamba T, Fujiyama Y (2004) Neutralization of interleukin-17 aggravates dextran sulfate sodium-induced colitis in mice. Clin Immunol. 1: 55-62.

[131] Yang XO, Chang SH, Park H, Nurieva R, Shah B, Acero L, Wang YH, Schluns KS, Broaddus RR, Zhu Z, Dong C (2008) Regulation of inflammatory responses by IL-17F. J Exp Med. 5: 1063-75.

[132] O'Connor W, Jr., Kamanaka M, Booth CJ, Town T, Nakae S, Iwakura Y, Kolls JK, Flavell RA (2009) A protective function for interleukin 17A in T cell-mediated intestinal inflammation. Nat Immunol. 6: 603-9.

[133] Wei G, Wei L, Zhu J, Zang C, Hu-Li J, Yao Z, Cui K, Kanno Y, Roh TY, Watford WT, Schones DE, Peng W, Sun HW, Paul WE, O'Shea JJ, Zhao K (2009) Global mapping of H3K4me3 and H3K27me3 reveals specificity and plasticity in lineage fate determination of differentiating CD4+ T cells. Immunity. 1: 155-67.

[134] Bernstein BE, Mikkelsen TS, Xie X, Kamal M, Huebert DJ, Cuff J, Fry B, Meissner A, Wernig M, Plath K, Jaenisch R, Wagschal A, Feil R, Schreiber SL, Lander ES (2006) A bivalent chromatin structure marks key developmental genes in embryonic stem cells. Cell. 2: 315-26.

[135] Azuara V, Perry P, Sauer S, Spivakov M, Jorgensen HF, John RM, Gouti M, Casanova M, Warnes G, Merkenschlager M, Fisher AG (2006) Chromatin signatures of pluripotent cell lines. Nat Cell Biol. 5: 532-8.

[136] Kamanaka M, Huber S, Zenewicz LA, Gagliani N, Rathinam C, O'Connor W, Jr., Wan YY, Nakae S, Iwakura Y, Hao L, Flavell RA (2011) Memory/effector (CD45RB(lo)) CD4 T

cells are controlled directly by IL-10 and cause IL-22-dependent intestinal pathology. J Exp Med. 5: 1027-40.

[137] Powrie F, Leach MW, Mauze S, Menon S, Caddle LB, Coffman RL (1994) Inhibition of Th1 responses prevents inflammatory bowel disease in scid mice reconstituted with CD45RBhi CD4+ T cells. Immunity. 7: 553-62.

[138] Chaudhry A, Samstein RM, Treuting P, Liang Y, Pils MC, Heinrich JM, Jack RS, Wunderlich FT, Bruning JC, Muller W, Rudensky AY (2011) Interleukin-10 signaling in regulatory T cells is required for suppression of Th17 cell-mediated inflammation. Immunity. 4: 566-78.

[139] Witte E, Witte K, Warszawska K, Sabat R, Wolk K (2010) Interleukin-22: a cytokine produced by T, NK and NKT cell subsets, with importance in the innate immune defense and tissue protection. Cytokine Growth Factor Rev. 5: 365-79.

[140] Coombes JL, Siddiqui KR, Arancibia-Carcamo CV, Hall J, Sun CM, Belkaid Y, Powrie F (2007) A functionally specialized population of mucosal CD103+ DCs induces Foxp3+ regulatory T cells via a TGF-beta and retinoic acid-dependent mechanism. J Exp Med. 8: 1757-64.

[141] Elias KM, Laurence A, Davidson TS, Stephens G, Kanno Y, Shevach EM, O'Shea JJ (2008) Retinoic acid inhibits Th17 polarization and enhances FoxP3 expression through a Stat-3/Stat-5 independent signaling pathway. Blood. 3: 1013-20.

[142] Laurence A, Tato CM, Davidson TS, Kanno Y, Chen Z, Yao Z, Blank RB, Meylan F, Siegel R, Hennighausen L, Shevach EM, O'Shea J J (2007) Interleukin-2 signaling via STAT5 constrains T helper 17 cell generation. Immunity. 3: 371-81.

[143] Yang XP, Ghoreschi K, Steward-Tharp SM, Rodriguez-Canales J, Zhu J, Grainger JR, Hirahara K, Sun HW, Wei L, Vahedi G, Kanno Y, O'Shea JJ, Laurence A (2011) Opposing regulation of the locus encoding IL-17 through direct, reciprocal actions of STAT3 and STAT5. Nat Immunol. 3: 247-54.

[144] Pot C, Apetoh L, Awasthi A, Kuchroo VK (2011) Induction of regulatory Tr1 cells and inhibition of T(H)17 cells by IL-27. Semin Immunol. 6: 438-45.

[145] Saraiva M, O'Garra A (2010) The regulation of IL-10 production by immune cells. Nat Rev Immunol. 3: 170-81.

[146] Reboldi A, Coisne C, Baumjohann D, Benvenuto F, Bottinelli D, Lira S, Uccelli A, Lanzavecchia A, Engelhardt B, Sallusto F (2009) C-C chemokine receptor 6-regulated entry of TH-17 cells into the CNS through the choroid plexus is required for the initiation of EAE. Nat Immunol. 5: 514-23.

[147] Gagliani N, Huber S, Flavell RA (2012) The Intestine: where amazing things happen. Cell Res. 2: 277-9.

[148] Wang Y, Su MA, Wan YY (2011) An essential role of the transcription factor GATA-3 for the function of regulatory T cells. Immunity. 3: 337-48.

[149] Zheng Y, Chaudhry A, Kas A, deRoos P, Kim JM, Chu TT, Corcoran L, Treuting P, Klein U, Rudensky AY (2009) Regulatory T-cell suppressor program co-opts transcription factor IRF4 to control T(H)2 responses. Nature. 7236: 351-6.

[150] Koch MA, Tucker-Heard G, Perdue NR, Killebrew JR, Urdahl KB, Campbell DJ (2009) The transcription factor T-bet controls regulatory T cell homeostasis and function during type 1 inflammation. Nat Immunol. 6: 595-602.

[151] Chaudhry A, Rudra D, Treuting P, Samstein RM, Liang Y, Kas A, Rudensky AY (2009) CD4+ regulatory T cells control TH17 responses in a Stat3-dependent manner. Science. 5955: 986-91.

[152] Chen Y, Haines CJ, Gutcher I, Hochweller K, Blumenschein WM, McClanahan T, Hammerling G, Li MO, Cua DJ, McGeachy MJ (2011) Foxp3(+) regulatory T cells promote T helper 17 cell development in vivo through regulation of interleukin-2. Immunity. 3: 409-21.

[153] Gutcher I, Donkor MK, Ma Q, Rudensky AY, Flavell RA, Li MO (2011) Autocrine transforming growth factor-beta1 promotes in vivo Th17 cell differentiation. Immunity. 3: 396-408.

Chapter 4

T Cell Metabolism in Autoimmune Diseases

Dan Li, Miranda Piccioni, Zhimei Gao, Chen Chen,
Zuojia Chen, Jia Nie, Zhao Shan, Yangyang Li, Andy Tsun and Bin Li

Additional information is available at the end of the chapter

http://dx.doi.org/10.5772/47749

1. Introduction

Metabolism generates energy for organisms to sustain all kinds of biological functions, such as cell growth and cell apoptosis. The immune system requires an adequate energy supply for its optimal function [1]. During the activation and differentiation of T cells, the balance between glycolysis and lipid oxidation shifts in order to cater for the cell's energy requirements [2]. There is increasing evidence that shows how metabolism has an important role in regulating immunity, and a series of molecules have been described to play a functional role in both metabolism and the regulation of immune responses [3; 4; 5]. Uncovering the transcriptional regulation of the proteins participating in these metabolic processes allows us to understand how metabolism regulates T cell fate [6]. A set of non-coding RNAs called microRNA (miRNA), can also regulate these metabolic networks by binding to the 3'UTR of its target transcripts [7; 8; 9].

Autoimmune diseases were thought to be primarily caused by the immune response towards self-antigens. Organ-specific autoimmune diseases, such as multiple sclerosis, thyroiditis and type I diabetes, tend to arise due to T cell-mediated damage [10]. Abnormal metabolic changes may thus alter T cell function leading to the development of human diseases, including autoimmune diseases [11].

In this chapter, we highlight the recent research advances in metabolism, in particular to:

1. The role of metabolism in T cell differentiation and function.
2. The role of miRNAs in metabolic processes.
3. Dysregulation of metabolism during autoimmunity.

2. The role of metabolism in T cell differentiation and function

The role of cellular metabolism is to generate energy and supply biosynthetic demands in order to sustain normal biological functions. In the immune system, the control of cell numbers and activity of different T cell subsets is important for generating an appropriate immune response to combat foreign pathogens and prevent the risk of developing autoimmunity. The fate of T cells is strongly linked to metabolism by regulating cell growth, survival, function and differentiation.

Naive T cells, having undergone positive and negative selection in the thymus [12; 13], enter the periphery and encounter their specific cognate antigens in the context of major histocompatibility complexes to become activated, and differentiate into effector T (Teff) or induced regulatory T (Treg) cells. Metabolically, naive T cells consume glucose and other essential nutrients at a low rate, enough to supply energy to maintain normal housekeeping functions [14]. Importantly, naive T cells require extrinsic signals to maintain sufficient levels of glucose metabolism to prevent atrophy and apoptosis [15].

T cells are activated through the T cell receptor (TCR) and CD28 by the engagement of MHC-peptide complexes and B7 family members on antigen presenting cells. During this process, the physiological and phenotypic repertoire of the T cells develop in a way to support rapid cell growth, proliferation, and the generation of effector T cells, in which metabolism plays a critical role [16]. To drive enhanced glucose metabolism in activated T cells, the upregulation of expression and trafficking of glucose transporter 1 (Glut1) is crucial [17] (Fig. 1). The downregulation of Glut1 in lymphoid cell lines can decrease proliferation and cause cell cycle arrest or apoptosis [18; 19]. In contrast, the transgenic overexpression of Glut1 in T cells increases cell size, cytokine production, and proliferation upon activation [20].

The expression of Glut1 in T cells is induced by activation with a strong TCR agonist or through the cross-linking of the TCR-associated CD3 protein [21]. Both the MAPK pathway (p38) and Myc activation are upstream of Glut1 activation [22; 23] and may mediate the TCR dependent control of Glut1. TCR signaling can also activate AMP-activated protein kinase (AMPK) [24], which upregulates glucose uptake to promote energy generation [25] and may be due in part to the upregulation of Glut1 expression. Following the loss of the TCR, naive T cells downregulate the expression of Glut1 [26]. Mitochondrial potential and cellular ATP levels are also reduced, which suggests the loss of glucose metabolism. Beside the TCR, interleukin (IL)-7 is also a key regulator of glucose uptake in T lymphocytes. IL-7 maintains glucose metabolism by promoting Glut1 trafficking [27]. The tyrosine residue at position 449 of IL-7Rα is required for IL-7–mediated regulation of glucose uptake, which promotes rapid activation of signal transducer and activator of transcription 5 (STAT5) and a delayed yet sustained activation of Akt [28].

The intracellular trafficking of Glut1 is important for its localization to the cell surface to support glucose uptake. Co-stimulation through CD28 ligation can provide a strong signal to direct the trafficking of Glut1 to the cell surface through the activation of the phosphatidylinositol 3-kinase (PI3K)/Akt signaling pathway [29]. Akt can be activated through the ligation of its N-terminal pleckstrin homology (PH) to phosphatidylinositol (3,4,5)-triphosphate (PIP3) at the plasma membrane, generated by PI3K from PIP2, and its subsequent phosphorylation by 3'-phosphoinositide-dependent protein kinase-1 (PDK-1) [30]. Once activated, Akt can interact with and modulate the activity of different binding partners. The increased glucose uptake and augmented glycolysis observed upon CD28 co-stimulation can be prevented by LY294002-mediated PI3K inhibition [29], which induces a significant down-modulation of Glut1. Conversely, PI3K activation is inhibited by cytotoxic T lymphocyte antigen-4 (CTLA-4), results in Glut1 internalization where it is targeted to lysosomes for degradation and prevents the upregulation of glucose metabolism in activated T cells [31].

Although Glut1 plays a central role in T cell glucose metabolism, there are still other regulators downstream of the initial glucose uptake. For example, Akt increases hexokinase activity to increase glucose phosphorylation to prevent its transport out of the cell [32; 33]. In addition, Akt can also promote the activity of the key glycolytic enzyme, phosphofructokinase, by the phosphorylation of phosphofructokinase-2 and generation of the allosteric activator, 2,6-phospho-fructose [34]. Myc, better known as a regulator of proliferation and apoptosis [35], has also been shown to play a pivotal role in activation-induced glycolysis, being necessary for the upregulation of glycolytic enzymes and transporters. However, it still remains unclear as to how these pathways are integrated into T cell metabolism.

T cell activation induces a rapid elevation in oxygen consumption [36]; however, the most dramatic increase is in glycolysis. This results in the significant increase in the production of lactate, which can adequately guarantee an efficient but quick energy supply to the cell [1; 2; 37]. This glycolytic program supplies energy to T cells during their rapid differentiation, and the increase in intracellular glucose levels supports the pentose phosphate pathway required for the synthesis of nucleic acids, NADPH for producing ATP, and lipid synthesis [38]. This metabolism shift to high glycolysis can influence T cell function and survival. When glucose metabolism is limited in activated T cells, there is a decrease in the proliferation and production of interferon-γ (IFN-γ), and an increase in the expression and activation of pro-apoptotic Bcl-2 family proteins [39; 40].

Naive T cells can differentiate into different T cell subsets after stimulation, and during differentiation the metabolic program must match the demands of each cell function. Treg cells and T helper cells have different metabolic phenotypes: Treg cells prefer lipid oxidation and helper T (Th) cells prefer the glycolytic program. Different metabolic culture conditions can thus influence T cell differentiation *in vitro* [2]. The inhibition of mTOR and activation of AMPK can increase and decrease the percentage of Treg and Th cells, respectively [2]. Hypoxia-inducible factor 1α (HIF1α) is required for the upregulation of glycolytic activity, the promotion of Th17 differentiation and inhibition of Treg cell differentiation. HIF1α is a key metabolic factor in the mTOR-dependent upregulation of glycolysis observed under Th17-skewing conditions [5] and negatively regulates Forkhead Box P3 (FOXP3) to inhibit Treg cell differentiation [41].

Leptin, a 16-kDa non-glycosylated protein encoded by the *ob* gene, is classically considered a hormone, as it regulates the balance between food intake and energy expenditure. The level of serum leptin is levels is correlated directly with body-fat stores, increasing with fat accumulation and decreasing during fasting [4]. In recent years, leptin has been proved to be an immune response regulator. Mice with a genetic deficiency of leptin (*ob/ob*) or leptin receptor (*ObR*) have a reduced susceptibility to autoimmunity [42; 43]. Leptin has a specific effect on T cell responses partly by increasing Th1 and suppressing Th2 cytokine production. Also, leptin antibody can enhance the proliferation and suppress the function of Treg cells by down modulating the cyclin dependent kinase inhibitor p27 (p27kip1), and the phosphorylation of the extracellular-related kinases 1 (ERK1) and ERK2 [44].

There is still much unknown regarding the complete mechanisms of metabolism in T cell function in a physiological setting. These mechanisms could also be tissue specific, and the timing or strength of these signals could be crucial to the final fate of the T cell.

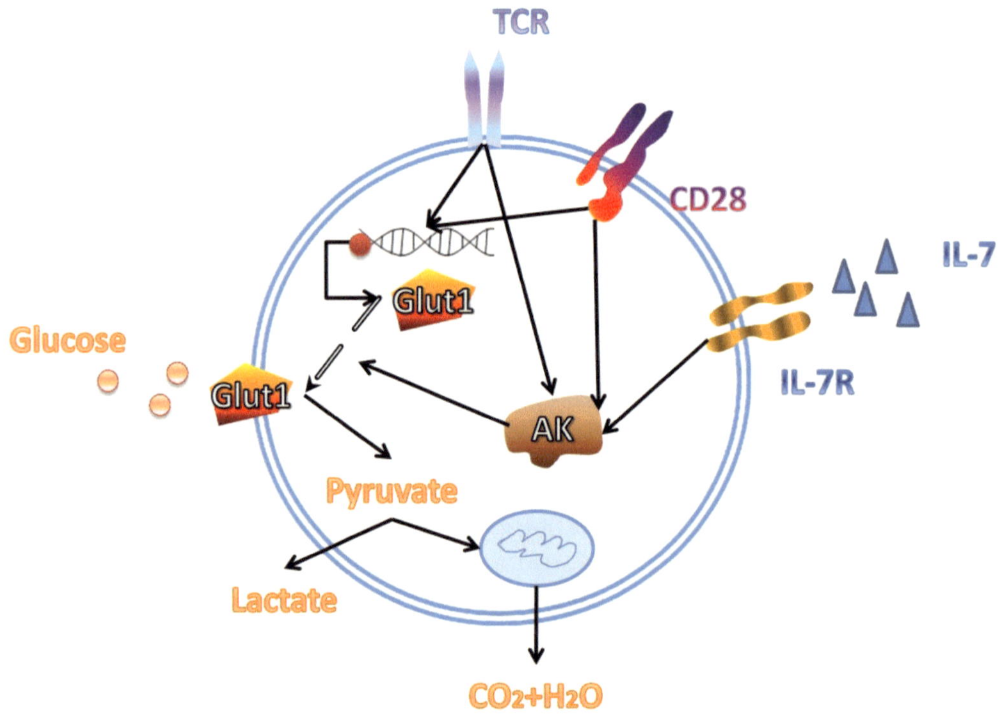

Figure 1. Glucose metabolism is activated by TCR, CD28 and cytokines in T cells. The increase in glycolysis is dramatic during T cell activation. In this process, the expression and intracellular trafficking of glucose transporter 1 (Glut1) is important as Glut1 controls the first step of glycolysis by facilitating the transport of glucose across the plasma membrane. The expression of Glut1 is upregulated by TCR and CD28 activation, while the trafficking to the cell surface is potentiated by signals from TCR, CD28 and IL-7 via Akt.

3. The role of miRNAs in metabolic processes

Metabolism interferes with the fate of T cells and plays a crucial role in the regulation of immunity. Cytokine/TCR signals and many growth factors have been reported to regulate metabolic processes [28; 29]. Moreover, microRNAs, a group of short non-coding RNA molecules that control gene expression by binding to the 3′ untranslated region (UTR) of complementary target mRNAs, are also involved in the regulation of metabolic networks [45; 46]. Here, we summarize the recent findings of metabolism regulating miRNAs and whether they currently play a role in T cell perturbation either directly or indirectly.

Insulin-related cell signal pathways regulate glucose metabolism and are related to the development of diabetes. The first miRNA identified in this program is the evolutionarily conserved and islet-specific miRNA, miR-375, which regulates glucose-induced insulin secretion by inhibiting the expression of Myotrophin (Mtpn) [47]. Further studies have indicated that miR-375 is regulated by glucose and that miR-375 inhibits glucose-induced INS-1E cell proliferation via the targeting of PDK-1 [48]. miR-375 has also been found to affect palmitate-induced lipoapoptosis in NIT-1 cells, a NOD-derived β-cell line [49]; here, mir-375 increases the susceptibility to palmitate-induced lipoapoptosis by targeting Mtpn. Thus, miR-375 emerges as a novel pharmacological target for the treatment of diabetes. Additionally, it has been shown that miR-375 can regulate the expression of thymic stromal lymphopoietin, a Th2-skewing cytokine in epithelia to help control parasitic infection [50].

miR-9 is another miRNA that has a possible role in insulin secretion by targeting Onecut-2 (OC-2) [51]. As OC-2 is a negative regulator of granuphilin, which is known as a key regulator of insulin secretion by repressing insulin exocytosis [52], miR-9 is proposed to negatively regulate insulin exocytosis. Furthermore, miR-9 expression is regulated during glucose-stimulated insulin secretion and modulates Sirtuin 1 (Sirt1) expression *in vivo* [53], a deacetylase that has been implicated in stabilizing Treg cells by stabilizing the expression of its master transcription factor FOXP3 [54].

The Lin-28/let-7 axis is also involved in glucose metabolism. Overexpression of Lin28a/B in mice results in insulin sensitivity, enhanced glucose tolerance, and resistance to diabetes, while overexpression of let-7 has the opposite effect [7]. The insulin-PI3K-mTOR signalling pathway, which regulates growth and glucose metabolism can be activated by Lin28a/B and suppressed by let-7. let-7 target genes in human are associated with type 2 diabetes, and it is suggested that enhancing Lin28 or abrogating let-7 may be therapeutically promising for treating diseases such as obesity and diabetes. Although the role of this axis has not been extensively investigated in T cells, it has been shown that let-7 is involved in regulating the sensitivity of T cells to Fas-mediated apoptosis [55]. The mTOR signalling pathway has also been shown to be regulated by miR-199a-3p, which alters the susceptibility of tumour cells to hypoxia [56].

In cardiomyocytes, miR-133 reduces insulin-mediated glucose uptake by decreasing GLUT4 expression. miR-133 is believed to be expressed specifically in adult cardiac and skeletal muscle tissues where it regulates the differentiation and proliferation of these cells [57]. It has been confirmed that the overexpression of miR-133 reduces the protein level of Kruppel-like factor 15 (KLF15) followed by its downstream target GLUT4. Silencing endogenous miR-133 *in vitro* increases the levels of KLF15 and GLUT4, which indicates a role of miR-133 in the metabolism of cardiac myocytes [8]. Insulin signalling can be regulated by miR-33a/b, which targets the insulin receptor substrate 2, an essential component of the insulin-signalling pathway in the liver [58]. miR-33a/b also regulates fatty acid metabolism by targeting several key enzymes involved in the regulation of fatty acid oxidation, including carnitine O-octaniltransferase, carnitine palmitoyltransferase 1A, hydroxyacyl-CoAdehydrogenase, Sirt6, and AMP kinase subunit-α [58]. Thus, mir-33a/b acts as a negative regulator of both insulin signalling and fatty acid oxidation in hepatic cell lines. There has yet to be any findings regarding the role of miR-133 and miR-33a/b in the modulation of T cells.

The liver specific miRNA, miR-122, is a key regulator of cholesterol and fatty-acid metabolism. Inhibition of miR-122 in the mouse liver results in reduced plasma cholesterol levels, increased hepatic fatty-acid oxidation, a decrease in hepatic fatty-acid and cholesterol synthesis rates, and the activation of AMPK [59]; interestingly, miR-122 can be induced by miR-370, which in turn induces lipogenic genes leading to the regulation of Cpt1α [60]. Although primarily thought to be expressed in the liver, miR-122 has been shown to be expressed in lymphoma cells. Its upregulation protects these cells towards chemotherapy-induced cytotoxicity [61]. AMPK is also regulated by miR-451. In glioma cells it has been found that increased glucose levels upregulates miR-451 which in turn regulates the AMPK pathway to promote cell growth [62].

HIF1, shown to promote Th17 but inhibit Treg cell differentiation [41], has been found to upregulate miR-210 in hypoxic cells. This increase is proposed to provide tumour cells the ability to survive under stressful conditions [63; 64]. The negative regulation of HIF1 itself has been found through the miR-17-92 cluster [65], miR-22 [66], miR-20b [67; 68], and miR-519c [69], and positively regulated indirectly through miR-31 [70] by the downregulation of factor-inhibiting hypoxia inducible factor and miR-130 through the P-body protein DDX6 [71]. In turn, miR-31 and miR-210 negatively regulates FOXP3 expression in Treg cells [72; 73], which would correlate with their roles in positively regulating HIF1 responses and Th17, but not Treg differentiation. Interestingly, HIF1α can also be negatively regulated by miR-155 [74], a miRNA that is highly upregulated in Treg cells induced by FOXP3 [75]. Also, miR-199a targets both HIF-1α and Sirt1, and thus may play a role in Treg cell differentiation [76; 77]. The miR-17-92 cluster also promotes Th1 responses and prevents induced Treg cell differentiation [78]. Finally miR-130, has also been found to be upregulated upon TCR stimulation of CD8+ T cells, and downregulates CD69 during differentiation [79]. Even with the wealth of information above, there is a lack of evidence that these miRNAs regulate HIF1 in T cells to contribute to the control of the differentiation of various T cell subsets.

Recent studies have demonstrated that miRNAs are pivotal in T cell development and function [80; 81; 82], which indicates that miRNAs are one of the important regulators of the immune system. miRNAs have also been implicated in regulating metabolic pathways, mostly identified thus far in non-immune cells in controlling blood glucose levels (Fig. 2). More research is required to identify whether miRNAs are also involved in the metabolic regulation of T cells. The identification of miRNA signatures in various T cell subtypes may provide clues towards the cross-regulation between metabolism and miRNA networks in lymphocytes [83].

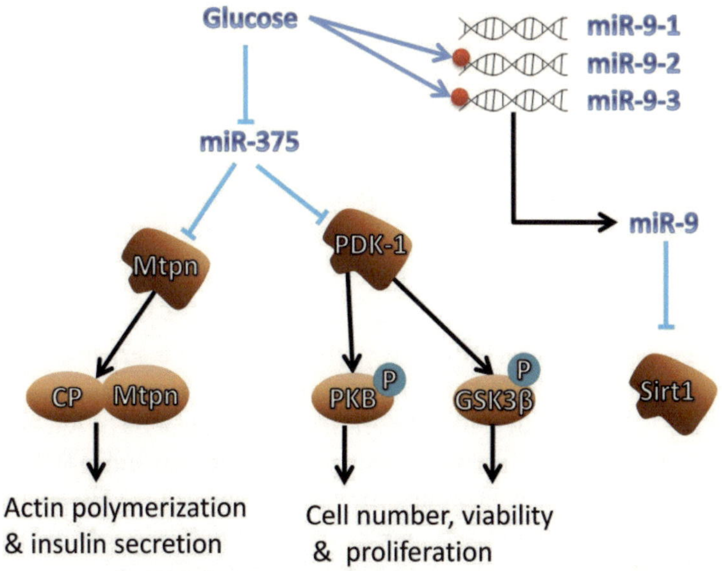

Figure 2. The regulatory network of microRNAs in pancreatic β-Cells. In pancreatic β-Cells some miRNAs participate in the insulin signal pathway. miR-375, which is downregulated by glucose, suppresses glucose-induced insulin secretion by inhibiting the expression of Myotrophin (Mtpn) and inhibits glucose-induced cell proliferation by targeting PDK-1. Glucose can enhance the expression of miR-9-2 and miR-9-3, which target Sirt1.

4. Dysregulation of metabolism during autoimmunity

The metabolic status of immune cells determines their fate and role in the immune system. The basic bioenergetic demands of resting lymphocytes can be essentially supplied by oxidative phosphorylation [84], while the increased amount of energy required during their activation implies a shift towards aerobic glycolysis. Much evidence exists regarding the role of Akt in the activation of mTOR, involved in a myriad of cellular processes, including translation, transcription, autophagy, growth and proliferation. mTOR is also known as a nutrient and energy "sensor", since it regulates the expression of multiple nutrient transporters [85]. Several studies have indicated that the Akt and mTOR pathways are intimately connected, given that the latter can be modulated by Akt, which in turn seems to be sensitive to mTOR inhibition by rapamycin [86; 87].

Autoimmune diseases comprises a large number of pathologies characterized by exacerbated immune responses against self-antigens. The mechanisms leading to autoimmunity are not yet fully understood, but their multifactorial basis is almost clear. Given the involvement of these pathways in the activation and differentiation of multiple T cell subsets, it is conceivable that alterations in the expression and/or function of one or more of the factors involved can lead to a breakdown in immune homeostasis.

Indeed, both systemic and organ-specific autoimmune diseases seem to rely on genetic, infectious and environmental predisposing factors [88]. Systemic lupus erythematosus (SLE) is the prototype of systemic autoimmune diseases. Subjects affected are characterized by a strong hyperactivation of autoreactive CD4+ T cells and a consequent aberrant expansion of B lymphocytes. Large amounts of autoantibodies are secreted, mostly targeting nuclear antigens and affecting skin, joints, blood vessels and the central nervous system (CNS) [89]. Glomerulonephritis can also occur, due to deposition of immunocomplexes in the kidney. Several studies have found in SLE patients marked deficiencies in the number and/or suppressive capacity of CD4+CD25^{high} Treg cells [90; 91], although early works also identified the abnormal resistance to suppression of Teff cells as a major issue in the loss of tolerance characterizing SLE [92].

From a molecular point of view, current hypotheses support a sustained activation of the Akt-mTOR axis in SLE. In a well known model of murine lupus, the New Zealand Black White (NZBW)/F1 hybrid has an elevated expression and activation of Akt and mTOR at the glomerular level. Treatment of mice with rapamycin inhibits Akt and mTOR activation, thus prolonging mice survival and ameliorating the clinical course of the disease [93]. The hyper-activation of the Akt pathway in CD4+ T cells from MRL/*lpr* mice, a model of spontaneous lupus, could also be inhibited by the use of specific PI3Kγ inhibitors [94]. An increase in Akt activation has been demonstrated in the peripheral blood from SLE patients, concurrently with an up-regulation of the phosphorylation of one of its downstream targets, GSK3β [95], known as a negative regulator of cell cycle progression [96]. An abnormal activation of mTOR has been demonstrated in human SLE [97], and promising results in the treatment of the disease have been obtained with rapamycin, which could act by facilitating the differentiation of Treg cells and promoting the expansion of other subsets able to limit the T cell stimulation of auto-reactive B cells [98]. Beyond Akt and mTOR, a dysregulation in leptin expression has also been found in SLE patients [99; 100], but further studies are required to unlock the mechanisms that control its secretion.

A role for the Akt-mTOR axis has also been demonstrated in the pathogenesis of multiple sclerosis (MS). MS is an inflammatory disease of the central nervous system, characterized by the presence of CD4+ autoreactive T cells able to target myelin-based antigens, thus causing the progressive formation of demyelinating lesions and neuronal degeneration [101]. Given the target of inflammation, MS is considered an organ-specific autoimmune disease. Several studies have tried to clarify the role of different T cell subsets in MS, but the complex network of immune cells in this pathology does not make this an easy task. In particular, the role of the Treg subsets has not yet been clearly addressed. No differences in numbers of Treg cells seem to exist between healthy subjects and MS patients, at least in the peripheral blood, and an increased number has been observed in the cerebrospinal fluid [102]. However, alterations in the Treg pool and function have been found [102; 103; 104]. Interestingly, gene-expression profile analysis of brains from post-mortem MS patients revealed a strong up-regulation of genes involved in cellular metabolism, such as Akt and HIF1α [105]. This is consistent with the findings that T cells from HIF$\alpha^{-/-}$ mice restimulated *ex vivo* with myelin oligodendrocyte glycoprotein (MOG) peptide display a reduced secretion of IL-17 and are poorly efficient to induce experimental autoimmune encephalomyelitis (EAE) in C57BL/6 mice [52]. Moreover, rapamycin administration is efficacious in treating EAE due to its dual action both on Treg and Teff cells [106]. The Akt-mTOR pathway seems to be subjected to leptin regulation during the development of EAE. Indeed, MOG-specific CD4+ T cells from leptin deficient (*ob/ob*) mice display a reduction in the activation of Akt and S6, downstream of mTOR. *Ob/ob* mice are resistant to adoptively transferred EAE [42; 107], a condition that can be restored by recombinant leptin administration [42]. In humans, increased levels of leptin has been detected in the CNS of MS patients [108].

Inhibitors of the mTOR pathway, such as sirolimus (rapamycin), are already used for the treatment of some autoimmune diseases, and many of its analogs constitute as promising candidates for a wide range of autoimmune diseases. Further study is required to reveal the metabolic signature of each disease in more depth, hence allowing the development of more specific and efficacious treatments.

A clear link has been established between Treg cells and type 1 diabetes (T1D), an inflammatory-autoimmune disease characterized by the inflammation and destruction of insulin-producing beta cells of the pancreas. This is particularly evident in individuals with IPEX (Immune Dysregulation, Polyendocrinopathy, Enteropathy, X-linked syndrome), in which the lack of Treg cells is associated with an increased susceptibility to diabetes [109]. The onset and progression of the pathology does not seem to be related to an altered number of Treg cells, since most works have demonstrated that there are no differences between T1D subjects and healthy controls in the peripheral blood [110; 111]. Most likely, a decreased suppressive capacity of Treg cells and an enhanced resistance to suppression of Teff cells seem to be the basis of the loss of self-tolerance observed in T1D [112; 113]. What really is hidden behind the alterations in T cell functions is still a matter of debate, but results from an early study have pointed out a strong activation of Akt in splenocytes from NOD mice, which could be prevented by the use of the PI3Kγ inhibitor AS605240 [114]. The amelioration observed in the clinical signs of diabetes after PI3K inhibition could be a consequence of the increase in Treg expansion as well as Teff suppression, probably due to the activation of cAMP response element-binding protein (CREB), a transcription factor shown to be involved in Foxp3 expression [115]. Anomalies in the number and function of T cell subsets have been also proved in other autoimmune diseases, such as rheumatoid arthritis (RA) [116] and psoriasis [117], but we are still far from clarifying the underlying molecular mechanisms behind their progression (Fig. 3).

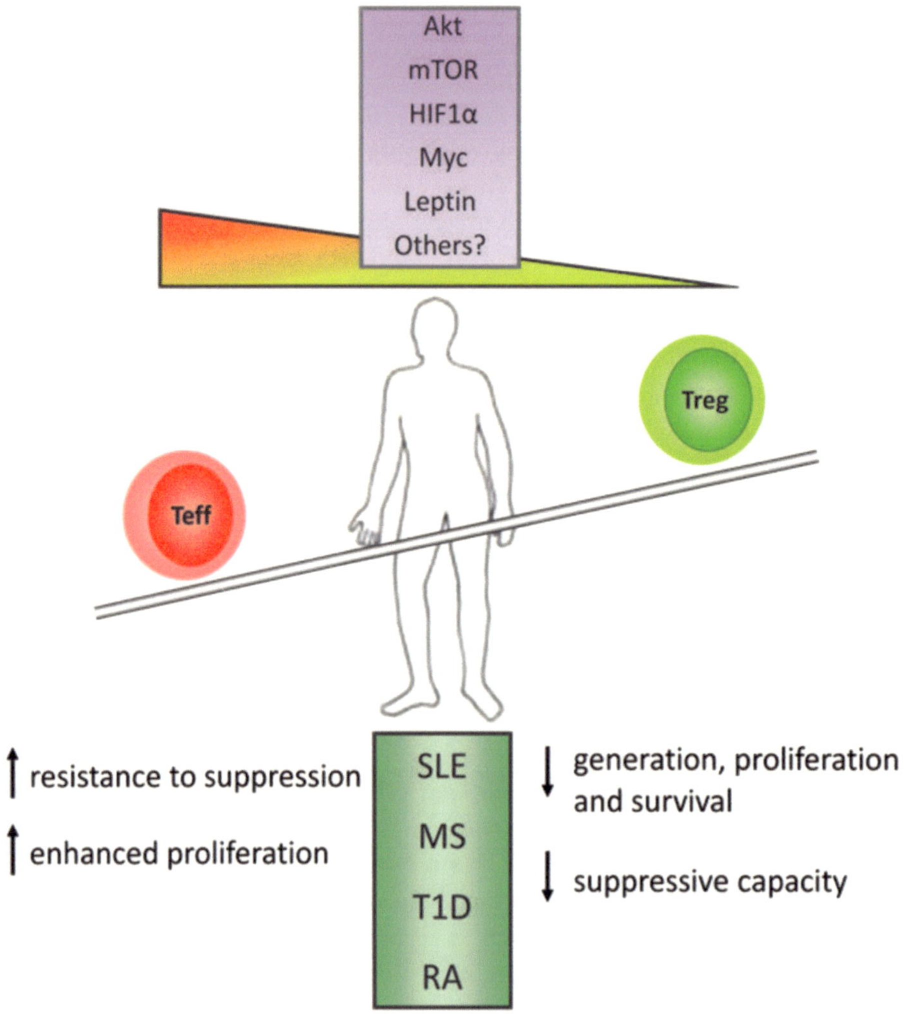

Figure 3. The metabolic factors influencing the immune system and autoimmune diseases. The balance between Treg and Teff function is crucial toward the maintenance of self tolerance. Akt, mTOR, HIF1α, Myc and Leptin are involved in tipping this balance, and the result of the dampening of Treg function or augmentation of Teff function could lead to the development of SLE, MS, T1D or RA.

Several studies have tried to highlight the genetic and metabolic background that predisposes individuals to autoimmune diseases preceding their onset, but this has been difficult due to the complex network of the different factors involved. A clear risk factor for the development of autoimmunity is represented by the presence of polymorphisms in the Human Leukocyte Antigen (HLA) class II locus, but non-HLA loci have also recently been identified. Some "autoimmune loci", such as *IL2RA, CTLA4, IL23R, IL10* and *PTPN22* are shared by a wide range of diseases, while others seem to be specific, such as the *VTCN1* (V-set domain containing T cell activation inhibitor 1) locus for SLE [118]. Allelic variants in the *PTPN22* locus, encoding for Lymphoid protein tyrosine phosphatase (Lyp), have been associated with a high predisposition to autoimmune diseases, including T1D, MS, SLE and RA. Protein tyrosine phosphatases (PTPs) catalyse the release of phosphate groups from tyrosine residues on signalling intermediates, thus playing a fundamental role in activating/deactivating specific transduction pathways. PTPs have been demonstrated to modulate the signalling events following T cell receptor (TCR) engagement with MHC-peptide complexes that lead to the activation and differentiation of T cells [119]. From a metabolic point of view, follow-up studies indicate that specific "lipidomic" profiles, such as low triglycerides, low levels of lysophosphatidylcholine and multiple phospholipids characterize the sera of children that later progress to T1D, as well as anomalies in the levels of glutamine, α-ketoglutarate and other amino acids [120; 121; 122; 123]. The adoption of metabolomics at a high-throughput level has also been useful to uncover these patterns [124]. Vitamin D deficiency has been associated with the increased likelihood of the development of autoimmune disease [125], including type 1 diabetes, and has been linked to key genes involved in the metabolism of 25(OH)D [126]. Despite the lack of direct evidence regarding the behaviour of different T cells subsets prior to the onset onset of autoimmune diseases, specific alterations in the levels of these modulators can be used to assess an individual's predisposing susceptibility to autoimmunity. Analysing specific T cell markers on a large scale and integrating them with certain genetic and metabolic biomarkers could become a powerful tool for predicting the risk and prognosis of specific autoimmune diseases.

5. Conclusion

Metabolism has an undoubtedly important role in the definition of the T cell repertoire. The constituents of the microenvironment or modulation of T cell responsiveness towards the environment controls the direction in which T cells differentiate. This, in turn, could lead to the development of autoimmune disease if the proinflammatory players prevail against opposing antiinflammatory cues. Although it is becoming clearer as to the role of metabolic networks in defining T cell fate and the development of autoimmunity—the molecular basis, especially the role of miRNAs in controlling T cell metabolism and sensitivity towards extracellular metabolic factors, remain unclear. Various drugs have been produced to tackle tumour growth from a metabolic point of view, and new strategies are emerging to target miRNAs as a therapy. Thus, the lessons learned from these fields may also contribute towards future therapeutic solutions against autoimmunity by specifically targeting T cells at the heart of metabolism.

Author details

Dan Li, Zhimei Gao, Chen Chen, Zuojia Chen,
Jia Nie, Zhao Shan, Yangyang Li, Andy Tsun* and Bin Li*
Key Laboratory of Molecular Virology & Immunology,
Unit of Molecular Immunology, Institut Pasteur of Shanghai,
Shanghai Institutes for Biological Sciences, Chinese Academy of Sciences, Shanghai, China

* Corresponding Author

Miranda Piccioni
Key Laboratory of Molecular Virology & Immunology,
Unit of Molecular Immunology, Institut Pasteur of Shanghai,
Shanghai Institutes for Biological Sciences, Chinese Academy of Sciences, Shanghai, China

Department of Experimental Medicine and Biochemical Sciences,
Microbiology Section, University of Perugia, Perugia, Italy

Acknowledgement

Our research is supported by the National Science Foundation of China (NSFC) 30972702, 31170825; NSFC-NIH 81161120417; Shanghai Pasteur Foundation; Shanghai 'Rising Star' program 10QA1407900; China-Germany PPP program; Novo Nordisk-Chinese Academy of Sciences Foundation; and the Chinese Academy of Sciences (CAS) network lab program. BL is a recipient of CAS '100-talent' program. AT is a recipient of CAS 'International Young Scientist Fellowship' and supported by NSFC 31150110337. We gratefully acknowledge the support of the Sanofi-Aventis-Shanghai Institutes for Biological Sciences scholarship program. We thank members in the Institut Pasteur of Shanghai for their critical comments and helpful discussions.

6. References

[1] [1] A. Perl, P. Gergely, Jr., G. Nagy, A. Koncz, and K. Banki (2004) Mitochondrial hyperpolarization: a checkpoint of T-cell life, death and autoimmunity. Trends Immunol. 25: 360-7.
[2] R.D. Michalek, V.A. Gerriets, S.R. Jacobs, A.N. Macintyre, N.J. MacIver, E.F. Mason, S.A. Sullivan, A.G. Nichols, and J.C. Rathmell (2011) Cutting edge: distinct glycolytic and lipid oxidative metabolic programs are essential for effector and regulatory CD4+ T cell subsets. J Immunol. 186: 3299-303.
[3] M. Munder, K. Eichmann, and M. Modolell (1998) Alternative metabolic states in murine macrophages reflected by the nitric oxide synthase/arginase balance: competitive regulation by CD4+ T cells correlates with Th1/Th2 phenotype. J Immunol. 160: 5347-54.
[4] G. Matarese, C. Procaccini, and V. De Rosa (2008) The intricate interface between immune and metabolic regulation: a role for leptin in the pathogenesis of multiple sclerosis? Journal of Leukocyte Biology. 84: 893-899.
[5] L.Z. Shi, R. Wang, G. Huang, P. Vogel, G. Neale, D.R. Green, and H. Chi (2011) HIF1alpha-dependent glycolytic pathway orchestrates a metabolic checkpoint for the differentiation of TH17 and Treg cells. J Exp Med. 208: 1367-76.
[6] J.D. Powell, and G.M. Delgoffe (2010) The mammalian target of rapamycin: linking T cell differentiation, function, and metabolism. Immunity. 33: 301-11.
[7] H. Zhu, N. Shyh-Chang, A.V. Segre, G. Shinoda, S.P. Shah, W.S. Einhorn, A. Takeuchi, J.M. Engreitz, J.P. Hagan, M.G. Kharas, A. Urbach, J.E. Thornton, R. Triboulet, R.I.

Gregory, D. Altshuler, and G.Q. Daley (2011) The Lin28/let-7 axis regulates glucose metabolism. Cell. 147: 81-94.

[8] T. Horie, K. Ono, H. Nishi, Y. Iwanaga, K. Nagao, M. Kinoshita, Y. Kuwabara, R. Takanabe, K. Hasegawa, T. Kita, and T. Kimura (2009) MicroRNA-133 regulates the expression of GLUT4 by targeting KLF15 and is involved in metabolic control in cardiac myocytes. Biochem Biophys Res Commun. 389: 315-20.

[9] R. Takanabe, K. Ono, Y. Abe, T. Takaya, T. Horie, H. Wada, T. Kita, N. Satoh, A. Shimatsu, and K. Hasegawa (2008) Up-regulated expression of microRNA-143 in association with obesity in adipose tissue of mice fed high-fat diet. Biochem Biophys Res Commun. 376: 728-32.

[10] E. Gambineri, T.R. Torgerson, and H.D. Ochs (2003) Immune dysregulation, polyendocrinopathy, enteropathy, and X-linked inheritance (IPEX), a syndrome of systemic autoimmunity caused by mutations of FOXP3, a critical regulator of T-cell homeostasis. Curr Opin Rheumatol. 15: 430-5.

[11] C. Morath, M. Zeier, B. Dohler, J. Schmidt, P.P. Nawroth, and G. Opelz (2008) Metabolic control improves long-term renal allograft and patient survival in type 1 diabetes. J Am Soc Nephrol. 19: 1557-63.

[12] K. Takada, and S.C. Jameson (2009) Naive T cell homeostasis: from awareness of space to a sense of place. Nat Rev Immunol. 9: 823-32.

[13] T.K. Starr, S.C. Jameson, and K.A. Hogquist (2003) Positive and negative selection of T cells. Annu Rev Immunol. 21: 139-76.

[14] R.G. Jones, and C.B. Thompson (2007) Revving the engine: signal transduction fuels T cell activation. Immunity. 27: 173-8.

[15] S.C. Jameson (2002) Maintaining the norm: T-cell homeostasis. Nat Rev Immunol. 2: 547-56.

[16] K.A. Frauwirth, and C.B. Thompson (2004) Regulation of T lymphocyte metabolism. J Immunol. 172: 4661-5.

[17] N.J. Maciver, S.R. Jacobs, H.L. Wieman, J.A. Wofford, J.L. Coloff, and J.C. Rathmell (2008) Glucose metabolism in lymphocytes is a regulated process with significant effects on immune cell function and survival. J Leukoc Biol. 84: 949-57.

[18] G.G. Guenther, E.R. Peralta, K.R. Rosales, S.Y. Wong, L.J. Siskind, and A.L. Edinger (2008) Ceramide starves cells to death by downregulating nutrient transporter proteins. Proc Natl Acad Sci U S A. 105: 17402-7.

[19] Y. Zhao, J.L. Coloff, E.C. Ferguson, S.R. Jacobs, K. Cui, and J.C. Rathmell (2008) Glucose metabolism attenuates p53 and Puma-dependent cell death upon growth factor deprivation. J Biol Chem. 283: 36344-53.

[20] C.M. Cham, and T.F. Gajewski (2005) Glucose availability regulates IFN-gamma production and p70S6 kinase activation in CD8+ effector T cells. J Immunol. 174: 4670-7.

[21] S.R. Jacobs, C.E. Herman, N.J. MacIver, J.A. Wofford, H.L. Wieman, J.J. Hammen, and J.C. Rathmell (2008) Glucose Uptake Is Limiting in T Cell Activation and Requires

CD28-Mediated Akt-Dependent and Independent Pathways. The Journal of Immunology. 180: 4476-4486.

[22] L.F. Barros, M. Young, J. Saklatvala, and S.A. Baldwin (1997) Evidence of two mechanisms for the activation of the glucose transporter GLUT1 by anisomycin: p38(MAP kinase) activation and protein synthesis inhibition in mammalian cells. J Physiol. 504 (Pt 3): 517-25.

[23] R.C. Osthus, H. Shim, S. Kim, Q. Li, R. Reddy, M. Mukherjee, Y. Xu, D. Wonsey, L.A. Lee, and C.V. Dang (2000) Deregulation of glucose transporter 1 and glycolytic gene expression by c-Myc. J Biol Chem. 275: 21797-800.

[24] P. Tamas, S.A. Hawley, R.G. Clarke, K.J. Mustard, K. Green, D.G. Hardie, and D.A. Cantrell (2006) Regulation of the energy sensor AMP-activated protein kinase by antigen receptor and Ca2+ in T lymphocytes. J Exp Med. 203: 1665-70.

[25] K. Barnes, J.C. Ingram, O.H. Porras, L.F. Barros, E.R. Hudson, L.G. Fryer, F. Foufelle, D. Carling, D.G. Hardie, and S.A. Baldwin (2002) Activation of GLUT1 by metabolic and osmotic stress: potential involvement of AMP-activated protein kinase (AMPK). J Cell Sci. 115: 2433-42.

[26] J.C. Rathmell, M.G. Vander Heiden, M.H. Harris, K.A. Frauwirth, and C.B. Thompson (2000) In the absence of extrinsic signals, nutrient utilization by lymphocytes is insufficient to maintain either cell size or viability. Mol Cell. 6: 683-92.

[27] J.C. Rathmell, E.A. Farkash, W. Gao, and C.B. Thompson (2001) IL-7 enhances the survival and maintains the size of naive T cells. J Immunol. 167: 6869-76.

[28] J.A. Wofford, H.L. Wieman, S.R. Jacobs, Y. Zhao, and J.C. Rathmell (2008) IL-7 promotes Glut1 trafficking and glucose uptake via STAT5-mediated activation of Akt to support T-cell survival. Blood. 111: 2101-11.

[29] K.A. Frauwirth, J.L. Riley, M.H. Harris, R.V. Parry, J.C. Rathmell, D.R. Plas, R.L. Elstrom, C.H. June, and C.B. Thompson (2002) The CD28 signaling pathway regulates glucose metabolism. Immunity. 16: 769-77.

[30] R.W. Matheny, Jr., and M.L. Adamo (2009) Current perspectives on Akt Akt-ivation and Akt-ions. Exp Biol Med (Maywood). 234: 1264-70.

[31] H.L. Wieman, S.R. Horn, S.R. Jacobs, B.J. Altman, S. Kornbluth, and J.C. Rathmell (2009) An essential role for the Glut1 PDZ-binding motif in growth factor regulation of Glut1 degradation and trafficking. Biochem J. 418: 345-67.

[32] K. Gottlob, N. Majewski, S. Kennedy, E. Kandel, R.B. Robey, and N. Hay (2001) Inhibition of early apoptotic events by Akt/PKB is dependent on the first committed step of glycolysis and mitochondrial hexokinase. Genes Dev. 15: 1406-18.

[33] D.R. Plas, S. Talapatra, A.L. Edinger, J.C. Rathmell, and C.B. Thompson (2001) Akt and Bcl-xL Promote Growth Factor-independent Survival through Distinct Effects on Mitochondrial Physiology. Journal of Biological Chemistry. 276: 12041-12048.

[34] J. Deprez, D. Vertommen, D.R. Alessi, L. Hue, and M.H. Rider (1997) Phosphorylation and activation of heart 6-phosphofructo-2-kinase by protein kinase B and other protein kinases of the insulin signaling cascades. J Biol Chem. 272: 17269-75.

[35] C.V. Dang, J.W. Kim, P. Gao, and J. Yustein (2008) The interplay between MYC and HIF in cancer. Nat Rev Cancer. 8: 51-6.
[36] D.A. Hume, J.L. Radik, E. Ferber, and M.J. Weidemann (1978) Aerobic glycolysis and lymphocyte transformation. Biochem J. 174: 703-9.
[37] D. Roos, and J.A. Loos (1973) Effect of phytohaemagglutinin on the carbohydrate metabolism of human blood lymphocytes after inhibition of the oxidative phosphorylation. Exp Cell Res. 77: 121-6.
[38] A.L. Sagone, Jr., A.F. LoBuglio, and S.P. Balcerzak (1974) Alterations in hexose monophosphate shunt during lymphoblastic transformation. Cell Immunol. 14: 443-52.
[39] E.F. Greiner, M. Guppy, and K. Brand (1994) Glucose is essential for proliferation and the glycolytic enzyme induction that provokes a transition to glycolytic energy production. Journal of Biological Chemistry. 269: 31484-31490.
[40] N.L. Alves, I.A. Derks, E. Berk, R. Spijker, R.A. van Lier, and E. Eldering (2006) The Noxa/Mcl-1 axis regulates susceptibility to apoptosis under glucose limitation in dividing T cells. Immunity. 24: 703-16.
[41] E.V. Dang, J. Barbi, H.Y. Yang, D. Jinasena, H. Yu, Y. Zheng, Z. Bordman, J. Fu, Y. Kim, H.R. Yen, W. Luo, K. Zeller, L. Shimoda, S.L. Topalian, G.L. Semenza, C.V. Dang, D.M. Pardoll, and F. Pan (2011) Control of T(H)17/T(reg) balance by hypoxia-inducible factor 1. Cell. 146: 772-84.
[42] G. Matarese, A. Di Giacomo, V. Sanna, G.M. Lord, J.K. Howard, A. Di Tuoro, S.R. Bloom, R.I. Lechler, S. Zappacosta, and S. Fontana (2001) Requirement for leptin in the induction and progression of autoimmune encephalomyelitis. J Immunol. 166: 5909-16.
[43] V. Sanna, A. Di Giacomo, A. La Cava, R.I. Lechler, S. Fontana, S. Zappacosta, and G. Matarese (2003) Leptin surge precedes onset of autoimmune encephalomyelitis and correlates with development of pathogenic T cell responses. J Clin Invest. 111: 241-50.
[44] V. De Rosa, C. Procaccini, G. Cali, G. Pirozzi, S. Fontana, S. Zappacosta, A. La Cava, and G. Matarese (2007) A key role of leptin in the control of regulatory T cell proliferation. Immunity. 26: 241-55.
[45] B.R. Wilfred, W.X. Wang, and P.T. Nelson (2007) Energizing miRNA research: a review of the role of miRNAs in lipid metabolism, with a prediction that miR-103/107 regulates human metabolic pathways. Mol Genet Metab. 91: 209-17.
[46] M.D. Walker (2008) Role of MicroRNA in pancreatic beta-cells: where more is less. Diabetes. 57: 2567-8.
[47] M.N. Poy, L. Eliasson, J. Krutzfeldt, S. Kuwajima, X. Ma, P.E. Macdonald, S. Pfeffer, T. Tuschl, N. Rajewsky, P. Rorsman, and M. Stoffel (2004) A pancreatic islet-specific microRNA regulates insulin secretion. Nature. 432: 226-30.
[48] A. El Ouaamari, N. Baroukh, G.A. Martens, P. Lebrun, D. Pipeleers, and E. van Obberghen (2008) miR-375 targets 3'-phosphoinositide-dependent protein kinase-1 and regulates glucose-induced biological responses in pancreatic beta-cells. Diabetes. 57: 2708-17.

[49] Y. Li, X. Xu, Y. Liang, S. Liu, H. Xiao, F. Li, H. Cheng, and Z. Fu (2010) miR-375 enhances palmitate-induced lipoapoptosis in insulin-secreting NIT-1 cells by repressing myotrophin (V1) protein expression. Int J Clin Exp Pathol. 3: 254-64.

[50] M. Biton, A. Levin, M. Slyper, I. Alkalay, E. Horwitz, H. Mor, S. Kredo-Russo, T. Avnit-Sagi, G. Cojocaru, F. Zreik, Z. Bentwich, M.N. Poy, D. Artis, M.D. Walker, E. Hornstein, E. Pikarsky, and Y. Ben-Neriah (2011) Epithelial microRNAs regulate gut mucosal immunity via epithelium-T cell crosstalk. Nat Immunol. 12: 239-46.

[51] V. Plaisance, A. Abderrahmani, V. Perret-Menoud, P. Jacquemin, F. Lemaigre, and R. Regazzi (2006) MicroRNA-9 controls the expression of Granuphilin/Slp4 and the secretory response of insulin-producing cells. J Biol Chem. 281: 26932-42.

[52] T. Kato, H. Shimano, T. Yamamoto, T. Yokoo, Y. Endo, M. Ishikawa, T. Matsuzaka, Y. Nakagawa, S. Kumadaki, N. Yahagi, A. Takahashi, H. Sone, H. Suzuki, H. Toyoshima, A.H. Hasty, S. Takahashi, H. Gomi, T. Izumi, and N. Yamada (2006) Granuphilin is activated by SREBP-1c and involved in impaired insulin secretion in diabetic mice. Cell Metab. 4: 143-54.

[53] D. Ramachandran, U. Roy, S. Garg, S. Ghosh, S. Pathak, and U. Kolthur-Seetharam (2011) Sirt1 and mir-9 expression is regulated during glucose-stimulated insulin secretion in pancreatic beta-islets. FEBS J. 278: 1167-74.

[54] J. van Loosdregt, Y. Vercoulen, T. Guichelaar, Y.Y. Gent, J.M. Beekman, O. van Beekum, A.B. Brenkman, D.J. Hijnen, T. Mutis, E. Kalkhoven, B.J. Prakken, and P.J. Coffer (2010) Regulation of Treg functionality by acetylation-mediated Foxp3 protein stabilization. Blood. 115: 965-74.

[55] S. Wang, Y. Tang, H. Cui, X. Zhao, X. Luo, W. Pan, X. Huang, and N. Shen (2011) Let-7/miR-98 regulate Fas and Fas-mediated apoptosis. Genes Immun. 12: 149-54.

[56] F. Fornari, M. Milazzo, P. Chieco, M. Negrini, G.A. Calin, G.L. Grazi, D. Pollutri, C.M. Croce, L. Bolondi, and L. Gramantieri (2010) MiR-199a-3p regulates mTOR and c-Met to influence the doxorubicin sensitivity of human hepatocarcinoma cells. Cancer Res. 70: 5184-93.

[57] J.F. Chen, E.M. Mandel, J.M. Thomson, Q. Wu, T.E. Callis, S.M. Hammond, F.L. Conlon, and D.Z. Wang (2006) The role of microRNA-1 and microRNA-133 in skeletal muscle proliferation and differentiation. Nat Genet. 38: 228-33.

[58] A. Davalos, L. Goedeke, P. Smibert, C.M. Ramirez, N.P. Warrier, U. Andreo, D. Cirera-Salinas, K. Rayner, U. Suresh, J.C. Pastor-Pareja, E. Esplugues, E.A. Fisher, L.O. Penalva, K.J. Moore, Y. Suarez, E.C. Lai, and C. Fernandez-Hernando (2011) miR-33a/b contribute to the regulation of fatty acid metabolism and insulin signaling. Proc Natl Acad Sci U S A. 108: 9232-7.

[59] C. Esau, S. Davis, S.F. Murray, X.X. Yu, S.K. Pandey, M. Pear, L. Watts, S.L. Booten, M. Graham, R. McKay, A. Subramaniam, S. Propp, B.A. Lollo, S. Freier, C.F. Bennett, S. Bhanot, and B.P. Monia (2006) miR-122 regulation of lipid metabolism revealed by in vivo antisense targeting. Cell Metab. 3: 87-98.

[60] D. Iliopoulos, K. Drosatos, Y. Hiyama, I.J. Goldberg, and V.I. Zannis (2010) MicroRNA-370 controls the expression of microRNA-122 and Cpt1alpha and affects lipid metabolism. J Lipid Res. 51: 1513-23.

[61] V. Manfe, E. Biskup, A. Rosbjerg, M. Kamstrup, A.G. Skov, C.M. Lerche, B.T. Lauenborg, N. Odum, and R. Gniadecki (2012) miR-122 regulates p53/Akt signalling and the chemotherapy-induced apoptosis in cutaneous T-cell lymphoma. PLoS One. 7: e29541.

[62] J. Godlewski, M.O. Nowicki, A. Bronisz, G. Nuovo, J. Palatini, M. De Lay, J. Van Brocklyn, M.C. Ostrowski, E.A. Chiocca, and S.E. Lawler (2010) MicroRNA-451 regulates LKB1/AMPK signaling and allows adaptation to metabolic stress in glioma cells. Mol Cell. 37: 620-32.

[63] X. Huang, L. Ding, K.L. Bennewith, R.T. Tong, S.M. Welford, K.K. Ang, M. Story, Q.T. Le, and A.J. Giaccia (2009) Hypoxia-inducible mir-210 regulates normoxic gene expression involved in tumor initiation. Mol Cell. 35: 856-67.

[64] T.J. Kelly, A.L. Souza, C.B. Clish, and P. Puigserver (2011) A hypoxia-induced positive feedback loop promotes hypoxia-inducible factor 1alpha stability through miR-210 suppression of glycerol-3-phosphate dehydrogenase 1-like. Mol Cell Biol. 31: 2696-706.

[65] A. Taguchi, K. Yanagisawa, M. Tanaka, K. Cao, Y. Matsuyama, H. Goto, and T. Takahashi (2008) Identification of hypoxia-inducible factor-1 alpha as a novel target for miR-17-92 microRNA cluster. Cancer Res. 68: 5540-5.

[66] M. Yamakuchi, S. Yagi, T. Ito, and C.J. Lowenstein (2011) MicroRNA-22 regulates hypoxia signaling in colon cancer cells. PLoS One. 6: e20291.

[67] Z. Lei, B. Li, Z. Yang, H. Fang, G.M. Zhang, Z.H. Feng, and B. Huang (2009) Regulation of HIF-1alpha and VEGF by miR-20b tunes tumor cells to adapt to the alteration of oxygen concentration. PLoS One. 4: e7629.

[68] S. Cascio, A. D'Andrea, R. Ferla, E. Surmacz, E. Gulotta, V. Amodeo, V. Bazan, N. Gebbia, and A. Russo (2010) miR-20b modulates VEGF expression by targeting HIF-1 alpha and STAT3 in MCF-7 breast cancer cells. J Cell Physiol. 224: 242-9.

[69] S.T. Cha, P.S. Chen, G. Johansson, C.Y. Chu, M.Y. Wang, Y.M. Jeng, S.L. Yu, J.S. Chen, K.J. Chang, S.H. Jee, C.T. Tan, M.T. Lin, and M.L. Kuo (2010) MicroRNA-519c suppresses hypoxia-inducible factor-1alpha expression and tumor angiogenesis. Cancer Res. 70: 2675-85.

[70] C.J. Liu, M.M. Tsai, P.S. Hung, S.Y. Kao, T.Y. Liu, K.J. Wu, S.H. Chiou, S.C. Lin, and K.W. Chang (2010) miR-31 ablates expression of the HIF regulatory factor FIH to activate the HIF pathway in head and neck carcinoma. Cancer Res. 70: 1635-44.

[71] K. Saito, E. Kondo, and M. Matsushita (2011) MicroRNA 130 family regulates the hypoxia response signal through the P-body protein DDX6. Nucleic Acids Res. 39: 6086-99.

[72] R. Rouas, H. Fayyad-Kazan, N. El Zein, P. Lewalle, F. Rothe, A. Simion, H. Akl, M. Mourtada, M. El Rifai, A. Burny, P. Romero, P. Martiat, and B. Badran (2009) Human

natural Treg microRNA signature: role of microRNA-31 and microRNA-21 in FOXP3 expression. Eur J Immunol. 39: 1608-18.

[73] H. Fayyad-Kazan, R. Rouas, M. Fayyad-Kazan, R. Badran, N. El Zein, P. Lewalle, M. Najar, E. Hamade, F. Jebbawi, M. Merimi, P. Romero, A. Burny, B. Badran, and P. Martiat (2012) MicroRNA Profile of Circulating CD4-positive Regulatory T Cells in Human Adults and Impact of Differentially Expressed MicroRNAs on Expression of Two Genes Essential to Their Function. J Biol Chem. 287: 9910-22.

[74] U. Bruning, L. Cerone, Z. Neufeld, S.F. Fitzpatrick, A. Cheong, C.C. Scholz, D.A. Simpson, M.O. Leonard, M.M. Tambuwala, E.P. Cummins, and C.T. Taylor (2011) MicroRNA-155 promotes resolution of hypoxia-inducible factor 1alpha activity during prolonged hypoxia. Mol Cell Biol. 31: 4087-96.

[75] S. Kohlhaas, O.A. Garden, C. Scudamore, M. Turner, K. Okkenhaug, and E. Vigorito (2009) Cutting edge: the Foxp3 target miR-155 contributes to the development of regulatory T cells. J Immunol. 182: 2578-82.

[76] S. Rane, M. He, D. Sayed, H. Vashistha, A. Malhotra, J. Sadoshima, D.E. Vatner, S.F. Vatner, and M. Abdellatif (2009) Downregulation of miR-199a derepresses hypoxia-inducible factor-1alpha and Sirtuin 1 and recapitulates hypoxia preconditioning in cardiac myocytes. Circ Res. 104: 879-86.

[77] S. Rane, M. He, D. Sayed, L. Yan, D. Vatner, and M. Abdellatif (2010) An antagonism between the AKT and beta-adrenergic signaling pathways mediated through their reciprocal effects on miR-199a-5p. Cell Signal. 22: 1054-62.

[78] S. Jiang, C. Li, V. Olive, E. Lykken, F. Feng, J. Sevilla, Y. Wan, L. He, and Q.J. Li (2011) Molecular dissection of the miR-17-92 cluster's critical dual roles in promoting Th1 responses and preventing inducible Treg differentiation. Blood. 118: 5487-97.

[79] N. Zhang, and M.J. Bevan (2010) Dicer controls CD8+ T-cell activation, migration, and survival. Proc Natl Acad Sci U S A. 107: 21629-34.

[80] L.F. Lu, M.P. Boldin, A. Chaudhry, L.L. Lin, K.D. Taganov, T. Hanada, A. Yoshimura, D. Baltimore, and A.Y. Rudensky (2010) Function of miR-146a in controlling Treg cell-mediated regulation of Th1 responses. Cell. 142: 914-29.

[81] D.F. Steiner, M.F. Thomas, J.K. Hu, Z. Yang, J.E. Babiarz, C.D. Allen, M. Matloubian, R. Blelloch, and K.M. Ansel (2011) MicroRNA-29 regulates T-box transcription factors and interferon-gamma production in helper T cells. Immunity. 35: 169-81.

[82] M. Yamamoto, E. Kondo, M. Takeuchi, A. Harashima, T. Otani, K. Tsuji-Takayama, F. Yamasaki, H. Kumon, M. Kibata, and S. Nakamura (2011) miR-155, a Modulator of FOXO3a Protein Expression, Is Underexpressed and Cannot Be Upregulated by Stimulation of HOZOT, a Line of Multifunctional Treg. PLoS One. 6: e16841.

[83] R.L. Rossi, G. Rossetti, L. Wenandy, S. Curti, A. Ripamonti, R.J. Bonnal, R.S. Birolo, M. Moro, M.C. Crosti, P. Gruarin, S. Maglie, F. Marabita, D. Mascheroni, V. Parente, M. Comelli, E. Trabucchi, R. De Francesco, J. Geginat, S. Abrignani, and M. Pagani (2011) Distinct microRNA signatures in human lymphocyte subsets and enforcement of the naive state in CD4+ T cells by the microRNA miR-125b. Nat Immunol. 12: 796-803.

[84] C.J. Fox, P.S. Hammerman, and C.B. Thompson (2005) Fuel feeds function: energy metabolism and the T-cell response. Nat Rev Immunol. 5: 844-52.

[85] M. Pierdominici, D. Vacirca, F. Delunardo, and E. Ortona mTOR signaling and metabolic regulation of T cells: new potential therapeutic targets in autoimmune diseases. Curr Pharm Des. 17: 3888-97.

[86] A.L. Edinger, and C.B. Thompson (2002) Akt maintains cell size and survival by increasing mTOR-dependent nutrient uptake. Mol Biol Cell. 13: 2276-88.

[87] M. Laplante, and D.M. Sabatini (2009) mTOR signaling at a glance. J Cell Sci. 122: 3589-94.

[88] J.H. Cho, and P.K. Gregersen Genomics and the multifactorial nature of human autoimmune disease. N Engl J Med. 365: 1612-23.

[89] J.C. Crispin, S.N. Liossis, K. Kis-Toth, L.A. Lieberman, V.C. Kyttaris, Y.T. Juang, and G.C. Tsokos Pathogenesis of human systemic lupus erythematosus: recent advances. Trends Mol Med. 16: 47-57.

[90] M. Miyara, Z. Amoura, C. Parizot, C. Badoual, K. Dorgham, S. Trad, D. Nochy, P. Debre, J.C. Piette, and G. Gorochov (2005) Global natural regulatory T cell depletion in active systemic lupus erythematosus. J Immunol. 175: 8392-400.

[91] X. Valencia, C. Yarboro, G. Illei, and P.E. Lipsky (2007) Deficient CD4+CD25high T regulatory cell function in patients with active systemic lupus erythematosus. J Immunol. 178: 2579-88.

[92] M.I. Vargas-Rojas, J.C. Crispin, Y. Richaud-Patin, and J. Alcocer-Varela (2008) Quantitative and qualitative normal regulatory T cells are not capable of inducing suppression in SLE patients due to T-cell resistance. Lupus. 17: 289-94.

[93] K. Stylianou, I. Petrakis, V. Mavroeidi, S. Stratakis, E. Vardaki, K. Perakis, S. Stratigis, A. Passam, E. Papadogiorgaki, K. Giannakakis, L. Nakopoulou, and E. Daphnis The PI3K/Akt/mTOR pathway is activated in murine lupus nephritis and downregulated by rapamycin. Nephrol Dial Transplant. 26: 498-508.

[94] D.F. Barber, A. Bartolome, C. Hernandez, J.M. Flores, C. Redondo, C. Fernandez-Arias, M. Camps, T. Ruckle, M.K. Schwarz, S. Rodriguez, A.C. Martinez, D. Balomenos, C. Rommel, and A.C. Carrera (2005) PI3Kgamma inhibition blocks glomerulonephritis and extends lifespan in a mouse model of systemic lupus. Nat Med. 11: 933-5.

[95] H. Tang, G. Tan, Q. Guo, R. Pang, and F. Zeng (2009) Abnormal activation of the Akt-GSK3beta signaling pathway in peripheral blood T cells from patients with systemic lupus erythematosus. Cell Cycle. 8: 2789-93.

[96] J. Liang, and J.M. Slingerland (2003) Multiple roles of the PI3K/PKB (Akt) pathway in cell cycle progression. Cell Cycle. 2: 339-45.

[97] A. Perl, D.R. Fernandez, T. Telarico, E. Doherty, L. Francis, and P.E. Phillips (2009) T-cell and B-cell signaling biomarkers and treatment targets in lupus. Curr Opin Rheumatol. 21: 454-64.

[98] D.R. Fernandez, T. Telarico, E. Bonilla, Q. Li, S. Banerjee, F.A. Middleton, P.E. Phillips, M.K. Crow, S. Oess, W. Muller-Esterl, and A. Perl (2009) Activation of mammalian

target of rapamycin controls the loss of TCRzeta in lupus T cells through HRES-1/Rab4-regulated lysosomal degradation. J Immunol. 182: 2063-73.

[99] C.P. Chung, A.G. Long, J.F. Solus, Y.H. Rho, A. Oeser, P. Raggi, and C.M. Stein (2009) Adipocytokines in systemic lupus erythematosus: relationship to inflammation, insulin resistance and coronary atherosclerosis. Lupus. 18: 799-806.

[100] M. Al, L. Ng, P. Tyrrell, J. Bargman, T. Bradley, and E. Silverman (2009) Adipokines as novel biomarkers in paediatric systemic lupus erythematosus. Rheumatology (Oxford). 48: 497-501.

[101] D.A. Hafler (2004) Multiple sclerosis. J Clin Invest. 113: 788-94.

[102] U. Feger, C. Luther, S. Poeschel, A. Melms, E. Tolosa, and H. Wiendl (2007) Increased frequency of CD4+ CD25+ regulatory T cells in the cerebrospinal fluid but not in the blood of multiple sclerosis patients. Clin Exp Immunol. 147: 412-8.

[103] J. Haas, B. Fritzsching, P. Trubswetter, M. Korporal, L. Milkova, B. Fritz, D. Vobis, P.H. Krammer, E. Suri-Payer, and B. Wildemann (2007) Prevalence of newly generated naive regulatory T cells (Treg) is critical for Treg suppressive function and determines Treg dysfunction in multiple sclerosis. J Immunol. 179: 1322-30.

[104] V. Viglietta, C. Baecher-Allan, H.L. Weiner, and D.A. Hafler (2004) Loss of functional suppression by CD4+CD25+ regulatory T cells in patients with multiple sclerosis. J Exp Med. 199: 971-9.

[105] U. Graumann, R. Reynolds, A.J. Steck, and N. Schaeren-Wiemers (2003) Molecular changes in normal appearing white matter in multiple sclerosis are characteristic of neuroprotective mechanisms against hypoxic insult. Brain Pathol. 13: 554-73.

[106] M. Esposito, F. Ruffini, M. Bellone, N. Gagliani, M. Battaglia, G. Martino, and R. Furlan Rapamycin inhibits relapsing experimental autoimmune encephalomyelitis by both effector and regulatory T cells modulation. J Neuroimmunol. 220: 52-63.

[107] M. Galgani, C. Procaccini, V. De Rosa, F. Carbone, P. Chieffi, A. La Cava, and G. Matarese Leptin modulates the survival of autoreactive CD4+ T cells through the nutrient/energy-sensing mammalian target of rapamycin signaling pathway. J Immunol. 185: 7474-9.

[108] C. Lock, G. Hermans, R. Pedotti, A. Brendolan, E. Schadt, H. Garren, A. Langer-Gould, S. Strober, B. Cannella, J. Allard, P. Klonowski, A. Austin, N. Lad, N. Kaminski, S.J. Galli, J.R. Oksenberg, C.S. Raine, R. Heller, and L. Steinman (2002) Gene-microarray analysis of multiple sclerosis lesions yields new targets validated in autoimmune encephalomyelitis. Nat Med. 8: 500-8.

[109] R.S. Wildin, and A. Freitas (2005) IPEX and FOXP3: clinical and research perspectives. J Autoimmun. 25 Suppl: 56-62.

[110] T. Brusko, C. Wasserfall, K. McGrail, R. Schatz, H.L. Viener, D. Schatz, M. Haller, J. Rockell, P. Gottlieb, M. Clare-Salzler, and M. Atkinson (2007) No alterations in the frequency of FOXP3+ regulatory T-cells in type 1 diabetes. Diabetes. 56: 604-12.

[111] A.L. Putnam, F. Vendrame, F. Dotta, and P.A. Gottlieb (2005) CD4+CD25high regulatory T cells in human autoimmune diabetes. J Autoimmun. 24: 55-62.

[112] S. Lindley, C.M. Dayan, A. Bishop, B.O. Roep, M. Peakman, and T.I. Tree (2005) Defective suppressor function in CD4(+)CD25(+) T-cells from patients with type 1 diabetes. Diabetes. 54: 92-9.

[113] A. Schneider, M. Rieck, S. Sanda, C. Pihoker, C. Greenbaum, and J.H. Buckner (2008) The effector T cells of diabetic subjects are resistant to regulation via CD4+ FOXP3+ regulatory T cells. J Immunol. 181: 7350-5.

[114] J. Azzi, R.F. Moore, W. Elyaman, M. Mounayar, N. El Haddad, S. Yang, M. Jurewicz, A. Takakura, A. Petrelli, P. Fiorina, T. Ruckle, and R. Abdi The Novel Therapeutic Effect of Phosphoinositide 3-Kinase-gamma Inhibitor AS605240 in Autoimmune Diabetes. Diabetes.

[115] H.P. Kim, and W.J. Leonard (2007) CREB/ATF-dependent T cell receptor-induced FoxP3 gene expression: a role for DNA methylation. J Exp Med. 204: 1543-51.

[116] K.M. Chavele, and M.R. Ehrenstein Regulatory T-cells in systemic lupus erythematosus and rheumatoid arthritis. FEBS Lett. 585: 3603-10.

[117] L. Chen, Z. Shen, G. Wang, P. Fan, and Y. Liu (2008) Dynamic frequency of CD4+CD25+Foxp3+ Treg cells in psoriasis vulgaris. J Dermatol Sci. 51: 200-3.

[118] P.S. Ramos, L.A. Criswell, K.L. Moser, M.E. Comeau, A.H. Williams, N.M. Pajewski, S.A. Chung, R.R. Graham, R. Zidovetzki, J.A. Kelly, K.M. Kaufman, C.O. Jacob, T.J. Vyse, B.P. Tsao, R.P. Kimberly, P.M. Gaffney, M.E. Alarcon-Riquelme, J.B. Harley, and C.D. Langefeld (2011) A comprehensive analysis of shared loci between systemic lupus erythematosus (SLE) and sixteen autoimmune diseases reveals limited genetic overlap. PLoS Genet. 7: e1002406.

[119] G.L. Burn, L. Svensson, C. Sanchez-Blanco, M. Saini, and A.P. Cope (2011) Why is PTPN22 a good candidate susceptibility gene for autoimmune disease? FEBS Lett. 585: 3689-98.

[120] M. Pflueger, T. Seppanen-Laakso, T. Suortti, T. Hyotylainen, P. Achenbach, E. Bonifacio, M. Oresic, and A.G. Ziegler (2011) Age- and islet autoimmunity-associated differences in amino acid and lipid metabolites in children at risk for type 1 diabetes. Diabetes. 60: 2740-7.

[121] M. Oresic, S. Simell, M. Sysi-Aho, K. Nanto-Salonen, T. Seppanen-Laakso, V. Parikka, M. Katajamaa, A. Hekkala, I. Mattila, P. Keskinen, L. Yetukuri, A. Reinikainen, J. Lahde, T. Suortti, J. Hakalax, T. Simell, H. Hyoty, R. Veijola, J. Ilonen, R. Lahesmaa, M. Knip, and O. Simell (2008) Dysregulation of lipid and amino acid metabolism precedes islet autoimmunity in children who later progress to type 1 diabetes. J Exp Med. 205: 2975-84.

[122] R. Madsen, V.S. Banday, T. Moritz, J. Trygg, and K. Lejon (2012) Altered Metabolic Signature in Pre-Diabetic NOD Mice. PLoS One. 7: e35445.

[123] M. Sysi-Aho, A. Ermolov, P.V. Gopalacharyulu, A. Tripathi, T. Seppanen-Laakso, J. Maukonen, I. Mattila, S.T. Ruohonen, L. Vahatalo, L. Yetukuri, T. Harkonen, E. Lindfors, J. Nikkila, J. Ilonen, O. Simell, M. Saarela, M. Knip, S. Kaski, E. Savontaus, and M. Oresic (2011) Metabolic regulation in progression to autoimmune diabetes. PLoS Comput Biol. 7: e1002257.

[124] T.J. Wang, M.G. Larson, R.S. Vasan, S. Cheng, E.P. Rhee, E. McCabe, G.D. Lewis, C.S. Fox, P.F. Jacques, C. Fernandez, C.J. O'Donnell, S.A. Carr, V.K. Mootha, J.C. Florez, A. Souza, O. Melander, C.B. Clish, and R.E. Gerszten (2011) Metabolite profiles and the risk of developing diabetes. Nat Med. 17: 448-53.

[125] A.L. Ponsonby, R.M. Lucas, and I.A. van der Mei (2005) UVR, vitamin D and three autoimmune diseases--multiple sclerosis, type 1 diabetes, rheumatoid arthritis. Photochem Photobiol. 81: 1267-75.

[126] J.D. Cooper, D.J. Smyth, N.M. Walker, H. Stevens, O.S. Burren, C. Wallace, C. Greissl, E. Ramos-Lopez, E. Hypponen, D.B. Dunger, T.D. Spector, W.H. Ouwehand, T.J. Wang, K. Badenhoop, and J.A. Todd (2011) Inherited variation in vitamin D genes is associated with predisposition to autoimmune disease type 1 diabetes. Diabetes. 60: 1624-31.

Chapter 5

Apoptosis and Autoimmune Disorders

Reginald Halaby

Additional information is available at the end of the chapter

http://dx.doi.org/10.5772/48164

1. Introduction

Apoptosis, or programmed cell death, comes from a Greek term meaning "the falling off of the leaves." Apoptosis is also known as cell suicide and is a mechanism that is present in most eukaryotic cells to regulate cell numbers. It can be considered as the opposite of mitosis. Apoptosis is a normal part of development and is required during development, creation of the central nervous system, degeneration of the tadpole tail during metamorphosis, and the loss of certain appendages during the larval to pupal metamorphosis in holometabolous insects.

Apoptosis is a major aspect of development and homeostasis. Apoptosis contributes to the sculpting of developing structures in vertebrate and invertebrate embryos. Deletion of interdigital webs in developing limbs (Hammar & Mottet, 1971), development of the fetal intestinal mucosa (Harmon et al., 1984), and retinal development (Penfold & Provis, 1986) all involve apoptosis. Apoptosis serves as a major mechanism for the regulation of cell numbers. For example, in the visual system of developing vertebrates, apoptosis preferentially eliminates neurons that form improper connections (Cowan et al., 1984). In the mammalian embryonic central nervous system, over 1/3 of newly formed cells die (Oppenheim et al., 1982) and during development of *Caenorhabditis elegans* 131 of the 1090 somatic cells die (Ellis & Horvitz, 1986). Some cells seem to die because they have no apparent function, such as the Mullerian duct in male embryos (Price et al., 1977). Apoptosis can serve as a defense mechanism to remove unwanted and potentially dangerous cells, such as self-reactive lymphocytes (Smith et al., 1989).

During development, the survival of lymphocytes is mediated by both active signaling and passive processes that regulate survival. These processes are extremely selective resulting in the elimination of the majority of developing lymphocytes (Owen & Jenkinson, 1992). Both T- and B-lymphocytes undergo developmental stages and appear to share many regulatory mechanisms. For example, the early survival of lymphocyte precursors is mediated primarily by cytokines, which both regulate the numbers of progenitors and play critical roles in initiating the rearrangement of the antigen receptor genes (Baird et al., 1999). Developing lymphocytes must create unique antigen receptors by rearrangement to generate the incredible diversity characteristic of an adaptive immune response (Jung et al., 2006). A consequence of the stochastic nature of this process is that only 1/3 of rearrangements are joined appropriately and give rise to a functional antigen receptor (Jung et al., 2006). Although several mechanisms (use of alternative antigen receptor gene loci and receptor editing) exist to allow further opportunities for successful rearrangement, the majority of lymphocytes fail to generate functional antigen receptors and are thus eliminated by programmed cell death (Berg & Kang, 2001; Nemazee, 2006).

2. Apoptosis and disease

The suppression of apoptosis increases the susceptibility of an individual to malignancy whereas uncontrolled apoptosis is associated with degenerative diseases. These include acquired immunodeficiency syndrome (AIDS; Ameison & Capron, 1991), cancer (Ling et al., 1993), Parkinson's disease (Walkinshaw & Waters, 1995), and Alzheimer's disease (Landfield et al., 1992). Abnormally elevated levels of apoptosis have been found in the lymph nodes of HIV-infected persons (Muro-Cacho et al., 1995). Indeed a clearer understanding of the regulation of apoptosis may result in better therapies.

In this chapter, we will examine how inappropriate or excessive apoptosis can lead to autoimmune disorders, such as type I diabetes, autoimmune thyroid disease, rheumatoid arthritis, lupus and others. Furthermore, we present data demonstrating that apoptosis-related treatments can be effective against various autoimmune disorders.

3. Type I Diabetes

Type I diabetes (T1D; also known as insulin-dependent or juvenile-onset diabetes) results from a presumed T-cell attack on the insulin-secreting β-cells of the pancreas. Controlled apoptotic cell death contributes to normal T-cell selection and education. Among the regulatory T-cells that actively suppress effector T-cells, the $FOXP3^{+}CD4^{+}CD25^{high}$ T-cells (T_{regs}) represent one of the best characterized sub-populations. There is accumulating evidence of a deficiency in either the frequency or function of T_{regs} in various human autoimmune diseases (Bacchetta et al., 2007), as well as in the pathogenesis of T1D (Brusko et al., 2005; Putnam et al., 2005). An increase in T_{reg} apoptosis was found to correlate with a decline in suppressive potential of these cells. The fact that both hyperglycemic T1D subjects and normoglycemic *at-risk* subjects showed this phenomenon suggests that T_{reg} apoptosis is more a precursor to, rather than a consequence of diabetes (Jailwala et al., 2009). Although T_{reg} apoptosis is likely to be one of the peripheral imbalances in T1D, there is very little known about the pathways and genes that make T_{regs} sensitive to apoptosis during the period right after the onset of disease. Understanding the mechanism by which cytokine deprivation in T1D induces expression of apoptotic genes should identify potential targets for novel treatments.

Therefore, interruption of normal T-cell selection can result in the generation of autoreactive cells (Takuma & Faustman, 2003). However, the mechanisms by which most candidate genes predispose to type 1 diabetes remain unclear. A recent study reports that *PTPN2*, a candidate gene for type 1 diabetes, modulates β-cell apoptosis after exposure to type I and II interferons (IFNs), cytokines that contribute to β-cell loss in early type 1 diabetes (Santin et al., 2011). The *PTPN2* gene encodes a phosphatase that is ubiquitously expressed (Doody et al., 2009). This phosphatase is induced by IFNγ and a synthetic dsRNA, polyinosinic-polycitidilic acid (PIC), in β-cells and exacerbates IFNγ- and PIC-induced β-cell apoptosis by modulating STAT1 activation (Coli et al., 2010; Moore et al., 2009). However, the mechanisms connecting this candidate gene to actual β-cell death remain unclear. Inhibition of *PTPN2* sensitizes pancreatic β-cells to apoptosis induced by both type I and II IFNs (Santin et al, 2011).

4. Autoimmune Thyroid Diseases

The Fas and TRAIL pathways are present and functional in the thyroid, and there is evidence suggesting their involvement in autoimmune diseases of the thyroid (Bretz et al., 1999; Kawakami et al 2000). Giordano et al. (1997) reported the constitutive expression of FasL (Fas ligand) on normal and Hashimoto's thyroiditis (HT) thyrocytes using immunohistochemistry, flow cytometry, and RT-PCR. The percentage of FasL-positive thyrocytes in Graves' thyroid was less than in normal thyroids (Sera et al., 2000). In contrast, another study was unable to detect FasL in thyrocytes (Xerri et al., 1997).

Although it is widely accepted that thyrocytes express the death receptor Fas, little is known about how this expression is modulated. It has been demonstrated that there is increased expression of Fas in the thyrocytes of patients with Hashimoto's thyroiditis (Hammond et al., 1997). Fas was also upregulated in the thyrocytes of patients with Graves' disease (Sera et al., 2000). The thyroid gland of Graves' disease patients contains TUNEL-positive thyrocytes and PCNA-positive thyrocytes, together with monocuclear cell infiltration (Sera et al., 2000). These data suggest that apoptosis and proliferation of thyrocytes may be abnormally accelerated, however, the proliferation of thyrocytes may outweigh their apoptosis, resulting in hyperplasia. IL-1β-treated thyrocytes become sensitive to apoptosis by anti-Fas IgM and activated T cells (Eguchi, 2001). Moreover, IL-1β-stimulated thyrocytes show reduced cytotoxic activity toward activated T cells. These results indicate that the IL-1β produced in the thyroid gland of Graves' disease patients might act on the thyroctyes to reduce their resistance to Fas-mediated apoptosis and lose their cytotoxic activity against activated T-cells, thus abolishing the immune-privilege status of the thyroid (Eguchi, 2001). This may provide an explanation for the accumulation of activated T cells in the of Graves' disease patients.

TSH receptor (TSHR) antibodies may be stimulating, blocking, or neutral in their functional influences and are found in patients with autoimmune thyroid disease, especially Graves' disease (Morshed et al., 2010). Although neutral TSHR antibodies failed to generate cAMP via Gαs effectors, they initiated unique molecular signaling, possibly via recruitment of multiple G proteins (Laugwitz et al., 1996; Büch et al., 2008), and thus influenced multiple downstream signal transduction cascades including PKC/MAPK, mTOR/S6K, NF-κB, certain cytokines, and oxidative stress signaling and ultimately caused rat thyroid cell apoptosis on chronic exposure. These findings suggest that oxidative stress may play a significant role in such antibody-induced thyrocyte death and thus exacerbate the chronic inflammatory process via antigen-driven mechanisms seen in autoimmune thyroid disease.

Bcl-2 is mitochondiral protein that inhibits apoptosis (Park & Hockenbery, 1996). Increased serum Bcl-2 may be linked to accelerated apoptosis and was observed in patients with malignancies (Tas et al., 2006). In euthyroid Hashimoto's thyroiditis patients compared with controls and euthyroid Graves' disease, increased serum Bcl-2 has been reported (Myśliwiec et al., 2006). In a recent study, a tendency towards higher Bcl-2 in Hashimoto's thyroiditis patients was found (Jiskra et al., 2009). Jiskra et al. (2009) further showed that there was no difference in serum Bcl-2 between hyperthyroid Graves' disease and when the euthyroid state was achieved.

5. Systemic Lupus Erythematosus

A common feature of autoimmune diseases such as systemic lupus erythematosus (SLE), systemic sclerosis, and mixed connective tissue disease is the breakdown of tolerance of self antigens, a consequence of which is the production of antibodies reactive with multiple self proteins (von Mühlen & Tan, 1995). In patients with SLE, increased numbers of apoptotic lymphocytes and macrophages have been observed (Emlen et al., 1994). Other proteins have been implicated to play a contributing role in the pathogenesis of SLE. Protein phosphatase 2A (PP2A) is an abundant and ubiquitously expressed, highly conserved enzyme (Janssens et al., 2008). It regulates a variety of cellular processes, including cell cycle progression and cell division, cell death, cytoskeleton dynamics, and signaling pathways (Janssens & Goris, 2001; Sontag, 2001). PP2A is composed of a scaffold subunit (A), a catalytic subunit (C), and a regulatory (B) subunit. A recent study showed that the subunit Bβ is involved in the regulation of programmed cell death triggered by IL-2 deficiency and identified a subset of patients with SLE in which altered regulation of PP2A Bβ is associated with resistance to IL-2 deprivation-induced apoptosis (Crispín et al., 2011). Apoptosis is an essential phenomenon that modulates the duration of immune responses and maintains the diversity of the lymphoid armamentarium. The importance of this process is well known, and the deficiency of central molecules involved in lymphocyte apoptosis causes lymphoproliferative and autoimmune diseases in mice and humans (Turbyville & Rao, 2010; Cohen, 2006). Apoptosis induced by IL-2 deprivation is triggered by intrinsic cellular signals (Lenardo et al., 1999). The balance between anti- and pro-apoptotic Bcl-2 family proteins determines the maintenance of the mitochondrial membrane potential. In the presence of IL-2, Bad is phosphorylated and sequestered in the cytoplasm by 14-3-3 proteins (Zha et al., 1996; Pastorino et al., 1999). Bim, another pro-apoptotic molecule, is absent, and levels of anti-apoptotic Bcl-2 and Bcl-x are high. During IL-2 deprivation, Bad becomes dephosphorylated, dissociates from 14-3-3, and translocates to the mitochondrial membrane where it binds to Bcl-2 and Bcl-x and neutralizes their anti-apoptotic capacity (Zha et al., 1996; Yang et al., 1995). This process results in the loss of the mitochondrial membrane potential and leads to apoptosis. The regulation of T-cell death following activation is known to be altered in patients with SLE (Gergely et al., 2002; Xu et al., 2004). Recent results indicate that the kinetics of apoptosis following IL-2 deprivation is affected in a fraction of patients with SLE (Crispín et al., 2011). Importantly, induction of PP2A Bβ upon IL-2 withdrawal was suboptimal or completely absent in these patients, which confirms the importance of PP2A Bβ as a molecule induced in cytokine withdrawal apoptosis and suggests that its faulty expression may underlie the observed phenotype. Mitochondrial hyperpolarization (MHP) could also contribute to the apoptosis resistance observed in SLE patients upon IL-2 deprivation (Gergely et al., 2002; Fernandez et al., 2006).

6. Apoptosis in rheumatoid arthritis

Fas and FasL both exist in membrane (mFas, mFasL) and soluble (sFas, sFasL) forms, but only engagement of mFas leads to the activation of caspase-8 via the Fas-associated death domain protein (FADD; Okamoto et al., 2000). Activated caspase-8 may lead to apoptosis via at least two well-described pathways: direct activation of caspase-3; and alteration of mitochondrial transmembrane potentials via Bcl-2 homology 3 (BH3)-interacting death-domain agonist (BID), leading to the cytoplasmic translocation of cytochrome c, which leads to activation of caspase-9, which in turn activates caspase-3 (Peng, 2006). Both pathways are regulated at the level of caspase-8 activation by the endogenous inhibitor FADD-like IL-1β-converting enzyme (FLICE)-inhibitory protein (FLIP), which may also be recruited by FADD. Interestingly, FLIP may also participate in an alternate signalling pathway, recruiting tumour necrosis factor-associated factor (TRAF) 1, TRAF2, the MAP kinase kinase kinase Raf1 and receptor-interacting protein (RIP) to activate extracellular signal-regulated kinase (ERK) and nuclear factor κB (NF-κB) pathways, leading to proliferation and/or inflammation (Peng, 2006).

Apoptotic cells are uncommonly observed in rheumatoid arthritis (RA) tissues *in vivo*, but synoviocytes, synovial T cells and macrophages have often been observed to express high levels of Fas and/or FasL, and are highly susceptible to Fas/FasL-induced apoptosis *in vitro*. This contrasts with osteoarthritis, in which such abnormalities in Fas/FasL expression and susceptibility to Fas-induced apoptosis are generally not observed (Firestein et al., 1995; Nakajima et al., 1995). The discrepancy between an absence of apoptotic cells *in situ* and enhanced susceptibility to Fas-induced apoptosis *in vitro* probably reflects multiple anti-apoptotic processes and/or phenomena in the rheumatoid synovium (Peng, 2006). For instance, increased intrasynovial and/or serum sFas appears to compete with mFas and prevent apoptosis of synoviocytes (Hasunuma et al., 1997). Also, in some studies, invading T cells have been found to be defective in FasL expression, which may account for ineffective clearance of activated (Fas-expressing) cells (Cantwell et al., 1997). In addition, synoviocyte- and/or stromal cell-derived cytokines [including transforming growth factor (TGF) β1 (Kawakami et al., 1996), basic fibroblast growth factor, TNF-α ,and interleukin-1

(Kobayashi et al., 2000a; Tsuboi et al., 1996)] protect RA synoviocytes from Fas-induced apoptosis, and such factors may account for the ability of RA T cells to be protected from apoptosis via their close interactions with fibroblast-like synoviocytes (Salmon et al., 1997). Furthermore, rheumatoid synovial fluid contains high levels of nitric oxide, which inhibits caspase-3 (Migita et al., 2001), as well as stromelysin-1 (matrix metalloproteinase-3), which can cleave mFasL to produce sFasL, which can compete with death-inducing mFasL (Matsuno et al., 2001). Thus, multiple pathways, both intra- and extracellular, impair Fas-induced apoptosis in RA joints. Still, whether these phenomena actually underlie the disease etiology or simply result from the initial inflammatory pathways of RA itself remains undetermined.

7. Sjogren's Syndrome

Sjogren's syndrome (SS) is an autoimmune disorder that affects multiple exocrine glands, particular those that produce moisture to coat exposed epithelia such as the oral and ocular surfaces. The role of apoptosis in loss of glandular tissue in SS is less clear (Wang et al., 2006). Environmental and genetic factors appear to contribute to the etiology of SS, although the evidence is relatively premature (Bolstad & Jonsson, 2002; Yamamoto, 2003). T-cell-mediated cytotoxicity (Manganelli & Fietta, 2003; Hayashi et al., 2004) and autoantibodies are important in loss of gland function. There is also a failure to remove autoimmune T-cells at the level of thymic selection, resistance of T-cells within the gland to undergo apoptosis, aberrant expression of increased levels of cell adhesion molecules on glandular epithelial cells (facilitating infiltration of autoimmune lymphocytes to glands), up regulation of human leukocyte antigen (HLA)-DR, and polyclonal activation of B-lymphocytes (Rehman, 2003). Glandular epithelial cells contribute to the autoimmune process by secreting pro-inflammatory cytokines. Specifically, pro-inflammatory cytokines, such as tumor necrosis factor (TNF)-α, interleukin (IL)-1β and 6 (Roescher et al., 2010) and (Muraki et al., 2004) in the exocrine glands in response to immune-mediated inflammation, are found over-expressed in the SS patients. IL-6, a potent inflammatory cytokine, is involved in acute phase reactions and both B and T-cell responses and the formation of germinal center-like structure (Roescher et al., 2010). It was found to be consistently high in saliva and serum and in the salivary glands of SS patients, not in subjects with xerostomia (dry mouth) only (Roescher et al., 2009). Furthermore, IL-1β is an effective inducer of other inflammatory cytokines such as IL-6, IL-8, TNF-α, and granulocyte-macrophage colony-stimulating factor (Fibbe et al., 1989; Chrousos, 1995). Dry-eye disease is accompanied by an increase in the proinflammatory forms of IL-1 (IL-1 α and mature IL-1 β) and a decrease in the biologically inactive precursor IL-1 β in tear fluid of SS patients (Solomon et al., 2001).

Several studies have analyzed the role of the Fas/FasL system in salivary gland lesions of patients with SS. Bolstad et al. (2003) demonstrated a substantial increase in the salivary gland tissue expression of the negative regulator molecules PD-1 and CTLA-4 and the apoptotic signal molecules Fas and FasL in SS patients compared with controls, suggesting the involvement of the Fas/FasL system in the apoptosis of ductal and acinar epithelial cells.

Abu-Helu et al. (2001) showed that salivary gland epithelial cell lines (SGEC) constitutively expressed more membranous Fas and intracellular FasL than controls, while Shibata et al. (2002) detected Fas/FasL expression in ductal and acinar cells of SS patients but not in controls. Other studies have suggested that Fas may accelerate the apoptotic death of peripheral CD4 T cells in SS patients (Zeher et al., 1999; Ohashi et al., 1996). However, Ohlsson et al. (2001) found Fas-induced epithelial cell apoptosis to be a rare event, with a frequency of less than 1% in salivary glands from 18 SS patients.

Loss of p53 activity allows the survival and proliferation of cells that should otherwise be eliminated. In primary SS, the expression of p53 and p21 was analyzed in salivary glands from 10 patients and 10 controls (Mariette et al., 2002). The p53 antigen was detected in the ductal cells of nine SS patients and only one control, and the p21 antigen in eight patients and two controls. Both antigens were located in the ductal cells of SS patients, but not in acinar cells. The expression of p53 and p21 in the ductal cells located around lymphoid infiltrates may represent a defense mechanism allowing DNA repair and thus preventing apoptosis, while the lack of over-expression of p53 and p21 in acinar cells could be one of the mechanisms responsible for acinar destruction by apoptosis in SS salivary glands.

Kong et al. (1997) demonstrated in SS that the expression of Bcl-2 makes them resistant to apoptotic cell death. Nakamura et al. (2000a) showed that Bcl-2 and Bcl-x were preferentially expressed in infiltrating mononuclear cells rather than in the acinar and ductal epithelial cells from salivary glands of 17 SS patients, while Ohlsson et al. (2002) detected Bcl-2 (but rarely Bax) in the infiltrating lymphocytes of salivary glands from SS patients. However, Abu-Helu et al. (2001) found that SGEC cell lines constitutively expressed antiapoptotic proteins, such as Bcl-2 and cFLIP, that might protect them from both spontaneous and anti-Fas mAb-mediated apoptosis. Kamachi et al. (2002) found an inhibitory effect of IFN-γ in Bcl-2 expression, which was enhanced by coadministration of TNFα, leading to an increase in the apoptosis of salivary gland cells. It seems that apoptosis of the epithelial acinar and ductal cells may depend on the imbalance between up-regulated death-promoters (Fas and Bax) and down-regulated apoptosis-suppressor signals (Bcl-2).

A stronger expression of activated caspase-3 and cleaved PARP in the acinar and ductal cells of salivary glands was found in 13/15 (87%) SS patients, while staining for activated caspase-9 was negative. Nakamura et al. (2000b) analyzed the role of the X chromosome-linked inhibitor of apoptosis (XIAP), a member of the IAP family that inhibits the activation of caspases, and found a strong expression in the acinar and ductal epithelial cells of SS patients but not in those of controls. Because caspase-3 and caspase-7 are effector enzymes, XIAP might protect salivary epithelial cells from apoptotic death in SS (Nakamura et al., 2000b). Hayashi et al. (2003) suggested that treatment with caspase inhibitors might prevent the development of the inflammatory process in salivary glands, and Inoue et al. (2001) found that caspase-inhibiting agents could inhibit the cleavage of α-fodrin. Increased caspase cascade activity may be involved in the progression of autoantigen proteolysis and tissue destruction in primary SS. The presence of activated caspase-3 in salivary glands indicates that excessive apoptosis may contribute to epithelial destruction in primary SS.

From the studies above, it can be concluded that the extrinsic apoptotic pathway as well as the intrinsic apoptotic pathway are involved in the pathogenesis of SS. FasL and its receptor, Fas, are essential in the homeostasis of the peripheral immune system. It can be considered that a defect in activation-induced cell death of effector T cells may result in the development of autoimmune exocrinopathy in Sjogren syndrome (Hayashi et al., 2004). Conversely, the increased rate of apoptosis of in epithelial cells in SS may result from either the imbalance between the down-regulated apoptosis-inhibitor Bcl-2 and the up-regulated apoptosis-inducer Bax, via the intrinsic pathway (Manganelli P & Fietta, 2003).

8. Apoptosis-related therapies for autoimmune disorders

Injection of high doses of soluble peptides leads to a state of T-cell unresponsiveness (referred to as anergy) owing to a block in T-cell proliferation and/or IL-2 production, or results in activation-induced cell death (AICD) after T-cell re-stimulation with the cognate peptide (Burstein et al., 1992; Critchfield et al., 1994). It is thought that tolerance induced by soluble peptides may be useful for antigen-specific immunotherapy for the treatment of human autoimmune diseases. Non-obese diabetic (NOD) mice spontaneously develop type 1 diabetes, which is characterized by T-cell-mediated inflammation of the pancreatic islets (insulitis) and the eventual destruction of the insulin-producing β-cells7. Prevention of type 1 diabetes in NOD mice can be achieved by inducing specific T-cell tolerance to pancreatic β-cell autoantigens prior to the total destruction of all the islet β-cells (Miller et al., 2007).

One of the more promising methods to induce tolerance for the prevention and treatment of autoimmune diseases, and the prevention of transplant rejection, is intravenous treatment with antigen-coupled, ethylene carbodiimide (ECDI)-fixed splenocytes (referred to here as antigen coupled cells). Treatment with antigen-coupled cells can induce anergy *in vitro* and peripheral tolerance *in vivo* (Miller et al., 1979; Sriram et al., 1983). The induction of tolerance by antigen-coupled cell treatment has also been shown to be an effective therapy in other disease models, including experimental autoimmune thyroiditis (Braley-Mullen et al., 1980) and in the NOD mouse model of diabetes (Fife et al., 2006). Unlike soluble-peptide therapy, in which (depending on the disease-inducing autoantigen) the tolerizing antigen can induce an anaphylactic response that results in the death of treated mice, antigen-coupled-cell therapy does not induce an allergic response, regardless of the antigen used, and appears to be well tolerated at all stages of disease (Smith et al., 2005; Pedotti et al., 2001).

Zauli et al. (2010) showed that recombinant human tumor necrosis factor (TNF)-related apoptosis-inducing ligand (TRAIL) ameliorated the severity of streptozotocin (STZ)-induced type 1 diabetes in a mouse model. Specifically, exogenous recombinant TRAIL, co-injected with STZ, significantly reduced the levels of islet damage with respect to animals injected with STZ alone (Zauli et al., 2010). Of note, treatment with recombinant TRAIL does not impair the viability of pancreatic islets, even when overexpressed (Dirice et al., 2009).

Thyroid arterial embolization was shown to effectively enhance the positive expression of pro-apoptotic genes of Fas, FasL, Bax, Bcl-2 and P53 in Grave's disease (GD) thyroid, thus promoting apoptosis of GD thyroid and restoring the thyroid size and function to normal conditions (Zhao et al., 2009). Furthermore, T lymphocytes from GD patients treated with thyroid hormones accompany reduction of Bcl-2 protein expression, production of reactive oxygen species, and reduction of mitochondrial delta psi, resulting in apoptotic lymphocyte death (Mihara et al., 1999). In a study of patients with Hashimoto's thyroiditis treated with Simvastatin, it was shown that CD4+ cells and B lymphocytes increased while CD8+ cells, natural killer cells, and activated T lymphocytes decreased significantly (Gullu et al., 2005). This effect is probably mediated via lymphocyte apoptosis as demonstrated with in vitro experiments and is not confined to Simvastatin since Mevastatin, Pravastatin and Cerivastatin also induced apoptosis in lymphocytes (Gullu et al., 2005). Thyroid cells can be sensitized to die via apoptosis by a unique combination of interferon-gamma and IL-1beta cytokines. Interferon-gamma/IL-1beta pretreatment sensitizes human thyroid cells to Fas-mediated apoptosis in a complex manner that overcomes the blockade of initiator caspases through increased expression of cell surface Fas receptor, increases in proapoptotic molecules that result in mitochondrial activation, and late caspase cleavage (Mezosi et al., 2005).

Lupus-prone (NZB x NZW)F1 mice spontaneously develop elevated titers of anti-DNA Abs that contain T cell determinants in their V(H) regions. It has been shown that tolerization with an artificial peptide based on these T cell determinants (pConsensus (pCons)) can block production of anti-DNA Abs and prolong survival of the mice (Singh et al., 1995). These data indicate that clinical suppression of autoimmunity after administration of pCons depends in part on the generation of CD8+ Ti cells that suppress secretion of anti-DNA Ig using mechanisms that include Foxp3, TGFβ, and resistance to apoptosis (Hahn et al., 2005). It is postulated that in the $CD8^+$ Ti cells, secretion of TGFβ, expression of *Foxp3*, and reduced apoptosis may likely be linked (Hahn et al., 2005).

The above studies strongly suggest that modulation of the Fas pathway may serve as attractive therapeutic targets. Many current RA therapies are in fact known to induce apoptosis in synovial cells, such as methotrexate and TNF-directed therapies, and appear to do so at least in part via Fas, at least in some pathogenic cell populations, such as T cells and/or synovial macrophages (Oshima et al., 2000; Genestier et al., 1998; Catrina et al., 2005). Thus, approaches targeted more specifically against Fas/FasL may be of benefit.

More direct evidence includes one study demonstrating the ability of anti-sense oligonucleotides against FLIP to sensitize RA synoviocytes strongly to Fas-induced apoptosis (Palao et al., 2005). Furthermore, in a model in which severe combined immunodeficient (*scid*) mice are engrafted with RA synovium, treatment with an apoptosis-inducing anti-Fas antibody, as well as gene therapy with FasL or FADD, induces apoptosis in both synoviocytes and mononuclear cell populations, diminishing cellular infiltrates (Okamoto et al., 1998; Kobayashi et al., 2000b; Matsuno et al., 2002). Thus, if apoptotic strategies are to be used therapeutically in inflammatory arthritis, current evidence altogether strongly supports activation of the apoptotic Fas pathway as a primary objective, at least in RA.

A recent study evaluated whether cholinergic autoantibodies contained in IgG purified from Sjogren sera could trigger apoptosis of A253 cell line (Reina et al., 2012). The use of A253 cell lines has revealed that salivary gland epithelial cells are particularly susceptible to Fas-mediated as well as Fas-independent apoptotic death after stimulation with IFN-γ, probably via the downregulation of the apoptosis inhibitor protein c-FLIP (Abu-Helu et al., 2001). Reina et al. (2012) demonstrated that anti-cholinergic autoantibodies in IgG purified from primary SS patient's sera mediates apoptosis of the A253 cell line in an inositol phosphate, caspase-3 and metalloproteinase-3 dependent manner.

9. Summary

The research reviewed in this chapter clearly demonstrates that there is a delicate balance between death and survival signals in the pathogenesis of autoimmune disorders. The apoptotic pathways involved may be disease-specific or shared in common. Although the precise mechanisms by which apoptosis modulates autoimmune disorders in not fully understood, deciphering the role played by apoptosis in these disorders will lead to improved treatment modalities for patients.

Author details

Reginald Halaby
Montclair State University, Montclair, New Jersey, USA

Acknowledgement

This work was supported by a grant from the National Institute of General Medical Sciences (T34 GM 079079) to R.H.

10. References

Abu-Helu RF, Dimitriou ID, Kapsogeorgou EK, Moutsopoulos HM, Manoussakis MN. Induction of salivary gland epithelial cell injury in Sjogren's syndrome: in vitro assessment of T cell-derived cytokines and Fas protein expression. J Autoimmun. 2001;17:141-153.

Ameison JC, Capron A. Cell dysfunction and depletion in AIDS: the programmed cell death hypothesis. Immunol Today. 1991;12:102-105.

Bacchetta R, Gambineri E, Roncarolo MG. Role of regulatory T cells and FOXP3 in human diseases. J Allergy Clin Immunol. 2007;120:227-235.

Baird AM, Gerstein RM, Berg LJ. The role of cytokine receptor signaling in lymphocyte development. Curr Opin Immunol. 1999;11:157–166.

Bolstad AI, Eiken HG, Rosenlund B, Alarcón-Riquelme ME, Jonsson R. Increased salivary gland tissue expression of Fas, Fas ligand, cytotoxic T lymphocyte-associated antigen 4, and programmed cell death 1 in primary Sjögren's syndrome. Arthritis Rheum. 2003;48:174-185.

Bolstad AI. Jonsson R. Genetic aspects of Sjögren's syndrome. Arthritis Res. 2002;4:353-359.

Braley-Mullen H, Tompson JG, Sharp GC, Kyriakos M. Suppression of experimental autoimmune thyroiditis in guinea pigs by pretreatment with thyroglobulin-coupled spleen cells. Cell Immunol. 1980;51:408-413.

Bretz JD, Rymaszewski M, Arscott PL, Myc A, Ain KB, Thompson NW, Baker JR Jr. TRAIL death pathway expression and induction in thyroid follicular cells. J Biol Chem. 1999;274:23627-23632.

Brusko TM, Wasserfall CH, Clare-Salzler MJ, Schatz DA, Atkinson MA. Functional defects and the influence of age on the frequency of CD4+ CD25+ T-cells in type 1 diabetes. Diabetes. 2005;54:1407–1414.

Büch TR, Biebermann H, Kalwa H, Pinkenburg O, Hager D, Barth H, Aktories K, Breit A, Gudermann T. G13-dependent activation of MAPK by thyrotropin. J Biol Chem. 2008;283:20330-20341.

Burstein HJ, Shea CM, Abbas AK. Aqueous antigens induce in vivo tolerance selectively in IL-2- and IFN-gamma-producing (Th1) cells. J Immunol. 1992;148:3687-3691.

Cantwell MJ, Hua T, Zvaifler NJ, Kipps TJ. Deficient Fas ligand expression by synovial lymphocytes from patients with rheumatoid arthritis. Arthritis Rheum. 1997;40:1644-1652.

Catrina AI, Trollmo C, af Klint E, Engstrom M, Lampa J, Hermansson Y, Klareskog L, Ulfgren AK. Evidence that anti-tumor necrosis factor therapy with both etanercept and infliximab induces apoptosis in macrophages, but not lymphocytes, in rheumatoid arthritis joints: extended report. Arthritis Rheum. 2005;52:61-72.

Chrousos GP. The hypothalamic-pituitary-adrenal axis and immune-mediated inflammation. N Engl J Med. 1995;332:1351-1362.

Cohen PL. Apoptotic cell death and lupus. Springer Semin Immunopathol. 2006;28:145-152.

Colli ML, Moore F, Gurzov EN, Ortis F, Eizirik DL. MDA5 and PTPN2, two candidate genes for type 1 diabetes, modify pancreatic beta-cell responses to the viral by-product double-stranded RNA. Hum Mol Genet. 2010;19:135-146.

Cowan WM., Fawcett JW, O'Leary DDM, Stanfield BB. Regressive events in neurogenesis. Science 1984;225:1258-1265.

Crispín JC, Apostolidis SA, Finnell MI, Tsokos GC. Induction of PP2A Bβ, a regulator of IL-2 deprivation-induced T-cell apoptosis, is deficient in systemic lupus erythematosus. Proc Natl Acad Sci U S A. 2011;108:12443-12448.

Critchfield JM, Racke MK, Zúñiga-Pflücker JC, Cannella B, Raine CS, Goverman J, Lenardo MJ. T cell deletion in high antigen dose therapy of autoimmune encephalomyelitis. Science. 1994;263:1139-1143.

Dirice E, Sanlioglu AD, Kahraman S, Ozturk S, Balci MK, Omer A, Griffith TS, Sanlioglu S. Adenovirus-mediated TRAIL gene (Ad5hTRAIL) delivery into pancreatic islets prolongs normoglycemia in streptozotocin-induced diabetic rats. Hum GeneT her. 2009;20:1177-1189.

Doody KM, Bourdeau A, Tremblay ML. T-cell protein tyrosine phosphatase is a key regulator in immune cell signaling: lessons from the knockout mouse model and implications in human disease. Immunol Rev. 2009;228:325-341.

Ellis HM, Horvitz HR. Genetic control of programmed cell death in the nematode *C.elegans*. Cell. 1986;44:817-829.

Emlen W, Niebur J, Kadera R. Accelerated in vitro apoptosis of lymphocytes from patients with systemic lupus erythematosus. J Immunol. 1994;152:3685-3692.

Eguchi K. Apoptosis in autoimmune diseases. Intern Med. 2001;40:275-284.

Fernandez D, Bonilla E, Mirza N, Niland B, Perl A. Rapamycin reduces disease activity and normalizes T cell activation-induced calcium fluxing in patients with systemic lupus erythematosus. Arthritis Rheum. 2006;54:2983-2988.

Fibbe WE, Daha MR, Hiemstra PS, Duinkerken N, Lurvink E, Ralph P, Altrock BW, Kaushansky K, Willemze R, Falkenburg JH. Interleukin 1 and poly(rI).poly(rC) induce production of granulocyte CSF, macrophage CSF, and granulocyte-macrophage CSF by human endothelial cells. Exp Hematol. 1989;17:229-234.

Firestein GS, Yeo M, Zvaifler NJ. Apoptosis in rheumatoid arthritis synovium. J Clin Invest. 1995;96:1631-1638.

Genestier L, Paillot R, Fournel S, Ferraro C, Miossec P, Revillard JP. Immunosuppressive properties of methotrexate: apoptosis and clonal deletion of activated peripheral T cells. J Clin Invest. 1998;10:322-328.

Gergely P Jr, Niland B, Gonchoroff N, Pullmann R Jr, Phillips PE, Perl A. Persistent mitochondrial hyperpolarization, increased reactive oxygen intermediate production, and cytoplasmic alkalinization characterize altered IL-10 signaling in patients with systemic lupus erythematosus. J Immunol. 2002;169:1092-1101.

Giordano C, Stassi G, De Maria R, Todaro M, Richiusa P, Papoff G, Ruberti G, Bagnasco M, Testi R, Galluzzo A. Potential involvement of Fas and its ligand in the pathogenesis of Hashimoto's thyroiditis. Science. 1997;275:960-963.

Gullu S, Emral R, Bastemir M, Parkes AB, Lazarus JH. In vivo and in vitro effects of statins on lymphocytes in patients with Hashimoto's thyroiditis. Eur J Endocrinol. 2005;153:41-48.

Hahn BH, Singh RP, La Cava A, Ebling FM. Tolerogenic treatment of lupus mice with consensus peptide induces Foxp3-expressing, apoptosis-resistant, TGFbeta-secreting CD8+ T cell suppressors. J Immunol. 2005;175:7728-7737.

Hammar SP, Mottet NK. Tetrazolium salt and electronmicroscopic studies of cellular degeneration and necrosis in the interdigital areas of the developing chick limb. J Cell Sci.1971; 8:229-251.

Harmon B, Bell L, Williams L. An ultrastructural study on the "meconium corpuscles" in rat foetal intestinal epithelium with particular reference to apoptosis. Anat Embryol. 1984;169:119-124.

Hammond LJ, Lowdell MW, Cerrano PG, Goode AW, Bottazzo GF, Mirakian R. Analysis of apoptosis in relation to tissue destruction associated with Hashimoto's autoimmune thyroiditis. J Pathol. 1997;182:138-144.

Hasunuma T, Kayagaki N, Asahara H, Motokawa S, Kobata T, Yagita H, Aono H, Sumida T, Okumura K, Nishioka K. Accumulation of soluble Fas in inflamed joints of patients with rheumatoid arthritis. Arthritis Rheum. 1997;40:80-86.

Hayashi Y, Arakaki R, and Ishimaru N. Apoptosis and estrogen deficiency in primary Sjögren's syndrome. Curr. Opin Rheumatol. 2004;16:522-526.

Hayashi T, Faustman DL. Role of defective apoptosis in type 1 diabetes and other autoimmune diseases. Recent Prog Horm Res. 2003;58:131-153.

Hayashi Y, Arakaki R, Ishimaru N. The role of caspase cascade on the development of primary Sjögren's syndrome. J Med Invest. 2003;50:32-38.

Inoue H, Tsubota K, Ono M, Kizu Y, Mizuno F, Takada K, Yamada K, Yanagi K, Hayashi Y, Saito I. Possible involvement of EBV-mediated alpha-fodrin cleavage for organ-specific autoantigen in Sjogren's syndrome. J Immunol. 2001;166:5801-5809.

Jailwala P, Waukau J, Glisic S, Jana S, Ehlenbach S, Hessner M, Alemzadeh R, Matsuyama S, Laud P, Wang X, Ghosh S. Apoptosis of CD4+ CD25(high) T cells in type 1 diabetes may be partially mediated by IL-2 deprivation. PLoS One. 2009;4:e6527.

Janssens V, Longin S, Goris J. PP2A holoenzyme assembly: in cauda venenum (the sting is in the tail). Trends Biochem Sci. 2008;33:113-121.

Janssens V, Goris J. Protein phosphatase 2A: a highly regulated family of serine/threonine phosphatases implicated in cell growth and signalling. Biochem J. 2001;353:417-439.

Jiskra J, Antosová M, Límanová Z, Telicka Z, Lacinová Z. The relationship between thyroid function, serum monokine induced by interferon gamma and soluble interleukin-2 receptor in thyroid autoimmune diseases. Clin Exp Immunol. 2009;156:211-216.

Kamachi M, Kawakami A, Yamasaki S, Hida A, Nakashima T, Nakamura H, Ida H, Furuyama M, Nakashima K, Shibatomi K, Miyashita T, Migita K, Eguchi K. Regulation of apoptotic cell death by cytokines in a human salivary gland cell line: distinct and synergistic mechanisms in apoptosis induced by tumor necrosis factor alpha and interferon gamma. J Lab Clin Med. 2002;139:13-19.

Kawakami A, Matsuoka N, Tsuboi M, Koji T, Urayama S, Sera N, Hida A, Usa T, Kimura H, Yokoyama N, Nakashima T, Ishikawa N, Ito K, Kawabe Y, Eguchi K. CD4+ T cell-mediated cytotoxicity toward thyrocytes: the importance of Fas/Fas ligand interaction inducing apoptosis of thyrocytes and the inhibitory effect of thyroid-stimulating hormone. Lab Invest. 2000;80:471-484.

Kawakami A, Eguchi K, Matsuoka N, Tsuboi M, Kawabe Y, Aoyagi T, Nagataki S. Inhibition of Fas antigen-mediated apoptosis of rheumatoid synovial cells in vitro by transforming growth factor beta 1. Arthritis Rheum. 1996;39:1267-1276.

Kobayashi T, Okamoto K, Kobata T, Hasunuma T, Kato T, Hamada H, Nishioka K. Differential regulation of Fas-mediated apoptosis of rheumatoid synoviocytes by tumor necrosis factor alpha and basic fibroblast growth factor is associated with the expression of apoptosis-related molecules. Arthritis Rheum. 2000;43:1106-1114.

Kobayashi T, Okamoto K, Kobata T, Hasunuma T, Kato T, Hamada H, Nishioka K. Novel gene therapy for rheumatoid arthritis by FADD gene transfer: induction of apoptosis of rheumatoid synoviocytes but not chondrocytes. Gene Ther. 2000;7:527-533.

Kong L, Ogawa N, Nakabayashi T, Liu GT, D'Souza E, McGuff HS, Guerrero D, Talal N, Dang H. Fas and Fas ligand expression in the salivary glands of patients with primary Sjögren's syndrome. Arthritis Rheum. 1997;40:87-97.

Landfield PW, Thibault, O, Mazzanti ML, Porter NM, Kerr, DS. 1992. Mechanisms of neuronal death in brain aging and Alzheimer's disease; role of endocrine-mediated calcium dyshomeostasis. J Neurobiol. 1992;23:1247-1260.

Laugwitz KL, Allgeier A, Offermanns S, Spicher K, Van Sande J, Dumont JE, Schultz G. The human thyrotropin receptor: a heptahelical receptor capable of stimulating members of all four G protein families. Proc Natl Acad Sci U S A. 1996;93:116-120.

Lenardo M, Chan KM, Hornung F, McFarland H, Siegel R, Wang J, Zheng L. Mature T lymphocyte apoptosis--immune regulation in a dynamic and unpredictable antigenic environment. Annu Rev Immunol. 1999;17:221-253.

Ling YH, Waldemar P, Perez-Soler R. Apoptosis induced by anthracycline in P388 parent and multidrug-resistant cells. Cancer Res. 1993;53:1845-1852.

Manganelli P, Fietta P. Apoptosis and Sjögren's syndrome. Semin Arthritis Rheum. 2003;33: 49-65.

Matsuno H, Yudoh K, Nakazawa F, Sawai T, Uzuki M, Nishioka K, Yonehara S, Nakayama J, Ohtsuki M, Kimura T. Antirheumatic effects of humanized anti-Fas monoclonal antibody in human rheumatoid arthritis/SCID mouse chimera. J Rheumatol. 2002;29:1609-1614.

Mariette X, Sibilia J, Roux S, Meignin V, Janin A. A new defensive mechanism to prevent apoptosis in salivary ductal cells from patients with Sjögren's syndrome: over-expression of p53 and p21. Rheumatology (Oxford). 2002;41:96-99.

Matsuno H, Yudoh K, Watanabe Y, Nakazawa F, Aono H, Kimura T. Stromelysin-1 (MMP-3) in synovial fluid of patients with rheumatoid arthritis has potential to cleave membrane bound Fas ligand. J Rheumatol. 2001;28:22-28.

Messina ME Jr, Halaby R. Does triptolide induce lysosomal-mediated apoptosis in human breast cancer cells? Med Hypotheses. 2011;77:91-93.

Mezosi E, Wang SH, Utsugi S, Bajnok L, Bretz JD, Gauger PG, Thompson NW, Baker JR Jr. Induction and regulation of Fas-mediated apoptosis in human thyroid epithelial cells. Mol Endocrinol. 2005;19:804-811.

Migita K, Yamasaki S, Kita M, Ida H, Shibatomi K, Kawakami A, Aoyagi T, Eguchi K. Nitric oxide protects cultured rheumatoid synovial cells from Fas-induced apoptosis by inhibiting caspase-3. Immunology. 2001;103:362-367.

Mihara S, Suzuki N, Wakisaka S, Suzuki S, Sekita N, Yamamoto S, Saito N, Hoshino T, Sakane T. Effects of thyroid hormones on apoptotic cell death of human lymphocytes. J Clin Endocrinol Metab. 1999;84:1378-1385.

Miller SD, Turley DM, Podojil JR. Antigen-specific tolerance strategies for the prevention and treatment of autoimmune disease. Nat Rev Immunol. 2007;7:665-677.

Miller SD, Wetzig RP, Claman HN. The induction of cell-mediated immunity and tolerance with protein antigens coupled to syngeneic lymphoid cells. J Exp Med. 1979;149:758-773.

Moore F, Colli ML, Cnop M, Esteve MI, Cardozo AK, Cunha DA, Bugliani M, Marchetti P, Eizirik DL. PTPN2, a candidate gene for type 1 diabetes, modulates interferon-gamma-induced pancreatic beta-cell apoptosis. Diabetes. 2009;58:1283-1291.

Morshed SA, Ando T, Latif R, Davies TF. Neutral antibodies to the TSH receptor are present in Graves' disease and regulate selective signaling cascades. Endocrinology. 2010;151:5537-5549.

Muraki Y, Tsutsumi A, Takahashi R, Suzuki E, Hayashi T, Chino Y, Goto D, Matsumoto I, Murata H, Noguchi E, Sumida T. Polymorphisms of IL-1 beta gene in Japanese patients with Sjögren's syndrome and systemic lupus erythematosus. J Rheumatol. 2004;31:720-725.

Muro-Cacho CA, Pontaleo G, Fauci AS. Analysis of apoptosis in lymph nodes of HIV-infected persons. J Immunol. 1995;154:5555-5556.

Myśliwiec J, Okota M, Nikołajuk A, Górska M. Soluble Fas, Fas ligand and Bcl-2 in autoimmune thyroid diseases: relation to humoral immune response markers. Adv Med Sci. 2006;51:119-122.

Nakajima T, Aono H, Hasunuma T, Yamamoto K, Shirai T, Hirohata K, Nishioka K. Apoptosis and functional Fas antigen in rheumatoid arthritis synoviocytes. Arthritis Rheum. 1995;38:485-491.

Nakamura H, Kawakami A, Tominaga M, Hida A, Yamasaki S, Migita K, Kawabe Y, Nakamura T, Eguchi K. Relationship between Sjögren's syndrome and human T-lymphotropic virus type I infection: follow-up study of 83 patients. J Lab Clin Med. 2000;135:139-144.

Nakamura H, Kawakami A, Yamasaki S, Nakashima T, Kamachi M, Migita K, Kawabe Y, Nakamura T, Koji T, Hayashi Y, Eguchi K. Expression and function of X chromosome-linked inhibitor of apoptosis protein in Sjögren's syndrome. Lab Invest. 2000;80:1421-1427.

Ohashi H, Ogawa N, Goto Y, Karahashi T, Akamine N. Elevated Fas (CD95) and bcl-2 protein expression on T cells from patients with primary Sjogren's syndrome. Arthritis Rheum. 1996;39:S288.

Ohlsson M, Szodoray P, Loro LL, Johannessen AC, Jonsson R. CD40, CD154, Bax and Bcl-2 expression in Sjögren's syndrome salivary glands: a putative anti-apoptotic role during its effector phases. Scand J Immunol. 2002;56:561-71.

Ohlsson M, Skarstein K, Bolstad AI, Johannessen AC, Jonsson R. Fas-induced apoptosis is a rare event in Sjögren's syndrome. Lab Invest. 2001;81:95-105.

Ohshima S, Mima T, Sasai M, Nishioka K, Shimizu M, Murata N, Yoshikawa H, Nakanishi K, Suemura M, McCloskey RV, Kishimoto T, Saeki Y. Tumour necrosis factor alpha (TNF-alpha) interferes with Fas-mediated apoptotic cell death on rheumatoid arthritis (RA) synovial cells: a possible mechanism of rheumatoid synovial hyperplasia and a clinical benefit of anti-TNF-alpha therapy for RA. Cytokine. 2000;12:281-288.

Okamoto K, Kobayashi T, Kobata T, Hasunuma T, Kato T, Sumida T, Nishioka K. Fas-associated death domain protein is a Fas-mediated apoptosis modulator in synoviocytes. Rheumatology (Oxford). 2000;39:471-480.

Okamoto K, Asahara H, Kobayashi T, Matsuno H, Hasunuma T, Kobata T, Sumida T, Nishioka K. Induction of apoptosis in the rheumatoid synovium by Fas ligand gene transfer. Gene Ther. 1998;5:331-338.

Oppenheim RW, Maderdrut JL, Wells DJ. Cell death of motoneurons in the chick embryo spinal cord. VI. Reduction of naturally occurring cell death in the thoracolumbar column of Terni by nerve growth factor. J Comp Neurol. 1982;210:174-189.

Owen JJ, Jenkinson EJ. Apoptosis and T-cell repertoire selection in the thymus. Ann NY Acad Sci. 1992;663:305–310.

Park JR, Hockenbery DM. BCL-2, a novel regulator of apoptosis. J Cell Biochem. 1996;60:12-17.

Pastorino JG, Tafani M, Farber JL. Tumor necrosis factor induces phosphorylation and translocation of BAD through a phosphatidylinositide-3-OH kinase-dependent pathway. J Biol Chem. 1999;274:19411-19416.

Pedotti R, Mitchell D, Wedemeyer J, Karpuj M, Chabas D, Hattab EM, Tsai M, Galli SJ, Steinman L. An unexpected version of horror autotoxicus: anaphylactic shock to a self-peptide. Nat Immunol. 2001;2:216-222.

Penfold PL, Provis JM. Cell death in the development of the human retina: phagocytosis of pyknotic and apoptotic bodies by retinal cells. Graefe's Arch Clin Exp Opthalmol. 1986;224:549-553.

Peng SL. Fas (CD95)-related apoptosis and rheumatoid arthritis. Rheumatology (Oxford). 2006 Jan;45(1):26-30.

Price JM, Donahoe PK, Ito Y, Hendren WH 3rd. Programmed cell death in the Mullerian duct induced by Mullerian inhibiting substance. Am J Anat. 1977;149:353-375.

Putnam AL, Vendrame F, Dotta F, Gottlieb PA. CD4+CD25high regulatory T cells in human autoimmune diabetes. J Autoimmun. 2005;24:55–62.

Rehman HU. Sjögren's syndrome. Yonsei Med J. 2003;44:947-954.

Reina S, Sterin-Borda L, Borda E. Anti-M(3) peptide IgG from Sjögren's syndrome triggers apoptosis in A253 cells. Cell Immunol. 2012 Apr 3. [Epub ahead of print]

Roescher N, Tak PP, Illei GG. Cytokines in Sjogren's syndrome: potential therapeutic targets. Ann Rheum Dis. 2010;69:945-948.

Roescher N, Tak PP, Illei GG. Cytokines in Sjögren's syndrome. Oral Dis. 2009;15:519-526.

Salmon M, Scheel-Toellner D, Huissoon AP, Pilling D, Shamsadeen N, Hyde H, D'Angeac AD, Bacon PA, Emery P, Akbar AN. Inhibition of T cell apoptosis in the rheumatoid synovium. J Clin Invest. 1997;99:439-446.

Santin I, Moore F, Colli ML, Gurzov EN, Marselli L, Marchetti P, Eizirik DL. PTPN2, a candidate gene for type 1 diabetes, modulates pancreatic β-cell apoptosis via regulation of the BH3-only protein Bim. Diabetes. 2011;60:3279-88.

Sera N, Kawakami A, Nakashima T, Nakamura H, Imaizumi M, Koji T, Abe Y, Usa T, Tominaga T, Ejima E, Ashizawa K, Yokoyama N, Ishikawa N, Ito K, Eguchi K. Fas/FasL mediated apoptosis of thyrocytes in Graves' disease. Clin Exp Immunol. 2001;124:197-207.

Shibata Y, Hishikawa Y, Izumi S, Fujita S, Yamaguchi A, Koji T. Involvement of Fas/Fas ligand in the induction of apoptosis in chronic sialadenitis of minor salivary glands including Sjögren's syndrome. Hum Cell. 2002;15:52-60.

Singh RR, Ebling FM, Sercarz EE, Hahn BH. Immune tolerance to autoantibody-derived peptides delays development of autoimmunity in murine lupus. J Clin Invest. 1995;96:2990-2996.

Smith CE, Eagar TN, Strominger JL, Miller SD. Differential induction of IgE-mediated anaphylaxis after soluble vs. cell-bound tolerogenic peptide therapy of autoimmune encephalomyelitis. Proc Natl Acad Sci U S A. 2005;102:9595-9600.

Smith CA, Williams GT, Kingston R, Jenkinson SJ, Owen JJT. Antibodies to CD3/T-cell receptor complex induce death by apoptosis in immature T cells in thymic cultures. Nature 1989;337:181-184.

Sontag E. Protein phosphatase 2A: the Trojan Horse of cellular signaling. Cell Signal. 2001;13:7-16.

Tas F, Duranyildiz D, Oguz H, Camlica H, Yasasever V, Topuz E. Serum vascular endothelial growth factor (VEGF) and bcl-2 levels in advanced stage non-small cell lung cancer. Cancer Invest. 2006;24:576-580.

Tsuboi M, Eguchi K, Kawakami A, Matsuoka N, Kawabe Y, Aoyagi T, Maeda K, Nagataki S. Fas antigen expression on synovial cells was down-regulated by interleukin 1 beta. Biochem Biophys Res Commun. 1996;218:280-285.

Turbyville JC, Rao VK. The autoimmune lymphoproliferative syndrome: A rare disorder providing clues about normal tolerance. Autoimmun Rev. 2010;9:488-493.

von Mühlen CA, Tan EM. Autoantibodies in the diagnosis of systemic rheumatic diseases. Semin Arthritis Rheum. 1995;24:323-358.

Walkinshaw G, Waters CM. Induction of apoptosis in catecholaminergic PC12 cells by L-DOPA. Implications for the treatment of Parkinson's disease. J Clin Invest. 1995;95:2458-2464.

Wang Y, Virji AS, Howard P, Sayani Y, Zhang J, Achu P, McArthur C. Detectionof cleaved alpha-fodrin autoantigen in Sjögren's syndrome: apoptosis and co-localisation of cleaved alpha-fodrin with activated caspase-3 and cleaved poly(ADP-ribose) polymerase (PARP) in labial salivary glands. Arch Oral Biol. 2006;51:558-566.

Xerri L, Devilard E, Hassoun J, Mawas C, Birg F. Fas ligand is not only expressed in immune privileged human organs but is also coexpressed with Fas in various epithelial tissues. Mol Pathol. 1997;50:87-91.

Xu L, Zhang L, Yi Y, Kang HK, Datta SK. Human lupus T cells resist inactivation and escape death by upregulating COX-2. Nat Med. 2004;10:411-415.

Yamamoto K. (2003) Pathogenesis of Sjögren's syndrome. Autoimmun Rev. 2003;2:13-18.

Yang E, Zha J, Jockel J, Boise LH, Thompson CB, Korsmeyer SJ. Bad, a heterodimeric partner for Bcl-XL and Bcl-2, displaces Bax and promotes cell death. Cell. 1995;80:285-291.

Zauli G, Toffoli B, di Iasio MG, Celeghini C, Fabris B, Secchiero P. Treatment with recombinant tumor necrosis factor-related apoptosis-inducing ligand alleviates the severity of streptozotocin-induced diabetes. Diabetes. 2010;59:1261-1265.

Zeher M, Szodoray P, Gyimesi E, Szondy Z. Correlation of increased susceptibility to apoptosis of CD4+ T cells with lymphocyte activation and activity of disease in patients with primary Sjögren's syndrome. Arthritis Rheum. 1999;42:1673-1681.

Zha J, Harada H, Yang E, Jockel J, Korsmeyer SJ. Serine phosphorylation of death agonist BAD in response to survival factor results in binding to 14-3-3 not BCL-X(L). Cell. 1996;87:619-628.

Zhao W, Gao BL, Yi GF, Jin CZ, Yang HY, Shen LJ, Tian M, Yu YZ, Li H, Song DP. Apoptotic study in Graves disease treated with thyroid arterial embolization. Endocr J. 2009;56:201-211.

Section 2

Specific Autoimmune Diseases

Chapter 6

Immune Complex Deposits as a Characteristic Feature of Mercury-Induced SLE-Like Autoimmune Process in Inbred and Outbred Mice

Alla Arefieva, Marina Krasilshchikova and Olga Zatsepina

Additional information is available at the end of the chapter

http://dx.doi.org/10.5772/47806

1. Introduction

Systemic autoimmune diseases, such as systemic lupus erythematosus (lupus, SLE), rheumatoid arthritis and systemic sclerosis (scleroderma), occur in up to 5-8% of the human population. Based on frequency of occurrence, they are the third most common diseases after cardiovascular pathologies and cancers. The overwhelming majority of cases of autoimmune diseases are in women (Fairweather & Rose, 2004).

Nowadays, great attention is paid to studying the impact of environment on the development of autoimmunity and autoimmune diseases. This is due to the increased influence of anthropogenic factors on the quality of human life. There is a good reason to suppose that repeated exposure of people to low doses of heavy metal compounds may promote the development of such diseases (Havarinasab et al., 2009). Humans can be exposed to these noxious substances from atmospheric pollution, food, cosmetics (Bagenstose et al., 1999; Bigazzi, 1998; Pelletier et al., 1994; Rowley & Monestier, 2005), dental amalgams (Eneström & Hultman, 1995; Guzzi et al., 2008; Pigatto & Guzzi, 2010), thimerosal-containing vaccines (Mutter & Yeter, 2008) and through the regular contacts with materials in manufacturing processes (da Costa et al., 2008).

Mercury is one of the most global environmental pollutants, with human exposure to organic, inorganic, and elemental species of mercury occurring in many diverse settings. Relatively few studies exist in the literature on the relationship of mercury exposure and biomarkers of autoimmunity or autoimmune diseases in humans. Cases of mercury-induced autoimmune kidney disease mediated by immune complex (IC) deposition have been noted historically in highly exposed populations (Gardner et al., 2010). A case-control study of scleroderma patients found an association between urinary mercury level and severity of the disease (Arnett et al., 1996). It is notable that the great artists who used paints containing mercury, suffered from autoimmune pathologies. Thus, P. Rubens, P.-A. Renoir, Robert O. Duffy suffered from rheumatoid arthritis, while P. Klee had systemic scleroderma (Pedersen & Permin, 1988).

Anti-nuclear (ANA) and anti-nucleolar (ANoA) autoantibodies presence in serum are used in the clinical diagnosis of lupus and scleroderma (Ho & Reveille, 2003; Kurien & Scofield, 2006), and some similarities have been noted between ANA/ANoA profiles in mercury-induced autoimmunity (HgIA) models and in some patients with scleroderma (Takeuchi et al., 1995). The possible influence of mercury on the human population was confirmed by the results obtained from the experiments with people exposed by mercury on the gold mine sites in Amazonian Brazil (Silbergeld et al., 2005; Silva et al., 2004). Exposure to mercury in these populations is related to the use of mercury in riverine small-scale artisanal gold mining operations, in which miners are directly exposed to inorganic and elemental mercury, and downstream communities can be exposed by consumption of fish contaminated by methylmercury in impacted watersheds (Gardner et al., 2010). Exposure to either methyl or inorganic mercury in such populations is associated with elevated titers of detectable ANA and ANoA (Alves et al., 2006).

Furthermore, through the use of rodent models, awareness of the direct effects of mercury on the immune system has increased. It is well known that the chronic administration of subtoxic doses of $HgCl_2$ (mercuric chloride) induces a SLE-like autoimmune disease in genetically susceptible inbred mice with $H\text{-}2^s$, $H\text{-}2^q$, and $H\text{-}2^f$ haplotypes or their hybrids (Hansson & Abedi-Valugerdi, 2003; Hultman et al., 1999; Reuter et al., 1989; Roether et al., 2002; Rowley & Monestier, 2005; Takeuchi et al., 1995). This HgIA is characterized by T-cell-dependent polyclonal activation of B-lymphocytes (Abedi-Valugerdi, 2008; Johansson et al., 1998), increased level of serum immunoglobulins (IgG1 and IgE) (Abedi-Valugerdi et al., 2000, 2008), production of ANoA and by the formation of IC in different organs impaired their functions (Arefieva et al., 2010; Bagenstose et al., 1999; Eneström et al., 1984; Havarinasab et al., 2008; Hultman et al., 1989; Robinson et al., 1997). Female mice tend to be more susceptible to HgIA, consistent with sex differences observed in autoimmune diseases in humans (Fairweather et al., 2008). It is important to notice, that thimerosal (constituent part of some vaccines for human) is equipotent to inorganic mercury in eliciting a lupus-like immune response in susceptible animals, but mice treated with methylmercury do not develop renal or systemic IC deposition (Haggqvist et al., 2005; Havarinasab et al., 2005, 2007; Havarinasab & Hultman, 2005).

The interesting thing is that the nucleolar 34-kDa protein fibrillarin is the major autoantigen in such autoimmune disorders either in mice or in human. Fibrillarin is one of the most evolutionarily conserved proteins and is involved in the early stages of maturation of ribosomal RNA (rRNA). This protein can often be a target of autoantibodies in various autoimmune disorders (Ho & Reveille, 2003; Rhodes & Vyse, 2007; van

Eenennaam et al., 2002; Yang et al., 2003): systemic scleroderma (58% of cases), SLE (39% of cases), rheumatoid arthritis (60% of cases). The presence of autoantibodies to fibrillarin in patients' blood is a suitable diagnostic marker for the early stages of autoimmune diseases development (Tormey et al., 2001). In addition, a recent case-control study reported that severely affected scleroderma patients with anti-fibrillarin antibodies (AFA) were more likely to have higher levels of mercury in urine as compared either to less severely affected cases without AFA or controls suggesting an etiologic role for mercury in this autoimmune disease (Arnett et al., 2000).

It is worth noting that, along with mercury which can induce the production of AFA among the genetically predisposed animals, some heavy metals such as silver (Abedi-Valugerdi, 2008; Hansson & Abedi-Valugerdi, 2003; Suzuki et al., 2011) and gold (Havarinasab et al., 2007, 2009) have the same ability. In addition, cadmium (Leffel et al., 2003), platinum (Chen et al., 2002) and lead (Tabata et al., 2003) are also known to have a negative impact on humans and animals. They induce/exacerbate the autoimmune processes in human and murine models of autoimmune diseases. However, unlike mercury, they do not cause such strong lymphoproliferation, polyclonal activation of lymphocytes and deposition of IC in kidneys - the most important features of autoimmune diseases.

Taken all the foregoing into account, it becomes clear why HgIA in mice is used as a model of human systemic autoimmune disorders for testing of immunosuppressive agents and for investigating of the molecular mechanisms of heavy metal-induced autoimmunity.

Following the modern hypothesis of a strong genetical predisposition to autoimmune diseases, the majority of animal experiments are conducted on inbred and genetically modified mice prone to mercury-induced or spontaneous autoimmunity. However, results obtained on such susceptible homozygous mice cannot be fully extrapolated on genetically heterogenous human population. That is why it is more correct to use different genetically heterogenous (outbred) mouse stocks as laboratory model in analysis of mercury exposure and consequences of it on humans. But, there are only a few studies supporting the idea that outbred mice are also susceptible to mercury and produce ANoA. It is earlier affirmed that development of ANoA production is controlled strictly by the class II of H-2 genes, i.e. only certain mouse strains with specific H-2 genotypes (e.g. H-2s and H-2q) produce ANoA upon exposure to mercury. Therefore, it was expected that mice carrying the heterozygous H-2 genotype will be highly resistant to mercury-induced ANoA production. In controversial, it has been recently found that chronic treatment with mercury induces production of ANoA in a large number of outbred ICR, NMRI and Black Swiss mice (Abedi-Valugerdi, 2008). Regarding this matter Dr. Abedi-Valugerdi has spoken his hypothesis about the absence of the particular genetical susceptibility to HgIA. It means that unlike in inbred mouse strains, H-2 heterozygosity does not confer resistance to mercury-induced ANoA production. In other words, environmental factors can induce autoimmunity in the absence of specific susceptible genes in members of a genetically heterogenous population. Thus, it allows to use outbred mice as suitable model for research of HgIA.

As mentioned above, one of the most significant features of $HgCl_2$-induced autoimmune process along with appearance of AFA is deposition of immune complexes in kidneys. It is necessary to notice that formation of IC in human kidneys is one of the consequences of heavy metals exposure or autoimmune diseases (Ohsawa, 1997; Markowitz & D'Agati, 2009). However, the exact localization and composition of the IC in kidneys, mechanisms of its formation and possible cytotoxic effects still remain poorly understood. We have performed this work to elucidate these questions and in order to examine whether IC are present in other organs of inbred mice. Another goal of our study was to discover whether AFA production and IC deposition, which are typical for mercury-induced autoimmunity in H-2s and H-2q inbred mouse strains, could be reproduced in outbred mice.

2. Material and methods

2.1. Mice

All studies presented were carried out in female inbred SJL/J and outbred CFW mice, which were 8 weeks old at the beginning of each experiment. Animals were obtained from Animal Breeding Facility-Branch of Shemyakin-Ovchinnikov Institute of Bioorganic Chemistry (AAALAC accredited). All animals obtained were axenic at the time of arrival. The health status for these mice was confirmed by monitoring in the AnLab laboratory (Czech Republic). The mice were housed at the Animal Facilities of the Shemyakin-Ovchinnikov Institute of Bioorganic Chemistry of the Russian Academy of Sciences (Moscow, Russian Federation) under specific pathogen-free (SPF) conditions with access to tap water and standard chow *ad libitum*. All animal experiments described here were conducted in accordance with the "Good Laboratory Practice in Russian Federation" (Decree of the Minister of Health of RF #267, dated June 19, 2003), Section 11 of the Declaration of Helsinki of the World Medical Association (1964) and the International Guiding Principles for Biomedical Research Involving Animals (1985).

2.2. $HgCl_2$ treatment

A solution of 0.4 mg/mL $HgCl_2$ (Sigma-Aldrich, St. Louis, MO, USA) was prepared in sterile 0.9% NaCl solution (OJSC Biochemist, Saransk, Russia). Groups of mice were injected subcutaneously (s.c.) with either 0.1 mL of $HgCl_2$ (1.6 mg/kg body weight) or 0.1 mL of sterile 0.9% NaCl every third day for 6 weeks.

2.3. Blood and tissue sampling

Before the experiment and after 6 weeks of $HgCl_2$ treatment, blood was obtained by retro-orbital puncture under ether anesthesia. The collected blood was allowed to clot for 30 min at 37ºC, centrifuged (800g, 10 min) and the serum obtained was used or stored at -70ºC.

Then, the mice were euthanized in a CO_2 chamber. Their kidneys, liver and spleen were dissected out aseptically during the autopsy. The organ pieces were used for cryotomy or stored in liquid nitrogen until used.

2.4. Detection of anti-nucleolar antibodies

The presence of serum ANoA was determined by indirect immunofluorescence (IIF) using murine NIH/3T3 cells as a substrate. The cells were grown on glass coverslips in DMEM supplemented with 10% FCS, glutamine, penicillin, and streptomycin (Paneco, Moscow, Russia) at 37ºC in a 5% CO_2 / 95% air atmosphere. Coverslips with attached cells were washed in PBS and fixed with 4% paraformaldehyde (PFA) in PBS for 15 min at room temperature, rinsed in PBS three times for 10 min, and permeabilized with 0.1% Triton X-100 in PBS for 10 min on ice, then washed in PBS four times for 5 min. The cells were incubated with the primary antibodies (murine sera from autoimmune and control mice) diluted 1:100 to 1:10000 in PBS and kept in the dark in a moist chamber for 45 min. Then, the cells were washed in PBS three times for 10 min, and incubated with Cy2-conjugated goat anti-mouse immunoglobulin G (IgG) antibodies (Jackson ImmunoResearch Lab., West Grove, PA, USA), diluted 1:200, for 45 min under the same conditions. Control cells were processed at the same time and in the same way, except that PBS was used instead of the murine sera. No stained structures were seen in the controls. Then, the cells were washed again three times for 10 min, incubated in 1 μg/mL DAPI (4′,6′-diamidino-2′-phenyindole) (Sigma-Aldrich, St. Louis, MO, USA) solution at room temperature for 10 min and then mounted on slides with Mowiol containing DABCO (1,4-diazabicyclo[2.2.2]octane) (Sigma-Aldrich, St. Louis, MO, USA). During the experimental period, slides were stored at 4ºC in the dark. The titer of ANoA was defined as the highest serum dilution that gave specific nucleolar staining (Havarinasab et al., 2008).

The cells were examined using an Axiovert 200 epifluorescence microscope (Carl Zeiss, Oberkochen, Germany) with PlanNeoFluar 40×/NA 0.75, Fluar 100×/NA 1.25, and AchroPlan 100×/NA 1.3 objectives. Images were obtained using a 13-bit monochrome camera (CoolSnap$_{cf}$; Roper Scientific, Tucson, AZ, USA).

2.5. Analysis of immune complexes in kidneys

The presence of renal IC in kidneys of inbred and outbred mice was detected by direct immunofluorescence (DIF). The slides with attached 5-μm thick cryosections (Microm HM 525, ThermoFisher Scientific, Waltham, MA, USA) were washed in cold PBS and then air-dried or fixed under various conditions: in absolute acetone/methanol for 5 min or in 4% PFA in PBS for 15 min. Some sections were then air-dried after fixation in absolute acetone or methanol. After incubation in 4% PFA, slides were washed three times for 10 min and permeabilized with 0.1% Triton X-100 in PBS for 10 min on ice, then washed in PBS four times for 5 min. After that, the sections were incubated with serial dilutions of either a fluorescein isothiocyanate (FITC)-conjugated goat anti-mouse total Ig (IgG + IgA + IgM) antibodies (Imtek, Moscow, Russia) and/or rabbit anti-mouse complement factor C3 primary antibodies (Abcam, Cambridge, UK), diluted 1:10, and Texas Red-conjugated donkey anti-rabbit IgG secondary antibodies (Jackson ImmunoResearch Lab, West Grove, PA, USA), diluted 1:400, in the dark in the moist chamber for 45 min. The initial dilution for FITC-conjugated antibodies was 1:50. The end-point titer for total immunoglobulins (Ig) was defined as the highest dilution that gave specific staining. Then, the slides were washed three times for 10 min, incubated in DAPI solution, as described above, and then mounted with Mowiol containing DABCO. During the experimental period, the slides were stored at 4ºC in the dark.

To visualize renal blood vessels varying in size and colocalize them with IC we used additional staining of organs with special dye Col-F (kindly furnished by Dr. Jerzy Dobrucki), which reveals collagen and elastin fibers that are part of the coats and elastic membranes of blood vessels. Halves of organs were washed in DMEM and put in Col-F dye solution in DMEM at 37ºC for 1 h. Then, the pieces of kidney were rapidly washed again, and cut for cryosections as described previously. To remove damaged/non-specifically stained tissue, the first 50-μm thick section was discarded. Fixed in 4% PFA cryosections were then washed and incubated according to the DIF method described above.

With the aim of distinguishing between proximal and distal renal tubules and colocalizing them with IC, we performed a staining assay using phalloidin-tetramethylrhodamine B isothiocyanate (TRITC; Sigma-Aldrich, St. Louis, MO, USA). This is a fluorescent phallotoxin that can be used to detect actin-rich structures, such as the brush border of the proximal renal tubules. After fixation cryosections were incubated with a mix of 5 μg/mL TRITC-conjugated phalloidin solution and FITC-conjugated goat anti-mouse total Ig antibody in the dark in a moist chamber for 45 min, washed, incubated in DAPI and mounted with Mowiol.

The slides were examined using Axiovert 200 epifluorescence and confocal LSM510 microscopes (Carl Zeiss, Oberkochen, Germany). Images were obtained using a 13-bit monochrome camera (CoolSnap$_{cf}$, Roper Scientific, Tucson, AZ, USA).

2.5.1. Detection of immunoglobulin isotypes as components of renal IC

Presence of IgG1, IgG2a and IgM immunoglobulins in kidneys of mercury-treated and control mice were determined using DIF, as described previously. To distinguish between IgG and IgM classes, we used fluorescein isothiocyanate (FITC)-conjugated goat anti-mouse total Ig (IgG + IgA + IgM) antibodies (Imtek, Moscow, Russia) in combination with TRITC-conjugated goat anti-mouse IgM secondary antibodies (Jackson ImmunoResearch Lab, West Grove, PA, USA).

To evaluate the presence of IgG1 and IgG2a immunoglobulin isotypes, we used TRITC-conjugated goat anti-mouse IgG antibodies (Jackson ImmunoResearch Lab, West Grove, PA, USA) in combination with FITC-conjugated goat anti-mouse IgG1 or IgG2a secondary antibodies (SouthernBiotech, Birmingham, AL, USA). The dilution for all the antibodies mentioned was 1:50.

2.5.2. Glomerular cell death assessment

The terminal deoxynucleotidyl transferase biotin-dUTP nick end labeling (TUNEL) method was performed on the kidney cryosections to visualize apoptotic glomerular cells to assess the cytotoxicity of immune deposits. It is widely known that the most common biochemical property of apoptosis is the endonucleolytic cleavage of chromatin. This method identifies apoptotic cells *in situ* using terminal deoxynucleotidyl transferase (TdT) to transfer biotin-dUTP to the free 3′-OH of cleaved DNA. The biotin-labeled cleavage sites were then visualized by reaction with fluorescein-conjugated avidin (avidin-FITC). TUNEL staining was conducted with a kit (TUNEL Apoptosis Detection Kit, Upstate Biotechnology, Lake Placid, NY, USA) according to the manufacturer's protocol. Next, the slides were incubated in DAPI solution, then mounted with Mowiol containing DABCO. The cells were then observed using a fluorescence microscope. Sections treated with 1 μg/mL bovine DNase I were used as a positive control for the TUNEL assay and DNA fragmentation.

2.6. Analysis of immune complexes in liver and spleen

The presence of IC in liver and spleen of inbred and outbred mice was also detected by DIF. The slides with attached cryosections were washed in cold PBS and then fixed in 4% PFA in PBS for 15 min. After that, the slides were prepared as described above.

For the blood vessels detection we used the same technique as it was described for kidneys.

2.7. Assay for *in vivo* binding of mercury-induced ANoA to the nucleoli of living cells

The colocalization of the mercury-induced ANoA with nucleolar protein fibrillarin within the cell nucleoli in mercury-treated outbred mice was detected by the IIF method. Briefly, the sections were fixed in 4% PFA, washed, permeabilized and incubated with 1:50 dilution of the primary rabbit polyclonal anti-fibrillarin antibodies (Abcam, Cambridge, UK) in the dark in the moist chamber for 45 min and washed again. FITC-conjugated goat anti-mouse total Ig (IgG + IgA + IgM) antibodies (Imtek, Moscow, Russia) in combination with Texas Red-conjugated donkey anti-rabbit IgG secondary antibodies (Jackson ImmunoResearch Lab, West Grove, PA, USA), diluted 1:100 and 1:200 respectively, were used as secondary antibodies. Then the slides were washed again, stained with DAPI and mounted with Mowiol according the IIF technique.

2.8. Statistical analysis

Serum levels of ANoA and IC titers are all expressed as means±standard deviation. Differences between these parameters for the control and Hg-treated groups were analyzed for statistical significance using the Mann-Whitney U-test. P values < 0.05 were considered to indicate statistical significance.

3. Results

3.1. $HgCl_2$ induces ANoA production in inbred and outbred mice

To test the ability of mercury to induce ANoA production in inbred and outbred mice, sera obtained from experimental and control mice were tested using an IIF technique. Analysis of sera obtained from mice at the end of the experiment (after 6 weeks of $HgCl_2$ treatment) showed that mercury was able to induce ANoA, in contrast to the saline-injected controls. The mean titer of ANoA in group of mercury-treated inbred mice was about 1520, in group of outbred mice - 10545 (Table 1). The pre-bleed sera from all groups of animals were ANoA-negative.

Mouse stock	Treatment	No. of mice	Titer of ANoA	Titer of IC		
				Glomerular mesangium	Blood vessel walls	Proximal tubules
Inbred **SJL/J**	6 weeks of **$HgCl_2$**	5	1520±1772[1,2]	17600±7838[2]	14400±3200[2]	4000[2]
	6 weeks of NaCl	4	0	1400±400	0	1400±400
Outbred **CFW**	6 weeks of **$HgCl_2$**	12	10545±3236[2]	6083±2018[2]	4750±1868[2]	13167±8462[2]
	6 weeks of NaCl	12	0	1700±249	0	2000±1083

[1] The numbers refer to mean reciprocal titer ± standard deviation; [2] $P < 0.05$, vs. saline-treated controls (Mann-Whitney U-test).

Table 1. Titers of serum ANoA and IC in kidneys of autoimmune and control mice.

Sera were incubated on NIH/3T3 cells followed by incubation with FITC-conjugated anti-mouse immunoglobulin antibodies; they characteristically stained nucleoli of interphase cells and peripheral chromosomal material (PCM) in mitotic cells (Fig. 1). Such stained regions matched the areas in which the major autoantigen in HgIA, fibrillarin, was revealed.

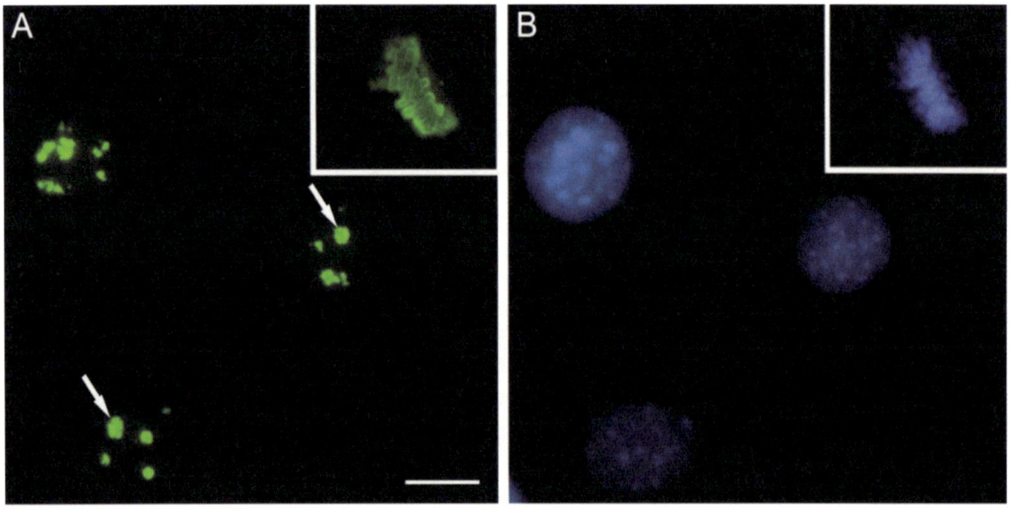

Figure 1. The nucleolar protein fibrillarin in murine NIH/3T3 cells is identified by serum from SJL/J autoimmune mouse treated with $HgCl_2$. A - indirect immunocytochemistry reveals fibrillarin in the nucleoli of interphase cells (*arrows*) and in the peripheral chromosomal material of metaphase cells (*insert*); sera from CFW autoimmune mice reveal the same staining patterns. B - DAPI staining of interphase nuclei and metaphase chromosomes. Scale bar - 10 μm.

So, we have concluded that six weeks of $HgCl_2$ treatment to female SJL/J and CFW mice resulted in strong ANoA production.

3.2. $HgCl_2$ induces heavy immune complex deposition in kidneys of inbred and outbred mice

3.2.1. Identification of glomerular IC in murine kidneys

Glomerular IC were revealed with all variants of tissue treatment (Table 2). However, on fixed cryosections, the general tissue morphology was better than on unfixed sections. In all cases, immune deposits were seen in the form of granules, which in places with the highest congestion merged and looked like brightly fluorescing spots (Fig. 2). Under epifluorescence and confocal microscopes, immune deposits often repeated the form of the mesangial cells and were clearly visible in the plane of the nuclei, as revealed using the dye DAPI or phase contrast (Fig. 2, 3). Additionally, only fixing with 4% paraformaldehyde strongly reduced the background fluorescence and increased clarity when looking at a tissue; the borders of the immune deposits appeared to be much sharper than with the other fixing techniques. Additionally, fixed sections could be stored for about 3 months at -70ºC without any appreciable loss of staining ability.

Localization	**Type of fixation**					
	Air-drying	Acetone	Acetone/ air-drying	Methanol	Methanol/ air-drying	**4% PFA**
Glomerular mesangium	+[1]	+	+	+	+	**+**
Blood vessel walls	+	+	+	+	+	**+**
Proximal tubules	-[2]	-	-	-	-	**+**

[1] Presence of IC; [2] absence of IC.

Table 2. IC in kidneys of $HgCl_2$-treated mice, revealed with various fixing conditions.

Our results showed a significantly increased titer of immunoglobulins in the glomerular mesangium in kidneys of $HgCl_2$-treated animals compared with control mice (Table 1). The $HgCl_2$-treated groups of mice showed a mean titer of mesangial Ig of about 17600 (inbred mice) and 6083 (outbred mice). The saline-injected control groups showed only 1400 (inbred) and 1700 (outbred) mean titers of secondary antibodies.

Moreover, we also have found the deposition of C3 component of complement system as part of glomerular IC (Fig. 4). It is necessary to notice that such C3 deposits do not always colocalize with regions containing immunoglobulins. This means that there are such areas in glomeruli where only C3 is revealed, but at the same time immunoglobulins are not seen. The saline-injected control mice were completely devoid of C3 deposits.

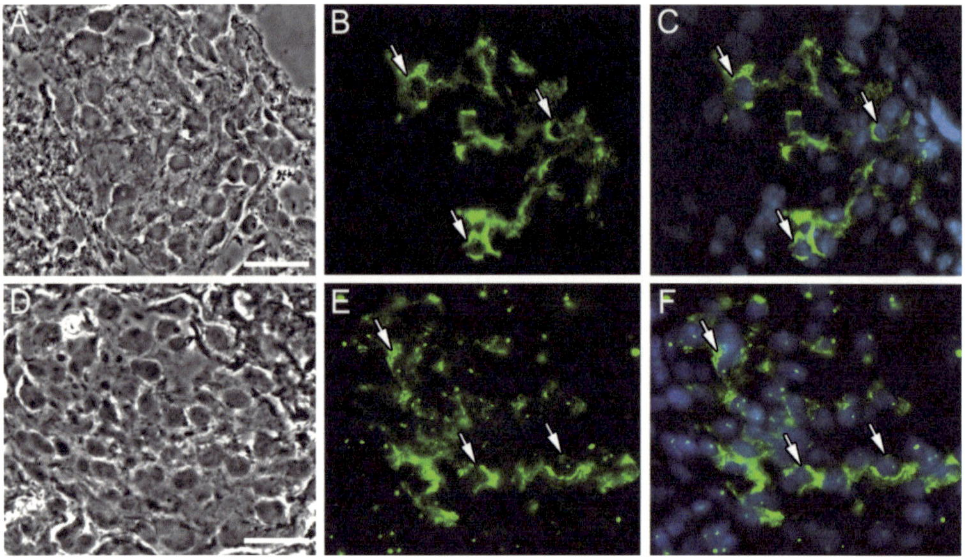

Figure 2. Immunohistochemical detection of immunoglobulins in glomeruli of autoimmune inbred (A-C) and outbred (D-F) mice. *Left column* - phase contrast, *middle column* - total immunoglobulin staining, *right column* - merge of immunoglobulin staining and nuclear chromatin DAPI–staining. *Arrows* point to glomerular cells in which it can be clearly seen that immunoglobulins are located in the cytoplasm around the cell nucleus. Immunoglobulins in the nuclei of outbred mice are also clearly seen. Scale bar - 30 μm.

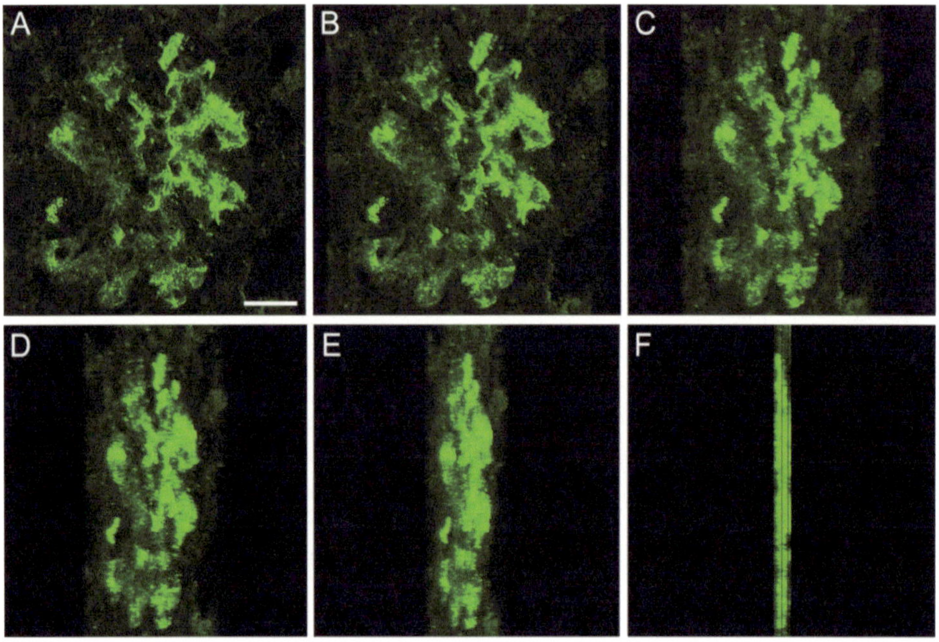

Figure 3. Visualization of immunoglobulins in glomerulus of autoimmune mouse under confocal laser scanning microscope. A–E: glomerular area reconstructed on the base of serial optical sections (counter-clockwise rotation model); F: side-view of the reconstructed area (thickness of this area is about 7 μm). Scale bar - 30 μm.

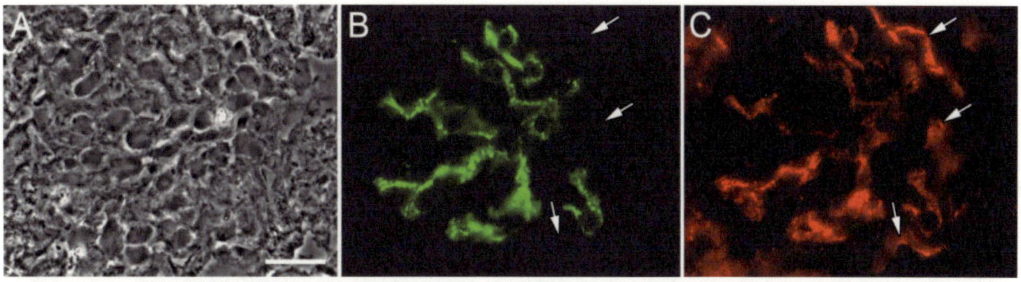

Figure 4. Localization of immunoglobulins and the C3 component of the complement system as components of immune deposits in glomerulus of autoimmune mouse after $HgCl_2$ treatment. A - phase contrast, B - total immunoglobulin staining, C - staining of C3 component of the complement system. *Arrows* show the C3-containing areas without immunoglobulins. Scale bar - 30 μm.

3.2.2. Identification of vascular IC in murine kidneys

Additionally, only the mercury-treated mice, not the control groups (Table 1), showed IC (Ig + C3) in the walls of renal blood vessels with all variants of tissue treatment (Table 2). This finding was confirmed by colocalization of IC with collagen and elastin fibers that are part of the coats and elastic membranes of blood vessels, which we revealed using the Col-F dye (Fig. 5). Comparison of places with immune deposit localization with collagen and elastin staining allowed us to conclude that IC were present in both the endothelial zone of vessels and in different layers of the basement of the vessel walls. Using the Col-F dye allowed us to conclude that deposits were present in all renal vessel walls, regardless of their size. Moreover, Col-F revealed even vessels that were not seen clearly with phase contrast. Similarly, glomerular IC could be seen in the form of granules, which in places with the highest concentration merged and looked like brightly fluorescing spots.

The mean titer of vascular Ig in the kidneys of the $HgCl_2$-treated groups of mice reached 14400 (inbred mice) and 4750 (outbred mice). The saline-injected control groups were completely devoid of deposits (Table 1).

3.2.3. Identification of tubular IC in murine kidneys

Immune deposits in renal tubules were seen out only when using 4% PFA as a fixative (Table 2). IC were seen in discrete granules of approximately equal size (about 1 μm) located in tubular epithelial cells (Fig. 6B, C).

We note that part of the renal tubules contained immune deposits whereas another part had none. To determine in which type(s) of renal tubules IC were present, we performed a combination of IHC analysis and staining with phalloidin-TRITC. As is well-known, phalloidin binds to actin, the basic structural component of the brush border, which is present in proximal renal tubules and is not expressed in distal parts. These results suggest that immune deposits were seen only in the proximal renal tubules, with a brush border, and not in the distal tubules, without a brush border (Fig. 6A, B).

Interestingly, the tubular IC consisted of immunoglobulins, but not the C3 component of complement. The mean titer of such deposits in proximal tubules was nearby 4000 (inbred) and 13167 (outbred). Besides, elevated titer of IC in the proximal tubules in outbred mice (compared with inbred mice) correlated with elevated titer of ANoA in their blood. Furthermore, the control group exhibited a lower mean titer of IC - 1400 for inbred mice and 2000 for outbred mice (Table 1). To our knowledge, this is the first report of immune deposits in the proximal renal tubules.

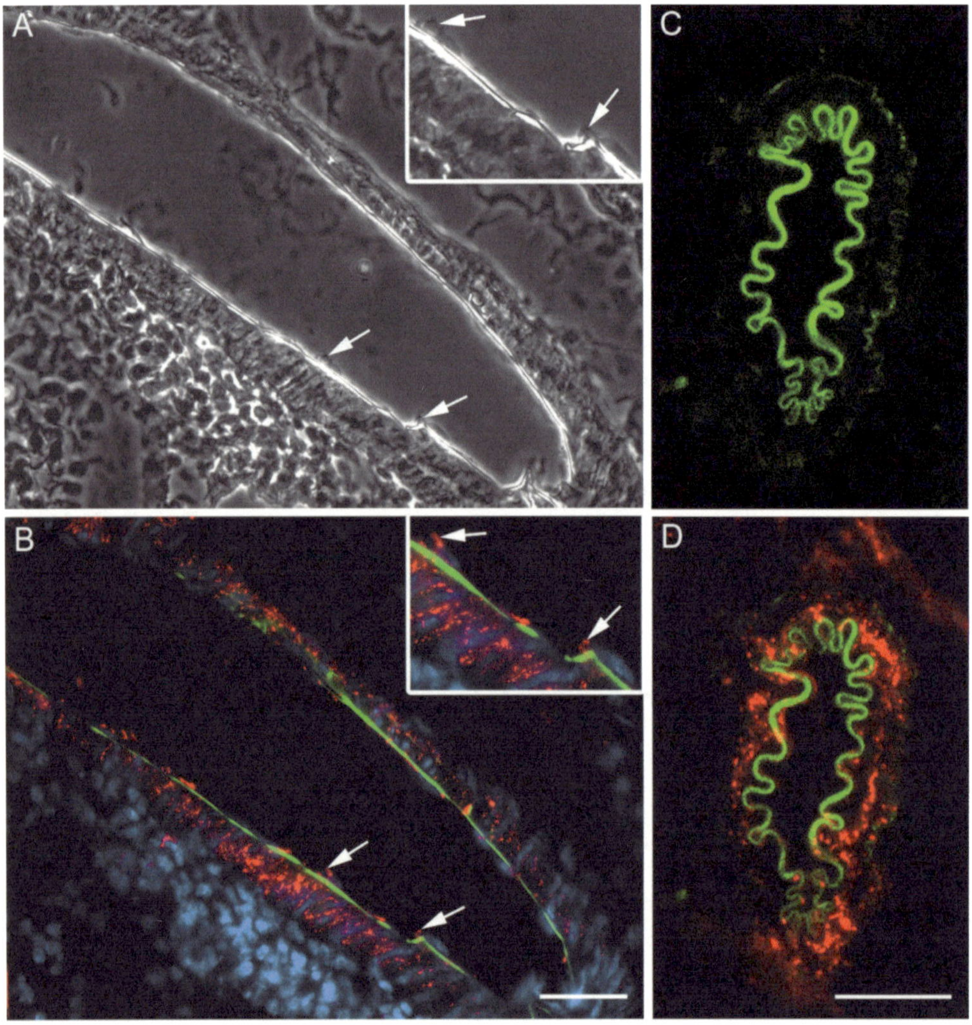

Figure 5. Immunoglobulins in renal blood vessels of varying sizes in autoimmune mice revealed with Col-F - a dye specific for collagen and elastic fibers. A, B - immunoglobulins in the blood vessel, which is clearly seen under phase contrast: A - phase contrast, B - staining with antiimmunoglobulin antibodies (*red*), Col-F dye (*green*) and nuclear chromatin staining with DAPI (*blue*); *inserts, arrows* - immunoglobulins in the endothelial part of this vessel. C, D - immunoglobulins in the blood vessel, revealed only by the Col-F dye: C - Col-F dye, D - staining with anti-immunoglobulin antibodies (*red*) and Col-F dye (*green*). Scale bar - 50 μm.

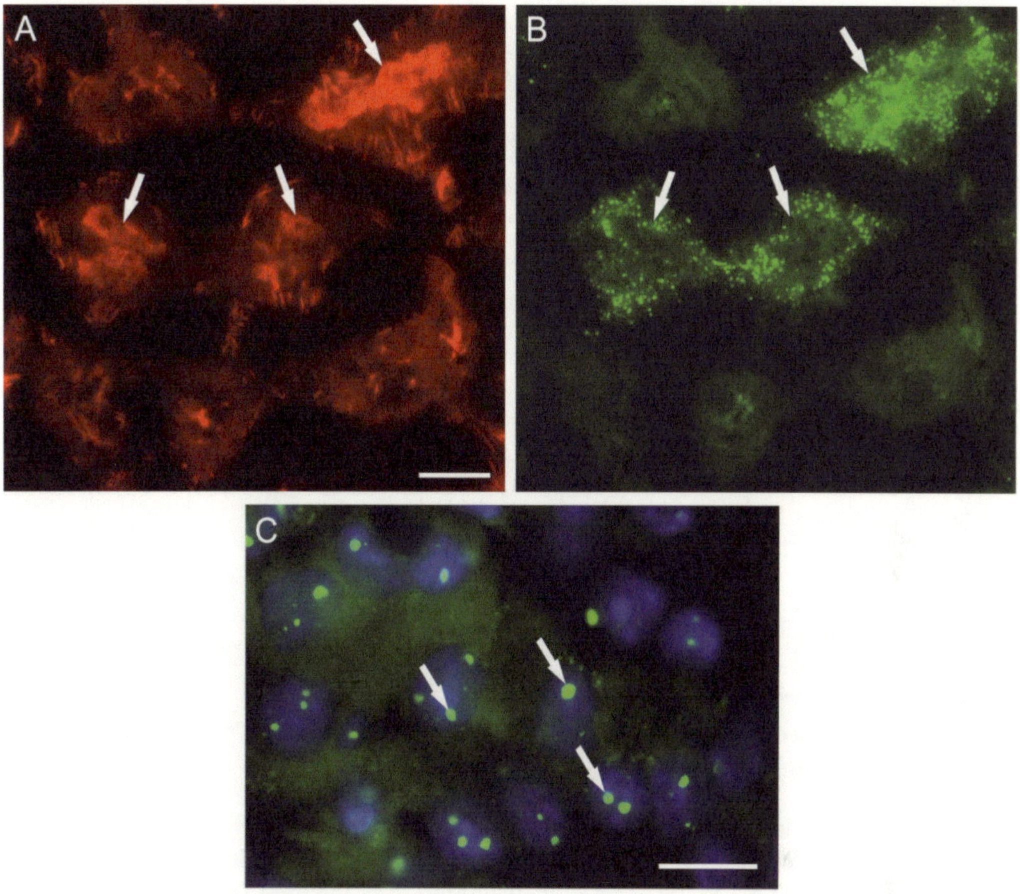

Figure 6. Localization of immunoglobulins in proximal renal tubules in inbred (A, B) and outbred (C) mice. A - revealing of brush border (*arrows*) in proximal tubules of inbred mice with the help of Phalloidin-TRITC staining, B - revealing of immunoglobulins in cytoplasm of epithelial cells in proximal tubules (*arrows*) of inbred mice; scale bar - 30 μм. C - revealing of immunoglobulins in cytoplasm and nuclei (*arrows*) of epithelial cells in outbred mice; scale bar - 20 μm.

3.2.4. Identification of immunoglobulin isotypes as components of IC in kidneys of inbred and outbred mice after $HgCl_2$ treatment

To understand which classes and isotypes of immunoglobulins are found in IC in different parts of murine kidneys, we performed combined multicolor DIF. Our results showed that immunoglobulin class G (IgG) occurred in all locations of IC: in glomeruli, blood vessel walls, and proximal tubules of autoimmune mice, and in glomeruli and proximal tubules of control mice. Immunoglobulin class M (IgM) was seen in glomeruli, proximal tubules, vessel walls of outbred autoimmune mice, and only in the glomeruli of both inbred autoimmune and control mice (Table 3). We did not assess whether immunoglobulin class A (IgA) was part of the immune complexes.

Mouse stock	Localization	IgG + IgM + IgA		IgG1		IgG2a		IgM	
		control	$HgCl_2$	control	$HgCl_2$	control	$HgCl_2$	control	$HgCl_2$
Inbred SJL/J	Glomerular mesangium	+[1]	+	+	+	-[2]	±[3]	+	+
	Blood vessel walls	-	+	-	+	-	-	-	-
	Proximal tubules	+	+	+	+	-	+	-	-
	Nucleoli	-	-	-	-	-	-	-	-
Outbred CFW	Glomerular mesangium	±	+	±	+	-	-	±	+
	Blood vessel walls	-	+	-	+	-	-	-	±
	Proximal tubules	+	+	±	+	-	±	-	+
	Nucleoli	-	+	-	+	-	+	-	-

[1] Presence of IC; [2] absence of IC; [3] slight deposits.

Table 3. Occurrence of different immunoglobulin isotypes as components of IC in kidneys of autoimmune and control mice.

Next, we tried to determine the IgG isotypes in IC. The results showed that the mesangial IgG deposits were dominated by the IgG1 isotype, but also contained IgG2a, consistent with Havarinasab et al. (2008). At the same time, we found only the IgG1 isotype in renal vessel wall deposits and both IgG1 and IgG2a isotypes in proximal tubule deposits (Table 3). The saline-injected control mice showed an absence of IgG2a deposits.

3.2.5. Assessment of possible IC toxicity in murine kidneys

To analyze the possible cytotoxicity of renal IC, we used the TUNEL method, which reveals fragmentation of DNA, a sign of cell destruction, *in situ*. The results showed that in glomeruli of both experimental and control animal groups, there was no significant increase in TUNEL-positive (i.e., apoptotic) cells.

3.3. Identification of IC in liver and spleen of inbred and outbred mice after $HgCl_2$ treatment

In the liver, a granular fixation of the anti-Ig antibodies was observed in the blood vessel walls of mercury-treated mice and, in contrast with earlier studies, in the liver hepatocytes in all groups of mice (Fig. 7). As in the kidneys, our results showed a significantly increased titer of Ig in the hepatocytes of $HgCl_2$-treated animals compared with control mice (not shown).

In the spleen, an intense granular pattern of the anti-Ig antibodies fixation was observed in the blood vessel walls and in the cells of lymphoid follicles, germinal centers, marginal zones and periarterial lymphatic sheaths (PALS) in mercury-treated mice (Fig. 8A, B).

White pulp of control animals had very rare and small germinal centers (these centers are known to appear during the Th2-dependent immune reactions). In contrast, germinal centers after the mercury chloride treatment were enlarged, prominent and quite frequent in all mice. Therefore, clear morphological attributes of Th2-antibody-producing immune response had been induced by the mercury chloride treatment in spleen.

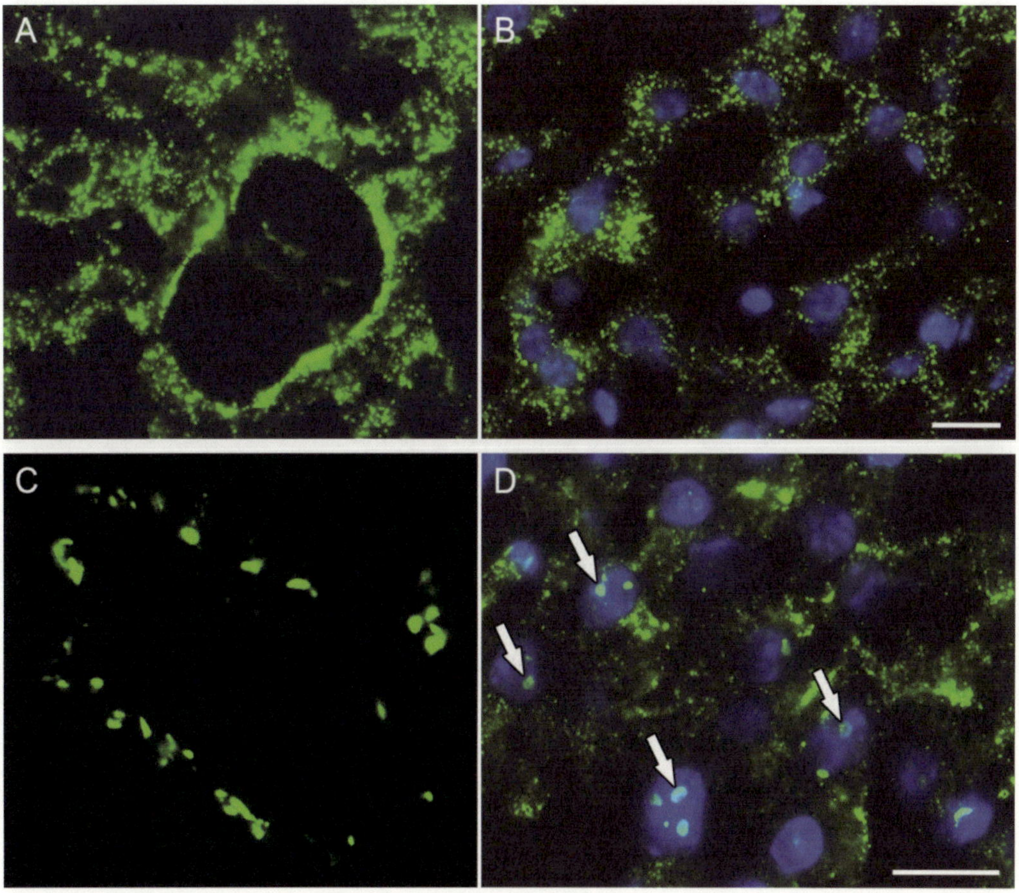

Figure 7. Immunohistochemical detection of immunoglobulins in liver of autoimmune inbred (A-B) and outbred (C-D) mice. A, C - immunoglobulins in liver blood vessels (total immunoglobulin staining); B, D - immunoglobulins in hepatocytes (merge of immunoglobulin staining and nuclear chromatin DAPI–staining), a*rrows* point to nuclei in which immunoglobulins can be clearly seen. Scale bar - 20 μm.

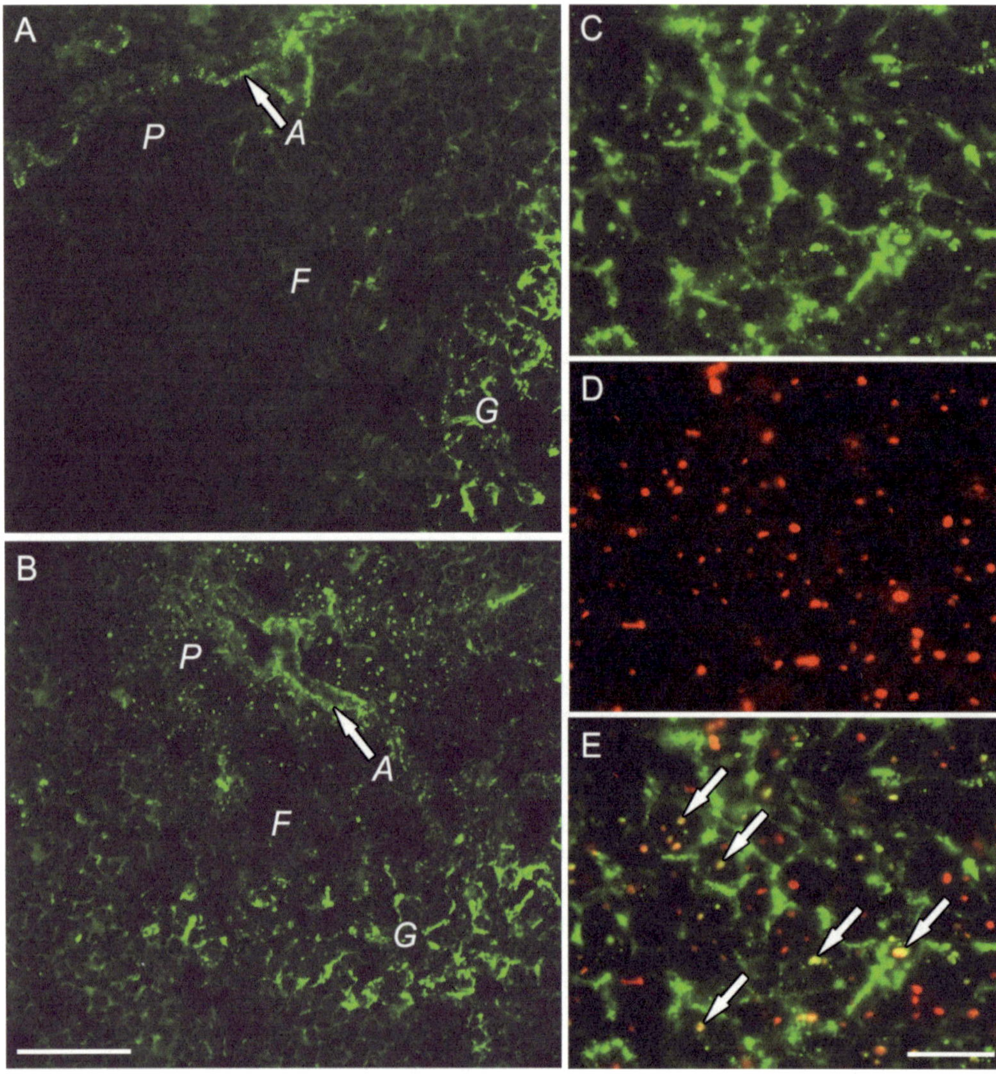

Figure 8. Immunohistochemical detection of immunoglobulins in spleen of autoimmune inbred (A) and outbred (B-E) mice. A, B - immunoglobulins in spleen blood vessels (*A-central artery, arrows*) and white pulp (*F-follicle, G-germinal center, P-PALS*), scale bar - 50 μm. C-E - results of colocalizing procedure: C - total immunoglobulin staining, D - staining with antifibrillarin antibodies, E - merge of immunoglobulin and fibrillarin staining patterns (yellow - *arrows*), scale bar - 20 μm.

3.4. Mercury-induced ANoA bind to the nucleoli of the kidney, liver and spleen cells in outbred mice *in vivo*

After analyzing the organs such as kidney, liver and spleen in all animals after 6 weeks of $HgCl_2$ treatment, we noticed some differences in the staining patterns in tissues from inbred and outbred mice following the method of DIF. As shown in Fig. 2, 6, 7, 8 most of the cells in the kidney, liver and spleen sections of mercury-treated outbred mice exhibited a strong nucleolar staining pattern with high titers of IgG1 and IgG2a immunoglobulins (Table 3). A nucleolar green fluorescence was found in the cells of the tissue sections prepared from the mercury- but not saline-injected mice. It should be noted that such intranucleolar staining was absent in nucleoli of inbred mercury-treated mice.

In a purpose of better understanding of autoantigen specificity, we colocalized such nucleolar patterns recognized by FITC- conjugated anti-Ig antibodies with loci recognized by commercial antibodies to nucleolar protein fibrillarin. The colocalizing procedure showed the whole coincidence of regions containing immunoglobulins with sites of nucleolar protein fibrillarin localization (Fig. 8C, D, E), allowing us to offer the hypothesis about different capability of autoantibodies to penetrate the cells in inbred and outbred mice after $HgCl_2$ treatment.

These results demonstrate for the first time that injection of mercury into the genetically geterogenous outbred mice induced autoantibodies which are able to penetrate into the cells of certain organs and react with their corresponding nucleolar antigens *in vivo*.

4. Discussion

The main hallmark of mercury-induced autoimmunity in genetically susceptible mice is the production of ANoA against the 34 kDa nucleolar protein fibrillarin (Abedi-Valugerdi, 2008). Because lots of studies have demonstrated that only homozygous mouse strains with susceptible H-2 genotypes are able to produce ANoA after mercury treatment, we next performed this work to test the ability of such heavy metal to induce ANoA production and IC deposition in heterozygous mouse population.

As demonstrated in Table 1 , 6 weeks of $HgCl_2$ treatment induced the ANoA production in both inbred and outbred mice in variable titers, whereas control saline-treated mice did not show any ANoA production. Moreover, it should be noted that magnitude of mercury-induced ANoA in outbred mice was even higher than that induced in inbred mice.

Another characteristic feature of HgIA we tested was the deposition of immune complexes in the kidney. According to literature reports, revealing IC in different parts of the kidney in autoimmune animals is usually done in two basic ways: on air-dried and acetone-fixed cryosections or on formaldehyde-fixed and paraffin-embedded sections (Chowdhury et al., 2005; Gobe & Nikolic-Paterson, 2005). Each of these procedures has its own advantages and disadvantages. Immunofluorescence (IF) staining of renal biopsies for the deposition of immunoglobulins and complement components is often the primary approach for a differential diagnosis of glomerular disease. However, a limitation of such IF applications is that they require frozen sections, which can suffer a loss of structural integrity during the process of tissue freezing (Gobe & Nikolic-Paterson, 2005). On the other hand, the problem with formaldehyde-fixed and paraffin-embedded sections is that tissue antigens are often denatured or masked (Chowdhury et al., 2005).

Thus, in the present work we tried to combine these approaches by fixing renal cryosections with formaldehyde under standard conditions along with routine clinical air-drying or acetone-fixing. This allowed us to use the highly informative IF method.

We showed that treatment of the cryosections with organic fixatives (acetone and methanol) led to appreciable damage of the renal tissue, but did not interfere with revealing IC in kidneys. These observations correlate well with scanning electron microscopy data, which showed damage to the plasma membrane of cells by fixing with acetone and methanol (Hoetelmans et al., 2001). We do not favor the air-drying of sections; despite its simplicity, preservation of cells on such cryosections was poor. Thus, the best choice of fixative for cell preservation was paraformaldehyde; it also appeared to be best in the context of information in that using it, we found out IC in renal proximal tubules in kidneys in all groups of mice. To our knowledge, there is no previous report on the presence of IC in proximal renal tubes.

In view of the fact that treatment with the organic fixatives leads to dehydration of the tissue, removing many water-soluble intracellular proteins, we suggest that the IC in proximal renal tubules consist largely of water-soluble complexes. Further, it does not seem strange that only the proximal tubules contained IC, while the distal tubules lacked them. It is known that molecules as big as immunoglobulins can be reabsorbed only in the proximal tubules, while the main function of the distal parts of the nephron is reabsorbtion of electrolytes.

In contrast to deposits in proximal renal tubules, glomerular IC in kidneys of autoimmune animals have been mentioned in the literature many times (Abedi-Valugerdi et al., 1997; Bigazzi, 1999; Havarinasab et al., 2008; Hultman et al., 1987, 1992, 1993; Kono et al., 2001). However, there is a question as to where (in mesangial cells and/or on their surface) they are located. Our results, merging areas with IC and DAPI staining by epifluorescence and confocal microscopy, suggest that, at least, the major part of deposits is localized inside the cells. Nevertheless, we cannot exclude the possibility that some part of the deposits is situated on the cell surface. For a definitive conclusion about the localization of glomerular IC, a study using electron IHC is necessary.

In addition to renal IC, we have found immune deposits in increased titers in liver hepatocytes and the white pulp spleen cells, suggesting in favor that HgIA is a comprehensive process involving many organs.

Furthermore, the development of HgIA is accompanied by the occurrence of IC in blood vessel walls (Hultman et al., 1993). It was recently shown that the dye Col-F binds selectively with the collagen and elastin fibrils in coats and elastic membranes of blood vessels in native tissues. However, the possibility of using Col-F in combination with the IHC analysis has not been reported previously. Thus, an original protocol for the simultaneous staining of collagen and elastin fibrils and immunolabeling of immune deposits was developed. Our observations, based on specific staining of collagen and elastic fibers as a part of vessel walls with the dye Col-F, allowed us to localize the IC in both the endothelial zone and across the whole width of the vessel walls in kidney, liver and spleen of mercury-treated mice. Additionally, revealing fibers using Col-F allowed us to visualize even the small vessels that were poorly identified with phase contrast because of elastic membrane thinning and luminal occlusion after tissue freezing.

According to our results, IC were present not only in organs of autoimmune mice, but also in the glomeruli, renal proximal tubules, hepatocytes and in the cells of spleen lymphoid follicles of control animals, although at a much lower level. This does not seem strange, because it is well-known in medicine that autoantibodies are found not only in the blood of autoimmune patients, but also in healthy individuals. In particular, sera from healthy people are capable of staining different cells (e.g., Hep-2) in an IIF reaction (Koelsch et al., 2007). However, the concentration (titer) of such antibodies is at least an order of magnitude less than in autoimmune patients. So, it seems possible that such antibodies in renal glomeruli, hepatocytes and proximal tubules could be derived from blood by filtration and primary urine by reabsorbtion, respectively, and become deposited in the cells. And the presence of immunoglobulins in cells of lymphoid follicles in the spleen is a sign of the normal functioning of the immune system.

Our investigation shows that immune complex deposits can differ not only in quantity, but also in composition. The C3 component of the complement system was seen as part of the renal IC only in the glomeruli and blood vessel walls, but not in the proximal tubules. In contrast with earlier studies (Hultman et al., 1987), the present investigation showed that some areas of the glomeruli containing C3 lacked Ig. Reasons for these features of IC composition can be a subject of future research. For these purposes, use of a laser microdissector with subsequent mass-spectrometric analysis of the cut areas may be useful.

Moreover, as described in the Results, renal IC consist of not only different classes but also different immunoglobulin isotypes. We demonstrated that glomerular IC include IgG, IgM, and, possibly, IgA immunoglobulins, while the vessel wall and proximal tubules contain almost no IgM.

More interesting is the occurrence of IgG immunoglobulin isotypes in the immune complexes. Results from initial studies suggested that HgIA in mice is mediated by a T helper type 2 (Th2) response (i.e., polyclonal B cell activation with hyper-IgE and -IgG1 production) (Abedi-Valugerdi, 2008; Gillespie et al,. 1995, 1996; Goldman et al., 1991; Ochel et al., 1991). However, further studies have revealed that the development of mercury-induced autoimmune manifestations cannot be explained simply by Th2-based immune response (Abedi-Valugerdi, 2008). In particular, IFN-ɣ, a key cytokine produced by activated T helper type 1 (Th1) cells, induces IgG2a response in the mouse and is absolutely required for the induction of ANoA production in this autoimmune condition (Abedi-Valugerdi 2008; Kono et al., 1998). Our results are consistent with this. Despite the Th2-dependent appearing of germinal centers in spleen after $HgCl_2$-treatment and the prevalence of the Th2-mediated IgG1 isotype as a component of IC, we also saw some IgG2a in the deposits, arguing in favor of Th1 activation too.

With all that the most important result of our research is the discovery of the ability of $HgCl_2$-induced ANoA to transverse the plasma and nuclear membrane of living cells and translocate to the nucleoli of different cells in outbred mice in vivo. We found that mercury-induced ANoA penetrated into the cells of certain organs (kidney, liver and spleen) and colocalized with special nucleolar protein fibrillarin - the major autoantigen in HgIA. This fact once again place outbred mice in close quarters with humans. As is well known from the literature, the autoantibodies from SLE patients are able to penetrate into the nuclei of cells in certain organs (Foster et al., 1994; Vlahakos et al., 1992; Yanase et al., 1997; Zack et al., 1996). It is likely that mercury-induced ANoA contain basic amino acid-rich sequences similar to those seen in anti-DNA autoantibodies derived from lupus-prone mice, allowing them to penetrate into the cell nuclei (Abedi-Valugerdi et al., 1999). Several studies have shown that penetrating autoantibodies cause cellular dysfunction after entering the cell and reacting with their intracellular antigens (Abedi-Valugerdi et al., 1999; Koscec et al., 1997; Reichlin, 1995). Therefore, it has been suggested that these antibodies might have pathogenic roles. However, our results do not confirm this, at least, at the beginning of the development of such mercury-induced autoimmune response. Formation of IC in different parts of the kidney was not accompanied by visible destruction or cell death, at least as evidenced by the TUNEL assay. The article of Abedi-Valugerdi et al. (1999) offers two possible explanations of this fact. First of all, the main target for mercury-induced ANoA is fibrillarin, which is known to be associated with snRNAs. In mammals the exact function of fibrillarin is not known, but it has been suggested that this nucleolar protein possibly participates in ribosomal biosynthesis. Based on this suggestion, it is likely that fibrillarin does not have a crucial role in the DNA synthesis and interfering with its function/structure by ANoA would not impair the cell proliferation. Second, since besides fibrillarin, several other nucleolar proteins (nucleolin, Surf-6, etc.) are also present in the mammalian nucleoli, it is likely that if fibrillarin is required for DNA synthesis and if binding of ANoA to fibrillarin impairs it's function, other nucleoproteins will take over fibrillarin's function. Since it has been suggested that fibrillarin is involved in the synthesis of ribosomal RNA, further studies are needed to test if nucleolar localization of ANoA would affect other cell functions such as protein synthesis. But, nevertheless, we cannot exclude the third possibility that destructive alterations could appear in later stages of disease development, because it is known that renal failure is one of the negative features associated with human autoimmune diseases (Tormey et al., 2001).

5. Conclusion

Thus, in our work we have shown that $HgCl_2$ induce very strong autoimmune process both in inbred and outbred mice, accompanied by ANoA production and heavy IC deposition. We have described novel localization and composition of such immune deposits in different organs. Also, we have come to conclusion about the higher penetrating capability of autoantibodies in outbred mice as compared with inbred mice. So, we have discovered that genetically heterogenous outbred CFW mice produce the same reaction on standard $HgCl_2$ treatment (1.6 mg/kg twice a week) as inbred SJL/J mice previously described to be most susceptible.

Our data thoroughly confirm and continue the findings of Dr. Abedi-Valugerdi suggesting that certain environmental factors, without requiring the presence of specific susceptibility genes, can induce some autoimmune manifestations in members of a genetically heterogenous population.

We think that outbred mice with $HgCl_2$-induced autoimmunity may also be used for testing of immunosuppressive drugs because they better reflect the human population then homozygous inbred mice. Thus, the present study could be very useful for further understanding, prediction and therapy of human systemic autoimmune diseases, in particular developing after the regular exposure of mercury compounds.

Author details

Alla Arefieva*, Marina Krasilshchikova and Olga Zatsepina
Shemyakin-Ovchinnikov Institute of Bioorganic
Chemistry of the Russian Academy of Sciences, Moscow, Russian Federation

Acknowledgement

Authors are grateful to Dr. K.A. Lukyanov (Shemyakin-Ovchinnikov Institute of Bioorganic Chemistry of the Russian Academy of Sciences, Moscow, Russian Federation) for the help in image recording and Dr. J.W. Dobrucki (Jagiellonian University, Krakow, Poland) for the provision of the dye ColF.

This work was supported by the Russian Foundation for Basic Research [grant number 08-04-00854]; the Ministry of Education and Science of the Russian Federation [Government Contracts numbers 14.740.11.0121, 14.740.11.0925].

6. References

Abedi-Valugerdi, M.; Hu, H. & Möller, G. (1997). Mercury-induced renal immune complex deposits in young (NZB x NZW) F1 mice: characterization of antibodies/autoantibodies. *Clinical and experimental immunology,*Vol.110, No.1, (October 1997), pp. 86-91

Abedi-Valugerdi, M.; Hu, H. & Möller, G. (1999). Mercury-induced anti-nucleolar autoantibodies can transgress the membrane of living cells in vivo and in vitro. *International immunology,* Vol.11, No.4, (April 1999), pp. 605-615

Abedi-Valugerdi, M. & Möller, G. (2000). Contribution of H-2 and non-H-2 genes in the control of mercury-induced autoimmunity. *International immunology,*Vol.12, No.10, (October 2000), pp. 1425-1430

Abedi–Valugerdi, M. (2008). Mercury and silver induce B cell activation and anti–nucleolar autoantibody production in outbred mouse stocks: are environmental factors more important than the susceptibility genes in connection with autoimmunity? *Clinical and experimental immunology,* Vol.155, No.1, (January 2008), pp. 117–124

* Corresponding Author

Alves, M.F.; Fraiji, N.A.; Barbosa, A.C.; De Lima, D.S.; Souza, J.R.; Dórea, J.G. & Cordeiro, G.W. (2006). Fish consumption, mercury exposure and serum antinuclear antibody in Amazonians. *International journal of environmental health research,* Vol.16, No.4, (August 2006), pp. 255–262

Aref'eva, A.S.; Dyban, P.A.; Krasil'shchikova, M.S.; Dobrucki, J.W. & Zatsepina, O.V. (2010). Localization and composition of renal immunodeposits in mice developing HgCl2-induced autoimmune process. *Tsitologiia,* Vol.52, No.6, (June 2010), pp. 477-486

Arnett, F.C.; Reveille, J.D.; Goldstein, R.; Pollard, K.M.; Leaird, K.; Smith, E.A.; Leroy, E.C. & Fritzler M.J. (1996). Autoantibodies to fibrillarin in systemic sclerosis (scleroderma). An immunogenetic, serologic, and clinical analysis. *Arthritis and rheumatism,* Vol.39, No.7, (July 1996), pp. 1151–1160

Arnett, F.C.; Fritzler, M.J.; Ahn, C. & Holian, A. (2000). Urinary mercury levels in patients with autoantibodies to U3-RNP (fibrillarin). *The Journal of rheumatology,* Vol.27, No.2, (February 2000), pp. 405-410

Bagenstose, L.M.; Salgame, P. & Monestier, M. (1999). Murine mercury-induced autoimmunity: a model of chemically related autoimmunity in humans. *Immunologic research,* Vol.20, No.1, pp. 67–78

Bigazzi, P.E. (1998). Mercury, In: *Immunotoxicology of Environmental and Occupational Metals,* J. Zelikoff, P. Thomas (Ed.), 131-161, Taylor & Francis, ISBN 978-074-8403-90-5, London, UK

Bigazzi, P.E. (1999). Metals and kidney autoimmunity. *Environmental health perspectives,* Vol.107, No.5, (October 1999), pp. 753-765

Chen, M.; Hemmerich, P. & von Mikecz, A. (2002). Platinum–induced autoantibodies target nucleoplasmicantigens related to active transcription. *Immunobiology,* Vol.206, No.5, (December 2002), pp. 474–483

Chowdhury, A.R.H.; Ehara, T.; Higuchi, M.; Hora, K. & Shigematsu, H. (2005). Immunohistochemical detection of immunoglobulins and complements in formaldehyde-fixed and paraffin-embedded renal biopsy tissues; an adjunct for diagnosis of glomerulonephritis. *Nephrology (Carlton),* Vol.10, No.3, (June 2005), pp. 298-304

da Costa, G.M.; dos Anjos, L.M.; Souza, G.S.; Gomes, B.D.; Saito, C.A.; Pinheiro, M.C.; Ventura, D.F.; da Silva, F.M. & Silveira, L.C. (2008). Mercury toxicity in Amazon gold miners: visual dysfunction assessed by retinal and cortical electrophysiology. Environmental research, Vol.107, No.1, (May 2008), pp. 98-107

Eneström, S. & Hultman, P. (1984). Immune-mediated glomerulonephritis induced by mercuric chloride in mice. *Experientia,* Vol.40, No.11, (November 1984), pp. 1234-1240

Eneström, S. & Hultman, P. (1995). Does amalgam affect the immune system? A controversial issue. *International archives of allergy and immunology,* Vol.106, No.3, (March 1995), pp. 180-203

Fairweather, D. & Rose, N.R. (2004). Women and autoimmune diseases. *Emerging infectious diseases,* Vol.10, No.11, (November 2004), pp. 2005–2011

Fairweather, D.; Frisancho-Kiss, S. & Rose, N.R. (2008). Sex differences in autoimmune disease from a pathological perspective. *The American journal of pathology,* Vol.173, No.3, (September 2008), pp. 600–609

Foster, M.H.; Kieber-Emmons, T.; Ohliger, M. & Madaio, M.P. (1994). Molecular and structural analysis of nuclear localizing anti-DNA lupus antibodies. *Immunologic research,* Vol.13, No.2-3, pp. 186-206

Gardner, R.M.; Nyland, J.F.; Silva, I.A.; Ventura, A.M.; de Souza, J.M. & Silbergeld, E.K. (2010). Mercury exposure, serum antinuclear/antinucleolar antibodies, and serum cytokine levels in mining populations in Amazonian Brazil: a cross-sectional study. Environmental research, Vol.110, No.4, (May 2010), pp. 345-354

Gillespie, K.M.; Qasim, F.J.; Tibbatts, L.M.; Thiru, S.; Oliveira, D.B. & Mathieson, P.W. (1995). Interleukin-4 gene expression in mercury-induced autoimmunity. *Scandinavian journal of immunology,* Vol.41, No.3, (March 1995), pp. 268-272

Gillespie, K.M.; Saoudi, A.; Kuhn, J.; Whittle, C.J.; Druet, P.; Bellon, B. & Mathieson, P.W. (1996). Th1/Th2 cytokine gene expression after mercuric chloride in susceptible and resistant rat strains. European journal of immunology, Vol.26, No.10, (October 1996), pp. 2388-2392

Gobe, G.C. & Nikolic-Paterson, D.J. (2005). Unmasking the secrets of glomerular disease for diagnosis. *Nephrology (Carlton),* Vol.10, No.3, (June 2005), pp. 296-297

Goldman, M.; Druet, P. & Gleichmann, E. (1991). TH2 cells in systemic autoimmunity: insights from allogeneic diseases and chemically-induced autoimmunity. *Immunology today,* Vol.12, No.7, (July 1991), pp. 223-227

Guzzi, G.; Fogazzi, G.B.; Cantù, M.; Minoia, C.; Ronchi, A.; Pigatto, P.D. & Severi, G. (2008). Dental amalgam, mercury toxicity, and renal autoimmunity. *Journal of environmental pathology, toxicology and oncology : official organ of the International Society for Environmental Toxicology and Cancer,* Vol.27, No.2, pp. 47-55

Häggqvist, B.; Havarinasab, S.; Björn, E. & Hultman, P. (2005). The immunosuppressive effect of methylmercury does not preclude development of autoimmunity in genetically susceptible mice. *Toxicology,*Vol.208, No.1, (March 2005), pp. 149–164

Hansson, M. & Abedi–Valugerdi, M. (2003). Xenobiotic metal–induced autoimmunity: mercury and silver differentially induce antinucleolar autoantibody production in susceptible H–2s, H–2q, H–2f mice. *Clinical and experimental immunology,*Vol.131, No.3, (March 2003), pp. 405–414

Havarinasab, S.; Häggqvist, B.; Björn. E.; Pollard, K.M. & Hultman, P. (2005). Immunosuppressive and autoimmune effects of thimerosal in mice. *Toxicology and applied pharmacology,* Vol.204, No.2, (April 2005), pp. 109–121

Havarinasab, S. & Hultman, P. (2005). Organic mercury compounds and autoimmunity. *Autoimmunity reviews,* Vol.4, No.5, (June 2005), pp. 270–275

Havarinasab, S.; Björn, E.; Ekstrand, J. & Hultman, P. (2007). Dose and Hg species determine the T–helper cell activation in murine autoimmunity. *Toxicology.* Vol.229, No.1–2, (January 2007), pp. 23–32

Havarinasab, S.; Björn, E.; Nielsen, J.B. & Hultman, P. (2007). Mercury species in lymphoid and non-lymphoid tissues after exposure to methyl mercury: correlation with autoimmune parameters during and after treatment in susceptible mice. *Toxicology and applied pharmacology,* Vol.221, No.1, (May 2007), pp. 21–28

Havarinasab, S.; Pollard, K.M. & Hultman, P. (2009). Gold– and silver–induced murine autoimmunity—requirement for cytokines and CD28 in murine heavy metal–induced autoimmunity. *Clinical and experimental immunology,* Vol.155, No.3, (March 2009), pp. 567–576

Ho, K.T. & Reveille, J.D. (2003). The clinical relevance of autoantibodies in scleroderma. *Arthritis research & therapy,* Vol.5, No.2, pp. 80-93

Hoetelmans, R.W.; Prins, F.A.; Cornelese-ten Velde, I.; van der Meer, J.; van de Velde, C.J. & van Dierendonck, J.H. (2001). Effects of acetone, methanol, or paraformaldehyde on cellular structure, visualized by reflection contrast microscopy and transmission and scanning electron microscopy. *Applied immunohistochemistry & molecular morphology : AIMM / official publication of the Society for Applied Immunohistochemistry,* Vol.9, No.4, (December 2001), pp. 346-351

Hultman, P. & Eneström, S. (1987). The induction of immune complex deposits in mice by peroral and parenteral administration of mercuric chloride: strain dependent susceptibility. *Clinical and experimental immunology,* Vol.67, No.2, (February 1987), pp. 283-292

Hultman, P.; Eneström, S.; Pollard, K.M. & Tan, E.M. (1989). Anti-fibrillarin autoantibodies in mercury-treated mice. *Clinical and experimental immunology,* Vol.78, No.3, (December 1989), pp. 470-477

Hultman, P.; Bell, L.J.; Eneström, S. & Pollard, K.M. (1992). Murine susceptibility to mercury. I. Autoantibody profiles and systemic immune deposits in hybrid, congenic, and intra-H-2 recombinant strains. *Clinical immunology and immunopathology,* Vol.65, No.2, (November 1992), pp. 98-109

Hultman, P.; Bell, L.J.; Eneström, S. & Pollard, K.M. (1993). Murine susceptibility to mercury. II. autoantibody profiles and renal immune deposits in hybrid, backcross, and H-2d congenic mice. *Clinical immunology and immunopathology,* Vol.68, No.1, (July 1993), pp. 9-20

Hultman, P. & Hansson-Georgiadis, H. (1999). Methyl mercury-induced autoimmunity in mice. *Toxicology and applied pharmacology,* Vol.154, No.3, (February 1999), pp. 203-211

Johansson, U.; Hansson-Georgiadis, H. & Hultman, P. (1998). The genotype determines the B-cell response in mercury-treated mice. *International archives of allergy and immunology,* Vol.116, No.4, (August 1998), pp. 295-305

Koelsch, K.; Zheng, N.Y.; Zhang, Q.; Duty, A.; Helms, C.; Mathias, M.D.; Jared, M.; Smith, K.; Capra, J.D. & Wilson, P.C. (2007). Mature B cells class switched to IgD are autoreactive in healthy individuals. *The* Journal of clinical investigation, Vol.117, No.6, (June 2007), pp. 1558-1565

Kono, D.H.; Balomenos, D.; Pearson, D.L.; Park, M.S.; Hildebrandt, B.; Hultman, P. & Pollard, K.M. (1998). The prototypic Th2 autoimmunity induced by mercury is dependent on IFN-gamma and not Th1/Th2 imbalance. *Journal of immunology (Baltimore, Md. : 1950),* Vol.161, No.1, (July 1998), pp. 234-240

Kono, D.H.; Park, M.S.; Szydlik, A.; Haraldsson, K.M.; Kuan, J.D.; Pearson, D.L.; Hultman, P. & Pollard, K.M. (2001). Resistance to xenobiotic-induced autoimmunity maps to chromosome 1. *Journal of immunology (Baltimore, Md. : 1950)*, Vol.167, No.4, (August 2001), pp. 2396-2403

Koscec, M.; Koren, E.; Wolfson-Reichlin, M.; Fugate, R.D.; Trieu, E.; Targoff, I.N. & Reichlin, M. (1997). Autoantibodies to ribosomal P proteins penetrate into live hepatocytes and cause cellular dysfunction in culture. *Journal of immunology (Baltimore, Md. : 1950)*, Vol.159, No.4, (August 1997), pp. 2033-2041

Kurien, B.T. & Scofield, R.H. (2006). Autoantibody determination in the diagnosis of systemic lupus erythematosus.

Scandinavian journal of immunology, Vol.64, No.3, (September 2006), pp. 227–235

Leffel, E.K.; Wolf, C.; Poklis, A. & White, K.L. Jr. (2003). Drinking water exposure to cadmium, an environmental contaminant, results in the exacerbation of autoimmune disease in the murine model. *Toxicology*, Vol.188, No.2–3, (June 2003), pp. 233–250

Markowitz, G.S. & D'Agati, V.D. (2009). Classification of lupus nephritis. *Current opinion in nephrology and hypertension*, Vol.18, No.3, (May 2009), pp. 220-225

Mutter, J. & Yeter, D. (2008). Kawasaki's disease, acrodynia, and mercury. *Current medicinal chemistry*, Vol.15, No.28, pp. 3000-3010

Ochel, M.; Vohr, H.W.; Pfeiffer, C. & Gleichmann, E. (1991). IL-4 is required for the IgE and IgG1 increase and IgG1 autoantibody formation in mice treated with mercuric chloride. *Journal of immunology (Baltimore, Md. : 1950)*, Vol.146, No.9, (May 1991), pp. 3006-3011

Ohsawa, M. (1997). Biomarkers for responses to heavy metals. *Cancer causes & control: CCC*, Vol.8, No.3, (May 1997), pp. 514-517

Pedersen, L.M. & Permin, H. (1988). Rheumatic disease, heavy-metal pigments, and the Great Masters. *Lancet.*, Vol.1, No.8597, (June 1988), pp. 1267-1269

Pelletier, L.; Castedo, M.; Bellon, B. & Druet, P. (1994). Mercury and autoimmunity, In: *Immunotoxicology and Immunopharmacology*, J.H. Dean, (Ed.), 539–552, Raven Press Ltd., ISBN 978-078-1702-19-5, New York, USA

Pigatto, P.D. & Guzzi, G. (2010). Linking mercury amalgam to autoimmunity. Trends in immunology, Vol.31, No.2, (February 2010), pp. 48-49

Reichlin, M. (1995). Cell injury mediated by autoantibodies to intracellular antigens. *Clinical immunology and immunopathology*, Vol.76, No.3, (September 1995), pp. 215-219

Reuter, R.; Tessars, G.; Vohr, H.V.; Gleichmann, E. & Luhrmann, R. (1989). Mercuric chloride induces autoantibodies against U3 small nuclear ribonucleoprotein in susceptible mice. *Proceedings of the National Academy of Sciences of the United States of America*, Vol.86, No.1, (January 1989), pp. 237-241

Rhodes, B. & Vyse, T.J. (2007). General aspects of the genetics of SLE. *Autoimmunity*, Vol.40, No.8, (December 2007), pp. 550-559

Robinson, C.J.; White, H.J. & Rose, N.R. (1997). Murine strain differences in response to mercuric chloride: antinucleolar antibodies production does not correlate with renal immune complex deposition. *Clinical immunology and immunopathology*, Vol.83, No.2, (May 1997), pp. 127-138

Roether, S.; Rabbani, H.; Mellstedt, H. & Abedi-Valugerdi, M. (2002). Spontaneous downregulation of antibody/autoantibody synthesis in susceptible mice upon chronic exposure to mercuric chloride is not owing to a general immunosuppression. *Scandinavian journal of immunology,* Vol.55, No.5, (May 2002), pp. 493-502

Rowley, B. & Monestier, M. (2005). Mechanisms of heavy metal-induced autoimmunity. *Molecular immunology,* Vol.42, No.7, (May 2005), pp. 833-838

Silbergeld, E.K.; Silva, I.A. & Nyland, J.F. (2005). Mercury and autoimmunity: implications for occupational and environmental health. *Toxicology and applied pharmacology,* Vol.207, No.2, (September 2005), pp. 282-292

Silva, I.A.; Nyland, J.F.; Gorman, A.; Perisse, A.; Ventura, A.M.; Santos, E.K.; Souza, J.M.; Burek, C.L.; Rose, N.R. & Silbergeld, E.K. (2004). Mercury exposure, malaria, and serum antinuclear/antinucleolar antibodies in amazon populations in Brazil: a cross-sectional study. *Environmental health : a global access science source,* Vol.3, No.1, (November 2004), p. 11

Suzuki, Y.; Inoue, T. & Ra, C. (2011). Autoimmunity-inducing metals (hg, au and ag) modulate mast cell signaling, function and survival. Current pharmaceutical design, Vol.17, No.34, (November 2011), pp. 3805-3814

Tabata, M.; Kumar Sarker, A. & Nyarko, E. (2003). Enhanced conformational changes in DNA in the presence of mercury(II), cadmium(II) and lead(II) porphyrins. *Journal of inorganic biochemistry,* Vol.94, No.1–2, (February 2003), pp. 50–58

Takeuchi, K.; Turley, S.J.; Tan, E.M. & Pollard, K.M. (1995). Analysis of the autoantibody response to fibrillarin in human disease and murine models of autoimmunity. *Journal of immunology (Baltimore, Md. : 1950),* Vol.154, No.2, (January 1995), pp. 961–971

Tormey, V.J.; Bunn, C.C.; Denton, C.P. & Black, C.M. (2001). Anti-fibrillarin antibodies in systemic sclerosis. *Rheumatology (Oxford),* Vol.40, No.10, (October 2001), pp. 1157-1162

Van Eenennaam, H.; Vogelzangs, J.H.; Bisschops, L.; Te Boome, L.C.; Seeling, H.P.; Renz, M.; De Rooij, D.J.; Brouwer, R.; Pluk, H.; Pruijn, G.J.; Van Venrooij, W.J. & Van Den Hoogen, F.H. (2002). Autoantibodies against small nucleolar ribonucleoprotein complexes and their clinical associations. *Clinical and experimental immunology,* Vol.130, No.3, (December 2002), pp. 532-540

Vlahakos, D.; Foster, M.H.; Ucci, A.A.; Barrett, K.J.; Datta, S.K. & Madaio, M.P. (1992). Murine monoclonal anti-DNA antibodies penetrate cells, bind to nuclei, and induce glomerular proliferation and proteinuria in vivo. *Journal of the American Society of Nephrology : JASN,* Vol.2, No.8, (February 1992), pp. 1345-1354

Yanase, K.; Smith, R.M.; Puccetti, A.; Jarett, L. & Madaio, M.P. (1997). Receptor-mediated cellular entry of nuclear localizing anti-DNA antibodies via myosin 1. *The Journal of clinical investigation,* Vol.100, No.1, (July 1997), pp. 25-31

Yang, J.M.; Hildebrandt, B.; Ludershmidt, C. & Pollard, K.M. (2003). Human scleroderma sera contain autoantibodies to protein components specific to the U3 small nucleolar RNP complex. *Arthritis and rheumatism,* Vol.48, No.1, (January 2003), pp. 210-217

Zack, D.J.; Stempniak, M.; Wong, A.L.; Taylor, C. & Weisbart, R.H. (1996). Mechanisms of cellular penetration and nuclear localization of an anti-double strand DNA autoantibody. *Journal of immunology (Baltimore, Md. : 1950)*, Vol.157, No.5, (September 1996), pp. 2082-2088

Abedi-Valugerdi, M.; Hu, H. & Möller, G. (1997). Mercury-induced renal immune complex deposits in young (NZB x NZW) F1 mice: characterization of antibodies/autoantibodies. *Clinical and experimental immunology,*Vol.110, No.1, (October 1997), pp. 86-91

Abedi-Valugerdi, M.; Hu, H. & Möller, G. (1999). Mercury-induced anti-nucleolar autoantibodies can transgress the membrane of living cells in vivo and in vitro. *International immunology,* Vol.11, No.4, (April 1999), pp. 605-615

Abedi-Valugerdi, M. & Möller, G. (2000). Contribution of H-2 and non-H-2 genes in the control of mercury-induced autoimmunity. *International immunology,*Vol.12, No.10, (October 2000), pp. 1425-1430

Abedi–Valugerdi, M. (2008). Mercury and silver induce B cell activation and anti–nucleolar autoantibody production in outbred mouse stocks: are environmental factors more important than the susceptibility genes in connection with autoimmunity? *Clinical and experimental immunology,* Vol.155, No.1, (January 2008), pp. 117–124

Alves, M.F.; Fraiji, N.A.; Barbosa, A.C.; De Lima, D.S.; Souza, J.R.; Dórea, J.G. & Cordeiro, G.W. (2006). Fish consumption, mercury exposure and serum antinuclear antibody in Amazonians. *International journal of environmental health research,* Vol.16, No.4, (August 2006), pp. 255–262

Aref'eva, A.S.; Dyban, P.A.; Krasil'shchikova, M.S.; Dobrucki, J.W. & Zatsepina, O.V. (2010). Localization and composition of renal immunodeposits in mice developing HgCl2-induced autoimmune process. *Tsitologiia,* Vol.52, No.6, (June 2010), pp. 477-486

Arnett, F.C.; Reveille, J.D.; Goldstein, R.; Pollard, K.M.; Leaird, K.; Smith, E.A.; Leroy, E.C. & Fritzler M.J. (1996). Autoantibodies to fibrillarin in systemic sclerosis (scleroderma). An immunogenetic, serologic, and clinical analysis. *Arthritis and rheumatism,* Vol.39, No.7, (July 1996), pp. 1151–1160

Arnett, F.C.; Fritzler, M.J.; Ahn, C. & Holian, A. (2000). Urinary mercury levels in patients with autoantibodies to U3-RNP (fibrillarin). *The Journal of rheumatology,* Vol.27, No.2, (February 2000), pp. 405-410

Bagenstose, L.M.; Salgame, P. & Monestier, M. (1999). Murine mercury-induced autoimmunity: a model of chemically related autoimmunity in humans. *Immunologic research,* Vol.20, No.1, pp. 67–78

Bigazzi, P.E. (1998). Mercury, In: *Immunotoxicology of Environmental and Occupational Metals,* J. Zelikoff, P. Thomas (Ed.), 131-161, Taylor & Francis, ISBN 978-074-8403-90-5, London, UK

Bigazzi, P.E. (1999). Metals and kidney autoimmunity. *Environmental health perspectives,* Vol.107, No.5, (October 1999), pp. 753-765

Chen, M.; Hemmerich, P. & von Mikecz, A. (2002). Platinum–induced autoantibodies target nucleoplasmicantigens related to active transcription. *Immunobiology,* Vol.206, No.5, (December 2002), pp. 474–483

Chowdhury, A.R.H.; Ehara, T.; Higuchi, M.; Hora, K. & Shigematsu, H. (2005). Immunohistochemical detection of immunoglobulins and complements in formaldehyde-fixed and paraffin-embedded renal biopsy tissues; an adjunct for diagnosis of glomerulonephritis. *Nephrology (Carlton),* Vol.10, No.3, (June 2005), pp. 298-304

da Costa, G.M.; dos Anjos, L.M.; Souza, G.S.; Gomes, B.D.; Saito, C.A.; Pinheiro, M.C.; Ventura, D.F.; da Silva, F.M. & Silveira, L.C. (2008). Mercury toxicity in Amazon gold miners: visual dysfunction assessed by retinal and cortical electrophysiology. Environmental research, Vol.107, No.1, (May 2008), pp. 98-107

Eneström, S. & Hultman, P. (1984). Immune-mediated glomerulonephritis induced by mercuric chloride in mice. *Experientia,* Vol.40, No.11, (November 1984), pp. 1234-1240

Eneström, S. & Hultman, P. (1995). Does amalgam affect the immune system? A controversial issue. *International archives of allergy and immunology,* Vol.106, No.3, (March 1995), pp. 180-203

Fairweather, D. & Rose, N.R. (2004). Women and autoimmune diseases. *Emerging infectious diseases,* Vol.10, No.11, (November 2004), pp. 2005–2011

Fairweather, D.; Frisancho-Kiss, S. & Rose, N.R. (2008). Sex differences in autoimmune disease from a pathological perspective. *The American journal of pathology,* Vol.173, No.3, (September 2008), pp. 600–609

Foster, M.H.; Kieber-Emmons, T.; Ohliger, M. & Madaio, M.P. (1994). Molecular and structural analysis of nuclear localizing anti-DNA lupus antibodies. *Immunologic research,* Vol.13, No.2-3, pp. 186-206

Gardner, R.M.; Nyland, J.F.; Silva, I.A.; Ventura, A.M.; de Souza, J.M. & Silbergeld, E.K. (2010). Mercury exposure, serum antinuclear/antinucleolar antibodies, and serum cytokine levels in mining populations in Amazonian Brazil: a cross-sectional study. Environmental research, Vol.110, No.4, (May 2010), pp. 345-354

Gillespie, K.M.; Qasim, F.J.; Tibbatts, L.M.; Thiru, S.; Oliveira, D.B. & Mathieson, P.W. (1995). Interleukin-4 gene expression in mercury-induced autoimmunity. *Scandinavian journal of immunology,* Vol.41, No.3, (March 1995), pp. 268-272

Gillespie, K.M.; Saoudi, A.; Kuhn, J.; Whittle, C.J.; Druet, P.; Bellon, B. & Mathieson, P.W. (1996). Th1/Th2 cytokine gene expression after mercuric chloride in susceptible and resistant rat strains. European journal of immunology, Vol.26, No.10, (October 1996), pp. 2388-2392

Gobe, G.C. & Nikolic-Paterson, D.J. (2005). Unmasking the secrets of glomerular disease for diagnosis. *Nephrology (Carlton),* Vol.10, No.3, (June 2005), pp. 296-297

Goldman, M.; Druet, P. & Gleichmann, E. (1991). TH2 cells in systemic autoimmunity: insights from allogeneic diseases and chemically-induced autoimmunity. *Immunology today*, Vol.12, No.7, (July 1991), pp. 223-227

Guzzi, G.; Fogazzi, G.B.; Cantù, M.; Minoia, C.; Ronchi, A.; Pigatto, P.D. & Severi, G. (2008). Dental amalgam, mercury toxicity, and renal autoimmunity. *Journal of environmental pathology, toxicology and oncology : official organ of the International Society for Environmental Toxicology and Cancer,* Vol.27, No.2, pp. 47-55

Häggqvist, B.; Havarinasab, S.; Björn, E. & Hultman, P. (2005). The immunosuppressive effect of methylmercury does not preclude development of autoimmunity in genetically susceptible mice. *Toxicology,*Vol.208, No.1, (March 2005), pp. 149–164

Hansson, M. & Abedi–Valugerdi, M. (2003). Xenobiotic metal–induced autoimmunity: mercury and silver differentially induce antinucleolar autoantibody production in susceptible H–2s, H–2q, H–2f mice. *Clinical and experimental immunology,*Vol.131, No.3, (March 2003), pp. 405–414

Havarinasab, S.; Häggqvist, B.; Björn. E.; Pollard, K.M. & Hultman, P. (2005). Immunosuppressive and autoimmune effects of thimerosal in mice. *Toxicology and applied pharmacology,* Vol.204, No.2, (April 2005), pp. 109–121

Havarinasab, S. & Hultman, P. (2005). Organic mercury compounds and autoimmunity. *Autoimmunity reviews,* Vol.4, No.5, (June 2005), pp. 270–275

Havarinasab, S.; Björn, E.; Ekstrand, J. & Hultman, P. (2007). Dose and Hg species determine the T–helper cell activation in murine autoimmunity. *Toxicology.* Vol.229, No.1–2, (January 2007), pp. 23–32

Havarinasab, S.; Björn, E.; Nielsen, J.B. & Hultman, P. (2007). Mercury species in lymphoid and non-lymphoid tissues after exposure to methyl mercury: correlation with autoimmune parameters during and after treatment in susceptible mice. *Toxicology and applied pharmacology,* Vol.221, No.1, (May 2007), pp. 21–28

Havarinasab, S.; Pollard, K.M. & Hultman, P. (2009). Gold– and silver–induced murine autoimmunity—requirement for cytokines and CD28 in murine heavy metal–induced autoimmunity. *Clinical and experimental immunology,* Vol.155, No.3, (March 2009), pp. 567–576

Ho, K.T. & Reveille, J.D. (2003). The clinical relevance of autoantibodies in scleroderma. *Arthritis research & therapy,* Vol.5, No.2, pp. 80-93

Hoetelmans, R.W.; Prins, F.A.; Cornelese-ten Velde, I.; van der Meer, J.; van de Velde, C.J. & van Dierendonck, J.H. (2001). Effects of acetone, methanol, or paraformaldehyde on cellular structure, visualized by reflection contrast microscopy and transmission and scanning electron microscopy. *Applied immunohistochemistry & molecular morphology : AIMM / official publication of the Society for Applied Immunohistochemistry,* Vol.9, No.4, (December 2001), pp. 346-351

Hultman, P. & Eneström, S. (1987). The induction of immune complex deposits in mice by peroral and parenteral administration of mercuric chloride: strain dependent susceptibility. *Clinical and experimental immunology,* Vol.67, No.2, (February 1987), pp. 283-292

Hultman, P.; Eneström, S.; Pollard, K.M. & Tan, E.M. (1989). Anti-fibrillarin autoantibodies in mercury-treated mice. *Clinical and experimental immunology,* Vol.78, No.3, (December 1989), pp. 470-477

Hultman, P.; Bell, L.J.; Eneström, S. & Pollard, K.M. (1992). Murine susceptibility to mercury. I. Autoantibody profiles and systemic immune deposits in hybrid, congenic, and intra-H-2 recombinant strains. *Clinical immunology and immunopathology,* Vol.65, No.2, (November 1992), pp. 98-109

Hultman, P.; Bell, L.J.; Eneström, S. & Pollard, K.M. (1993). Murine susceptibility to mercury. II. autoantibody profiles and renal immune deposits in hybrid, backcross, and H-2d congenic mice. *Clinical immunology and immunopathology,* Vol.68, No.1, (July 1993), pp. 9-20

Hultman, P. & Hansson-Georgiadis, H. (1999). Methyl mercury-induced autoimmunity in mice. *Toxicology and applied pharmacology,* Vol.154, No.3, (February 1999), pp. 203-211

Johansson, U.; Hansson-Georgiadis, H. & Hultman, P. (1998). The genotype determines the B-cell response in mercury-treated mice. *International archives of allergy and immunology,* Vol.116, No.4, (August 1998), pp. 295-305

Koelsch, K.; Zheng, N.Y.; Zhang, Q.; Duty, A.; Helms, C.; Mathias, M.D.; Jared, M.; Smith, K.; Capra, J.D. & Wilson, P.C. (2007). Mature B cells class switched to IgD are autoreactive in healthy individuals. *The* Journal of clinical investigation, Vol.117, No.6, (June 2007), pp. 1558-1565

Kono, D.H.; Balomenos, D.; Pearson, D.L.; Park, M.S.; Hildebrandt, B.; Hultman, P. & Pollard, K.M. (1998). The prototypic Th2 autoimmunity induced by mercury is dependent on IFN-gamma and not Th1/Th2 imbalance. *Journal of immunology (Baltimore, Md. : 1950),* Vol.161, No.1, (July 1998), pp. 234-240

Kono, D.H.; Park, M.S.; Szydlik, A.; Haraldsson, K.M.; Kuan, J.D.; Pearson, D.L.; Hultman, P. & Pollard, K.M. (2001). Resistance to xenobiotic-induced autoimmunity maps to chromosome 1. *Journal of immunology (Baltimore, Md. : 1950),* Vol.167, No.4, (August 2001), pp. 2396-2403

Koscec, M.; Koren, E.; Wolfson-Reichlin, M.; Fugate, R.D.; Trieu, E.; Targoff, I.N. & Reichlin, M. (1997). Autoantibodies to ribosomal P proteins penetrate into live hepatocytes and cause cellular dysfunction in culture. *Journal of immunology (Baltimore, Md. : 1950),* Vol.159, No.4, (August 1997), pp. 2033-2041

Kurien, B.T. & Scofield, R.H. (2006). Autoantibody determination in the diagnosis of systemic lupus erythematosus.

Scandinavian journal of immunology, Vol.64, No.3, (September 2006), pp. 227–235

Leffel, E.K.; Wolf, C.; Poklis, A. & White, K.L. Jr. (2003). Drinking water exposure to cadmium, an environmental contaminant, results in the exacerbation of autoimmune disease in the murine model. *Toxicology,* Vol.188, No.2–3, (June 2003), pp. 233–250

Markowitz, G.S. & D'Agati, V.D. (2009). Classification of lupus nephritis. *Current opinion in nephrology and hypertension,* Vol.18, No.3, (May 2009), pp. 220-225

Mutter, J. & Yeter, D. (2008). Kawasaki's disease, acrodynia, and mercury. *Current medicinal chemistry,* Vol.15, No.28, pp. 3000-3010

Ochel, M.; Vohr, H.W.; Pfeiffer, C. & Gleichmann, E. (1991). IL-4 is required for the IgE and IgG1 increase and IgG1 autoantibody formation in mice treated with mercuric chloride. *Journal of immunology (Baltimore, Md. : 1950),* Vol.146, No.9, (May 1991), pp. 3006-3011

Ohsawa, M. (1997). Biomarkers for responses to heavy metals. *Cancer causes & control: CCC,* Vol.8, No.3, (May 1997), pp. 514-517

Pedersen, L.M. & Permin, H. (1988). Rheumatic disease, heavy-metal pigments, and the Great Masters. *Lancet.,* Vol.1, No.8597, (June 1988), pp. 1267-1269

Pelletier, L.; Castedo, M.; Bellon, B. & Druet, P. (1994). Mercury and autoimmunity, In: *Immunotoxicology and Immunopharmacology,* J.H. Dean, (Ed.), 539–552, Raven Press Ltd., ISBN 978-078-1702-19-5, New York, USA

Pigatto, P.D. & Guzzi, G. (2010). Linking mercury amalgam to autoimmunity. Trends in immunology, Vol.31, No.2, (February 2010), pp. 48-49

Reichlin, M. (1995). Cell injury mediated by autoantibodies to intracellular antigens. *Clinical immunology and immunopathology*, Vol.76, No.3, (September 1995), pp. 215-219

Reuter, R.; Tessars, G.; Vohr, H.V.; Gleichmann, E. & Luhrmann, R. (1989). Mercuric chloride induces autoantibodies against U3 small nuclear ribonucleoprotein in susceptible mice. *Proceedings of the National Academy of Sciences of the United States of America*, Vol.86, No.1, (January 1989), pp. 237-241

Rhodes, B. & Vyse, T.J. (2007). General aspects of the genetics of SLE. *Autoimmunity*, Vol.40, No.8, (December 2007), pp. 550-559

Robinson, C.J.; White, H.J. & Rose, N.R. (1997). Murine strain differences in response to mercuric chloride: antinucleolar antibodies production does not correlate with renal immune complex deposition. *Clinical immunology and immunopathology*, Vol.83, No.2, (May 1997), pp. 127-138

Roether, S.; Rabbani, H.; Mellstedt, H. & Abedi-Valugerdi, M. (2002). Spontaneous downregulation of antibody/autoantibody synthesis in susceptible mice upon chronic exposure to mercuric chloride is not owing to a general immunosuppression. *Scandinavian journal of immunology*, Vol.55, No.5, (May 2002), pp. 493-502

Rowley, B. & Monestier, M. (2005). Mechanisms of heavy metal-induced autoimmunity. *Molecular immunology*, Vol.42, No.7, (May 2005), pp. 833-838

Silbergeld, E.K.; Silva, I.A. & Nyland, J.F. (2005). Mercury and autoimmunity: implications for occupational and environmental health. *Toxicology and applied pharmacology*, Vol.207, No.2, (September 2005), pp. 282-292

Silva, I.A.; Nyland, J.F.; Gorman, A.; Perisse, A.; Ventura, A.M.; Santos, E.K.; Souza, J.M.; Burek, C.L.; Rose, N.R. & Silbergeld, E.K. (2004). Mercury exposure, malaria, and serum antinuclear/antinucleolar antibodies in amazon populations in Brazil: a cross-sectional study. *Environmental health : a global access science source*, Vol.3, No.1, (November 2004), p. 11

Suzuki, Y.; Inoue, T. & Ra, C. (2011). Autoimmunity-inducing metals (hg, au and ag) modulate mast cell signaling, function and survival. Current pharmaceutical design, Vol.17, No.34, (November 2011), pp. 3805-3814

Tabata, M.; Kumar Sarker, A. & Nyarko, E. (2003). Enhanced conformational changes in DNA in the presence of mercury(II), cadmium(II) and lead(II) porphyrins. *Journal of inorganic biochemistry*, Vol.94, No.1–2, (February 2003), pp. 50–58

Takeuchi, K.; Turley, S.J.; Tan, E.M. & Pollard, K.M. (1995). Analysis of the autoantibody response to fibrillarin in human disease and murine models of autoimmunity. *Journal of immunology (Baltimore, Md. : 1950)*, Vol.154, No.2, (January 1995), pp. 961–971

Tormey, V.J.; Bunn, C.C.; Denton, C.P. & Black, C.M. (2001). Anti-fibrillarin antibodies in systemic sclerosis. *Rheumatology (Oxford)*, Vol.40, No.10, (October 2001), pp. 1157-1162

Van Eenennaam, H.; Vogelzangs, J.H.; Bisschops, L.; Te Boome, L.C.; Seeling, H.P.; Renz, M.; De Rooij, D.J.; Brouwer, R.; Pluk, H.; Pruijn, G.J.; Van Venrooij, W.J. & Van Den Hoogen, F.H. (2002). Autoantibodies against small nucleolar ribonucleoprotein complexes and their clinical associations. *Clinical and experimental immunology*, Vol.130, No.3, (December 2002), pp. 532-540

Vlahakos, D.; Foster, M.H.; Ucci, A.A.; Barrett, K.J.; Datta, S.K. & Madaio, M.P. (1992). Murine monoclonal anti-DNA antibodies penetrate cells, bind to nuclei, and induce glomerular proliferation and proteinuria in vivo. *Journal of the American Society of Nephrology : JASN,* Vol.2, No.8, (February 1992), pp. 1345-1354

Yanase, K.; Smith, R.M.; Puccetti, A.; Jarett, L. & Madaio, M.P. (1997). Receptor-mediated cellular entry of nuclear localizing anti-DNA antibodies via myosin 1. *The Journal of clinical investigation,* Vol.100, No.1, (July 1997), pp. 25-31

Yang, J.M.; Hildebrandt, B.; Ludershmidt, C. & Pollard, K.M. (2003). Human scleroderma sera contain autoantibodies to protein components specific to the U3 small nucleolar RNP complex. *Arthritis and rheumatism,* Vol.48, No.1, (January 2003), pp. 210-217

Zack, D.J.; Stempniak, M.; Wong, A.L.; Taylor, C. & Weisbart, R.H. (1996). Mechanisms of cellular penetration and nuclear localization of an anti-double strand DNA autoantibody. *Journal of immunology (Baltimore, Md. : 1950),* Vol.157, No.5, (September 1996), pp. 2082-2088

Chapter 7

Celiac and Inflammatory Bowel Diseases in Children with Primary Humoral Immunodeficiency

Anna Pituch-Noworolska and Katarzyna Zwonarz

Additional information is available at the end of the chapter

http://dx.doi.org/10.5772/50219

1. Introduction

The co-existence of immunodeficiency and autoimmunity called as "old couple" is known from the clinics, but the background and mechanism responsible for this phenomenon is far from explanation. The both; immunodeficiency and autoimmune diseases belong to group of rare diseases. The population of children with immunodeficiency of humoral immunity demonstrating clinical symptoms of deficiency is small and only a part of them develops autoimmune disease which means these patients are really very small group. Because of low number of such patients there is a lack of standards of diagnostic procedures and therapeutic approach.

The clinical observations and analysis of co-existence of these two different pathomechanisms lead to questions –

1. why, in diseases with impaired function of immune system, the antibodies and autoantibodies are produced,
2. why the prolonged inflammation develops leading to tissue and organ damage,
3. why these autoimmune diseases are different in clinical features, course and response to therapy,
4. why we are not able to find the factors helping in selection of patients with high risk of autoimmune disease within immunodeficiency group.

The develop of autoimmune diseases is a result of many factors occurring in sequence or at the same time what seems to be the puzzle with hundreds of pieces. In the immune deficiency some of these pieces are missed at the beginning but despite this the puzzle is fulfilled and the autoimmunity develops. It is why, this phenomenon is still fascinating….

2. The role of antibodies in pathomechanism of celiac and inflammatory bowel diseases

2.1. The production of autoantibodies

The autoantibodies are produced by B-1 subpopulation of B lymphocytes, plasma cells localized in lymph nodes and bone marrow, similarly to production of specific antibodies to pathogens; bacterial, viral or parasitic. They react with autoantigens e.g. determinants, receptors present on cell surface, products of cells (e.g. hormones, cytokines, insulin, enzymes), nuclei, DNA and organelles released after cells death. In healthy people the autoantibodies (e.g. antinuclear, rheumatoid factor) are noted in the serum in low titer what is probably an effect of persist low affinity self-reacting T and B lymphocytes in the thymus and bone marrow. The increase of occurrence and amount of autoantibodies with age in the healthy people is supporting the view that this small population of self-reactive lymphocytes is present during whole life [1].

The induction of autoantibodies production is not fully elucidated and the hypothesis about trigger by chronic inflammation, molecular mimicry with microbial antigens, aberrant expression of HLA-DR on cell surface as facilitating factor, are postulated. In systemic autoimmune diseases like lupus the antigens are intracellular so the above suggestions are not very suitable. The possible explanations of anti-DNA antibodies production includes the process of apoptosis and formation of nucleosomes containing pure DNA. It is highly probable, that dying cells e.g. within inflammatory infiltrations of tissues release many different organelles, proteins and enzymes induce production of antibodies to them. The antibodies against structure of nucleus (e.g. histones, centromers, centriols, nucleoli), Golgi apparatus, mitochondria, peroxidase, specific proteins (e.g. Scl-70, RNP), enzymes are associated with different types of autoimmune diseases. Delayed clearing of dying cells and abundance, stability, resistance to degradation of some nucleoproteins are stimulating the immune response through activation of Toll-like receptors. This hypothesis might apply to some of systemic autoimmune diseases [1].

The presence of autoantibodies in high titer is generally associated with damage of target cells or organs and occurrence of clinical symptoms of disease. The deposits of immune complexes (autoantibodies – antigens – complement) in the vessels or located directly in the tissue expressing the autoantigen are injurious for the surrounding tissue. These complexes bind the complement, activate the cascade, stimulate the production of pro-inflammatory cytokines, chemotactic factors for infiltrating cells leading to support of autoantibodies production and amplification of the inflammation (self-perpetuating inflammatory process). In animal models this damaging effect of autoantibodies and immune complexes was showed for systemic autoimmune diseases. In celiac disease, the anti transglutaminase antibodies are associated with reduction of intestinal epithelial cells endocytosis, differentiation and proliferation. In general, they lead to decrease of intestinal/epithelial barrier function. The studies demonstrated the reduction of the epithelial cells adhesion in experimental model with CaCo cell line and anti-transglutaminase antibodies implicated the role of these antibodies in pathogenesis of celiac disease. In histology of mucous membrane from patients with untreated celiac disease, the epithelium tends to blister or totally detach from the basement membrane. The antibodies mediated inhibition of epithelial cells adhesion might be an explanation for the detachment [2]. The mechanism of tissue damage and role of autoantibodies in IBD (Leśniowski-Crohn's disease and ulcerative colitis) are not fully described [3-5].

3. Primary deficiency of humoral immunity

3.1. Isolated IgA deficiency (IgAD)

IgAD is the most common immunodeficiency of humoral immunity. The frequency of this deficiency is variable in different regions e.g. 1:400 in Finland, 1:600 in USA and 1:15000 children in Japan. The environmental factors, diet and food type, climate are suggested as explanation for this wide range of IgAD frequency [6-8]. The diagnosis of IgAD is based on low level (often below detection) of IgA, normal or compensatory high level of IgG, normal level of IgM in child older than 4 years of life. In this defect the majority of affected children (70-80%) is asymptomatic [6,7]. The remaining (20-30%) IgAD patients suffer from recurrent infections, allergies and autoimmune diseases. The respiratory and gastrointestinal tract are mainly involved. Recurrent infections of upper respiratory tract caused by different bacterias, often encapsulated are noted in younger children, the prolonged sinusitis is typical for older children and teenagers. Within IgAD patients the incidence of allergies is 20 times higher then in healthy population. The asthma, allergic rhinitis, conjunctivitis, food allergy, atopic dermatitis and urticaria are common. The autoimmunity is represented by hematological symptoms e.g. thrombocytopenia, neutropenia, hemolytic anemia and gastrointestinal disease like celiac disease, IBD. In adults with IgAD the lupus erythematodes, rheumatoid arthritis, thyroid diseases and chronic active hepatitis are noted [6,9-12]. In gastrointestinal tract, besides the autoimmune chronic inflammatory disease, the infestation with *Giardia lamblia,* bacterial infections, nodular hyperplasia are very often observed within IgAD patients [6,12]. The occurrence of clinical symptoms like abdominal pain, discomfort, diarrhea, constipation is 10-20 times higher within IgAD than within healthy children. The most probable explanation is deficient production of secretory IgA [9,13].

The pathogenesis of IgAD is based on defective terminal maturation of B cells into IgA secreting plasma cells leading to reduced level of serum and secretory (mucosal) IgA [13]. The IgA exists in both monomeric and polymeric (mainly dimeric) forms. In humans two subclasses are distinguished – IgA1 and IgA2. The dimeric IgA is formed with joining (J)-chain. The secretory IgA (sIgA) is produced locally within lymphoid tissue under the mucous membrane and released at the luminal surface of jejunum [14]. sIgA composed of IgA2 molecules characterizes high resistance to enzymatic digestion by bacterial proteases. This immunoglobulin plays an important role in protection of mucous membranes lining the gastrointestinal, respiratory and urinary tracts from pathogens present within the lumen. It is the first line of defense against microorganisms based on agglutinating activity and facilitating the clearance of pathogens [12]. The role of sIgA in selection of antigens entering through the mucous membrane is also postulated. Functions of sIgA include direct neutralization of pathogens, intracellular neutralization of viruses during transepithelial transport and inhibition of receptors mediated activation of immune system [12]. The lack of sIgA is compensated by IgG and IgM [12]. The chronic inflammatory diseases as celiac disease, Leśniowski-Crohn's disease, ulcerative colitis are only a part of gastrointestinal symptoms seen in IgAD patients. The other causes of clinical symptoms (abdominal pain, discomfort, constipation or diarrhea) include bacterial infections e.g. *Helicobacter pylori, Campylobacter jejuni* (preferentially in adults) and parasitic *Giardia lamblia* infestation. In jejunum biopsy the type of mucosal damage, villous flattening are suggesting celiac disease. After therapy eliminating *Giardia lamblia* the damage of mucous is repaired, however, in some cases this damage may be irreversible. The deep mucous damage difficult to repair is also an effect of the prolonged infection and diarrhea. sIgA is necessary for clearance of jejunum surface from e.g. parasites, bacterias and yeasts so the lack of this immunoglobulin facilitates attachment and proliferation of the organism on the surface of intestinal epithelium [6,9,11,12,15].

The frequency of Leśniowski-Crohn's disease, ulcerative colitis (mainly in adults) is not well recognized in IgAD [13,16]. Moreover, in adult patients with IgAD and gastrointestinal symptoms the nodular lymphoid hyperplasia (NLH) is observed and diagnosed as a separate clinical entity. In histology, the nodules contain the large amount of IgM-bearing cells. There are found in lamina propria, superficially in submucosa of small intestine, occasionally in large bowel, rectum or stomach. Massive occurrence of these nodules and/or large size are associated with malabsorption, flattening of villi and with obstruction in some cases [16]. The differential diagnosis of Leśniowski-Crohn's disease, nodular lymphoid hypertrophy (NLH) or celiac disease is difficult because the clinical symptoms and histological changes are overlapping.

3.2. Common variable immunodeficiency (CVID)

The common variable immunodeficiency is a heterogeneous disease with the frequency of 1:25000 to 1:66000 diagnosed first in adults. Following this, the description of clinical features and course of disease was based on observations of adult patients. CVID is diagnosed after exclusion all other known causes of hypogammaglobulinemia in adults and in children older than 4 years of life. The criteria of CVID include hypogammaglobulinemia (IgG only or IgG and IgA, IgM), low production of specific antibodies in response to vaccination and, in reasonable amount of patients, disorders of cellular response e.g. low number of T cells, reverse CD4:CD8 ratio, low response of T lymphocytes to stimulation *in vitro* [7,12,17-20]. The hypogammaglobulinemia is a result of deregulation of B-cell differentiation process and disturbances of T-cell regulatory function [18]. Impaired T-cell function (e.g. proliferation) and signaling have also been reported, including abnormalities in expression and function of T cell receptor. Number of B lymphocytes in peripheral blood and in lymph nodes are within normal range usually but the amount of plasma cells is diminished. However, in 12% of CVID patients the number of B lymphocytes in peripheral blood is below detection level [21]. Analysis of B cell subpopulation showed the reduction of memory B cells (CD19+CD27+IgD-) number in majority of CVID patients. The reduction of memory B cells is associated with more severe clinical course of CVID (e.g. splenomegaly, bronchiectases, autoimmunity). Up to now, it is the one and only parameter with predictive value for the clinical course of CVID [22,23]. However, the reduction of memory B cells did not correlate with genetic mutation described in CVID patients [17]. In subset of CVID patients (5-10%) mutation in TACI (transmembrane activator and calcium-modulator) gene was discovered. TACI is a member of TNF-like receptor family involved in transduction of signals associated with cell survival, apoptosis and isotype switching. The ligands for TACI expressed on peripheral B cells include BAFF (B-cell activating factor) and APRIL (a proliferation-inducing ligand) both in TNF ligand family expressed on monocytes and dendritic cells. BAFF and APRIL can induce isotype switching but in the absence of TACI (their receptor) plasma cell maturation and immunoglobulins production is inhibited [18]. The heterogeneity of clinical features noted within CVID patients might resembled defects like TACI deficiency, BAFF deficiency, APRIL deficiency, loss of inducible co-stimulator and others diagnosed as one disease although named "variable" [18].

The observations of CVID in children showed the difference between these patients and adults in clinical symptoms and course of disease [24]. Within patients diagnosed as adults, the chronic sinusitis, bronchiectases, chronic lung disease are more common than in CVID diagnosed in childhood (Table 1). The level of IgG (before substitution) is not predictive for type, severity and clinical course of infections [21,28]. The bacterial cultures showed *Haemophilus influenzae, Streptococcus pyogenes, Staphylococcus aureus* and *Streptococcus pneumoniae* in european population of CVID patients [16,25-26]. Moreover, the susceptibility of CVID patients to specific type of microorganism is noted so *Ureaplasma uraelyticum, Mycoplasma* (different species), enteroviruses are leading to infections and destructive chances of organs (e.g. fibrotic process in bladder). Despite the cumulating data about deficiencies of humoral immunity, the diagnosis of CVID is delayed 6 to 8 years an average, what lead to sequelae of recurrent infections e.g. lung fibrosis, bronchiectases, chronic sinusitis, underweight, inhibition of growth, anemia [20-21,25-27]. In a large study of 248 CVID patients (children and adults) the severe and recurrent infections, mostly in respiratory system, were noted in 90% of patients [19]. The chronic lung disease was noted in 27% of adult patients. The recurrent infections of lower respiratory tract may be associated with the bronchiectases. However, the bronchiectases often are a consequence of few but severe lung infections. In children, the chronic lung disease and bronchiectases are rare and seen in group of teenagers (the time of disease seemed to be an important factor). Moreover, in children with CVID the lymphoid interstitial pneumonia (LIP); unusual and rare type of lung disease is seen. In our group of 52 children with CVID the histology of lung biopsy showed LIP in 2 patients (boy and girl). In both cases the prolonged therapy with steroids was effective but adverse reactions to steroids limited this therapy. The lung fibrosis was slowed down although still progressing what lead to respiratory insufficiency despite of regular IgG substitution [personal observations]. The chronic sinusitis, LIP or bronchiectases are developing independently to regular substitution of IgG, even in higher dose [28].

Common variable immunodeficiency	Adults	Children
Infections before the diagnosis	Chronic sinusitis, chronic lung disease, bronchiectases	Recurrent acute infections of respiratory tract, ORL and sinuses (90% of patients)
Autoimmunity:hematology	thrombocytopenia, leukopenia (neutropenia), hemolytic anemia	thrombocytopenia, leukopenia (neutropenia), hemolytic anemia
gastrointestinal tract	atrophic gastritis, pernicious anemia, ulcerative colitis, primary biliary cirrhosis, autoimmune hepatitis, Leśniowski-Crohn's disease	celiac disease, Leśniowski-Crohn's disease, atrophic gastritis (teenagers)
systemic	rheumatoid arthritis, sclerodermia, systemic lupus erythematosus, Sjogren syndrome	juvenile rheumatoid arthritis (rare, teenagers)
other	lymphomas, gastric cancer, granulomas formation	LIP (lymphoid interstitial pneumonia), lymphomas

Table 1. The differences between CVID in adults and children

The autoimmunity is associated with CVID in about 20-30% of patients and the hematological symptoms are most common [10,16,17,19,21,29-34]. The dysregulation of immune system in CVID seemed to be paradoxical; while antibody production in response to pathogens and vaccines is impaired, at the same time the production autoantibodies might be excessive [32]. In large study of 311 adult patients with CVID the autoimmunity was diagnosed in 37% (116 patients). The cytopenias were noted in 55 patients including thrombocytopenia (41 patients), hemolytic anemia (17 patients) and neutropenia (10 patients) [30]. The slightly lower percentage of autoimmunity (22%) was noted within other studied group of 248 CVID adult patients but the thrombocytopenia was most frequent [19,32]. In reasonable number of patients the autoimmune symptoms preceded the diagnosis of CVID [17,19,21,34].

The autoimmune/inflammatory diseases of gastrointestinal tract (IBD) including Leśniowski-Crohn's disease, celiac disease, pernicious anemia, autoimmune liver disease, ulcerative colitis and nodular lymphoid hyperplasia (NLH) are the second group of complications (coexisting symptoms/diseases) noted in 20-50% of CVID patients [9,13,16,18-19,21,28-29,34-36]. The clinical symptoms of IBD in CVID are similar to patients without CVID but often more discrete, milder and unspecific. In children unspecific abdominal pain, weight loss and inhibition of growth are prominent. The typical symptoms like diarrhea, constipation and dyspepsia, disturbances of jejunum motility, weakness are present too but they could be often neglected and explained by school stress, problems of diet, life style and maturation. In both groups of CVID patients the results of malabsorption are observed [13,16,19].

The diagnosis of autoimmune diseases is based on presence of antibodies and autoantibodies in serum. In CVID there are two problems: low production of specific antibodies as a marker of immune system dysfunction and lack of antibodies of given immunoglobulin class e.g. IgA in cases of CVID with IgA deficiency. The second problem is associated with histology of tissues involved in autoimmune process. The disturbances of B cell ontogeny seen as abnormal maturation, impaired somatic hypermutation and lack of memory B cell are associated with different histology of jejunum in IBD in CVID [13,36]. In biopsy of jejunum mucous of patients with celiac or Leśniowski-Crohn's disease the low number, even lack of B cells and plasma cells in infiltrations are observed. This atypical pattern of infiltrating cells in CVID became a reason for named the celiac disease as celiac-like, similar – Crohn's-like instead Crohn's disease [13,37].

3.3. Substitution of immunoglobulins in CVID

The main goal of regular substitution of immunoglobulin IgG (intravenous or subcutaneous) in CVID is replacing the specific antibodies. These antibodies produced by healthy blood donors after vaccinations and contact with common pathogens prevent the infections with spectrum of common pathogens. The dose for substitution is wide (0.4 - 0.8 g/kg body weight) with the suggestion for higher dose in first period of IgG substitution to obtained patient's stabilization ("steady-state"). After 6-8 months of regular substitution, the maintaining dose is usually about 0.4 g/kg body weight. The half-life of IgG is 21-24 days indicating intravenous infusion of IgG (IVIG) in every 3-4 weeks [16-17,20,28,38-40]. The modifications of dose are possible in two ways – higher (or lower) dose for singular infusion and shorter (or longer) distance between infusions. The bacterial infections, wounds healing after injuries or surgery are consuming immunoglobulins so higher dose of IgG is recommended. Moreover, the individual variations in half-life of administered IgG, shorter half-time in patients with chronic lung disease or gastrointestinal disease need the modifications of IVIG substitution (patient-tailored), precise monitoring of IgG level and clinical status of patient [20]. The purpose of substitution is to prevent infections, at least, to decrease their frequency and moderate their clinical course. Moreover, the regular substitution of IgG in replacing dose is effective in some autoimmune disease like chronic thrombocytopenia, chronic neutropenia [16]. This effect is probably associated with anti inflammatory activity of IgG, although the precise mechanisms are not described. The different mechanisms responsible for anti-inflammatory activity on IgG preparation are defined for the high dose of immunoglobulins used in autoimmune diseases. It might be that; the regularity, long time of substitution and accumulation of small repeated effects are responsible for anti-inflammatory activity of IVIG in low dose, similar to anti-inflammatory effects of IVIG high dose (1.0-2.0 g/kg b.w.) [20,38]. The adverse reactions of IVIG occurred immediately during the infusion or after up to 4 days. They are mild or sever including anaphylactic shock [16,41]. Most often the fever, chills, pain (headache, abdominal pain) are noted in children during the infusion. The most severe, late reactions are the consequence of tissue distribution of immunoglobulin particularly into central nervous system. Heavy and progressive headache, vomiting, disturbances of vision, speech and balance keeping are typical. The therapy with intensive hydration and steroids given intravenously are usually effective. In a case of occurrence of severe adverse reactions the subcutaneous (SCIG) form of substitution is recommended. The amount of immunoglobulins given monthly is divided in four portions (0.1 g/kg of body weight per week) administered with special pomp. The effectiveness is similar to intravenous substitution, the adverse reaction are very rare and limited to the place of injection. SCIG is form of home therapy very comfortable for patients, offering the independence from the hospital.

3.4. Antibiotics in prophylaxis of infections

In part of children with CVID the effect of IVIG or SCIG is weak and the infections occurred despite regular substitution. In this group of patients, especially with chronic inflammation (sinusitis, lymphocyte infiltrating pneumonia – LIP), bronchiectases, lung fibrosis and (in some cases) permanent leukopenia; the prophylaxis with antibiotics is suggested. The 3-4 months' periods of antibiotics or trimetoprim introduced in prophylactic dose help in control of infections and improve the patient's comfort. The therapy with antibiotics is still a matter of discussion and approaches to this therapy varies depending of clinical centre, severity of cases. The recommendation for antibiotics prophylaxis is prevention of the endocarditis during invasive procedures [28].

4. Diagnostic procedures in celiac disease and inflammatory bowel diseases

4.1. The standards of IBD and celiac disease diagnosis

Standard of IBD diagnosis includes the clinical symptoms, laboratory tests (e.g. antibodies detection), imaging procedures (gastroscopy, colonoscopy, other radiological methods) and histological examination of jejunum biopsy [4,42-49]. The laboratory markers are helpful in early diagnosis preceding the onset of severe clinical symptoms in many patients. In last years the detection of antibodies associated with autoimmune process in gastrointestinal tract are commonly used as screening in risk group of children including immunodeficiencies (IgAD, CVID).

4.1.1. The immunological markers

The typical clinical symptoms of celiac disease (periods of diarrhea or constipation, abdominal pain, cramps, feeling of discomfort, low weight with difficulty to gain) in small children are noted in about 20% of all patients diagnosed as celiac [51]. The remaining patients demonstrate the results of jejunum functional disorders leading to sideropenic anemia, osteopenia, afts, enamel damage, delay of puberty, concentrations problems and hypoproteinemia or many others without direct association with gastrointestinal tract. The latent, silent or asymptomatic forms of celiac disease are diagnosed in older children, teenagers and adults. The familiar predisposition is associated with expression of HLA-DQ2 and HLA-DQ8 determinants [43,48-50].

For celiac disease the serological assays include antibodies to: endomysium, transglutaminase and gliadin. The antibodies against gliadin (deamidated form – GAF) are tested in IgA and IgG class with indirect immunofluorescence in serum diluted 1:10 [52]. The sensitivity and specificity is declared as 100% in IgG class and 95-99% in IgA class [53]. The endomysial antibodies (EMA) are associated with reticulin-gliadin complex and transglutaminase as enzyme active in formation of this complex. Antibodies are tested with indirect immunofluorescence in serum (dilution 1:10) with tissue slides of monkey's jejunum or smooth muscles (endomysium contains reticulin type 1 (R1) - basic antigen for endomysial antibodies). The serial dilution of serum is helpful in monitoring the results of Gluten Free Diet (GFD). The sensitivity and specificity of these antibodies in IgA class is up to 100% [48,50]. The test performed in IgG class is valid and clinically significant for IgAD patients.

The discovery of role of tissue transglutaminase (tTg) in pathomechanism of celiac disease helped in understanding the induction of immune response to gliadin. This enzyme deamidated and/or transamidated gliadin proteins increasing their immunogenicity. Moreover, tTg is facilitating the formation of gliadin-reticulin complex and location of these complexes deposits on subepithelial basic membrane. The role of tTg in reduction of intestinal epithelial cell adhesion and in detachment of epithelium was described recently [2]. Antibodies against tTg are tested with ELISA commercially available kits for IgA and IgG class of immunoglobulins. The sensitivity of this test is 96%, the specificity – 98% [48,50]. The results of detection tTg antibodies are showed as optical density recalculated to standard curve. Results above 20 units are recognized as positive. High specificity of tTg antibodies and occurrence in level above 200 units seemed to be satisfactory for celiac disease diagnose without further biopsy of jejunum [50]. These antibodies are clinically significant in IgA class preferentially; with exception for IgAD when antibodies in IgG class are considered [52]. The introduction of GFD leads to decrease of antibodies production below detection level in 3-6 months in majority of patients [48,50]. Persistent high level of antibodies to tTg is observed in celiac disease refractory to GFD (RCD type I and RCD type II)[54]. Moreover, antibodies against tTg are observed in about 20% of patients with Leśniowski-Crohn's disease. The clinical significance of these antibodies in Leśniowski-Crohn's disease is unknown. It might be thought; that the inflammation and lymphocytic infiltrates are spreading from region typical for celiac disease to another part of jejunum. However, the localization of Leśniowski-Crohn's disease in other parts of gastrointestinal tract like esophagus or large bowel and presence of anti tTg antibodies is not supporting this idea [50].

The antibodies against *Saccharomyces cerevisiae* (ASCA) antigens are observed in 60-80% of Leśniowski-Crohn's disease patients [5,55]. Occurrence of these antibodies is explained by increased permeability of barrier between jejunum lumen:submucosal tissue and loss of precise selective role of this barrier. The direct contact between yeast and immunocompetent cells is possible and uncontrolled what stimulates production of antibodies. In healthy people this yeast is normally seen in distal region of jejunum (Bauchin' valve) without the induction of antibodies production. ASCA in IgA class are clinically significant in patients with normal IgA level as for IgAD patients the IgG class antibodies are assayed. For both class IgG and IgA the level above 20 RU/ml is considered as positive. However, comparison of ASCA in IgA and IgG in Leśniowski-Crohn's patients showed ASCA in both immunoglobulin's classes in majority of patients what suggested (according the author) that both IgA and IgG ASCA should be measured [5]. The diagnostic specificity of ASCA is 99% and sensitivity in Leśniowski-Crohn's patients is 80%, positive predictive value - 88% [5]. The new tests (for ELISA) are based on eluated singular proteins of *Saccharomyces cerevisiae* membrane with the similar specificity for Leśniowski-Crohn's disease.

The immunofluorescence indirect test offers detection of antibodies to exocrine pancreas cells cytoplasm (PAB) and their products as useful for diagnosis of Leśniowski-Crohn's disease [55]. Two distinct patterns were noted with the patients' sera tested on human pancreas tissue. The following pancreatic autoantigens were identified; glycoproteins expressed as glycosyl phosphoinositol (GP1) and membrane-anchored protein (GP2) [4]. GP2 is a glycosylated protein accounting for more than half of the zymogen granule membrane proteins in acinar cells. Recent studies showed the expression of GP2 is not limited to pancreatic acinar cells but is noted on epithelial cells follicle-associated or in Peyer's patches too [4]. In the follicle-associated epithelial cells GP2 is restricted to M cells. These cells are located mainly in distal part of ileum being a site of original inflammation in reasonable percentage of patients with Leśniowski-Crohn's disease [4]. The frequency of PAB antibodies in patients with Leśniowski-Crohn's disease is rather low (14%-30%)[4,55-56] however, the specificity of this assay is 93%, positive predictive value is 77% and negative predictive value – 45% [55-56]. The clinical observations indicated the association of PAB with stricturing or penetrating form of the Leśniowski-Crohn's disease [4] but this data were not supported by others. It means, that PAB are independent to disease activity, localization, clinical course and response to therapy with corticosteroids and/or immunosuppression [4,55].

The antinuclear (ANA), antimyeloperoxidase antibodies (pANCA) and against goblet cells (mucins are autoantigen, GAB) antibodies are commonly used for immunological diagnosis of ulcerative colitis (UC). Presence of these antibodies is detected with immunofluorescence and ELISA. The antibodies against neutrophils cytoplasmic antigens (ANCA) are recognized as cytoplasmic (proteins 3 - cANCA) and perinuclear (myeloperoxidase - pANCA) based on microscopic pattern [5,56]. pANCA prevalence in UC is estimated as 71.4%, in comparison to Leśniowski-Crohn's patients – 2.3% and healthy control – 4.8% of positive seras. Comparison of IgA and IgG class of pANCA in group of 28 UC patients showed higher titer for IgA but in majority of patients pANCA were present in both classes of immunoglobulins. The results of ELISA assay for ANCA with different eluated antigens showed lower percentage of patients with positive results than immunofluorescence. Probably the antigens used for ELISA are not covering all possible neutrophil cytoplasmic antigens reacting with patients serum [56]. The antigens identified as responsible for pANCA immune response in UC patients are localized not only in cytoplasm of neutrophils but also inside nucleus (histone 1, nonhistone chromosomal protein, high mobility group of proteins) [56].

The presence of antibodies against goblet cells (GAB) is tested with immunofluorescence (normal jejunum slides) or ELISA. In study of 28 UC patients GAB was detected in 46.4%

[56] in both classes of immunoglobulins with much higher titer for antibodies in IgA class. The sensitivity of GAB is estimated as 46%, specificity – 100% predictive positive value – 100% and predictive negative value – 73% [56]. Studies of reactivity of GAB with different tissue slides from gastrointestinal tract showed the best reactivity in appendix tissue [3]. The reaction with ileum, sigmoid and rectum tissue was from weak to strong with the tendency to resemble clinically affected intestinal segments [3].

The antibodies to enterocytes were described as clinically significant marker for autoimmune enteropathy [43,57]. The detection of these antibodies with indirect immunofluorescence showed a linear pattern most frequently along the apex or brush border of enterocyte on frozen section of human small bowel. These antibodies are predominantly IgG class and have been reported to occur after the mucosal damage onset [57].

4.1.2.The histology of jejunum in celiac disease and Leśniowski-Crohn's disease

The typical changes in celiac disease are classified according Marsh, Oberhuber and Corazza [48]. The classification according Marsh (4 types) is commonly used and number of intraepithelial lymphocytes (IEL), ratio crypts:villi heights, villi structure and height are basic parameters. In advanced stage (Marsh type 3) severe inflammation, flat villi and hyperplastic crypts are noted. In other classification e.g. Oberhuber the mucous of jejunum damage is divide into 8 stages including stage 0 of normal mucous structure, without changes. Classification proposed by Corazza is simplest and described only 3 stages – grade A – normal architecture of mucous, grade B1 and grade B2 – with atrophic villi up to flat mucous. The problem of celiac disease diagnosis arises when patients with clinical symptoms and serology tests results suggesting celiac disease have no visible changes in histology of mucous membrane (Marsh type 0, Oberhuber type 0, Corazza grade A) [48,58]. For these patients, electron microscopy assay is useful for detection of submicroscopical changes of enterocytes which support celiac disease diagnosis or suggest the diagnosis of microscopic enteritis [48,51,57-59]. However, observations of patients with typical clinical symptoms of celiac disease without changes of mucous showed improvement on GFD supporting the clinical diagnosis of latent type of celiac disease [50].

The infiltrations and formation of new lymphoid nodules, increase of IEL number are typical for chronic inflammation of jejunum. Infiltration in celiac disease consists lymphocytes (T and B), plasma cells and some monocytes. Within the lymphocytes present in mucous membrane the cells with TCRγ/δ characteristic are observed. In Leśniowski-Crohn's disease the infiltration contains lymphocytes, monocytes, neutrophils and plasma cells. The similar pattern with increased number of neutrophils is noted in UC. The proportion between the cells within infiltrate is associated with profile of proinflammatory cytokines released locally and induction of antibodies production as effect of contact of antigen presenting cells (APC) with e.g. MPO from neutrophils or the nuclei debris after cell death in situ [45-46].

The nature and function of T regulatory (Treg) subpopulation of T lymphocytes was extensively studied in relation to IBD. Natural Treg (CD4+/CD25+/FoxP3+) from thymus and iTreg (inducible Treg) are involved in monitoring the immune response, maintaining the immune balance, prevention of excessive and potentially harmful immune activation within mucous of gastrointestinal tract [47,61-62]. The study of Treg lymphocytes (CD4/CD25/FoxP3) within the lamina propria patients with Leśniowski-Crohn's disease and UC showed increased number of these cells; whereas the number in peripheral blood was decreased as compare to healthy people. It suggested central role of this population in local regulation of prolonged inflammatory process within jejunum wall [44]. Immunohistochemistry is the basic method for detection of Treg lymphocytes in biopsy specimens, the flow cytometry is used for assay of Treg number in peripheral blood. The immunohistochemistry is commonly used for analysis of proportion and characteristics of different cells within inflammation e.g. macrophages, T and B lymphocytes, plasma cells and others. This approach based on histopathology of jejunum helps to classify the subgroups of IBD patients. It will create specific "biological signature" unique to each patient so this patient can be treated with rational, individual therapy targeting the specific defect or aberrations underlying intestinal inflammatory pathway [47].

5. Problems of gastrointestinal autoimmune diseases in children with PID

5.1. Celiac disease in IgAD and CVID patients

Celiac disease diagnosed as latent, silent or untypical form in children older than infants comprises about 80% of celiac patients. The clinical symptoms are discrete or absent so the diagnosis is often delayed. There have been more than 200 symptoms reported in association with gluten sensitivity [51]. The effects of jejunum dysfunction (malabsorption) presented as low level of iron resistant to oral therapy, vitamins, calcium, zinc and other minerals deficiency are suggesting celiac disease in children and teenagers [63]. The problem of celiac disease diagnosis in CVID and IgAD children lays in paucity and unspecificity of symptoms and overlapping with symptoms typical for IgAD or CVID with lack of IgA (e.g. abdomen pain, episodes of diarrhea, chronic diarrhea, food allergy).

High prevalence of celiac disease in IgAD patients (10-20 times higher risk than in population) suggested the common genetic background for these two diseases. It was demonstrated that ancestral haplotype HLA-A1,Cw7,B8,DR3,DQ2 is important for association between IgA and celiac disease [6,12-13]. However, the observations of frequency of celiac disease within IgAD population did not support this correlation because the observed frequency of celiac disease is still lower than expected based on genetic background [13]. Other hypothesis indicated that abnormal handling of gluten and gliadin in absence of IgA might induce the mucous damage and onset of clinical symptoms of celiac disease. The study of B lymphocyte stimulator (BLyS) and a proliferation-inducing ligand (APRIL) in patients with IgAD and celiac disease showed increased of both factors in IgAD as compared to healthy persons but differences between IgAD with celiac disease and without celiac disease were below significance. Increase of APRIL level might be interpreted as part of the mechanism of compensation leading to overproduction of IgG and IgM [64]. The analysis of IEL TCRγ/δ showed highest level in IgAD with celiac disease, increased number in IgAD - higher than control [60].

The production of antibodies to gliadin, endomysium and to transglutaminase are preserved in IgAD patients but in IgG class. However, in some cases of IgAD the presence and high level of anti transglutaminase antibodies in IgA class is seen. In these cases the trace level of IgA (below detection in nephelometry) is enough to show antibodies to tTg with high sensitive technique of ELISA (personal observations). Within our 47 children with IgAD antibodies for celiac disease were noted in 11 patients (23%) – antibodies for gliadin – in 9 patients, for endomysium and for tTg in one patient each. Celiac disease was diagnosed based on anti tTg antibodies (in IgA and IgG class) in one patient without clinical symptoms. The histology of jejunum is typical for the celiac disease including cases diagnosed early with no changes (Marsh type 0) and similar to changes observed in children without IgAD. It is obvious, that in IgAD plasma cells producing IgA are missing, although total number of plasma cells is preserved. In majority of IgAD patients the gluten-free diet (GFD) is effective [16].

In CVID the problem of serological diagnosis of celiac diseases is more complex because of low production of antibodies and IgA deficiency in part of CVID patients. In consequence of these the possibility of serological diagnosis of autoimmune disease in CVID is excluded by many authors [9,13,37]. However, the permanent stimulation with autoantigens is leading to production of antibodies despite of decreased function of immune system. Level of autoantibodies is detectable but lower than in patients without immune deficiency [personal observation, 36]. In our study of 40 children with CVID antibodies for gliadin were noted in 3 patients (7.5%), for endomysium and tTg in 2 patients followed with diagnosis of celiac disease. Algorithm for celiac disease diagnosis is shown in Table 2. In jejunum biopsy the mucous contains excess of IEL (mainly T), lymphoid aggregates, granulomas, crypts distortion. Within this group of patients the celiac disease is often refractory to GFD (RCD) leading to malabsorption syndrome and severe clinical conditions [20]. Poor response to GFD suggests the distinct pathogenesis of celiac disease with 2 forms recently recognized [13]. In type I of RCD the IEL expressed normally CD3 and CD8 determinants as well as polyclonal T-cell receptor (TCR) arrangement. In RCD type II the aberrant lymphocyte population is expanded with loss of surface expression of CD3 and CD8, intracellular presence of CD3 determination and monoclonal TCR arrangement. Type II of RCD is associated with poor prognosis, increased mortality due to progressing malabsorption syndrome and due to T-cell lymphoma in reasonable number of patients [54]. Therapy includes supplementation with proteins, vitamins and microelements, parenteral nutrition, probiotics, steroids (given intravenously in high dose) and antibiotics for bacterial overgrowth in jejunum [16]. The second line of therapy offers immunosuppression (azathioprine) and/or monoclonal antibodies against TNF (infliximab, etanercept, humira) in patients with active, progressive disease [65].

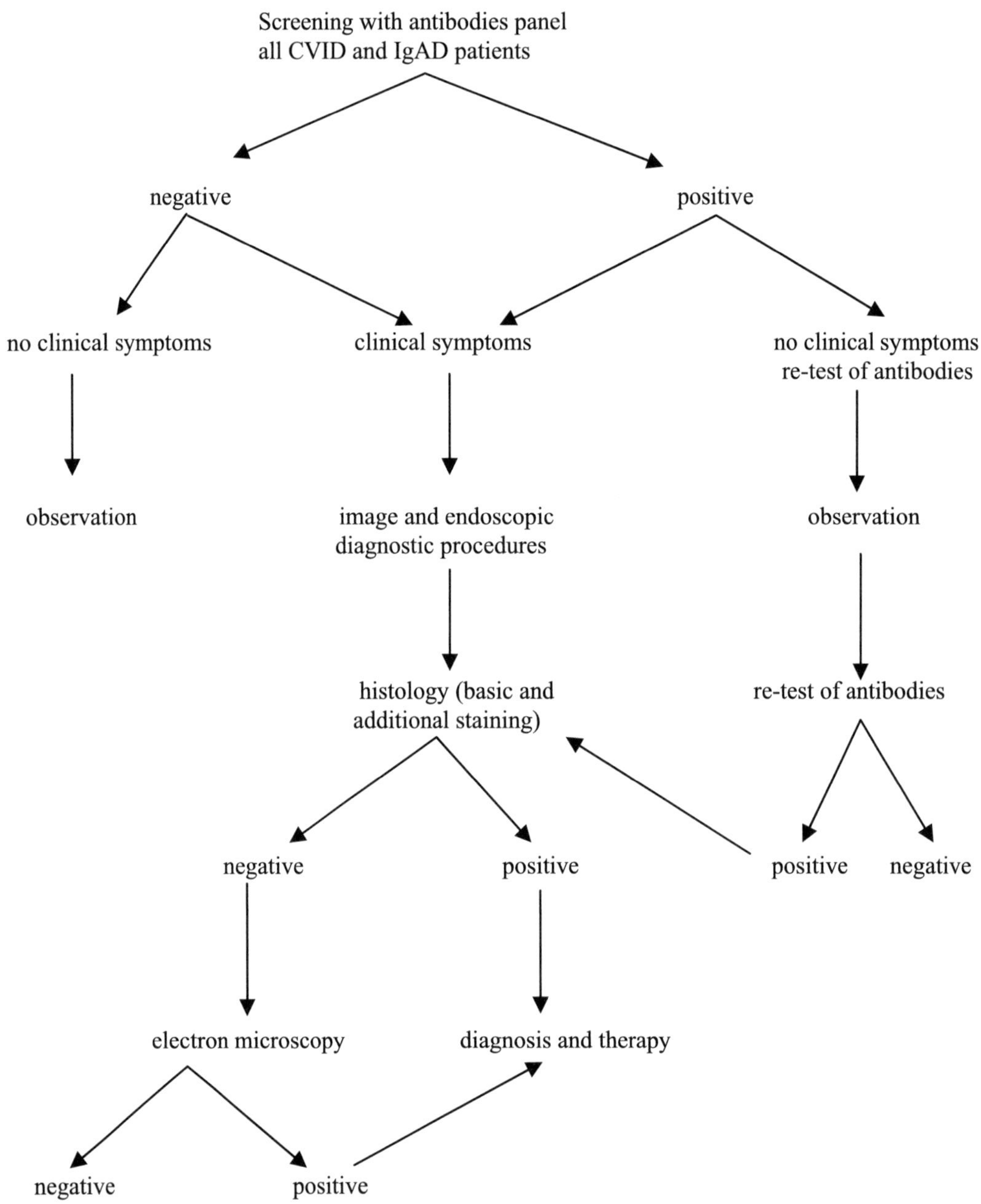

Table 2. Algorithm of the diagnostic procedures for celiac disease and IBD in CVID and IgAD patients

5.2. Leśniowski-Crohn's disease and UC in IgAD and CVID patients

Chronic diarrhea is noted as a typical clinical symptom of gastrointestinal involvement seen in wide range of adult patients (10% - 50%) with CVID [13,16,18,20]. In children with CVID and IgAD the chronic diarrhea is much less frequent but data are based on relatively small number of patients. IBD are sporadic in IgAD children with clinical course similar to children without IgAD. Within CVID patients IBD remain a significant problem in 19-32% of patients [20]. Moreover, IBD in patients with CVID is recognized as distinct form sharing histological features consistent more with lymphocytic colitis, collagenous colitis than classic IBD [13,37]. In patients, mainly adults, with Leśniowski-Crohn's disease and CVID the formation of granuloma within jejunum wall is observed. Furthermore, the substitution of immunoglobulins does not inhibit and/or reverse symptoms of chronic colitis [13,15]. The different explanations are proposed but hypothesis that IgG from immunoglobulin preparations are not able to reach the lumen of intact jejunum particularly in CVID patients without IgA seemed to be interesting. Other possible explanations include Treg defects, T cell driven inflammation, different patterns of locally produced cytokines as compared to Leśniowski-Crohn's disease in patients without CVID [13]. The special role of T lymphocytes in CVID patients with gastrointestinal symptoms was indicated by different histology of jejunum. Despite the lack of plasma cells in biopsy specimens as typical and characteristic; the villi flattening, increased number of IEL and lymphocytes in lamina propria, increased epithelial apoptosis were observed in CVID patients [13,15,20]. The study of cytokines produced locally in lamina propria showed decreased production of IL-23, IL-17 and TNF in CVID patients with Leśniowski-Crohn's disease as compare to patients without CVID, what suggest alternative pathway of inflammation [13].

Therapy of Leśniowski-Crohn's disease in CVID is generally similar as for patients without immunodeficiency although inflammation in CVID might be more difficult to control. Immunosuppression (e.g.azathioprine, cyclosporine) is used when anti inflammatory drugs and steroids (rapidly metabolized budesonide) are without results and process of inflammation is still active. Induction of remission with anti cytokine monoclonal antibodies (infliximab, etanercept) is effective in CVID patients but the very careful monitoring of infections, particularly fungal, is necessary due to T cell defects [13].

The frequency of UC within CVID and IgAD patients is not known. The large study of 248 patients with CVID including children and adults showed the UC only in 7 patients [19]. In this study ten patients was described as having a significant malabsorption but without specific gastrointestinal diagnosis what showed the problems of establishing the diagnosis in immune deficiency patients [19].

5.3. Differential diagnosis – Collagenous sprue and autoimmune enteropathy

The difficulties in diagnosis of celiac disease, poor response to GFD, IBD with different histology of jejunum seen in patients with CVID, IgAD and gastrointestinal symptoms suggested searching for other diseases overlapping clinical features. The collagenous sprue is severe malabsorptive disorder with histology similar to celiac disease. It is rare disorder characterized by small intestinal villi and crypts atrophy, increased IEL number, subepithelial collagen deposit entrapping cellular components of lamina propria [49]. The clinical and histological similarities (villi atrophy, poor response to GFD during one year) might suggest the refractory or poorly controlled celiac disease. However, in collagenous sprue the serological test and HLA-DQ2 or HLA-DQ8 are negative what indicate separate entity. The relation between celiac disease, refractory sprue and collagenous sprue is still a matter of discussion but collagenous sprue seemed to be a part of refractory sprue based on poor response to GFD [49]. In histology in collagenous sprue; the subepithelial collagen layer thicker than 12 μm, embedding small capillaries and lamina propria entrapping cells e.g. lymphocytes, fibroblasts are typical. These entrapped cellular elements are a mandatory criterion for this disease. Celiac disease is characterized by increased number of IEL whereas in collagenous sprue these lymphocytes are absent. The precise diagnosis is important because the collagenous sprue is progressing with high ratio of death due to malabsorption and malnutrition. The aggressive therapy includes steroids, immunosuppression and total parenteral nutrition. Up to now, the collagenous sprue was not observed in CVID and IgAD patients but the occurrence of RCD, progressing malabsorption syndrome might suggest existence of this disease within immune deficiency patients.

The term of microscopic enteritis was used for patients with symptoms of malabsorption without prominent inflammation, villous effacement or ulceration seen in conventional light microscopy [59]. This observation may explain the co-existence of symptomatic gluten sensitivity, malabsorption and normally looking mucosa (Marsh 0) [48,58-59]. In patients with RCD the electron microscopy assay seemed to be useful for diagnosis of microscopic enteritis what helps to recognize celiac disease with mild or minimal mucosal abnormalities.

The autoimmune enteropathy is not associated with celiac disease but represents heterogeneous entity consisting protracted diarrhea in young children with circulating antibodies. Affected patients appear to fall into 2 groups: with or without immune deficiency. The syndrome of intractable or protracted diarrhea of infancy was associated with high mortality. Now, the parenteral nutrition, symptomatic therapy of complications, improvement of diagnostic modalities has permitted prolonged survival of these children [57]. Immune deficiency seen in these patients were X-linked syndrome of neonatal diabetes with polyendocrinopathy, IPEX (Immunodysregulation, Polyendocrinopathy, Enteropathy, X-linked), T-cell defects, CVID and IgAD. The immunological tests showed a variety of antibodies but most important for diagnosis are antibodies against enterocyte circulating in patients serum. Other antibodies were typical for autoimmune disease of endocrine glands (anti thyroid peroxidase - TPO, Langerhan's islet) and kidney, liver diseases (anti tubular basement membrane, antinuclear, anti-smooth muscles, liver-kidney antigen). Antigens for enterocyte antibodies were characterized as 50 kD and 75 kD proteins present in enterocyte cytoplasm. Diagnosis in neonate and infants with chronic severe diarrhea is based on small jejunum biopsy and immunological tests. The antibodies anti enterocyte are suggesting the autoimmune enteropathy. Symptomatic therapy include diet, parenteral nutrition, "immunological" therapy include steroids (but with no great success), immunosuppression with different drugs e.g. azathioprine, cyclophosphamide and cyclosporine. The second line of therapy offers tacrolimus with a good response. IPEX syndrome patient has been treated with hematopoietic stem cell transplantation [57].

6. General remarks

The diagnosis of IBD and celiac disease is based on clinical symptoms, laboratory tests and endoscopic procedures. Antibodies are the markers of these diseases despite that their role in pathomechanism of chronic inflammation is not fully recognized. The weak production of antibodies in response to vaccine antigens in humoral immunity deficiency seemed to be overestimated since the prolonged stimulation with antigens persistent in contact with immunocompetent cells induce production of antibodies. The antibodies detection used as screening is helpful in early diagnosis due to predictive value of these antibodies. From the other side, in patients with immunodeficiency clinical symptoms might be mild, unspecific and suggesting the association with basic disease (CVID or IgAD) not the concomitant autoimmunity. The high risk of autoimmune diseases in CVID and IgAD is an indication for antibodies screening in these patients but the results should be analyzed with caution. Patients with immunodeficiency are different in all aspects of their immune system function including response to infections, chronic inflammations, autoimmunity prevalence and high risk of tumours. The replacement of specific antibodies with substitution of immunoglobulin for CVID patients is covering only a small part from the complex defect in function of immune system.

Author details

Anna Pituch-Noworolska and Katarzyna Zwonarz
Department of Clinical Immunology,
Polish-American Institute of Pediatrics, Medical College, Jagiellonian University, Kraków, Poland

7. References

[1] Elkon K, Casali P (2008) Nature and function of autoantibodies. Nat. Clin. Pract. Rheumatol. 4; 491-498.

[2] Lindfors K, Kaukinen K (2012) Contribution of celiac disease autoantibodies to the disease process. Expert Rev. Clin. Immunol. 8; 151-154.

[3] Ardesjo B, Portela-Gomez GM, Rorsman F, Gerdin E, Loof L, Grimelius L, Kampe O, Ekwall O (2008) Immunoreactivity against goblet cells in patients with inflammatory bowel disease. Inflamm. Bowel Dis. 14; 652-661.

[4] Bogdanos DP, Rigopoulou EI, Smyk DS, Roggenbuck D, Reinhold D, Forbes A, Laass MW, Conrad C (2011) Diagnostic value, clinical utility and pathogenic significance of reactivity to the molecular targets of Crohn's disease specific-pancreatic autoantibodies. Autoimmunity Reviews 11; 143-148.

[5] Papp M, Norman GL, Altorjay I, Lakatos PL (2007) Utility of serological markers in inflammatory bowel diseases: gadget or magic?. World J. Gastroenterol. 14; 2028-2036.

[6] Aghamohammadi A, Cheragi T, Gharagozlou M, Movahedi M, Rezaei N, Yeganeh M, Parvaneh N, Abolhassani H, Pourpak Z, Moin M (2009) IgA deficiency:

correlation between clinical and immunological phenaotypes. J. Clin. Immunol. 29; 130-136.

[7] Fried AJ, Bonilla FA (2009) Pathogenesis, diagnosis, and management of primary antibody deficiencies and infections. Clin. Microbiol. Rev. 22; 396-414.

[8] Vries de E, Driessen G (2011) Primary immunodeficiency in children: a diagnostic challenge. Eur. J. Pediatr. 170; 169-177.

[9] Arkwright PD, Abinun M, Cant AJ (2002) Autoimmunity in human primary immunodeficiency diseases. Blood 99; 2694-2702.

[10] Cunningham-Rundles C (2002) Hematologic complications of primary immune deficiencies. Blood Reviews 16; 61-64.

[11] Diez R, Garcia MJ, Vivas S, Arias L, Rascarachi G, Pozo E, Vaquero LM, Miguel A, Sierra M, Calleja S, De Morales RJM (2010) Gastrointestinal manifestations in patients with primary immunodeficiencies causing antibody deficiency. Gastroenterol. Hepatol. 33; 347-351.

[12] Jacob CMA, Pastorino AC, Fahl K, Carneiro-Sampaio M, Monteiro RC (2008) Autoimmunity in IgA deficiency. J. Clin. Immunol. 28; S56-S61.

[13] Agarwal S, Mayer L (2009) Pathogenesis and treatment of gastrointestinal disease in antibody deficiency syndromes. J. Allergy Clin. Immunol. 124; 658-664.

[14] Vale AM, Schroeder HW (2010) Clinical consequences of defects in B-cell development. J. Allergy Clin. Immunol. 125; 78-787.

[15] Kobrynski LJ, Mayer L (2011) Diagnosis and treatment of primary immunodeficiency disease in patients with gastrointestinal symptoms. Clin. Immunol. 139; 238-248.

[16] Agarwal S, Cunningham-Rundles C (2009) Autoimmunity in common variable immunodeficiency. Current Allergy and Asthma Reports. 9; 347-352.

[17] Blanco-Quiros A, Solis-Sanchez P, Garrote-Adrados JA, Arranz-Sanz E (2006) Common variable immunodeficiency. Old questions are getting clearer. Allergol. Immunopathol. 34; 263-275.

[18] Daniels JA, Lederman HM, Maitra A, Montgomery EA (2007) Gastrointestinal tract pathology in patients with common variable immunodeficiency (CVID). Am. J. Surg. Pathol. 31; 1800-1812.

[19] Cunningham-Rundles C, Bodian C (1999) Common variable immunodeficiency. Clin. Immunol. 92; 34-48.

[20] Cunningham-Rundles C (2010) How I treat common variable immune deficiency. Blood 116; 7-15.

[21] Chapel H, Cunningham-Rundles C (2009) Update in understanding common variable immunodeficiency disorders (CVIDs) and the management of patients with these conditions. Brit. J. Haematol. 145; 709-727.

[22] Alachkar H, Taubenheim N, Haenay MR, Dyrandy A, Arkwright PD (2006) Memory switched B cell percentage and not serum immunoglobulin concentration is associated with clinical xcomplications in children and adults with specific

antibodiy deficiency and common variable immunodeficiency. Clin. Immunol. 120; 310-318.

[23] Huck K, Feyen O, Ghost S, Beltz K, Bellert S, Niehues T (2009) Memory B-cells in healthy and antibody deficient children. Clinical Immunol. 131; 50-59.

[24] Glocker E, Ehl S, Grimbacher B (2007) Common variable immunodeficiency in children. Curr. Opinion Pediatr. 19; 685-692.

[25] Llobet MP, Soler-Palacin P, Detkova D, Hernandez M, Caragol I, Espanol T (2009) Common variable immunodeficiency: 20-years experience at a single centre. Ped. Allergy Immunol. 20; 113-118.

[26] Oksenhendler E, Gerard L, Fieschi C, Malphettes M, Moulliot G, Jaussaud R, Viallard J-F, Gardembas M, Galicier L, Schleinitz N, Suarez F, Soulas-Sprauel P, Hachulla E, Jaccard A, Gardeur A, Theodorou I, Rabian C, Debre P (2008) Infections in 252 patients with common variable immunodeficiency. Clin. Infectious Dis. 46; 1547-1554.

[27] Urschel S, Kaykci L, Wintergerst U, Nothes G, Jansson A, Bolechradfsky BH (2009) Common variable immunodeficiency disorders in children: delayed diagnosis despite typical clinical presentation. J. Pediatr. 154; 888-894.

[28] Bethune CA, Spickett GP (2000) Common variable immunodeficiency. BioDrug 13; 243-253.

[29] Arason GJ, Jorgensen GH, Ludviksson BR (2010) Primary immunodeficiency and autoimmunity. Scand. J. Immunol. 71; 317-328.

[30] Boileau J, Mouillot G, Gerard L, Carmagnat M, Rabian C, Oksenhendler E, Pasquali J-L, Korganow A-S (2011) Autoimmunity in common variable immunodeficiency. J. Autoimmunity 36; 25-32.

[31] Brandt D, Gershwin ME (2006) Common variable immunodeficiency and autoimmunity. Autoimmunity Rev. 5; 465-470.

[32] Bergbreiter A, Salzer U (2009) Common variable immunodeficiency: a multifaceted and puzzling disorder. Expert Review Clin. Immunol. 5; 167-180.

[33] Giannouli S, Anagnostou D, Soliotis F, Voulgarelis M (2004) Autoimmune manifestations in common variable Immunodeficiency. Clin. Rheumatol. 23; 449-452.

[34] Knight AK, Cunningham-Rundles C (2006) Inflammatory and autoimmune complications of common variable immune deficiency. Autoimmunity Rev. 5; 156-159.

[35] Al-Muhsen SZ (2010) Gastrointestinal and hepatic manifestations of primary immune deficiency diseases. Saudi J. Gastroenterol. 16; 66-74.

[36] Malamut G, Verkarre V, Suarez F, Viallard J-F, Lascaux A-S, Cosnes J, Bouhnik Y, Lambotte O, Bechade D, Ziol M, Lavergne A, Hermine O, Cerf-Bensussan N, Cellier C (2010) The enteropathy associated with common variable immunodeficiency. Amer. J. Gastroenterol. 105; 2262-2275.

[37] Agarval S, Smereka P, Harpaz N, Cunnigham-Rundles Ch, Mayer L (2011) Characterization of immunologic defects in patients with common variable immunodeficiency (CVID) with intestinal disease. Inflamm. Bowel Dis. 17; 251-259.

[38] Nimmerjahn F, Ravetch JV (2008) Anti-inflammatory actions of intravenous immunoglobulin. Ann. Rev. Immunol. 26; 513-533.

[39] Nimmerjahn F, Ravetch JV (2010) Antibody-mediated modulation of immune responses. Immunological Rev. 236; 265-275.

[40] Pituch-Noworolska A, Błaut-Szlósarczyk A (2010) Immunoglobulins: characteristics, indications for use and clinical effectiveness. Int. Review Allergology Clin. Immunol. 16; 94-101.

[41] Pituch-Noworolska A, Błaut-Szlósarczyk A, Zwonarz K (2010) Stosowanie preparatów immunoglobulin ludzkich – objawy niepożądane. In polish. (The use of human immunoglobulins – adverse reactions). Polski Merkuriusz Lekarski 29; 202-205.

[42] Akobeng AK (2008) Crohn's disease: current treatment options. Arch. Dis. Child. 93; 787-792.

[43] Barton SH, Murray JA (2008) Celiac disease and autoimmunity in the gut and elsewhere. Gastroenterol. Clin. North Am. 37; 411-428.

[44] Kaser A, Zeissig S, Blumberg RS (2010) Inflammatory bowel disease. Ann. Rev. Immunol. 28; 573-621.

[45] Stange EF, Travis SPL, Vermeiere S, Reinisch W, Geboes K, Barakauskiene A, Feakis R, Flejou JF, Herfarth H, Hommes DW, Kupcinskas L, Lakatos PL, Mantzaris GJ, Schreiber S, Villanacci V, Warren BF (2008) European evidence based consensus on the diagnosis and management of ulcerative colitis. J. Crohn's Colitis 2; 1-23.

[46] Stange EF, Travis SPL, Vermeiere S, Verlinger C, Kupcinskas L, Geboes K, Barakauskiene A, Villanacci V, von Herbay A, Warren BF, Gasche C, Tilg H, Schreiber SW, Scholmerich J, Reinisch W (2006) European evidence based consensus on the diagnosis and management of Crohn's disease. Gut 55; suppl.1, i1 1- i1 5.

[47] Schirbel A, Fiocchi C (2010) Inflammatory bowel disease: established and evolving considerations on its etiopathogenesis and therapy. J. Digestive Diseases 11; 266-276.

[48] Walker MM, Murray JA (2011) An update in the diagnosis of celiac disease. Histopathology 59;166-179.

[49] Zhao X, Johnson RL (2011) Collagenous sprue. Arch. Pathol. Lab. Med. 135; 803-809.

[50] Evans KE, Sanders DS (2011) What is the use of biopsy and antibodies in celiac disease. J. Internal. Med. 269; 572-581.

[51] Nejad AR, Rostami K, Pourhoseingholi MA, Mojarad EN, Habibi M, Dabiri H, Zali Mr (2009) Atypical presentation is dominant and typical for celiac disease. J. Gastrointestin. Liver Dis. 18; 285-291.

[52] Beyazit Y, Sayilir A, Kekilli M, Tas A (2010) IgA and IgG antibody testing for coeliac disease. Eur. J. Int. Medicine 21; 467-468.

[53] Villalta D, Tonutti E, Prause Ch, Koletzko S, Uhling HH, Vermeersch P, Bossuyt X, Stern M, Laass MW, Ellis JH, Ciclitira PJ, Richter T, Daehnrich C, Schlumberger W, Mothes T (2010) IgG antibodies against deamidated gliadin peptides for diagnosis of celiac disease in patients with IgA deficiency. Clin. Chemistry 56; 464-468.

[54] Tennyson Ch, Green PHH (2011) The role of capsule endoscopy in patients with nonresponsive celiac disease. Gastrointestinal Endoscopy 74; 1323-1324.

[55] Demirsoy H, Ozdil K, Ersoy O, Kesici B, Karaca C, Alkim C, Akbayir N, Erdem LK, Onuk MD, Beyzadeoglu T (2010) Anti-pancreatic antibody in Turkish patients with inflammatory bowel disease and first-degree relatives. World. J. Gastroenterology 7; 5732-5738.

[56] Homsak E, Micetic-Turk D, Bozic B (2010) Autoantibodies pANCA, GAB and PAB in inflammatory bowel disease: prevalence, characteristics and diagnostic value. Wien. Klin. Wochenschr. 122; 19-25.

[57] Russo P, Alvarez F (2002) Autoimmune enteropathy; a review. Clin. Applied Immunol. Rev. 2; 203-206.

[58] Sbarbati A, Valletta E, Bertini M, Cipolli M, Morroni M, Pinelli L, Tato L (2003) Gluten sensitivity and "normal" histology. Digestive Liver Disease 35; 768-773.

[59] Rostami K, Villanacci V (2009) Microscopic enteritis: novel prospect in celiac disease clinical and immuno-histogenesis. Digestive Liver Disease 41; 245-252.

[60] Borrelli M, Maglio M, Agnese M, Paparo F, Gentile S, Colicchio B, Tosco A, Auricchio R, Troncone R (2009) High density of intraepithelial γ/δ lymphocytes and deposits of immunoglobulin (Ig)M anti tissue transglutaminase antibodies in the jejunum of celiac patients with IgA deficiency. Clin. Exp. Immunol. 160; 199-206.

[61] Glocker E, Grimbacher B (2012) Inflammatory bowel disease. Cell. Mol. Life Sci. 69; 41-48.

[62] Genre J, Errante PR, Kokron CM, Toledo-Barros M, Camara NOS, Rizzo LV (2009) Reduced frequency of CD4+CD25highFoxP3+ cells and diminished FoxP3 expression in patients with common variable immunodeficiency: a link to autoimmunity? Clin. Immunol. 132; 215-221.

[63] Valletta E, Fornaro M, Pecori S, Zanoni G (2011) Selective immunoglobulin A deficiency and celiac disease. J. Invest. Allergol Clin. Immunol. 21; 242-244.

[64] Fabris M, De Vita S, Visentini D, Fabro C, Picierno A, Lerussi A, Villalta D, Alessio MG, Tampoia MA, Tonutti E (2009) B-lymphocyte stimulator and a proliferation-inducting ligand serum levels in IgA-deficient patients with and without celiac disease. Ann. NY Acad. Sci. 1173; 268-273.

[65] Sandhu BK, Fell JME, Beattie RM, Mitton SG, Wilson DC, Jenkins H (2010) Guidelines for the management of inflammatory bowel disease in children in the United Kingdom. J. Ped. Gastroenterol. Nutrition 50; S1-S13.

[66] Damen GM, van Krieken H, Hoppenreijs E, van Os E, Tolboom JJM, Warris A, Yntema J-B, Nieuwenhuis EES, Escher JC (2010) Overlap, common features and essential differences in pediatric granulomatous inflammatory bowel disease. J. Ped. Gastroenterol. Nutrition 51; 690-697.

Chapter 8

Central Nervous System Resident Cells in Neuroinflammation: A Brave New World

J.P.S. Peron, D. Oliveira, W. N. Brandão, A. Fickinger,
A. P. Ligeiro de Oliveira, L. V. Rizzo and N.O.S. Câmara

Additional information is available at the end of the chapter

http://dx.doi.org/10.5772/48161

1. Introduction

Neuroinflammatory and central nervous system (CNS) demyelinating diseases have most of its pathological features based on immune cells infiltrating brain parenchyma and leading to neuronal death and focal or diffuse destruction of the CNS architecture, as extensively reviewed (Rodriguez 2007; Weiner 2008; Shie FS 2011). In this context, the role for resident and infiltrating inflammatory cells is very relevant, as they may be both the trigger and the maintainers of the neuroinflammatory process (Almolda B 2011). The combination of interesting concepts of neurology to the immunology laboratory, has rendered glial cells with a more dynamic and immunological shape.

Stroke and Multiple Sclerosis (MS) are on the opposite sides of the coin of the neuroimmune diseases, depending on innate and adaptive immunity, respectively. That is the main reason why stroke is denominated as a neuroinflammatory rather than an autoimmune disease, and the opposite for MS. Despite this difference, which relies on the fact that cognate antigens for T cells were described for MS but not for stroke, central nervous system resident cells play a pivotal role on both cases. This greatly evidences the importance of brain parenchymal cells in the pathogenesis of neuroinflammatory and neurodegenerative diseases.

Innate immune system greatly differs from adaptive immune system in many ways. Innate immunity is much older concerning its phylogeny, whereas adaptive immunity is relatively recent. It is interesting to mention that the first lymphocytes appeared with the gnatus cartilaginous fish, such as sharks and rays (Matsunaga T 1998), whereas in 1882 Metchikoff E demonstrated that starfish had singular phagocytic cells which are now believed to be the macrophage ancestral, as reviewed (Janeway CA Jr 2001). Besides its phylogenetic discrepancies, innate and adaptive immune systems also greatly differ in function and recognition. One important difference is that lymphocytes express Recombinase Activating Genes (RAG), conferring unique T and B cell receptors. Further differences between innate and adaptive immunity are described in Table 1 (adapted from (Abbul K Abbas 2006).

Specific Feature	Innate Immunity	Adaptive Immunity
Specificity	Macrophages, dendritic cells, neutrophils recognize Pathogen Associated Molecular Patterns (PAMPs) as Lipopolissacharide, peptidoglycan, ssRNA, dsRNA, unmethylated CpG nucleotides, mannose rich glycans among many others.	T lymphocytes recognize by its T cell receptor (TCRs), peptides presented by antigen presenting cells in the context of the MHC molecules. B cells recognize through the B cell receptor (BCRs) several different molecules, such as DNA, RNA, Lipids, Carbohydrates that may or may not be associated to carrier proteins.
Receptors	Pattern Recognition Receptors (PRRs) such as Toll-like receptors 1-12, NOD, Dectin-1, NLRPs.	T cell receptor (TCRs) and B cell receptor (BCRs)
Clonality	No	Yes. Each cell expresses only one type of TCR or BCR.
Self-tolerance	No mechanism to maintain tolerance to self.	T and B lymphocytes undergo selection mechanisms in the thymus and bone marrow, respectively.

Table 1. Table one pinpoints some important differences between innate and adaptive immune system.

In this sense, the discrepancy between stroke and MS pathology is mainly due to the fact that Multiple Sclerosis (MS) and its murine model Experimental Autoimmune Encephalomyelitis (EAE) are secondary to a peripheral still-to-be-defined activation of T CD4 cells specific for myelin derived epitopes. On the other hand, during stroke, no cognate antigens have been clearly established so far, and innate immune cells such as macrophages and neutrophils play the master role.

Acute stroke, defined as the occlusion or hemorrhage of brain blood vessels, culminates in neuronal and glial cell death and the local release of pro-inflammatory molecules (S Stoll G 2010). These molecules, named Danger Associated Molecular Patterns (DAMPs), such as Heat Shock Proteins (HSPs), degraded extracellular matrix, F-actin filaments (Ahrens S 2012), ATP and many others (Seong Seong 2004), may induce blood brain barrier (BBB) disruption and activation of resident cells (Ceulemans AG 2010; Stoll G 2010). This is followed by polymorphonuclear and mononuclear cells infiltration establishing the inflammatory foci (Stoll G 2010; Thiel A 2011). It is noteworthy that ischemic stroke comprises more than 80% of the cases, caused by embolus or thrombus (Stoll G 2010). Stroke is also considered a heavy burden for Public Health Policies as almost 80% of patients suffer from further disability [18]. Stroke lesions are time-dependent, and longer periods of ischemia induce greater lesions than shorter periods. This is intimately linked to the reminiscent blood supply offered to the tissue. After stroke, two well defined regions are described: i) the region with completely abolished blood supply is the core, with intense necrosis, and ii) peripherally to the core is the penumbra, with the presence of inflammatory infiltrate.

Acute lesions are immune independent, and most cell death is due to altered ionic balance, enhanced water input to the cell body resulting in edema, high calcium influx and secondary high glutamate release (Dirnagl U 1999; Ceulemans A 2010). For instance, glutamate release spreads early throughout brain parenchyma inducing neuronal death by a phenomenon called excitotoxicity, mediated by ionotropic glutamate receptors, such as NMDAR (N-methyl-D-aspartate) (Ceulemans A 2010). Besides biochemical alterations, the release of inflammatory molecules, as Heat-shock proteins (HSPs), histamine, prostaglandins, TNF-α, is also observed in the injured area. Altogether, these inflammatory factors released after necrotic cell death induce the activation of resident cells, such as astrocytes, microglia, endothelial cells and even neurons, to secrete more pro-inflammatory cytokines and chemokines, and not only recruiting but also favoring the migration of inflammatory cells to the ischemic site. These mechanisms will be discussed in this chapter.

Secondary to the acute phase, a leukocyte-dependent period emerges. Due to the disruption of the BBB, and the local secretion of chemokines and other leukocyte-recruiting factors, inflammatory cells such as neutrophils, macrophages and even lymphocytes arrive from the periphery and then interact with brain parenchymal cells establishing the inflammatory process itself. Neutrophils and macrophages secrete high amounts of innate immunity derived cytokines such as IL-1 , IL-6, IL-8, IL-12, IL-15, IL-17, IL-18, IL-23, TNF-α, LIF, and chemokines as CCL2, CCL6, CCL21 and many others (Charles A Janeway 2002; Ghiringuelli F 2007; Suzuki T. 2007; Song C 2008; Weiner 2008). Just to mention, several other inflammatory factors were also found in ischemic area, such as matrix metalloproteinases (MMPs) (Del Zoppo GJ 2012), Adenosine Triphosphate (ATPs) (Arbeloa J 2011), High Mobility Group-box 1 (HMGB1)(Wang H 1999), HSPs (Romi F 2011), leucotrienes, prostaglandins, glutamate (Dhawan J 2011), leptin (Avraham Y 2011), complement factors and many others (Dirnagl U 1999; Ceulemans AG 2010). However, it is interesting to mention that these factors may also be secreted by many resident cells, such as microglia, astrocytes and also endothelial cells, overlapping the role of resident Vs. infiltrating cells. To make an example, IL-1β, whose source may be both macrophages and astrocytes, greatly contributes to the activation of the vascular beds facilitating adherence and transmigration of circulating leukocytes, as well as to the increased intracellular calcium in neurons and astrogliosis (Stoll G 2010). To corroborate the importance of IL-1, recently the use of Anankira®, the recombinant IL-1Ra (IL-1 receptor antagonist) has been proposed to be used in therapy, as an attempt to abrogate the deleterious IL-1-derived features (Emsley HC 2005).

Thus, it is clear that during stroke, the importance of different cellular populations has been established; no matter these cells are infiltrating macrophages and neutrophils or resident astrocytes and microglia. Thus, therapeutic approaches whose mechanisms focus on the reduction of local inflammation and cellular recruitment may be consider as promising alternatives for reducing the overall disability so usually observed in these patients.

Very different from stroke, where the inflammatory process starts inside the CNS, during MS, self-reacting T CD4 cells are somehow activated in the periphery and further migrate to the target organ. In this context, there are two main differences between MS and stroke: i) the need for activated T cells to gain access to the CNS, and ii) the disease is autoimmune in nature, thus cognate antigens, such as myelin and proteolipoprotein epitopes are well described. Although it is a consensus that these self-reacting cells are specific for myelin-derived antigens (Weiner HL 1993; Korn T 2007; Rodriguez 2007), the trigger for these cells to be activated in the periphery is still matter of intense debate. Other possibilities related to MS incidence and prevalence range from association to certain HLA haplotypes, as for HLA-DRB1*1501 e HLA-DRB5*0101, HLA-DQB1 (Oksenberg Jr 2005), to genetic polymorphisms, and although not very accepted, even viral infections, as recently reviewed (Owens GP 2011).

MS is a neuroinflammatory and demyelinating disease of the CNS that leads to great disability in younger adults, and most of its incidence is observed in northern countries of Europe and also the United States (WHO 2006). Multiple Sclerosis stands for multiple scars, referring to the inflammatory plaques where myelin is lost mostly in perivascular regions of the white matter and whose observation by Magnetic Resonance Imaging (MRI) is considered the most reliable diagnostic approach. Myelin sheets are produced by neuron-surrounding oligodendrocytes, the main target cells during MS. Death of these cells results in axonal dissection, followed by neuronal lost and thus reduction in neuronal impulse transmission, resulting in weakness, fatigue, numbness and overall disability. Concerning its onset and evolution, MS may be separated in i) primary progressive ii) secondary progressive and also iii) the relapsing-remitting type. Usually the disease starts with a relapse-remitting pattern of the symptoms followed by a progressive stage of increasing disability, considered the more severe cases (Weiner 2008). Many patients evolve to a more chronic stage of the disease, with no relapses, but a more prominent progressive lost of motor coordination, sensory and autonomic function is observed. It is noteworthy that many of these symptoms are tightly regulated by the local inflammatory milieu in the CNS, as well as by the activation status of the resident cells.

Much of our understanding concerning the molecular and cellular mechanisms of MS was obtained after observations made on its murine model, Experimental Autoimmune Encephalomyelitis (EAE). With historical relevance, it is worthy to mention that the EAE model started after Prof. Thomas Rivers decided to understand why many years before,

Prof. Louis Pasteur experimental animals used to develop paralysis after vaccination against rabies. Rivers proceeded with the same protocol as Pasteur, immunizing rabbits with spinal cords extracts from rabbits that were inoculated with the rabies virus. At the same time he included a control group which consisted of extracts from non-contaminated animals. Interestingly, animals that received these extracts also developed paralysis, highlighting the fact that the secondary paralysis was not a rabies virus-dependent observation. Interestingly, the features develop by the animals was very similar to those observed by Pasteur many years earlier. It was also very exciting to recall that at that time Freund was describing its complete adjuvant (Complete Freund Adjuvant), what made Rivers research much easier, as the immunization for EAE induction changed from around 20 inoculations of brain extracts to only one injection. Then, one of the most used model to study not only neuroinflammation and neurodegeneration but also autoimmunity mechanisms had been brought to scientific community, as reviewed (Baxter 2007).

MS was previously considered to be the prototype of a Th1 type of autoimmune disease, where IFN-γ-secreting T CD4 (Kroenke MA 2007; Dardalhon V 2008) and CD8 (Michael P. Crawford 2004; Goverman J 2005) cells are greatly relevant and widely found in the periphery, liquor and brain parenchyma (Matusevicius D 1999). On the other hand, many contrasting data were obtained using the EAE model. In fact, it was known by a long date that mice deficient for IFN-γ were more susceptible to EAE induction when compared to control animals (Chu CQ 2000). This is in fact corroborated by other autoimmune disease model, the Experimental Autoimmune Uveitis (EAU) (Jones LS 1997). This was much unexpected, and for a great period of time a matter of intense speculation. Moreover, corroborating these findings, studies using animals deficient for p19, p35 and p40, the subunits for the heterodimers IL-12 (p35 + p40) and IL-23 (p19 + p40), had demonstrated that, unexpectedly, IL-23 was more relevant then IL-12 in these same models, raising still more questions in the field of EAE pathology (Cua DJ 2003). Thus, for many years there was a gap in the understanding on the actual role for IFN-γ-secreting Th1 cells in the EAE model. It is worthy to mention that much less was known for the human disease.

The final answer for that was obtained many years later when, using the EAE model, a new population of T cells was described as the main players in the pathogenesis of EAE The so-called Th17 cells secrete high amounts of the cytokines IL-17A, IL-17F (Ivanov I 2006), IL-21 (Zhou L 2007) and GM-CSF (Codarri L 2011), and its master regulator is the rorc gene which encodes the gene for the retinoic acid orphan receptor, RORγt (Ivanov I 2006). To further corroborate this hypothesis, it was demonstrated that IL-17 knockout mice are resistant to EAE induction, which was very contrasting with data obtained from IFN-γ knockout mice, as reviewed (Komiyama Y 2006). Besides, it became clear that these cells arise in the periphery in the dependence of two cytokines, IL-6 + TGF-β, whose activity was demonstrated to be inducers of rorc expression and thus Th17 commitment. Corroborating previous data, it was clarified that IL-23 is the maintenance factor for these cells to remain viable and active. In fact, IL-23r deficient cells are unable to be maintained viable and thus induce disease (Cua DJ 2003; Zhou L 2007). Thus, the findings in p19 KO mice highlighted the fact that these mice were resistant to EAE induction due to the reduced survival of encephalitogenic Th17 cells in the periphery. However, it is well accepted that both Th1 and Th17 cells are found in focal lesions in MS and EAE, comprising around 20-25% and 10-15% of the CNS infiltrating T CD4 cells respectively (Murphy AC 2010; Peron JP 2010). Moreover, it is well accepted the fact both populations intimately interact with CNS resident cells, as astrocytes, microglia and neurons.

Aside from the discussion whether this or that population of CD4 cells is more important, it is a fact that a mixed population is found in the inflamed brain parenchyma, and in most cases Th1 cells outnumber Th17 cells. Interestingly, it has now been established that each population possibly infiltrate the CNS through different mechanisms. Actually, infiltrating cells may reach the CNS by three separate routes: 1) by direct transmigration through the capillary and post-capillary venules of the BBB and 2) from the blood to the cerebrospinal fluid at the choroid plexus and 3) migration through meningeal vessels to the subarachnoid space (B. 2006). In this sense, it has been recently demonstrated that Th1 cells use the $\alpha4\beta1$ integrins (Very Late Antigen- 4 – VLA-4) to infiltrate the spinal cord during EAE. The blockade of VLA-4 did not block Th17 cells to infiltrate the brain, expressing both IL-23R and CCR6. Accordingly, T cell-conditional $\alpha4$-deficient mice were not resistant to actively induced EAE but showed an ataxic syndrome with predominantly supraspinal infiltrates of T cells (Rothhammer V 2011). Corroborating this idea, it was previously showed that Th17 cells constitutively express the chemokine receptor CCR6, whose ligand, CCL20 is also constitutively expressed by choroid plexus cells. Thus, it is clear that Th1 and Th17 cells differ not only in phenotype and function, but also in its ways to gain access to the CNS (Jäger A 2009; Murphy AC 2010).

It is well established that after the entry of Th1 and Th17 cells to the brain parenchyma, these cells need to be reactivated upon encounter with MHC-Ag bearing cells on a second hit phenomenon. After re-activation in situ, Th1 and Th17 lymphocytes release its contents, most of which are pro-inflammatory cytokines, such as IFN-γ, TNF-α and IL-6 for Th1, and IL-17A, IL-17F, IL-21 and IL-22 for Th17 cells. In this context, CNS resident cells play an important role, not only because of its capacity to second hit T cells, but also because they express cytokine receptors and Toll-like receptors (TLRs), very important for the amplification of the inflammation. Thus, studies on the biology of astrocytes, microglia, endothelial cells and also neurons during inflammatory processes will greatly contribute to the understanding of the pathogenesis of neuroinflammatory and neurodegenerative disease.

1.1. Central nervous system resident cells and stroke

Due to the high necessity for blood supply and oxygen, brain resident cells are very sensitive to hypoxic injury. Neurons are the most affected, followed by astrocytes, microglia and finally endothelial cells (Dirnagl U 1999). During stroke, necrotic cell death is followed by the release of intracellular content, such as pro-inflammatory cytokines, that greatly accounts for the initiation of the process. In fact, activation of astrocytes and microglial cells during stroke, either by the early necrotic cell death or by the later inflammatory cells-derived cytokines, is an important process directly involved with the disease pathology (Dirnagl U 1999; Ceulemans A 2010). However, we must not exclude the role for infiltrating macrophages, a rich source of cytokines and chemokines, found in the ischemic foci as soon as 10 hours.

Microglial cells are CNS resident phagocytic cells, with great resemblance to macrophages, however, it has been recently demonstrated that these macrophage-like cells in fact differ in ontogeny. Microglial cells were believed to derive from a myeloid precursor whose marker is the transcription factor PU.1. However, PU.1 knockout mice were absent not only of microglia but also macrophages, showing that microglial cells were in fact derived from a myeloid lineage, but PU.1 was a not a specific marker [1, 2]. Interesting results have demonstrated that bone marrow (BM) transplantation restored microglia presence in the central nervous system, what led to the interpretation that microglial cells do in fact derive from a common precursor in the BM [1] (Kettenmann H 2011). However, many of these experiments were performed after whole-body or central nervous system (CNS) irradiation. Using a parabiotic system, where the circulatory systems of two mice are connected, experiments demonstrated that no donor-derived cells are found in the CNS of parabiotic mice [3]. Recent reports using Green Fluorescent Protein (GFP) couple to the fractalkine receptor (CX3CR1- GFP) and Runt- related transcription factor 1 (Runx1) - Cre reporter mice described the presence of fetal yolk sac- derived microglial precursor cells at day E9.5. On day E10.5, microglial cells are already found in CNS, as circulatory system has been established. Thus, microglial are generated upon primitive haematopoiesis in the yolk sac, independent from bone marrow haematopoiesis [4]. Actually there is still a search for a reliable marker to indentify microglial cells by flow cytometry. One option is to use the markers CD45 and CD11b, where CD11b+CD45low cells are considered microglia and CD11b+CD45high are considered macrophages.

At resting state, microglial cells have a body shape very similar to dendritic cells, as they posses many dendrites or branches. Those are believed to be actively involved in the clearance of cellular debris as well as in the immunesurveillance, as some viruses and bacteria may reach the brain [13-14]. Moreover, it was already demonstrated that after ischemic brain injury, microglia migrate to the penumbra covering the remaining living neurons. As these neurons die by apoptosis, proper caping by microglia results in fast phagocytosis and thus avoiding more inflammation. This was demonstrated to be dependent on the expression of the LFA-1 integrin.

Non-activated microglia are described to be very quiescent with an anergic-like state. Resting microglia have very little capacity to prime naïve T cells as they express very low levels of MHC II molecules, and are negative for CD80, CD86 and CD40 (Kettenmann H 2011).This status seem to be maintained by several different mechanisms. For instance, it was recently demonstrated that, microglial cells express a high amount of the miRNA-124. This oligonucleotide directly inhibits the CCAAT/enhancer-binding protein-α (C/EBP-α) and also its target, the above mentioned PU.1. Further, this inhibition down-regulates CD45 and MHC II expression and also TNF-α secretion [15]. Interestingly, peritoneal macrophages do not express miRNA-124 and bone marrow derived macrophages are rendered less activated when transfected with miRNA-124 [15]. Thus, the specific expression of such miRNA greatly accounts for the anergic state of microglial cells.

The intimate contact with norepinephrine-releasing adrenergic neurons, as in the locus coeruleus may be also responsible for maintaining microglia hyporesponsive. Microglial cells express β2-adrenergic receptors associated to G stimulatory proteins. These proteins trigger the activity of adenilate cyclase increasing cAMP synthesis. Elevated intracellular cAMP concentrations activate Protein Kinase A (PKA) which may have many suppressive activities. PKA phosphorylates Csk and Ezhrin, whose kinase activity phosphorylates inhibitory proteins of Lck (Ruppelt A 2007). High cAMP levels also phosphorylates CREB (Cyclic AMP Responsive Elements Binding Protein) that translocates to the nucleus [16, 17]. CREB interacts with CREB Binding Protein (CBP) activating several promoters, such as IL-10. PKA is also able to phosphorylate the Nuclear Factor of Activated T Cells (NF-AT). It is worthy to remember that NF-AT is inactive at its phosphorylated state. Altogether these are some of the mechanisms that greatly contribute to the hyporesponsiveness of microglial cells.

Although at resting state microglial cells are very "polite", after activation they start to express a whole different set of genes, acquiring the capacity not only to secrete significant amounts of cytokines, chemokines and other inflammatory molecules, but also to present antigens and activate CNS infiltrating T cells. In fact, there are at least three acceptable ways to activate microglial cells: i) with pro-inflammatory cytokines, such as IFN-γ, TNF-α and IL-17; ii) engagement of TLRs ligands, such as LPS, PGN, HSPs, and iii) the phagocytosis of myelin debris from demyelinating regions. Altogether, these are the main mechanisms by which microglial cells subverts the anergic-induced state, and thus acquiring an active role in neuroinflammation, as observed during acute brain ischemia.

It was recently proposed that microglia posses all inflammasome derived machinery, thus conferring these cells positive for IL-1 / IL-18. IL-1β interacts with its receptor activating a signaling pathway that is shared with Toll-like receptors (TLRs) through MyD88 and culminating in NF-κB phosphorylation and translocation to the nucleus. IL-1R was shown to be widely found in rat hippocampus, but preferentially at synaptic sites. More interesting, it was also demonstrated that IL-1R co-localizes with the ionotropic glutamate receptor NMDA through its GluN2B subunit (Gardoni F 2011). Just to mention, a few overall effects of IL-1β are: induces rapid local inflammation and up-regulates the synthesis of other cytokines and costimulatory molecules, as CD80, CD86 and CD40. IL-1β also disturbs ionic balance, increases Ca^{2+} influx in neurons leading to degeneration, facilitates BBB disruption and most important, it is a potent stimuli for endothelial cells to express adhesion molecules which amplifies local inflammatory cells recruitment (Ceulemans AG 2010).

IL-6 is not found in the CNS at resting state. On the other hand, it is widely found after stroke, and may be secreted by many resident cells, as microglia, astrocytes, endothelial cells and also infiltrating monocytes and T cells. Interestingly, microglia are not only able to secrete IL-6 but also they express IL-6R, evidencing a positive feedback loop. IL-6 signaling in microglia phosphorylates STAT-1, STAT-3 and ERK, culminating in MHC II, CD40 and IL-12p70 up-regulation and increasing inflammation (Lin HW 2009). However it is also accepted a dichotomy for IL-6 function, as many reports have also demonstrated its protective role after stroke. In this concern, it is interesting to mention that IL-6 up-regulates the transcription of the suppressive molecule IL-1ra (IL-1 Receptor Antagonist), thus blocking some of the deleterious functions of IL-1. In fact, higher IL-6 levels may positively correlate with a better neuropathological outcome (Emsley HC 2005).

It is noteworthy that microglial cells secrete so many inflammatory factors, such as IL-1, IL-4, IL-6, IL-17, TNF-α, synthesize reactive oxygen and nitrogen species, secrete matrix metaloproteinase as MMP-2, MMP-9, and other factors. Microglia also express several membrane receptors, as TLR-2, TLR-4, NLRP3 (Nalp3), gp91 phox (Dohi K 2010), ciclooxinagenase-2 (Cox-2), oncostatin M, heme-oxigenase -1 (HO-1) [10, 15-17]. Onconstatin M shares the IL-6R beta chain and thus phosphorylates STAT-3 and also NF-κB transcription factors, up-regulating TNF-α secretion and iNOS expression (Baker BJ 2010). It is also known that activated microglia secrete high amounts of glutamate and TNF-α. These molecules are able to induce apoptosis of neurons but especially of oligodendrocytes, leading to demyelination, a hallmark of MS and EAE. For this reason, it has been more and more evidenced that microglial cells have a very important role in the pathogenesis of several different inflammatory diseases of the CNS, as stroke [13, 18], multiple sclerosis [17], Alzheimer disease, amyotrophic lateral sclerosis and also different types of brain and liquor infections, as reviewed [19].

The products of NADPH oxidase activation, the reactive oxygen species (ROIs), are also a very relevant source for cellular injuries. In this concern, ischemia can also induce this pathway whose importance in the pathogenesis of stroke is well established. The voltage-gated proton channel Hv1 counterbalances NADPH oxidase and subsequent cellular loss of electrons with protons. It has recently been shown that mouse and human brain microglia, but not neurons or astrocytes, expressed large Hv1-mediated currents and that Hv1 was required for NAPDH oxidase activity and ROI generation in brain microglia in situ and in vivo. Thus, Hv1 knockout mice are less prone to develop neuronal death and brain damage after stroke. These indicate that, aside the cytokine and glutamate burst, ROIs are responsible for a substantial fraction of brain damage at early time points after ischemia, and rendering Hv1 with a promising therapeutic approach (Wu LJ 2012).

In summary, there is a never ending list of features, such as released factors, receptors expressed, ROIs, membrane molecules, MMPs, that points out microglia as a very important resident cell population, with an unquestionable relevance in the mechanisms of triggering and perpetuating CNS inflammation. On the other hand, although mostly shown as an important pro-neuroinflammatory agent, it is conceivable that microglial cells may have a modulatory function, in an attempt to reduce neuroinflammation. In fact, it has been demonstrated that microglia may also secrete anti-inflammatory molecules such as IL-10 [20], TGF-β, IL-1Ra and express suppressive molecules as Suppressor of Cytokine Signaling

(SOCS-3) [21], the tryptophan depleting enzyme indoleamine-2,3-dioxigenase (IDO) [22] and also IL-4 (Ponomarev ED 2007). It has recently been accepted that, as observed in macrophages, microglial cells may also be divided in those with pro-inflammatory activity, called Microglia 1 (M1) and those with regulatory activity, called Microglia 2 (M2), as extensively reviewed (Martinez FO 2009). Such findings, much contributes towards the great relevance of microglial cells during neuroinflammatory diseases. However, further studies must be performed to a better understanding of the suppressive activities of microglial cells.

Activated astrocytes also play a significant role in the pathogenesis of stroke. Astrocytes may not only secret many cytokines, chemokines and MMPs but also undergo astrogliosis, which is an exacerbated proliferation of astrocytes as a wound-healing like process. Astrocytes may secrete significant amounts of TNF-α, interestingly with both neuroprotective and neurotoxic properties. TNF-α belongs to a great family of cytokines and also membrane bound molecules, such as Fas, FasL, Glucocorticoid Induced TNF Receptor (GITR) and several others (Abbul K Abbas 2006). It has been proposed that TNF-α follows a biphasic pattern of secretion after brain ischemia, and the first wave is detected as soon as 1-3 hours probably, and the second after 24-36 hours. This fluctuation may be a consequence of two separate sources for this cytokine, as it may be first derived by the tissular injury itself, and the second one derived from resident cells activation and also from infiltrating inflammatory cells (Ceulemans AG 2010). Moreover, TNF-α using its death domains, induces apoptosis of endothelial cells, and thus promoting CNS infiltration, as it disrupts BBB (Ceulemans AG 2010). However, contrasting data showing that previous treatment with TNF-α protect from neuronal death, although the mechanisms are still to be elucidated. AVC

Transglutaminase 2 (TG2) is a Ca(2+)-dependent transamidating enzyme ubiquitously expressed in the body. TG2 is the predominant form of transglutaminase expressed in the mammalian nervous system. Previously, it was shown that TG2 can affect both cell death and cell survival mechanisms depending on the cell type and the stressor. Intriguingly, infarct volumes in TG2 knockout mice were significantly reduced when compared to controls. Neurons from TG2 knockout mice showed decreased viability in response to oxygen-glucose deprivation, which was not observed in astrocytes, as they were resistant to oxygen-glucose deprivation in situ. Interestingly, wild type and knock out neurons were protected against oxygen glucose deprivation when they were co-cultured with astrocytes from TG2 knockout mice (Colak G 2012). Therefore, the decreased stroke volumes observed in TG2 knock out evidences that its expression is more important in astrocytes. Altogether, this serves to corroborate the idea that neuron-astrocyte crosstalk plays a significant role in mediating stroke pathogenesis.

Matrix metalloproteinases (MMPs) are extracellular matrix remodeling enzyme, very important for tecidual infiltration. Recent data on non-nervous system tissue showed intracellular and even intranuclear localizations for different MMPs. In this concern it was recently demonstrated that MMPs localization to the nucleus of neurons may correlate to apoptotic cell death. More interesting, cells expressing MMP-9 in the nuclear compartment also co-expressed activated-caspase 3, linking MMP-9 expression to neuronal and glial death (Del Zoppo GJ 2012). The research has shown for the first time the localization of MMP-9 to the nucleus of human neurons. Altogether this gives more relevance to MMPs secretion in the CNS as it correlates not only with facilitation of the cellular infiltration.

Moreover, the mechanisms through which astrogliosis is orchestrated is still considered to be unknown. However, it has been recently demonstrated that CD36 plays a pivotal role in astrocytic survival, and proliferation In fact, CD36 deficient and CD36 -siRNA treated animals had reduced astrogliosis and wound healing. Thus, it is now accepted that CD36 signaling intimately correlates with astroglial proliferation (Bao Y 2012).

The presence and the role of certain types of dendritic cells (DCs) in the CNS is constant matter of intense debate. Things get even darker when it concerns stroke pathogenesis. Some reports have shown that both resident and peripheral DCs may route to CNS after ischemic injury. Using CD11c-GFP animals, it was clearly shown that as soon as 24 hours after medial cerebral artery occlusion (MCAO), brain dendritic cells (bDCs) are found peripherally to the penumbra area. Using bone marrow chimeras, where both wild type and CD11c - GFP animals were irradiated followed by bone marrow reconstitution interestingly demonstrated that bDCs migrate to the penumbra, whereas peripherally recruited DCs are mostly found in the core. These cells were highly positive for the expression of the dendritic cells marker CD11c and several T cell activation-related molecules, as MHC II, CD80 and CD86. However, this was not observed early after MCAO occlusion, and thus, the initial activation observed in the CNS is most probably dependent on microglial activation rather than on bDCs (Felger JC 2010).

As professional antigen presenting cells as DCs are important in the pathogenesis of stroke, it is conceivable that T cells may also have a relevant role due to antigen recognition. However, one may not forget that, differently from MS, stroke is not an autoimmune disease, and the cognate epitopes recognized by T and B cells after ischemia are still matter of debate. However, elegant researches have demonstrated a pivotal role for T cells in stroke lesions, mostly on a later period after ischemia. In fact, IFN-γ deficient mice develop much smaller lesions than control animals. Although this IFN-γ may derive from different sources, it is accepted that Th1 cells play a relevant role in this phenomenon. Moreover, T CD4 deficient animals are much more resistant to ischemic injury and this may corroborate the role for these lymphocytes, as recently reviewed (Brait VH 2012). This only contributes to the hypothesis that T cells may have an important role in the ischemic brain lesions.

IL-17 is the hallmark of the T CD4 lymphocytes with Th17 phenotype (Ivanov I 2006; Iwakura Y 2006). It is now accepted that many other cell types may also secrete this cytokine, as microglia and astrocytes (Kawanokuchi J 2008), alveolar macrophages (Song C 2008), and many others. Several important roles for the biological function of IL-17 have been evidenced during neuroinflammation. For instance, it was demonstrated that human BBB endothelial cells express IL-17R constitutively. Thus, bioactive IL-17 facilitates the disruption of the BBB reducing the tight cellular interaction of endothelial cells through

GAP junctions (Kebir H 2007). Moreover, IL-17 is also considered a potent neutrophil recruiting factor, increasing cellular infiltrate. To further corroborate the importance of IL-17 on the pathogenesis of stroke, it was interestingly demonstrated that IL-17 deficient animals have smaller brain focal lesions when compared to wild-type controls. More interesting, using conditional deletion approaches, it was well established that this IL-17 was secreted by T γδ lymphocytes. The abrogation of IL-17 secretion only in this population resulted in an increased resistance in developing lesions. It is interesting to mention that these observations were performed on day seven after MCAO (Shichita T 2010). Thus, these observations pointed not only to the importance of the IL-17 cytokine but also to the pivotal role played by T γδ lymphocytes. It is worthy to mention that myelin sheets are lipid-rich structures and T γδ cells recognize lipidic antigens.

In summary, the importance of CNS resident cells during neuroinflammatory processess is out of question. The primary secretion of inflammatory factors that follows necrotic cell death is the first trigger for local inflammation. This greatly increases endothelial permeability resulting in the recruitment of inflammatory cells from the periphery. These cells will physically interact with CNS resident cells, and thus, perpetuating the process. It is interesting to mention that some anti-inflammatory factors may also be detected. However, the knowledge about its regulatory functions is just starting, at least after ischemic brain injury.

1.2. Central nervous system resident cells and MS/EAE

Most autoimmune diseases result from the peripheral activation of T CD4 cells against endogenous peptides, as is the case for arthritis, Systemic Lupus Erithematosus (SLE), myastenia gravis (MG), ankilosing spondilytis (AS), Vogt-Kainag-Harada Syndrome (VKH) and multiple sclerosis (MS). It is well accepted that in MS such antigens are myelin-derived epitopes. After activation in the periphery, these T cells migrate to the target organ where they need to be reactivated on a second hit phenomenon. Through this phenomenon a new set of genes are transcribed and translated. For instance, pro-inflammatory cytokines, chemokines, and T cell-activating membrane receptors are promptly up-regulated. MHC I and II, CD80, CD86, CD40, TLR-2, and many cytokines receptors, as IFN-γR and IL-17R are up-regulated in microglia after CNS infiltration of encephalitogenic T CD4 cells. In this concern, which population of CNS resident cells is indispensable for this in situ interaction with infiltrating T cells is still a matter of intense debate, and microglia and resident dendritic cells (DCs) are the main candidates.

Multiple sclerosis (MS) and its murine model, EAE, are characterized by an autoimmune response against myelin-derived epitopes, which culminates in inflammatory infiltrate, gliosis, damage of the myelin sheath and also neuronal death (Neumann 2003; Rebenko-Moll NM 2006; Rodriguez 2007). Many studies have focused on the correlation between different cell types infiltrating the CNS during EAE and the clinical features of the disease. For instance, it has been shown that T CD4+ (Kroenke MA 2007) and CD8+ (Goverman J 2005) cells, as well as macrophages and microglial cells are involved in EAE pathogenesis (Weiner 2008). It is worthy to remember that, as discussed in the introduction, MS pathogenesis is orchestrated by both Th1 and Th17 encephalitogenic cells.

The discovery of DCs by Ralph Steinman was considered a huge breakthrough in the immunology field, rendering Steinman with a Nobel Prize in 2011. Since then, DCs are widely studied and used in many different fields, and it is now accepted as CNS resident cells, as bDCs. In the search for resident DCs in the brain, the use of CD11c –GFP animals was very useful. It was clearly demonstrated that GFP+ cells were find in brain parenchyma of naïve animals, and thus called brain dendric cells or bDCs. More interesting, it was shown that bDCs were found in the circunventricular organs, whose characteristics are not to be isolated by the BBB. Thus, it seems clear that bDCs may have an important role in brain surveillance. Moreover, and corroborating this idea, bDCs have migrating abilities, as they route to lesions of kainic acid-induced neuronal death. Concerning bDCs, is established that they are important players in the second-hit of brain and spinal cord infiltrating T CD4 cells. Using the murine model for EAE, it was demonstrated that bDCs not only present CNS-derived antigens to T cells, but they also input both Th1 and Th17 phenotype to naïve T CD4 cells (Felger JC 2010). It is interesting to remember that, as discussed in the introduction, both populations play a very relevant role in MS pathogenesis. Corroborating this idea, another research has shown that CD14 infiltrating monocytes acquire the CD83+CD209+ dendritic cell phenotype with a significant capacity to prime T cells after passing the BBB. These cells were able to secrete IL-12p70, IL-6 and TGF-β and thus generating Th1 and Th17 cells .

Although questioned by some researchers, it is believed that under resting conditions microglial cells do not express significant levels MHC I and II molecules, impairing its ability to activate T cells. This, greatly differ from resident dendritic cells, what points out for a most likely role for bDCs in the activation of infiltrating T cells than microglial cells. However, further presentation of myelin-derived epitopes by microglia to T cells triggers T cells to release a great deal of pro-inflammatory cytokines, as IFN-γ and TNF-α for Th1, and IL-17, IL-22 and GM-CSF for Th17 cells, establishing focal inflammation (Murphy AC 2010; Almolda B 2011). Microglia also secrete significant amounts of IL-23, as observed from human samples. Moreover, besides Th17 cells, both microglia and astrocytes are able to secrete IL-17 (Kawanokuchi J 2008). It has also been established that these populations also constitutively express IL-17R. It is interesting to mention that in vitro activation of astrocytes and microglial with rIL-17 resulted in interesting outcomes, such as the up-regulation of MCP-1, MCP-5, MIP-2 and KC. Thus, it is unquestionable that IL-17 greatly contributes fort the amplification of the inflammatory infiltrate, and its source may be resident cells as well as Th17 infiltrating lymphocytes.

Interestingly, using a microglial paralysis approach, it was clearly shown that functional microglia are fully needed for the establishment of the CNS inflammation. CD11b-HSVTK transgenic mice, which express herpes simplex thymidine kinase in macrophages and microglia after ganciclovir treatment impairs microglial activation, as observed by the interruption on the release of nitrite, proinflammatory cytokines and chemokines. As a consequence, mice are more resistant to EAE induction, with reduced CNS lesions, myelin degradation, cellular infiltration and cytokine release (Heppner HL 2005).

Due to its resemblance with macrophages, it is conceivable that microglia expression all inflammasome associated molecules, which in fact happens to be true. Microglia secrete not only IL-1β, but also IL-18 and IL-33, all of them caspase-1 derived cytokines. As discussed in the stroke session, IL-1 β has a very important role in the initiation of the inflammatory infiltrate. NOD (Nucleotide-binding domain, Leucine-rich Repeat containing family) like receptors (NLRs) have also been reported as important DAMP receptors in the CNS, being easily found in microglia (Chakraborty S 2010). Altogether, inflammasome-derived cytokines as well as NLRs and TLRs activation greatly contributes for local inflammation and thus influencing overall outcome.

Although it was known that IL-17 had a very important role in the pathogenesis of MS and EAE, either from resident cells or from Th17 cells, it was not well established the target of IL-17. Thus, it was elegantly demonstrated that IL-17-derived action is mostly played by astrocytes. Using conditional deletion of the Act-1 gene, that encodes an adaptor molecule of the IL-17R, it was clearly demonstrated that astrocytes change into a much activated state after engagement with IL-17. It is interesting to mention that IL-17 induced the expression of CXCL1, CXCL2, CXCL9, CXCL-12, IL-6, MMP-3 and MMP-9 in vitro and in vivo. Thus, NesCre / Act-1flox/flox mice are very resistant to EAE induction, with reduced CD4, CD19 and monocytes infiltration of the CNS. More interesting, Act-1 abrogation from microglia/macrophage or endothelial cells did not show any difference (Kang Z 2010) .This points out not only the main target of IL-17 activity, but also the importance of the CNS resident cells as astrocytes in the pathogenesis of EAE. Moreover, using astrocytes cultures, researchers demonstrated that these cells are able to induce Th1 and Th17 cells (Li Y 2007).

In fact, neuroglia cells, as astrocytes, microglia constitutively express many cytokines and chemokines receptors, such as IL-1R, IL-4R, IL-10R, IL-12R, TNFR1, TNFR2, GM-CSFR, IFN-γR, IL-17RA, CCR2, CCR5, TLR-2, TLR-4 among many others (Sedjwick 1991; Lin HW 2009). The engagement of these cytokines with its receptors triggers a cascade of events resulting in the expression of molecules such as, MHC I and II, iNOS, CD45, CD80, CD86, IL-1, IL-6, MMP-2, MMP-9, CCL2, among many others. Thus, the direct interaction of infiltrating encephalitogenic Th1 and Th17 cells with CNS resident cells, as microglia and astrocytes, is of great importance for the understanding of the pathogenesis of MS and also other neuroinflammatory diseases.

At last but not least, it is interesting to mention the role of oligodendrocytes during MS. In fact, oligodendrocytes are the main targets of peripherally activated T CD8 cells, whose antigen recognition induces oligodendendrocyte death by apoptosis, and thus demyelination, the hallmark of MS and EAE (Neumann 2003). Oligodendrocytes may be killed by several distinct mechanisms, such as FasL – Fas interaction, granzymes from cytotoxic T CD8 cells and also high amounts of TNF-α (Neumann 2003). More recently it has also been demonstrated that during EAE, the neuroinflammatory process significantly reduces the amount of Connexins (Cx), such as Cx32, Cx43 and Cx47. This reduction is associated with a disturbance in the gap junctions of oligodendrocytes and altered ionic balance, inducing cell death (Markoullis K 2012). In this context, besides the aforementioned ways to induce demyelination, intercellular interaction among glial cells also seem to have a pivotal relevance. The integrity of the myelin sheet is mandatory for a well functioning CNS. However, this integrity is breached during MS, damaging and destroying neuronal ability to transmit information, leading to a severe overall impairment.

2. Conclusions

The term glia, stands for glue, referring to the architectural role of these populations, such as astrocytes and microglial cells. Nowadays however, much new information was obtained concerning their biology, not only at resting state but also during neuroinflammatory processes. In this concern, microglia and astrocytes had gained more and more attention in the neuroimmunology field, specially due to its great capacity to generate important inflammatory factors, and also to directly interact with infiltrating T cells or monocytes. This results in the amplification of neuroinflammatory process and establishing the lesions themselves. In fact, it has been recently proposed a shift from T cell to innate immune dependence during the chronic phase of multiple sclerosis. Overall, data pointed out to microglial cells and astrocytes as master players during neuroinflammation, and therapeutic approaches focusing on reducing it activation status may greatly contribute to the treatment of neurological diseases, such as MS and stroke.

	Relevance in Stroke	Relevance in EAE / MS
Microglia	Express several receptors as IL-1R, IL-4R, IL-10R, IL-12R, TNFR1, TNFR2, GM-CSFR, IFN-γR, IL-17RA, CCR2 and CCR5.	Express several receptors as IL-1R, IL-4R, IL-10R, IL-12R, TNFR1, TNFR2, GM-CSFR, IFN-γR, IL-17RA, CCR2 and CCR5.
	Migrate to the penumbra caping dying neurons to reduce inflammation.	After activation up-regulates MHC I and II, CD40, CD45, CD80 and CD86 to activate infiltrating T cells.
	Hv1 expression correlates with NADPH oxidase activity and neuronal injury.	Secrete MCP-1, MCP-5, MIP-2 and KC after IL-17 activation.
	Secrete IL-1, IL-6, IL-12, IL-17, IL-23, TNF-α.	Secrete IL-1, IL-6, IL-12, IL-17, IL-23, TNF-α.
Astrocytes	Transglutaminase expression up-regulates cell death.	Undergo intense proliferation orchestrated by CD36
	Secrete IL-6, IL-12, TNF-α, MMP-3 and MMP-9.	After activation by IL-17 secrete high amounts of CXCL1, CXCL2, CXCL9, CXCL-12, IL-6, MMP-3, MMP-9, MCP-1, MCP-5, MIP-2
bDCs	bDCs migrate to the penumbra whereas peripherally recruited DCs migrate to the core.	Activate infiltrating T cells.
	May be involved in the activation of Tγδ lymphocytes.	Induce both Th1 and Th17 cells.

Table 2. Features highlights the importance of separate features in stroke and EAE/MS.

Author details

J. P. S. Peron*, D. Oliveira, W. N. Brandão, A. Fickinger and N. O. S. Câmara
Transplantation Immunobiology Lab, Department of Immunology, Institute of Biomedical Sciences IV, University of São Paulo, Cidade Universitária, São Paulo-SP, Brazil

J. P. S. Peron and N. O. S. Câmara
Disciplina de Nefrologia Universidade Federal de Sao Paulo, Sao Paulo, Brazil

A.P. Ligeiro de Oliveira
Laboratoty of Lung Inflammation Post Graduate Program in Biophotonics Applied to Health Sciences Nove de Julho University, São Paulo-SP, Brazil

L. V. Rizzo
Instituto de Ensino e Pesquisa, Hospital Israelita Albert Einstein, Morumbi, Sao Paulo, SP, Brazil

3. References

Abbul K Abbas, Jordan S. Pober. Andrew H. Lichtman. (2006). Cellular and Molecular Immunology, 4th Edition. Saunders Editor.

Ahrens S, Sancho D, Hanč P, Kjær S, Feest C, Fletcher G, Durkin C, Postigo A, Skehel M, Batista F, Thompson B, Way M, Reis E Sousa C, Schulz O (2012). "F-Actin Is an Evolutionarily Conserved Damage-Associated Molecular Pattern Recognized by DNGR-1, a Receptor for Dead Cells." Immunity Immunity(36): 4.

Almolda B, Castellano B. (2011). "Antigen presentation in EAE: role of microglia, macrophages and dendritic cells." Front Biosci. 16: 1157-71.

Arbeloa J, Gottlieb M, Matute C. (2011). "P2X7 receptor blockade prevents ATP excitotoxicity in neurons and reduces brain damage after ischemia." Neurobiol Dis 45(3): 954-61.

Avraham Y, Lassri V, Vorobiev L, Kabesa M, Dayan M, Chernoguz D, Berry E, Leker RR. (2011). "Leptin induces neuroprotection neurogenesis and angiogenesis after stroke." Curr Neurovasc Res 8(4): 313-22.

Baker BJ, Qin H, Ma X, Benveniste EN. (2010). "IL-27 inhibits OSM-mediated TNF-alpha and iNOS gene expression in microglia." Glia 58(9): 1082-93.

Bao Y, Kim E, Bhosle S, Guo H, Febbraio M, Haskew-Layton RE, Ratan R, Cho S. (2012). "CD36 is involved in astrocyte activation and astroglial scar formation." J Cereb Blood Flow Metab. 2012 Apr 18. doi: 10.1038/jcbfm.2012.52. [Epub ahead of print].

Baxter, A. G. (2007). "The origin and application of experimental autoimmune encephalomyelitis." Nat Med 7(11): 904.

Brait VH, Drummond GR, Sobey CG. (2012). "Importance of T lymphocytes in brain injury, immunodeficiency, and recovery after cerebral ischemia." J Cereb Blood Flow Metab 32(4): 598-611.

---

* Corresponding Author

Ceulemans A, Kooijman R, Hachimi-Idrissi S, Sarre S, Michotte Y. (2010). "The dual role of the neuroinflammatory response after ischemic stroke: modulatory effects of hypothermia " Journal of Neuroinflammation(7): 74-92.

Ceulemans AG, Kooijman R, Hachimi-Idrissi S, Sarre S, Michotte Y. (2010). "The dual role of the neuroinflammatory response after ischemic stroke: modulatory effects of hypothermia." J Neuroinflammation 7: 74.

Chakraborty S, Gupta M, Basu A. (2010). "Inflammasome Signaling At The Heart Of Central Nervous System Pathology." Journal of Neuroscience Research 88: 1615–1631.

Janeway CA. (2002). "Innate Immune Recognition." Annu Rev Immunol(20): 197-216.

Chu CQ, Dalton DK. (2000). "Failure to suppress the expansion of the activated CD4 T cell population in interferon gamma-deficient mice leads to exacerbation of experimental autoimmune encephalomyelitis." J Exp Med 192(1): 123-128.

Codarri L, Tosevski V, Hesske L, Fontana A, Magnenat L, Suter T, Becher B. (2011). "RORγt drives production of the cytokine GM-CSF in helper T cells, which is essential for the effector phase of autoimmune neuroinflammation." Nat Immunol 12(6): 560-567.

Colak G. (2012). "Complete transglutaminase 2 ablation results in reduced stroke volumes and astrocytes that exhibit increased survival in response to ischemia." Neurobiol Dis 45(3): 1042-50.

Cua DJ, Chen Y, Murphy CA, Joyce B, Seymour B, Lucian L, To W, Kwan S, Churakova T, Wiekowski S, Lira S, Gormank SA, Kasteleink RA Sedgwick JD. (2003). "Interleukin-23 rather than interleukin-12 is the critical cytokine for autoimmune inflammation of the brain." Nature 421: 744-748.

Crawford MP, Sterling B. Ortega, Riyaz S. Mehta, Rachel E. Hewitt, David A. Price, Peter Stastny, Daniel C. Douek, Richard A. Koup, Michael K. Racke, and Nitin J. Karandikar. (2004). "High prevalence of autoreactive neuroantigen-specific $CD8^+$ T cells in multiple sclerosis revealed by novel flow cytometric assay." Blood(103): 4222-4231.

Dardalhon V, Kuchroo VK, Anderson AC. (2008). "Role of Th1 and Th17 cells in organ-specific autoimmunity." J Autoimmun 31(3): 252-256.

Del Zoppo GJ, Gu YH, Osada T, Kanazawa M, Milner R, Wang X, Hosomi N, Mabuchi T, Koziol JA. (2012). "Microglial cell activation is a source of metalloproteinase generation during hemorrhagic transformation." J Cereb Blood Flow Metab 2012 Feb 22. doi: 10.1038/jcbfm.2012.11. [Epub ahead of print]

Dhawan J, Luo Z, Nawrocky M, Smith SD, Biegon A. (2011). "A new look at glutamate and ischemia: NMDA agonist improves long-term functional outcome in a rat model of stroke." Future Neurol 6(6): 823-834.

Dirnagl U, Moskowitz MA. (1999). "Pathobiology of ischaemic stroke: an integrated view. ." Trends Neurosci 22: 391-397.

Dohi K, Nakamachi T, Yofu S, Satoh K, Miyamoto K, Song D, Tsunawaki S, Shioda S, Aruga T. (2010). "Gp91phox (NOX2) in classically activated microglia exacerbates traumatic brain injury." J Neuroinflammation 7: 41.

Emsley HC, Georgiou RF, Vail A, Hopkins SJ, Rothwell NJ, Tyrrell PJ. (2005). "A randomised phase II study of interleukin-1 receptor antagonist in acute stroke patients." J Neurol Neurosurg Psychiatry 76: 1366-1372.

Emsley HC, Georgiou RF, Vail A, Hopkins SJ, Rothwell NJ, Tyrrell PJ: (2005). "A randomised phase II study of interleukin-1 receptor antagonist in acute stroke patients. " J Neurol Neurosurg Psychiatry 76: 1366-1372.

Engelhardt B. (2006). "Mollecular mechanisms involved in T cell migration across the blood-brain barrier." J Neural Transm 113: 477-485.

Felger JC, Kaunzner UW, Gottfried-Blackmore A, Gal-Toth J, McEwen BS, Iadecola C, Bulloch K. (2010). "Brain dendritic cells in ischemic stroke: time course, activation state, and origin." Brain Behav Immun 24(5): 725-737.

Gardoni F, Zianni E, Corsini E, Galli CL, Cattabeni F, Marinovich M, Di Luca M, Viviani B. (2011). "Distribution of interleukin-1 receptor complex at the synaptic membrane driven by interleukin-1b and NMDA stimulation." J Neuroinflammation 8(1): 14.

Ghiringuelli F, Housseau F, Kroemer G, Zitvogel L. (2007). "Links between innate and cognate tumor immunity." Curr Opin Immunol(19): 224-231.

Goverman J, Huseby ES (2005). "The role of CD8(+) T cells in multiple sclerosis and its animal models." Curr Drug Targets Inflamm Allergy 4: 239-245.

Heppner HL, Marino D, Falsig J, Raivich G, Hövelmeyer N, Waisman Ari ,Rülicke, Prinz M, Priller J, Becher B, Aguzzi A. (2005). "Experimental autoimmune encephalomyelitis repressed by microglial paralysis." Nat Med 11(2): 146-152.

Ivanov I, Zhou B, Tadokoro CE, Leppeley A, Lafaille JJ, Cua DJ, Littman DR. (2006). "The Orphan Nuclear Receptor RORgt Directs the Differentiation Program of Proinflammatory IL-17+ T Helper Cells." Cell(126): 1121-1133.

Iwakura Y. (2006). "The IL-23/IL-17 axis in inflammation." J Clin Invest. 116(15): 1218-22.

Jäger A, Sobel RA, Bettelli E, Kuchroo VK. (2009). "Th1, Th17, and Th9 effector cells induce experimental autoimmune encephalomyelitis with different pathological phenotypes." J Immunol 183(11): 7169-7177.

Janeway CA. (2001). "Innate immune recognition." Annu Rev Immunol. 20: 197-216.

Jones LS, Agarwal RK, Tarrant TK, Chan CC, Wiggert B, Caspi R. (1997). "IFN-gamma-deficient mice develop experimental autoimmune uveitis in the context of a deviant effector response." J Immunol 15(158): 5997-605.

Kang Z, Gulen MF, Liu C,Giltiay N,Qin H, Liu L, Qian W, Ransohoff RM, Bergmann C, Stohlman S, Tuohy VK, Li X. (2010). "Astrocyte-Restricted Ablation of Interleukin-17-Induced Act1-Mediated Signaling Ameliorates Autoimmune Encephalomyelitis." Immunity 32: 415-422.

Kawanokuchi J, Nitta A, Yamada K, Mizuno T, Takeuchi H, Suzumura A. (2008). "Production and functions of IL-17 in microglia." J Neuroimmunol 194: 54-61.

Kebir H, Ifergan I, Dodelet-Devilers, Bernarsd M, Giuliani F, Arbour N, Becher B, Prat A. (2007). "Human Th17 lymphocytes, promote blood brain barrier disruption and central nervous sysyem inflamation." Nat Immunol 13(10): 1173-1175.

Kettenmann H, Noda M, Verkhratsky A. (2011). "Physiology of Microglia." Physiol Rev 91: 461–553.

Komiyama Y, Matsuki T, Nambu A, Ishigame H, Kakuta S, Sudo K, Iwakura Y. (2006). "IL-17 plays an important role in the development of experimental autoimmune encephalomyelitis." J Immunol. 177(1): 566-573.

Korn T, Gao W, Bettelli E, Awasthi A, Petersen TR, Bäckström BT, Sobel RA, Wucherpfennig KW, Strom TB, Oukka M, Kuchroo VK. (2007). "Myelin specific regulatory T cells accumulate in the CNS but fail to control autoimmune inflamation." Nat Med(13): 423-431.

Kroenke MA. (2007). "Th17 and Th1 Responses Directed Against the Immunizing Epitope, as Opposed to Secondary Epitopes, Dominate the Autoimmune Repertoire During Relapses of Experimental Autoimmune Encephalomyelitis." Journal of Neuroscience Research 85: 1685-1693.

Li Y, Hu A, Gran B, Rostami A, Zhang G. (2007). "Increased IL-23p19 expression in multiple sclerosis lesions and its induction in microglia." Brain 130: 490-451.

Lin HW. (2009). "Context-dependent IL-6 potentiation of interferon- gamma-induced IL-12 secretion and CD40 expression in murine microglia." J Neurochem 111(3): 808-818.

Markoullis K, Gardner C, Hadjisavvas A, Reynolds R, Kleopa KA. (2012). "Disruption of oligodendrocyte gap junctions in experimental autoimmune encephalomyelitis." Glia. 2012 Mar 27. doi: 10.1002/glia.22334. [Epub ahead of print].

Martinez FO, Gordon S. (2009). "Alternative activation of macrophages: an immunologic functional perspective." Annu Rev Immunol 27: 451-83.

Matsunaga T. (1998). "What brought the adaptive immune system to vertebrates? The jaw hypothesis and the sea horse." Immunolog Rev 166: 177-186.

Matusevicius D, He B, Kostulas N, Ozenci V, Fredrikson S, Link H. (1999). "Interleukin-17 mRNA expression in blood and CSF mononuclear cells is augmented in multiple sclerosis." Mult Scler(5): 101-104.

Murphy AC, Lynch MA, Mills KH. (2010). "Infiltration of Th1 and Th17 cells and activation of microglia in the CNS during the course of experimental autoimmune encephalomyelitis." Brain Behav Immun 24(4): 641-51.

Neumann, H. (2003). "Molecular mechanisms of axonal damage in inflamatory central nervous system diseases." Curr Opin Neurol 16(3): 267-273.

Oksenberg Jr. (2005). "Genetics of multiple sclerosis." Neurol Clin 1(23): 61-75.

Owens GP, Burgoon MP, Yu X, Bennett JL. (2011). "Viruses and multiple sclerosis." Neuroscientist 17(6): 659-676.

Peron JP, Yang K, Chen ML, Brandao WN, Basso AS, Commodaro AG, Weiner HL, Rizzo LV. (2010). "Oral tolerance reduces Th17 cells as well as the overall inflammation in the central nervous system of EAE mice." J Neuroimmunol 227(1-2): 10-17.

Ponomarev ED, Tan Y, Dittel BN. (2007). "CNS-derived interleukin-4 is essential for the regulation of autoimmune inflammation and induces a state of alternative activation in microglial cells." J Neurosci 27(40): 10714-21.

Rebenko-Moll NM, Cardona A, Ransohoff RM. (2006). "Chemokines, mononuclear cells and the nervous system: heaven (or hell) is in the details." Curr Opin Immunol 18: 683-689.

Rodriguez, M. (2007). "Effectors of demyelination and remyelination in the CNS: implications for multiple sclerosis." Brain Pathol(17): 219-229.

Romi F, Gilhus NE. (2011). "Heat-shock proteins in clinical neurology." Eur Neurol 66(2): 65-69.

Rothhammer V, Petermann F, Srivastava R, Claussen MC, Hemmer B, Korn T. (2011). "Th17 lymphocytes traffic to the central nervous system independently of $\alpha4$ integrin expression during EAE." J Exp Med 208(12): 2465-76.

Ruppelt A, Grönholm M, Aandahl EM, Tobin D, Carlson CR, Abrahamsen H, Herberg FW, Carpén O, Taskén K. (2007). "Inhibition of T cell activation by cyclic adenosine 5'-monophosphate requires lipid raft targeting of protein kinase A type I by the A-kinase anchoring protein ezrin." J Immunol 179(8): 5159-5168.

S Stoll G, Nieswandt B. (2010). "Combating innate inflammation: a new paradigm for acute treatment of stroke?" Ann N Y Acad Sci 1207: 1207: 149-54.

Sedjwick J, Schwender S, Dorries R, Butcher GW, ter Meulen V. (1991). "Isolation and direct characterization of resident microglial cells from the normal and inflamed central nervous system." Proc Natl Acad Sci USA 88: 7438-7442.

Seong S. (2004). "Hydrophobicity: an ancient damageassociated molecular pattern that initiates innate immune responses." Nat Rev Immunol 4: 469-479.

Shichita T, Ooboshi H, Sugimori H, Nakagawa R, Takada I, Iwaki T, Okada Y, Iida M, Cua DJ, Iwakura Y, Yoshimura A. (2010). "Pivotal role of cerebral interleukin-17-producing gammadeltaT cells in the delayed phase of ischemic brain injury." Nat Med 15(8): 946-950.

Shie FS, Chen CH, Ho IK. (2011). "Neuroimmune pharmacology of neurodegenerative and mental diseases." J Neuroimmune Pharmacol 6(1): 28-40.

Song C, Lei Z, Li B, Liang D, Liu G, Li D, Zhang G, Huang B, Feng ZH. (2008). "IL-17-producing alvolar macrophages mediate allergic ling inflammation related to asthma." J Immunol 181: 6117-6124.

Stoll G, Nieswandt B. (2010). "Combating innate inflammation: a new paradigm for acute treatment of stroke?" Ann N Y Acad Sci: 149-154.

Suzuki T, Toma C., Ashida H., Ogawa M., Yoshikawa Y., Mimuro H., Inohara N., Sasakawa C. and Nun ez G. (2007). "Differential regulation of caspase-1 activation, pyroptosis, and autophagy via Ipaf and ASC in Shigella-infected macrophages." PLoS Pathog 3(111).

Thiel A. (2011). "Imaging of microglia activation in stroke." Stroke 42(2): 507-512.

Wang H, Zhang M, Vishnubhakat JM, Ombrellino M, Che J, Frazier A, Yang H, Ivanova S, Borovikova L, Manogue KR, Faist E, Abraham E, Andersson J, Andersson U, Molina PE, Abumrad NN, Sama A, Tracey KJ. (1999). "HMG-1 as a late mediator of endotoxin lethality in mice." Science 285(5425): 248-251.

Weiner HL. (2008). "A shift from adaptive to innate immunity: a potential mechanism of disease progression in multiple sclerosis." J Neurol. 55(1): 3-11.

Weiner HL, Matsui M, Orav EJ, Khoury SJ, Dawson DM, Hafler DA. (1993). "Double-blind pilot trial of oral tolerization with myelin antigens in multiple sclerosis." Science 259(5099): 1321-1324.

WHO (2006). "Neurological Disorders: Public Health Challenge." WHO(1-18).

Wu LJ, Akhavan Sharif MR, Baker A, Jia Y, Fahey FH, Luo HR, Feener EP, Clapham DE. (2012). "The voltage-gated proton channel Hv1 enhances brain damage from ischemic stroke." Nat Neurosci. 15(4): 565-573.

Zhou L, Spolski R, Sherendoz K, Egawa T, Levy DE, Leonard WJ, Littmann DR (2007). "IL-6 programs Th17 cell differentiation by promoting sequential engagement of the IL-21 and IL-23 pathways." Nat Immunol 8(9): 1-8.

Chapter 9

Autoimmune Encephalitis in Rural Central Illinois

Reuben Mari Valenzuela, Paayal Patel and Jorge C. Kattah

Additional information is available at the end of the chapter

http://dx.doi.org/10.5772/48409

1. Introduction

Encephalitis may be defined as "An acute inflammatory global neurologic dysfunction", characterized by altered mental status with protracted clinical course and high risk of significant morbidity. Timely therapeutic intervention is paramount to insure a good outcome". The most common endemic infectious encephalitis in immune-competent hosts involves several types of herpes virus infections, frequently herpes simplex virus (HSV). We may add to this group the less common epidemic-regional, arbovirus encephalitis. In recent years however, identification of novel auto-antibodies lead to the classification of autoimmune encephalitis in two clinical settings: 1.A paraneoplastic disorder (PNS) with either an overt or an occult neoplasm driving the dysimmune response 2. Antibodies directed against specific neuronal receptor channels in patients without underlying malignancy. In both groups, the initial management involves search for a possible occult neoplasm as a trigger of the autoimmune response and the expeditious initiation of immunosuppressive therapy. Autoimmune non-paraneoplastic encephalitis is the focus in this chapter. We will discuss four cases with autoimmune encephalitis diagnosed on our service in recent years. The clinical phenotype, work up results and treatment will be reported. A management algorithm will also be proposed (Figure 1). All four patients were residents of either rural or small urban Illinois communities. These cases illustrate how familiarity with these disorders and increasing comfort with immune-suppression represent a needed skill in the practice of General Neurology.

2. Case reports

Case 1

A 19 year old previously healthy right-handed Caucasian male presented with recent onset generalized tonic-clonic seizure on September, 2011. A few days later, he developed confusion, automatism, blepharospasm, orofacial dyskinesia and dysautonomia. His pulse rate would vary from 30 to 120 per minute throughout the day. He did not have fever, chills, neck stiffness, headache or viral-like prodrome. Neurological examination on admission was non-focal. Signs of meningeal irritation or increased intracranial pressure were not present. Other than sustained ankle clonus, we did not find additional abnormalities. Initial and serial follow-up brain computed tomography (CT) and magnetic resonance imaging (MRI) were unremarkable. Cerebrospinal fluid (CSF) findings were non-specific, with a lymphocytic pleocytosis (WBC 25, >90% lymphocytes) and negative bacterial, viral, fungal and protozoal cultures. Herpes simplex virus polymerase chain reaction (HSV-PCR) was negative. An electroencephalogram (EEG) showed slowing of background activity in the delta range, without epileptiform discharges. Work up for an occult malignancy was unrevealing. Computed tomography of the chest, abdomen and pelvis as well as a testicular ultrasound were all normal. Tumor markers including alpha fetoprotein (AFP) and beta human chorionic gonadotropin (*B*-hCG) were all negative. An autoimmune study performed by the Mayo Clinic laboratory was positive for anti-N-methyl D-aspartate (NMDA) antibody and negative for other relevant auto-antibodies, in particular the anti-Ma antibody. Treatment with intravenous methylprednisolone (MP), 1 gram (gm) daily for 5 days and a 5-day course of human immunoglobulin (Ig) at 0.4 gm/kg daily for 5 days was initiated. This was repeated once weekly for two months, along with tapering oral prednisone and a single dose of Rituximab. The patient also began 500 mg of mycofenolate twice daily with gradual and eventually complete neurological improvement. The patient returned to the spring semester in College and doing well.

Case 2

A 61 year old previously healthy right-handed Caucasian female presented with sudden episodic involuntary rapid irregular movements and posturing of the right upper extremity, facial grimacing and declining short term memory. Physical examination revealed intermittent involuntary facial grimacing and right hemiballismus but otherwise unremarkable neurologic examination. Her initial basic metabolic panel (BMP) demonstrated sodium (Na) of 127 (normal range 137-145 mmol/l) and Chloride (Cl) of 87 (normal range 98-107 mmol/l) but was otherwise unrevealing. Thyroid stimulating hormone (TSH), Vitamin B12 (B12), antinuclear antibody (ANA) and Copper levels were all within normal limits. A CT of the head revealed a 3.5 mm right frontal gray and white matter hypodensity. Pre and post-contrast brain MRI showed abnormal signal and edema involving the right anterior caudate and lentiform nuclei (Figure 1), and the genu and anterior limb of the right internal capsule (Figure 1). Electroencephalogram showed diffuse background slowing in the theta and delta range without epileptiform discharges. Several involuntary hemibalismus events were video-captured and deemed non-epileptic in nature. Magnetic resonance angiography (MRA) of the head and neck and trans-thoracic echocardiography (TTE) were normal. Hyponatremia normalized with fluid restriction. Clinically, symptoms other than short term memory deficits appeared to spontaneously resolve. The initial presumed diagnosis was an atypical vascular event. Repeat brain imaging as her clinical course seemed to briefly stabilize, demonstrated no change in previously noted abnormality. Subsequently, she developed increased agitation, disorientation, confusion, impulsivity, upper extremity chorea along with fecal and urinary incontinence. Her serum sodium dropped to 112 meq/ml, hence a 3 % NaCl therapy was initiated. Patient continued to decline clinically and required endotracheal intubation. Electroencephalogram showed asymmetric diffuse background slowing at the theta and delta frequency range, right hemisphere worse than left. A spinal tap showed normal opening pressure with normal glucose, protein, cell count, culture, venereal disease research laboratory (VDRL), Cryptococcus, IgG/Albumin ratio, myelin basic protein and oligoclonal bands. Patient appeared to improve clinically in relation to correction of her serum sodium status. She was extubated within a few days of her initial decline. In her case, hyponatremia was thought to be secondary to syndrome of inappropriate anti-diuretic hormone secretion (SIADH) and responded well to demeclocycline. Neuropsychiatric evaluation revealed deficits in concentration and constructional apraxia with delayed memory speed and processing. Patient's behavioral presentation and scores on cognitive testing suggested primarily a subcortical dysfunction with relatively intact performance on tests related to cortical functioning. Frequent episodes of facial grimacing and automatisms were noted during clinical recovery. A repeat EEG captured multiple complex partial seizures emanating from the right temporal lobe, therefore anticonvulsant therapy was started. Two follow-up brain MRI studies showed resolution of previous lesions, consistent with a transient inflammatory process.

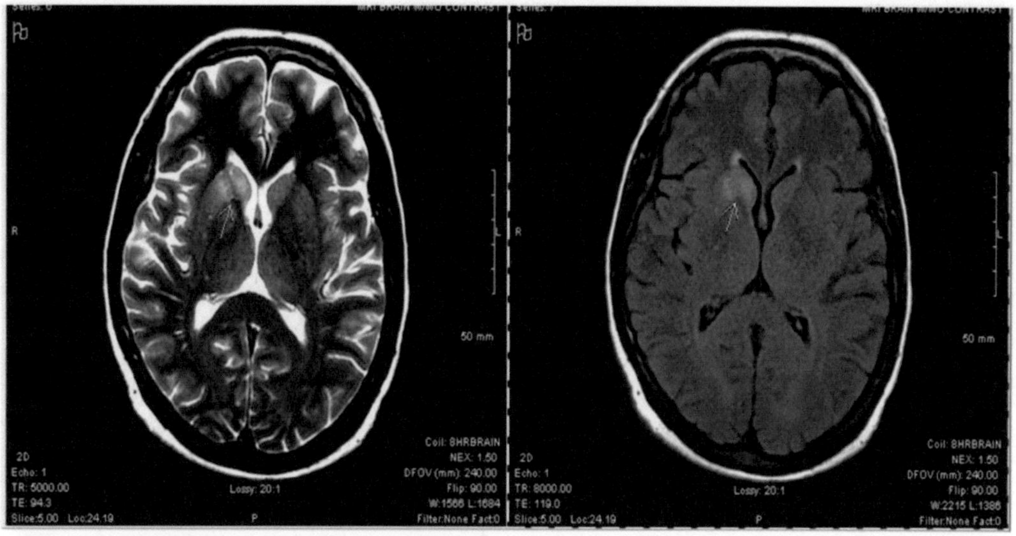

Figure 1. Brain MRI in Autoimmune Encephalitis
Axial T2 and FLAIR MRI of the brain in case 2. High signal intensity is present in the right caudate nucleus and adjacent anterior limb of the internal capsule.

Autoimmune encephalitis was suspected and patient was started on a 7-day course of human Ig at 0.4g/kg/24hours and leviteracetam therapy. In the ensuing week, despite normal neuroimaging, she suffered from frequent falls, orthostasis, hypothermia and bradycardia. Clinical suspicion of autoimmune encephalitis was confirmed by the presence of anti-voltage gated potassium channel antibodies. Computed tomography of the chest, abdomen and pelvis were unremarkable for malignancy making the diagnosis autoimmune limbic encephalitis most likely etiology. A 5-day course of human Ig at 0.4g/kg/24 hours was administered along with 1 gram IV MP. This was later followed by a slow taper of prednisone at 60 mg daily. Neurological exam remained non-focal, except for abnormal upper extremity movements which were persistent throughout hospitalization. Her dysautonomia, cognition and memory improved significantly. She begun tapering oral prednisone upon discharge for eight months and is presently back to normal.

Case 3

A 65 year old right-handed Caucasian male was admitted for evaluation of brief intermittent episodes of dysarthria, emotional lability and bizarre behavior. According to his wife, "crying spells" in recent months were not his usual nature. He had been a very healthy individual up until a very recent diagnosis of prostate cancer. Neurological examination was remarkable for astereognosia without other focal deficits. Mental status examination was normal without evidence of previously reported emotional lability. Initial brain MRI without contrast was normal. A comprehensive metabolic panel (CMP) requested on admission was remarkable for hyponatremia at 130 mmol/l. An EEG demonstrated independent epileptiform discharges from bilateral temporal lobes consistent with electrographic partial seizures. Oxcarbamazepine therapy was initiated at an oral dose of 300 mg twice daily with a recommendation to increase oral salt intake. Outpatient neuropsychological testing demonstrated prominent memory dysfunction characterized by global amnesia and semantic fluency deficiency consistent with left temporal lobe dysfunction. Generalized grand mal seizures and post-ictal confusion prompted readmission. Hyponatremia worsened at 126mmol/l, thus oxcarbamazepine was switched to leviteracetam. Despite the lack of clinical or electrographic seizure recurrence, the patient remained confused and disoriented. A repeat pre and post-contrast brain MRI demonstrated symmetric high T2 signal intensity involving bilateral mesial temporal lobes consistent with limbic encephalitis (Figure 2). Lumbar puncture (LP) revealed normal pressure, along with normal glucose and protein. Cells were not present and cytology was negative for malignant cells. Cerebrospinal fluid gram stain and cultures were negative. VDRL, HSV- PCR, cryptococcal antigen and lyme titers in the CSF were negative. Cerebrospinal fluid paraneoplastic panel was positive for neuronal voltage-gated potassium channel antibodies (0.60 nmol/l). Full body positron emission tomography (PET) scan was unremarkable for malignancy. Five days of MP at 1 gm/day and human Ig therapy at 0.4mg/kg/day were administered. Following these interventions, he demonstrated clinical improvement and was able to independently perform all activities of daily living. However, he continued to demonstrate severe long term memory impairment for nearly two months. He gradually improved on monthly human Ig and MP infusion therapy. In addition, he had episodic confusion and aphasia which required Video-EEG monitoring. No electrographic epileptiform activity was observed but lamotrigine therapy was initiated and maintained with successful outcome. Nearly 8 months from initial presentation, patient was noted to have complete resolution of symptoms. EEG and brain MRI returned to normal. Simultaneously, prostate cancer was characterized as adenocarcinoma, with a Gleason score of 5. He was treated successfully with external beam irradiation with subsequent decrease in his prostate specific antigen (PSA) levels. Human Ig and MP therapy was completed within a year and later discontinued. Thereafter, neurological and psychiatric examination remained normal.

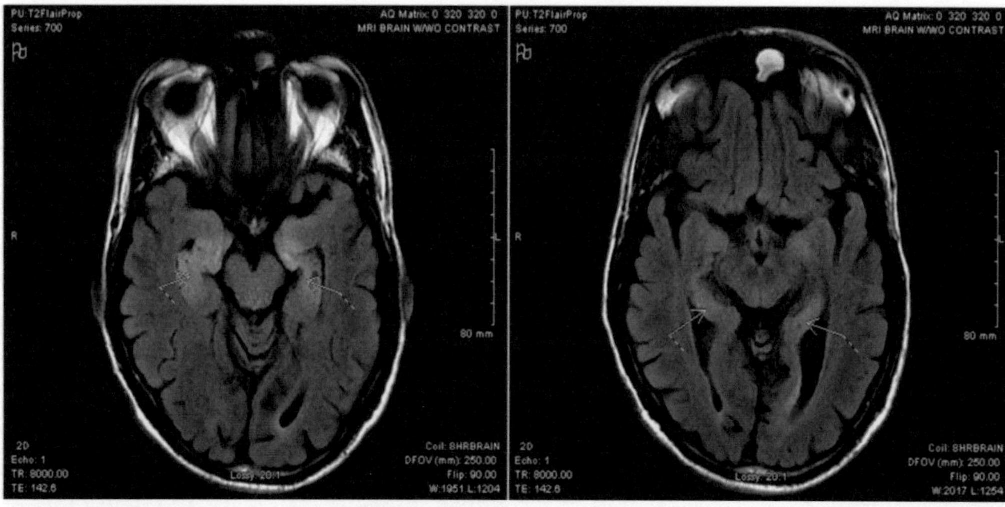

Figure 2. Brain MRI in Limbic Encephalitis
Axial FLAIR MRI of the brain in case 3. Areas of increased signal intensity are noted in the hippocampi. The right side is slightly thickened. CSF examination in this patient was normal and the Voltage-gated Potassium antibodies were present

Case 4

A 37 year old right-handed Caucasian female presented with an acute delirium associated with significant psychomotor agitation. Her past medical history was significant for acute polyendocrine autoimmune endocrine syndrome type 2 (APS 2) as well as Hashimoto's thyroiditis diagnosed in her early 20'. A few years later, she developed an acute autoimmune adrenal failure secondary to anti-21 hydroxylase antibodies (Titer: 27.3 U/ml; Normal :< 1 U/ml). Ovarian failure later ensued in her 30's. Her clinical and HLA picture (DR3 and DR4) were all diagnostic of an APS 2. Her neurologic examination was non-focal. A brain MRI and CSF were normal except for the presence of 6 white blood cells in the CSF. Herpes simplex virus-PCR was negative as well. An EEG demonstrated diffuse, generalized delta rhythm. Three years into her illness, a syndrome of recent memory loss occurred and a repeat MRI showed bilateral increased signal intensity involving the hippocampi. Anti-voltage-gated potassium channel (VGPC) antibody titers and a paraneoplastic panel were both unremarkable, and thus a diagnosis of recurrent autoimmune limbic encephalitis was made. She improved on high-dose MP followed by tapering oral steroids. Patient has done well for the last decade on 20 mg of methotrexate weekly. To our knowledge, this is the first description of autoimmune encephalitis associated with APS 2.

3. Discussion

The initial presentation of these patients consisted of an acute deterioration of mental status, agitation and sensorial changes with either a complex partial and or focal motor seizures. While initial dysfunction of the limbic system was seen in only one case, subsequent symptoms related to unilateral or bilateral medial temporal lobe dysfunction, complex partial seizures and memory loss developed in two additional patients, shortly after onset of symptoms. The term limbic was coined by Paul Broca from the Latin word meaning "ring" [26]. He used the word limbic to define structures located within the medial temporal lobes and diencephalon, which are involved in the formation and consolidation of short term memory. In addition, neurologic findings localized to this area frequently involve movement disorders and automatisms. We will review key pathogenic causes of autoimmune encephalitis, describe common clinical characteristics and propose a management algorithm.

4. Pathogenesis

A practical classification of autoimmune encephalitis can be based on pathogenic mechanism. In some instances, autoimmunity is triggered by a known or occult neoplasm, however in the absence of malignancy, auto-antibodies are directed against intracellular or neural membrane receptors. The cause of autoimmunity in non-PNS cases is unclear. Antibodies may be directed against intracellular antigens: (anti-Hu and anti-Ma), or antibodies against neuronal antigens (VGKC, NMDA receptor and Gamma-amino butyric acid (GABA) type b receptors) (1-25). Identification of these antibodies may provide a clue as to the possible associated neoplasm. For instance, anti-NMDA encephalitis is frequently associated with germ-cell tumors of the ovary and may rarely be seen in men, as was the case we reported. Anti-Ma antibodies are often present among patients with germ cell tumors of the testis. The anti-Hu is frequently present in small cell lung carcinoma (SCLC). Recent autoimmune encephalitis with antibodies against the alpha-amino-3 hydroxi-isoxazole propionic acid (AMPA) receptor have been reported reported [24]. Practically, the entire gamut of known auto-antibodies should be ordered in this group of patients as there is significant clinical overlap despite diverse neuronal antigenic targets. Once herpes virus encephalitis is ruled out, an investigation with auto-antibodies evaluation and immunosuppressive therapy can be initiated (Table 1). Given that reports from the immunologic testing usually take anywhere from two to three weeks, treatment should be initiated even before a diagnosis is confirmed. The initial therapy consists of high-dose intravenous Methyl-prednisolone, 1 gm daily for five days, followed by intravenous human Ig, usually at a dose of 0.4 gm/ kg per day for five additional days. Following a definitive diagnosis of autoimmune encephalitis, a plan of prolonged immunosuppressive treatment may be designed.

Importantly, Dalmau, et al recently reported serum reactivity to the leucine-rich glioma inactivated 1 protein (LGI1) among patients with VGKC antibodies [11,12]. It is unclear however, if anti-VGKC antibodies can be used to screen for this syndrome in every case. Hyponatremia is frequent and was found in two of our patients. We did not evaluate our patients for LGI1 antibodies because the above article by Dalmau et al was not in print when we evaluated these patients.

The neuropathologic findings in patients with paraneoplastic (PNS) autoimmune encephalitis include perivascular and interstitial lymphocytic cuffing, microglial proliferation, gliosis and neuronal degeneration. It is likely that non-PNS autoimmune encephalitis is associated with similar findings.

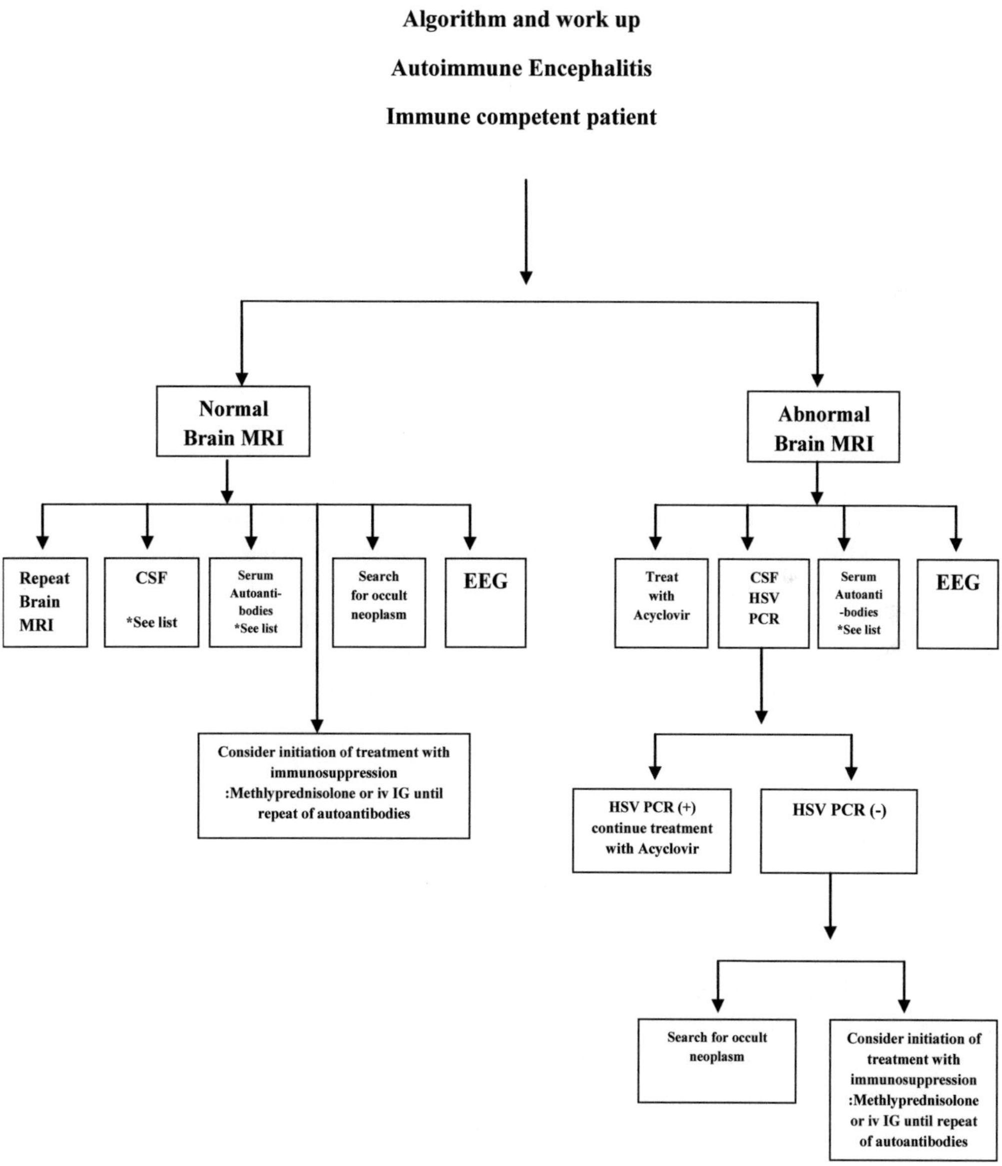

Table 1. Algorithm for autoimmune encephalitis

5. Clinical findings

The initial clinical manifestations of these disorders may suggest compromise of limbic structures and often precede global cerebral dysfunction. This sequence was observed in three of our patients (Table 2, cases 2, 3, 4). At times, a more rapid onset of symptoms may be observed. (Table2, case 1). Complex partial and Grand mal seizures are both common. Focal signs are otherwise infrequent, however confusion, agitation and delirium are present and maybe the initial presentation, particularly in anti-NMDA antibody mediated encephalitis. HSV encephalitis should be excluded and initiation of acyclovir therapy should not be delayed until CSF HSV-PCR result is available. Lack of improvement or worsening clinical picture despite treatment with acyclovir may suggest autoimmune encephalitis. Nutritional deficiency with Korsakoff's psychosis is usually evident from additional history and clinical findings. It is not possible from the clinical findings alone to determine if encephalitis represents a PNS. In fact, in greater than 65% of cases, PNS-related encephalitis is the first symptom of cancer. Occasionally, autoimmune encephalitis may mimic Creutzfeldt- Jacob disease (CJD) and both serum and CSF neuronal specific enolase, 14:3:3 protein and tau levels can be elevated. Consequently, a diagnosis of autoimmune encephalitis should be considered among possible CJD patients. Brain MRI is often abnormal in autoimmune limbic encephalitis; however a normal brain MRI in NMDA-associated encephalitis is not infrequent.

6. Neuroimaging

Brain MRI is generally abnormal. Unilateral or bilateral increased signal abnormalities involving mesial temporal lobes may be observed (Figure 2). Thickening of the hippocampi may be present without significant mass effect. Contrast enhancement is not frequent. Non-limbic MRI lesions may be found as well. The presence of susceptibility artifact if found would be suggestive of HSV encephalitis. In cases of anti-NMDA receptor encephalitis, imaging may be normal, thus making the diagnostic process even a greater challenge. The imaging abnormalities described may improve after initiation of treatment.

7. Additional testing

A work-up summary for patients with presumed autoimmune encephalitis is suggested in table 1. Electroencephalography would be abnormal in most cases. Generalized or focal slowing, epileptiform discharges emanating from temporal or frontal lobes are both frequent. Status epilepticus would be an unusual finding. Lumbar puncture frequently reveals a normal pressure and may show moderate lymphocytosis, increased protein and possibly oligoclonal bands, increased IgG and increased CNS IgG synthesis rate. HSV titers and PCR should be negative and neuronal specific enolase levels may be increased. Auto-antibodies may also be detected in CNS and titers can be monitored as a measure of treatment response. Comprehensive metabolic panels are generally normal with the exception perhaps of hyponatremia due to SIADH. Tumor markers may be present, suggesting PNS. We propose a work up algorithm that has been helpful in our experience. (table 1) A list of auto-antibodies, including PNS is listed in table 3

Patient	Clinical Presentation	MRI Findings	CSF Findings	Autoimmune Antibodies	Management
Case 1 19-year old male	Confusion Automatisms Oral dyskinesia Blepaharospasm Dysautonomia	Normal X 2	Lymphocytic Pleocytosis 25 WBC	Anti NMDA Receptor Antibodies	Mp Human IG Rituximab Cellcept
Case 2 61 year old female	Chorea Dystonia Hyponatremia Agitation Confusion	Increased Signal Caudate + Lentiform Nuclei + internal capsule	Normal	Anti –Voltage Gated K Channel Antibodies	MP Human IG Oral Prednisone
Case 3 65 year old male	Anxiety Crying spells Personality Change Hyponatremia Memory Loss Partial complex and grand mal seizures	Increased signal in bilateral temporal lobes	Normal	Anti-Voltage Gated K Channel Antibodies	MP Monthly Human IG
Case 4	Agitation Confusion Memory Loss Partial Complex seizures	Increased Signal bilateral temporal lobes	Mild CSF Lymphocytosis 6 WBC Increased Lactic Acid One OCB*	Anti-microsomal antibodies Antibodies against the 21-hydroxilase Polyendocrine Autoimmune failure type 2	MP Human IG Weekly Methotrexate Oral prednisone

Table 2. Clinical presentation, pertinent work-up and management of four cases

Neuronal Nuclear Antibodies
Antineuronal Nuclear Antibody- Type 1 (ANNA-1)
Antineuronal Nuclear Antibody- Type 2 (ANNA-2)
Antineuronal Nuclear Antibody- Type 3 (ANNA-3)
Neuronal and Muscle Cytoplasmic Antibodies
Purkinke Cell Cytoplasmic Antibody- Type 1 (PCA-1)
Purkinke Cell Cytoplasmic Antibody- Type 2 (PCA-2)
Purkinke Cell Cytoplasmic Antibody- Type Tr (PCA-Tr)

Amphiphysin Antibody
CRMP-5-IgG
Cation Channel Antibodies
N-Type Calcium Channel Antibody
P/Q Type Calcium Channel Antibody
Acetylcholine Receptor (Muscle) Binding Antibody
Acetylcholine Receptor Ganglionic Neuronal Antibody
Paraneoplastic Evaluation Algorithm
Aliases:
Acetylcholine Receptor (Muscle AChR) Binding Antibody
AChR (Acetylcholine Receptor)
AGNA
Amphiphysin Antibody, serum
ANNA (Antineuronal Nuclear Antibody)
AntiCV2
Anti-Enteric Neuronal Antibody
Anti-GAD65 (Anti-Glutamic Acid decarboxylase)
Anti-Glial Nuclear Antibody
Anti-Purkinke Cell Cytoplasmic Antibody
Anti-Ri
Anti-Skeletal Muscle Antibody
Anti-Yo
Antineuronal
APCA (Anti-Purkinke Cell Antibody
Calcium Channel Blockers
Cantoxin (Receptor Antibodies)
Cerebellar Antibodies
Syndrome and Antibody
Chorea
Collapsin Response-Mediator Protein 5 Antibody (CRMP-5), serum
Cramp-Fasciculation
CRMP-5-IgG
Dorsal Root Ganglion Antibody
Hu Antibody
ICab (Islet Cell Cytoplasmic Antibody)
Isaac's disease
Motor End-Plate Antibody
Motor Nerve Terminal Antibodies
Muscle Skeletal Antibodies
Muscle Culture Antibodies
Myoid Antibody
N-Type Calcium Channel Antibody

Neuromuscular hyperexcitability
Neuromyotonia
Neuronal Ganglionic Acetylcholine Receptor Antibody
Neuronal Nuclear Antibody
Neuronal Nuclear Antibody Panel
NMDA-Receptor Antibody (N-Methyl-D-Aspartate Receptor Antibodies)
Ovarian Cancer-Related Antibodies
P/Q Type Calcium Channel Antibody
Paraneoplastic Antibodies
Paraneoplastic Autoantibody Evaluation
Paraneoplastic Neurological Autoimmunity
Purkinke Cell Cytoplasmic Antibody- Type 1 (PCA-1)
Purkinke Cell Cytoplasmic Antibody- Type 2 (PCA-2)
Purkinke Cell Cytoplasmic Antibody- Type Tr (PCA-Tr)
Potassium Channel Antibodies (specify)
Ri, Antibody
Stiff-man Syndrome
Glutamic Acid Decarboxylase Antibody (Gad 65)
Striational (Striated Muscle) Antibodies
VGCC (Volatage Gated Calcium Channel Antibody)
Eaton Lambert Syndrome
Yo-Antibody
Ovarian Cancer

Table 3. Antibody testing among patients with autoimmune neurologic syndromes

8. Treatment

There is no evidence-based data to guide management of autoimmune encephalitis. Initially, a combination of intravenous high dose MP for 5 days and human Ig dose of 0.4 gm/kg for 5 days can be the first line of treatment. This may be followed by monthly injection of MP and human Ig. Rituximab may be helpful with 4 to 6 monthly doses. In some cases, additional on-going immunosuppression with mycofenolate or cyclophosphamide may be needed to treat either slow or non-improving cases. In addition, if the work up uncovers a neoplasm, surgical resection or chemotherapy should be initiated without delay. Considering that the initial identification of non-PNS autoimmune encephalitis is relatively recent, epidemiologic factors are now becoming apparent. Frequency and geographic distribution of these disorders will be available soon and this information could set the stage for future multicenter treatment trials.

Author details

Reuben Mari Valenzuela

PGY-2 Neurology Resident UICOMP, Illinois Neurologic Institute, University of Illinois College of Medicine, Peoria, USA

Paayal Patel
PGY-3 Neurology Resident UICOMP, Illinois Neurologic Institute, University of Illinois College of Medicine, Peoria, USA

Jorge C. Kattah
Department of Neurology UICOMP, Illinois Neurologic Institute, University of Illinois College of Medicine, Peoria, USA

9. References

[1] Vincent A, Buckley C, Schott JM, Baker I, Dewar BK, Detert N, Clover L, Parkinson A, Bien CG, Omer S, Lang B, Rossor MN, Palace J. Potassium channel antibody-associated encephalopathy: a potentially immunotherapy-responsive form of limbic encephalitis. Brain 2004; 127:701–712.
[2] Guletkin HS, Rosenfeld MR, Voltz R, Eichen J, Posner J, Dalmau J. Paraneoplastic limbic encephalitis: neurological symptoms, immunologic findings and tumor association in 50 patients. Brain.2000; 123:1481-1494.
[3] Geschwind MD, Tan KM, Lennon VA, Barajas RF Jr, Haman A, Klein CJ, Josephson SA, Pittock SJ (2008) Voltage-gated potassium channel autoimmunity mimicking Creutzfeldt-Jakob disease. Arch Neurol; 65:1341–1346
[4] Khan NL, Jeffree MA, Good C, Macleod W, Al-Sarraj S Histopathology of VGKC antibody-associated limbic encephalitis. Neurology 2009; 72:1703–1705
[5] Thieben MJ, Lennon VA, Boeve BF, Aksamit AJ, Keegan M, Vernino S. Potentially reversible autoimmune limbic encephalitis with neuronal potassium channel antibody. Neurology 2004; 62:1177–1182
[6] Cornelius JR, Pittock SJ, McKeon A, Lennon VA, Aston PA, Josephs KA, Tippmann-Peikert M, Silber MH.Sleep manifestations of voltage-gated potassium channel complex autoimmunity. Arch Neurol. 2011; 68:733-8
[7] Merchut MP. Management of voltage-gated potassium channel antibody disorders. Neurol Clin. 2010; 28:941-959.
[8] Gast H, Schindler K, Z'graggen WJ, Hess CW. Improvement of non-paraneoplastic voltage-gated potassium channel antibody-associated limbic encephalitis without immunosuppressive therapy. Epilepsy Behav. 2010;17:555-557.
[9] Rinaldi C, Russo CV, Filla A, De Michele G, Marano E. Course and outcome of a voltage-gated potassium channel antibody negative Morvan's syndrome. Neurol Sci. 2009; 30:237-239
[10] Iizuka T, Sakai F, Ide T, Monzen T, Yoshii S, Iigaya M, Suzuki K, Lynch DR, Suzuki N, Hata T, Dalmau J..Anti-NMDA receptor encephalitis in Japan: long-term outcome without tumor removal. Neurology. 2008. 70:504–511.
[11] Dalmau J, Tüzün E, Wu HY, Masjuan J, Rossi JE, Voloschin A, Baehring JM, Shimazaki H, Koide R, King D, Mason W, Sansing LH, Dichter MA, Rosenfeld MR, Lynch DR.

"Paraneoplastic anti-N-methyl-D-aspartate receptor encephalitis associated with ovarian teratoma. Ann. Neurol 2007; 61: 25–36.
[12] Dalmau J, Gleichman AJ, Hughes EG, Rossi JE, Peng X, Lai M, Dessain SK, Rosenfeld MR, Balice-Gordon R, Lynch DR. Anti-NMDA-receptor encephalitis: case series and analysis of the effects of antibodies. Lancet Neurol; 2011: 1091–8.
[13] Vincent A, Bien J Christian, Irani PS, Waters P. Autoantibodies associated with diseases of the CNS: new developments and future challenges. Lancet Neurol. 2011;10: 759-72
[14] Grisold W, Giometto B, Vitaliani R and Oberndorfer S Current approaches to the treatment of paraneoplastic Encephalitis. Ther Adv Neurol Disord (2011) 4(4) 237-248
[15] Titulaer J, R. Soffietti, J Dalmau, N.E. Gilhus, B. Giometto, FG, Raus, W. Grisold, J Honnorat, P. A. E. Sillevis Smith. R Tanasescu, C. A. Vedeler, R. Voltz and J. J. G. M. Verschuuren. Screening for tumors in paraneoplastic syndromes: report of an EFSN Task Force. European Journal of Neurology 2011, 18: 19-27.
[16] McNeill P. Kirkpatrick, Charles D. Clarke, Hasan H. Sonmezturk, Bassel Abou-Khalil. Rhythmic delta activity represents a form of non-convulsive status epilepticus in anti-NMDA receptor antibody encephalitis. Epilepsy and Behavior 20 (2011) 392-394
[17] Barry H, Hardiman O, Healy DG, Keogan M, Moroney J, Molnar PP, Cotter DR, Murphy KC. Anti- NMDA receptor encephalitis: an important differential diagnosis in psychosis. Psychiatry 2011; 199:508-9. Epub 2011 Oct 7.
[18] Zhang Q, Tanaka K, Sun P, Nakata M, Yamamoto R, Sakimura K, Matsui M, Kato N. Suppression of synaptic plasticity by cerebrospinal fluid from anti-NMDA receptor encephalitis patients. Neurobiol Dis. 2012; 45:610-615
[19] Lee M, Lawn N, Prentice D, Chan J. Anti-NMDA receptor encephalitis associated with ictal asystole. J Clin Neurosci. 2011:1716-1718
[20] Ham HP, Daniel-Johnson JA, Stotler BA, Stephens H, Schwartz J. Therapeutic plasma exchange for the treatment of anti-NMDA receptor encephalitis. J Clin Apher. 2011 Sep 5. doi: 10.1002/jca.20311. [Epub ahead of print]
[21] Gabilondo I, Saiz A, Galán L, González V, Jadraque R, Sabater L, Sans A, Sempere A, Vela A, Villalobos F, Viñals M, Villoslada P, Graus F. Analysis of relapses in anti-NMDAR encephalitis. Neurology. 2011; 77: 996-999.
[22] Kashyape P, Taylor E, Ng J, Krishnakumar D, Kirkham F, Whitney A. Successful treatment of two paediatric cases of anti-NMDA receptor encephalitis with Cyclophosphamide: The need for early aggressive immunotherapy in tumour negative paediatric patients. Eur J Paediatr Neurol. 2011 Aug 9. [Epub ahead of print]
[23] Irani SR, Vincent A. Autoimmune encephalitis -- new awareness, challenging questions. Discov Med. 2011; 11:449-58.
[24] Bataller L, Galiano R, Garcia Escrig M. Reversible paraneoplastic limbic encephalitis associated with antibodies to the AMPA receptor. Neurology, 2010; 74:265-267.
[25] Lai M, Huijbers MGM, Lancaster E, Dalmau J, Gordon BR. Investigation of the LGI1 as the antigen in limbic encephalitis previously attributed to potassium channels : a case series. 2010; 9: 776-785

[26] MacLean PD. Some psychiatric implications of physiological studies on frontotemporal portion of limbic system (visceral brain). Electroencephalography and Clinical Neurophysiology 4 (4): 407–418.

Chapter 10

The Role of the Antigen GAD 65 in Diabetes Mellitus Type 1: A Molecular Analysis

Marco Wiltgen and Gernot P. Tilz

Additional information is available at the end of the chapter

http://dx.doi.org/10.5772/48329

1. Introduction

Diabetes mellitus patients have a high blood sugar (glucose) level resulting either from the body's failure to produce enough insulin (Diabetes Mellitus Type 1) or because body cells do not properly respond to the produced insulin (Diabetes Mellitus Type 2) [1,2]. During the digestion, carbohydrates, contained in food, are converted within a few hours to glucose. Insulin is a hormone produced in the pancreas that enables body cells (primarily muscle and fat cells) to absorb glucose which is in turn transformed into energy needed for daily life [3,4]. The insulin production is triggered by the increase of the glucose concentration in blood (Figure 1).

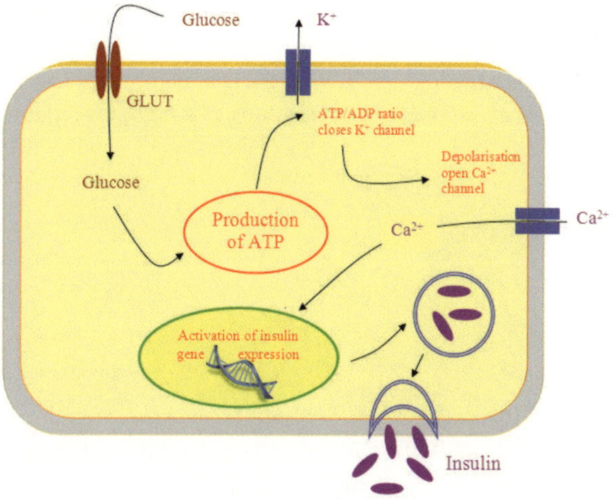

Figure 1. By the decomposition of glucose, ATP is produced in the beta cells. The increase of the ATP concentration closes the K^+ channel, leading to a depolarisation which in consequence opens the Ca^{2+} channel. Ca^{2+} activates the insulin gene expression via the Calcium Responsive Element Binding Protein (CREB). By exocytosis, the produced insulin is set free in the blood.

The regulatory function of insulin results in an instantly higher reception of glucose after the meals (Figure 2). Normally, insulin regulates the uptake of glucose from the blood during the course of a day (Figure 3). The inability of the body cells to absorb the glucose results in an accumulation (casual plasma glucose: 11.1 mmol/L) in the blood (hyperglycemia), leading to various potential medical complications and commonly leads to coma [5,6]. If the glucose concentration in the blood exceeds a certain amount it is discharged via the urine. Serious long-term complications of diabetes mellitus include cardiovascular disease, chronic renal failure and retinal damage [7-10]. Diabetes mellitus is currently a worldwide epidemic disease, sometimes referred as epidemic disease of the 21-th century [11,12]. Therefore an early diagnosis is desirable, enabling prevention at begin of this autoimmune disease.

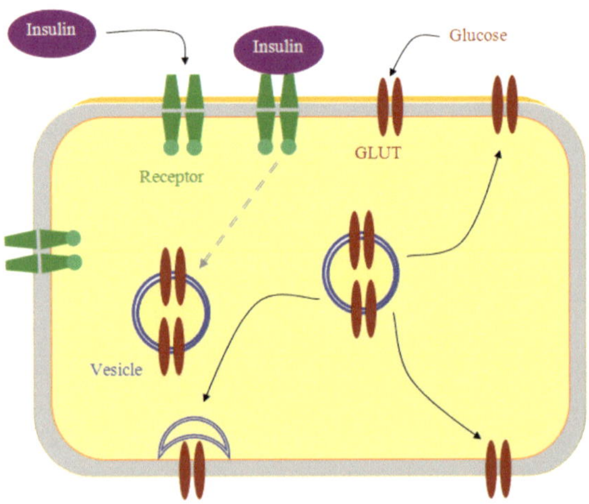

Figure 2. The hormone insulin induces the reception of glucose into the cells by a member of the transport protein GLUT. The binding of insulin at receptors, located at the cell surface, initiates the fusion of intracellular vesicles, containing GLUT, with the cell membrane. This increases instantly the number of the GLUT molecules at the cell surface, resulting in a higher reception of glucose.

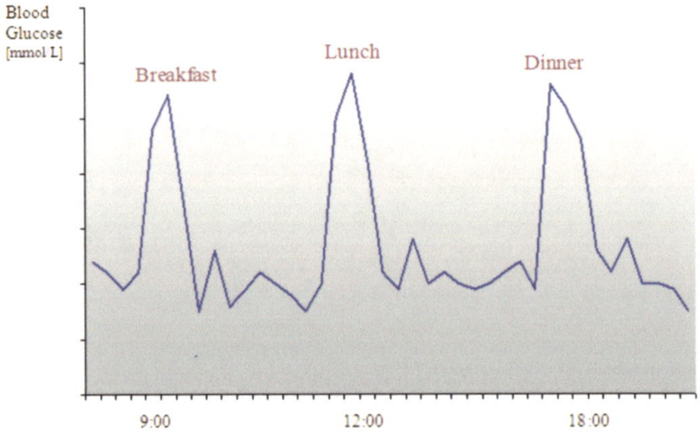

Figure 3. Qualitative view of the fluctuation of the blood sugar concentration in humans during the course of a day with 3 meals.

Diabetes mellitus type 1 result from the inability of the body to produce endogenous insulin; in consequence the patient must inject the required insulin, either manually or automatically via an insulin pump [13-14]. This is a major burden, because the insulin therapy, management and monitoring of diabetes is necessary for the rest of patient's life [15]. Goal of the insulin therapy is not the healing of the patient, but the replacement of the lack of endogenous insulin. Diabetes mellitus type 1 includes childhood-onset diabetes, juvenile diabetes, and insulin-dependent diabetes mellitus (IDDM) [16]. The type 1 diabetes causes approximately 10% of diabetes mellitus cases worldwide and represents a majority of diabetes in children [17]. Recent publications show that a doubling of diabetes mellitus type 1 in childhood (younger than 5 years) is expected by 2020, and in the juvenile age (younger than 15 years), the disease will rise by 70% [18]. Diabetes mellitus type 1 is characterized by a loss of the insulin-producing beta cells of the islets of Langerhans in the pancreas [19] (Figure 4). The majority of diabetes mellitus type 1 cases is of an immune-mediated nature, where the loss of beta cell results from a T-cell mediated autoimmune attack (antibodies: GADA, ICA, IA-2, IAA) [20]. After 80-90% of the beta cells are destroyed, the diabetes mellitus type 1 manifests. Therefore, at the start of the disease there is still a remaining insulin production. Mostly, at the onset of the disease, the affected people are otherwise healthy and of normal weight. In the early stages, the sensitivity and responsiveness to insulin are usually normal. The symptoms of diabetes mellitus are frequent urination (polyuria), increased thirst (polydipsia) and increased hunger (polyphagia) [21]. (Originally, the main symptom was excessive sweet urine, known as glycosuria). Diabetes mellitus type 1 may also cause a rapid weight loss and irreducible mental fatigue.

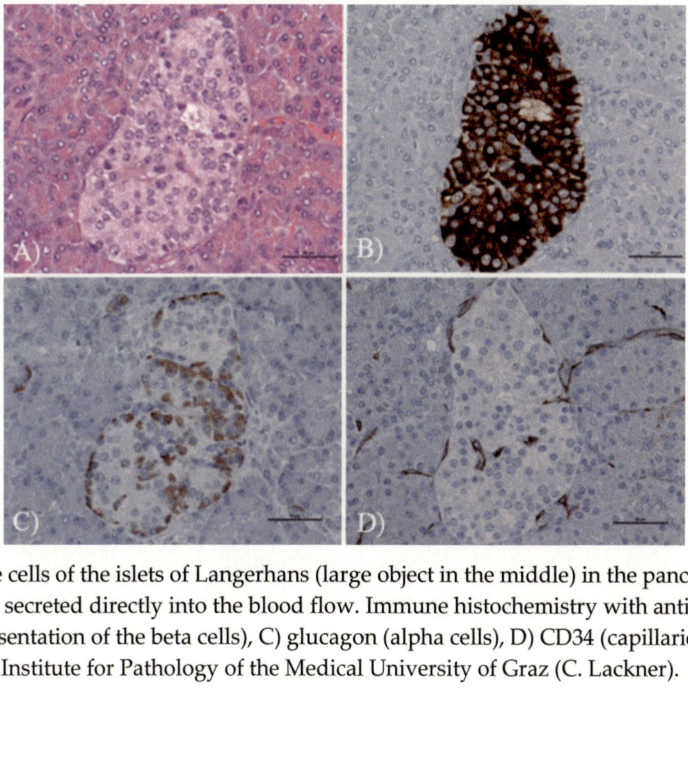

Figure 4. A) The cells of the islets of Langerhans (large object in the middle) in the pancrease produce insulin, which is secreted directly into the blood flow. Immune histochemistry with antibodies against: B) insulin (representation of the beta cells), C) glucagon (alpha cells), D) CD34 (capillaries). Picture provided by the Institute for Pathology of the Medical University of Graz (C. Lackner).

Whereas diabetes type 2 is mainly caused by lifestyle factors (such as smoking, elevated cholesterol levels, obesity, high blood pressure) and inheritance, diabetes type 1 seems to be only partly inherited, by mutations of the major histocompatibility complex (MHC) at chromosome 6, and requires an environmental trigger (possibly due to an infection). Certain infections, with some evidence pointing at Coxsackie B4 virus, rubella virus and others are considered risk factors [22-25]. Various nutritional risk factors, such as; the consumption of cow milk; early exposure to the protein gluten existing in some grass-related grains, notably wheat, rye, and barley, have been studied [26-28]. Bafilomycine, which is produced at decayed places in potatoes by streptomyces, leads to a glucose intolerance and damage to the islets of Langerhans in the pancreas. To explain the reaction of the autoimmune mechanism, it is assumed that certain bacteria and virus appears (from the point of view of the antibodies) similar to the cells of the pancreas (more precisely to a protein at the cell surface) and therefore the body destroys not only the infiltrated bacteria and virus but also attacks its own cells. Some sub structures of the antigens are similar to insulin and therefore trigger the autoimmune attack to the pancreas. Because insulitis, an inflammation of the islets of Langerhans of the pancreas, is considered to be a preliminary stage of diabetes mellitus type 1, an diminishing of the inflammation processes is considered to be a possible immune-therapeutically measure for the prevention of diabetes. The inflammation begins mostly in the childhood or at juvenile age.

For diabetes mellitus type 1, islet cell auto-antibodies (ICA) could be detected in 80% of the cases [29]. Other auto-antibodies are insulin-antibodies (IAA) and tyrosinphosphatase-antibodies (IA-2) [30]. The glutamic acid decarboxylase antibody (GADA) specifically attacks the enzyme glutamic acid decarboxylase (GAD 65) in the beta cells [31-34]. (65 refers to the molecular mass of 65kD). This antibody is an indication for diabetes type 1, although it is present in only 50-70% of the cases at the onset of the disease and at later stages successively more rarely. The GAD 65 gene is expressed in brain cells and in the beta cells of the pancreas. Inside the beta cells, the enzyme GAD 65 (EC 4.1.1.15) catalyzes the irreversible alpha-decarboxylation of L-glutamate into gamma-aminobutyrate (GABA) and carbon dioxide. (GABA is used as a neurotransmitter in the brain).

$$^{(-)}OOC-\underset{\displaystyle NH_3^{(+)}}{\overset{\displaystyle H}{\overset{|}{\underset{|}{C}}}}-CH_2-CH_2-COO^{(-)} \xrightarrow{GAD65} {}^{(+)}H_3N-CH_2-CH_2-COO^{(-)} + CO_2$$

GAD uses pyridoxal-phosphate (PLP) as a cofactor. GAD 65 is a homo dimer (it consists of two identical chains), characterized by successively 4 stranded β-sheets and 7 stranded β-sheets (Figure 5). The enzyme that can provoke an autoimmune reaction against the beta cells of the pancreas progressing to type 1 diabetes mellitus [35]. The GAD 65 antigen was considered to be strictly located intra-cytoplasmatic in the beta cells of the pancreas. But this hypothesis can not explain the procedure of immunization and therefore the occurrence of GAD 65 antibodies in the blood.

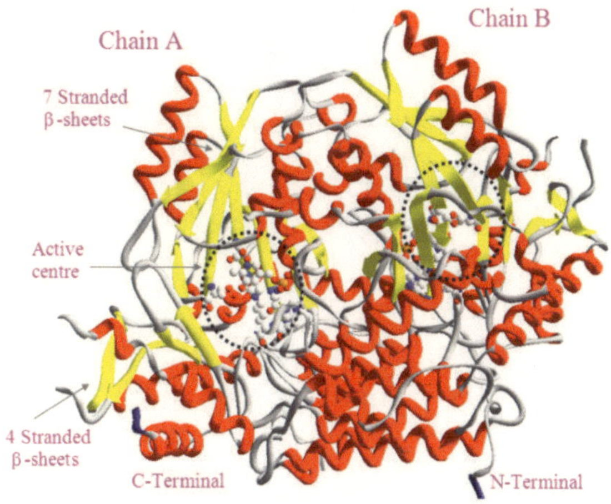

Figure 5. The enzyme GAD 65 is a dimer. Each chain contains 4 stranded β -sheets (yellow) surrounded by three α -helices (red) and 7 stranded β -sheets surrounded by eight α -helices. Every chain has an own active centre.

To understand the procedure and development of immunization, it was proposed that in an initial step the immune system is primed by the accessibility to GAD 65 [36,37]. The assumption is that the enzyme has to be in the human serum and should be found in higher concentrations before the onset of the disease. The proof and quantitative evaluation of GAD 65 in the human blood is done with the Fluorescence Correlation Spectroscopy (FCS), the Enzyme-Linked Immunosorbent Assay (ELISA) and the Surface enhanced laser desorption ionisation – time of flight (SELDI-TOF) system.

To illustrate the mechanism of autoimmunization, the visualization of the GAD 65 tertiary structure, together with its antigenic determinants and the associated electrostatic field, is essential. The 3-D molecular surface, derived from space filling models, visualizes the fitting of the GAD 65 epitopes to the paratopes of the antibodies and quantitative values for the GAD 65 antigenic properties are obtained by dual models. The electrostatic potential and details of the electronic structure of the GAD 65 epitopes are calculated by quantum theoretical methods. Readers, not interested in theoretical and mathematical details, can omit the corresponding chapters as the figures enable a pictorial understanding of the principles.

2. Measurement of GAD 65 in human sera

The GAD 65 molecules are detected by the binding with their unique and specific antibodies, which enables it to pick out the GAD 65 molecules in a mixture of different molecules (Figure 6). All detection methods, used in this work, are based on this principle. The monoclonal antibodies Z1 and Z2, provided by Phadia, Sweden-Diagnostics, Freiburg/Breisgau, Germany, were used for the detection of GAD 65 in all the assays. Antibody Z1 and antibody Z2 are reacting with different epitopes of the GAD 65 molecule.

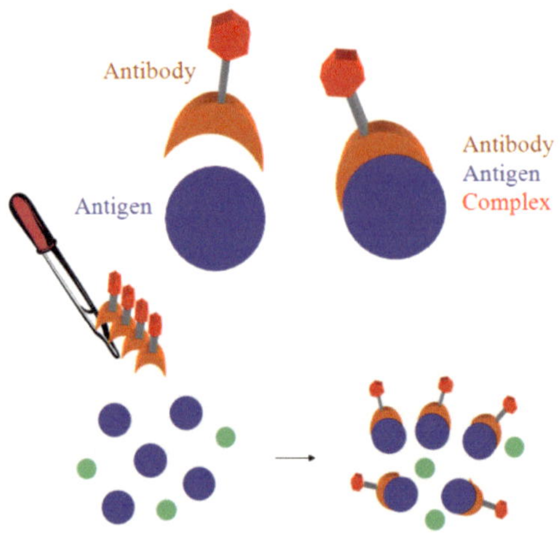

Figure 6. Antigens, like GAD 65, are detected by specific capturing with their corresponding antibodies. This enables it to pick up the antigen GAD 65 from a mixture of molecules.

Because very small concentrations of GAD 65 circulating in the human sera were expected, the ultra-sensitive fluorescence correlation spectroscopy (FCS) was used, at the beginning, for the search of free circulating GAD 65.

2.1. Fluorescence Correlation Spectroscopy (FCS)

FCS is a very sensitive analytical tool which enables the observation of a small number of molecules (up to picomolar concentrations) in a small volume element. By the FCS, the information about the molecules in the volume element is gained by evaluation of fluorescence fluctuations. FCS was developed by D. Magde, E. Elson, and W.W. Webb in 1972 [38]. The development of sensitive detectors such as avalanche photodiodes makes it possible to detect fluorescence signals coming from individual molecules in highly diluted samples. Improvements in the measurement techniques, notably by the introduction of confocal microscopy, enable a more precise separation of the measurement volume from the background. This improved the signal-to-noise ratio and allowed single molecule detection. In the 1990's began the practical application of FCS in molecular biology, ranging from the study of molecular dynamics, the determination of the size of proteins and the antigen-antibody coupling to the study of biochemical pathways in living cells.

2.1.1. Configuration and principle

With the FCS method, the GAD 65 molecules and their interaction with the corresponding monoclonal antibodies are measured by determining their diffusion times in a tiny volume element [39-43]. For this purpose the antibody molecules are labelled with fluorescent markers and excited by laser light. Because fluorochromes come in a variety of colours and can be specifically bound to particular molecules it is possible to study the behavior of individual molecules.

The FCS setup consists of a laser, an inverted microscope, a beam splitter (dichroic mirror), several optical units, a spectrometer with photo diode and an evaluation unit (Figure 7). The laser beam is directed by the beam splitter through the inverted microscope and focussed into a small focal volume of the sample. The labelled molecules in the sample are excited and emit fluorescence light. The emitted fluorescence light passes through the inverted microscope and the beam splitter. The beam splitter separates the excitation light from the emitted fluorescence light by transmitting the fluorescence light to the spectrometer and reflecting the excitation light back to the microscope. The transmitted fluorescence light then passes through a pinhole which blocks scattered excitation light and fluorescence light from outside the focal spot. The intensity of the filtered light is measured by avalanche photo diodes. The evaluation of the FCS measurement results is based on auto-correlation and cross-correlation analysis of the fluorescence fluctuations.

The optical unit of the FCS set up used in this study consists of a ConfoCor 2 (Zeiss) spectrometer and a confocal Zeiss Axiovert 100 microscope. An Argon ion-laser (458, 488, 514 nm) and 2 Helium neon lasers (543, 633 nm) are used for the excitation of the fluorescent molecules. The laser-light is concentrated by a C-Apochromat objective (x 40/1.2 W corr.) on small spots (diameter: 0.5 μm) in the sample solution. The GAD antibodies, were pipetted into a borosilicate chamber (Nalge Nunc, Lab Tek. chambered cover glass, German borosilicate cover glass, 8 chamber version), located on top of the inverted microscope.

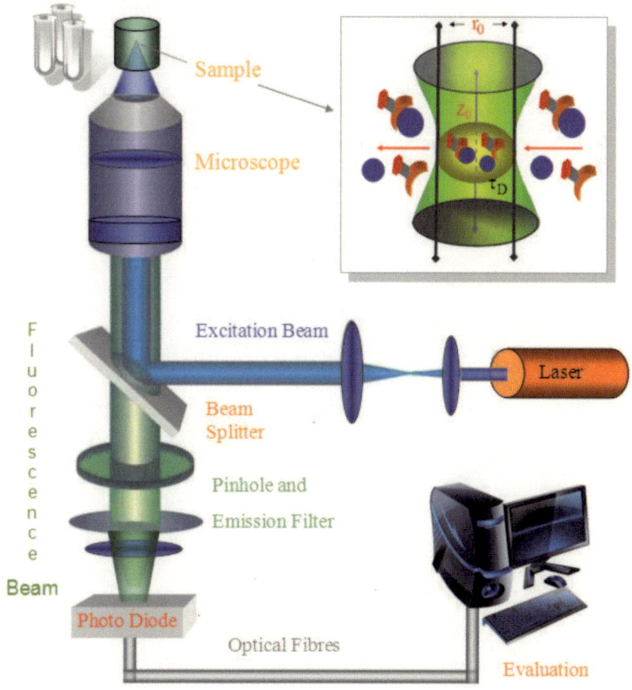

Figure 7. Set up and principle of the Fluorescence Correlation Spectroscopy (the radius r_0 is approximately 0.5 μm).

2.1.2. Evaluation of the fluorescence signal

The fluorescence intensity is fluctuating due to the Brownian motion of the molecules through the focal volume element, defined by the optical system, whereby the concentration of the particles $c(r,t)$ is randomly fluctuating around the average concentration $\langle C \rangle$:

$$\delta c(r,t) = c(r,t) - \langle C \rangle \tag{1}$$

The analysis gives the average number of fluorescent particles and average diffusion time, when the particle is passing through the volume. Since the relative fluctuations become smaller with increasing numbers of measured molecules, it is important to minimize the number of molecules in the focal volume. Changes in the diffusion times yield conclusions about the binding of GAD 65 to the corresponding antibody. The diffusion time of the labelled molecules depends on their size, therefore antigen-antibody compounds, which are bigger, show a slower diffusion time than the separated individual molecules. Modifications of the diffusion times give the required information on existence and concentration of GAD 65 in the specimens.

The fluorescence intensity fluctuations are recorded over time and quantified by temporally auto-correlation. From the auto-correlation and cross-correlation analysis of the fluorescence signal, results the characteristic diffusion times of the molecules. By the auto-correlation analysis, the measured fluorescence signal is compared with itself at some later time. The detected fluorescence signal intensity $I(t)$, at time step t, fluctuates around the mean intensity value $\langle I(t) \rangle$. The fluctuations of the emitted fluorescence signal are defined as the deviations from the temporal average of the signal:

$$\delta I(t) = I(t) - \langle I(t) \rangle \tag{2}$$

Whereby the mean intensity over the time period T is defined by:

$$\langle I(t) \rangle = \frac{1}{T} \int_0^T I(t')dt' \tag{3}$$

The auto-correlation function $G(\tau)$ combines the average fluctuation of the molecule at time step t with its fluctuation shifted by time τ (correlation time). The normalized auto-correlation function is defined as:

$$G(\tau) = \frac{\langle \delta I(t) \cdot \delta I(t+\tau) \rangle}{\langle I(t) \rangle^2} \tag{4}$$

The auto-correlation amplitude $G(0)$ is the normalized variance of the fluctuating fluorescence signal. If all fluctuations arise from changes in the local concentration of the molecules within the volume element of the focal spot, the variations in the fluorescence intensity can be written as:

$$\delta I(t) = \int_V W(r)\delta c(r,t)dV \tag{5}$$

The term $\delta(c(r,t))$ determines the dynamics of the molecules: $\delta c(r,t)$ describes the fluctuations in the local molecule concentration at time t .The function $W(r)$ describes the spatial distribution of the emitted fluorescence light. Substituting the expression for the intensity fluctuations into the auto-correlation function yields:

$$G(\tau) = \frac{\iint W(r)W(r')\langle\delta(c(r,t))\delta(c(r',t+\tau))\rangle dVdV'}{\left(\int W(r)\delta(c(r,t))dV\right)^2} \tag{6}$$

The auto-correlation function $G(\tau)$ is characterized by the correlation time τ and the correlation amplitude $G(0)$. Every process, producing fluctuations in the fluorescence intensity, has a characteristic correlation time. The FCS output by itself only represents a time spectrum. Interpretations on physical phenomena have to be extracted from the auto-correlation function by developing appropriate physical models. The parameters of interest are found after fitting the auto-correlation curve to modeled functional forms.

2.1.3. *Model of free diffusion*

If the model of free diffusion is used, the fluctuation signal is characterized by the diffusion time (in-out motion of the molecules in the volume element) and the average number of molecules in the volume element (Figure 8). The spatial and timely distribution of the molecule concentration in the model of free diffusion is given by the differential equation:

$$\frac{\partial}{\partial t}c(r,t) = D\left(\frac{\partial^2}{\partial x^2}+\frac{\partial^2}{\partial y^2}+\frac{\partial^2}{\partial z^2}\right)c(r,t) \tag{7}$$

This implies that the molecules are freely diffusing in three dimensions with the diffusion coefficient D. The larger the mass of the molecule, the larger is the diffusion time and in consequence the fluctuation is getting slower (Figure 8). The spatial distribution of the emitted fluorescence light $W(r)$ is approximated by a three dimensional Gaussian distribution:

$$W(r) = exp\left(-2\frac{x^2+y^2}{r_0^2}\right)exp\left(-\frac{z^2}{z_0^2}\right) \tag{8}$$

With:

$$r_0 = \sqrt{x_0^2+y_0^2} \tag{9}$$

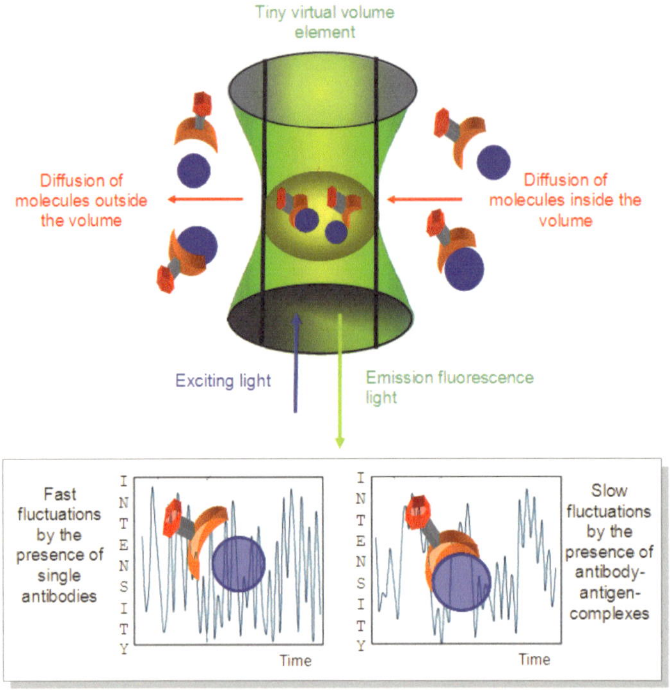

Figure 8. Shown is the diffusion of the labelled antibodies and the antigen-antibody complexes through the volume element, formed by the laser beam. The diffusion of the molecules through the volume element, due to their Brownian motion, is measured as fluctuations of the emitted fluorescence light. The different diffusion velocities give rise to different fluctuations lengths.

The function $W(r)$ is decayed to e^{-2} at r_0 in lateral direction and for $z = z_0$ in axial direction. By assuming the three dimensional Gaussian distribution of the emitted fluorescence light, the effective focal volume is calculated by:

$$V_{eff} = \int_V W(r)dV = \left(\frac{\pi}{2}\right)^{\frac{3}{2}} r_0^2 z_0 \qquad (10)$$

The dimensions r_0 and z_0 are determined by calibration measurements (Figure 7). Integrating out the differential equation for the free diffusion yields:

$$c(r,t) = \frac{c_0}{8(\pi Dt)^{\frac{3}{2}}} exp\left(-\frac{r^2}{4Dt}\right) \qquad (11)$$

This leads to a relation between the diffusion constant and the concentration fluctuation:

$$\langle \delta c(r,t)\delta c(r,t+\tau)\rangle = \langle C\rangle exp\left(-\frac{|r-r'|^2}{4D\tau}\right) \qquad (12)$$

For the model of free diffusion, the auto-correlation function (formula 6) can be calculated analytically (by use of formula 8 and formula 12) as:

$$G(\tau) = G(0)\frac{1}{\left(1+\frac{\tau}{\tau_D}\right)}\frac{1}{\sqrt{1+\left(\frac{r_0}{z_0}\right)^2\left(\frac{\tau}{\tau_D}\right)}} \tag{13}$$

τ_D is the diffusion time. This is the mean transit time of the molecule in the volume element (reciprocal of the average diffusion speed of the molecules). The relationship between the diffusion time τ_D and the diffusion coefficient D is given by:

$$\tau_D = \frac{r_0^2}{4D} \tag{14}$$

The auto-correlation amplitude $G(0)$ is proportional to the reciprocal of the average number of molecules $\langle N \rangle$ in the volume element:

$$G(0) = \frac{1}{\langle N \rangle} \tag{15}$$

Then, the local concentration of the fluorescent molecules in the effective focal volume element (formula 10) can be determinate from the amplitude $G(0)$ of the auto-correlation function:

$$\langle C \rangle = \frac{\langle N \rangle}{V_{eff}} = \frac{1}{V_{eff}G(0)} \tag{16}$$

Due to statistical averaging, the relative fluctuations of the fluorescent signal become weaker with an increasing concentration of molecules. Therefore it is important to minimize the concentration of molecules in the focal volume. The decay of the auto-correlation function is determined by the diffusion time (Figure 9). When the correlation time τ equals the diffusion time τ_D, then the auto-correlation takes the form:

$$G(\tau = \tau_D) = \frac{G(0)}{2}\frac{1}{\sqrt{1+\left(\frac{r_0}{z_0}\right)^2}} \tag{17}$$

The diffusion time τ_D is determined as fit parameter from the auto-correlation curve. Every augmentation of the mass of a biomolecule, resulting from the interaction with a second molecule, can be determined from the increase of the diffusion time. Molecular interactions are followed up by recording successive auto-correlation curves with shortest integration time. From those auto-correlation curves, changes in the diffusion time are determined (Figure 9).

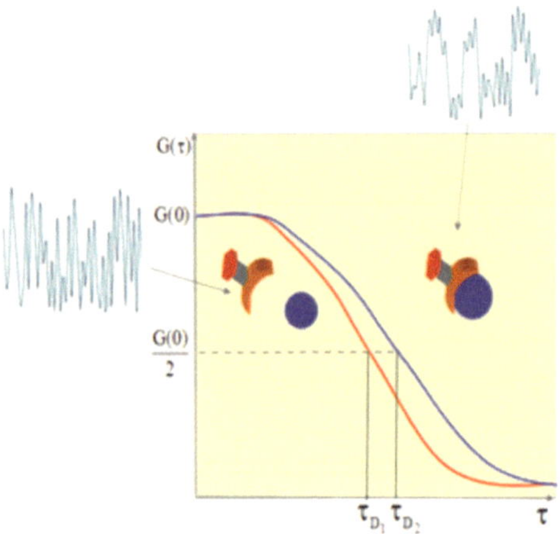

Reagents	Diffusion Time [microseconds]	
Antibody 1, labelled with Alexa 647	469	τ_1
Antibody 2, labelled with Alexa 488	230	
Antibody 1 in compound with GAD 65	985	τ_2
Antibody 2 in compound with GAD 65	630	

Figure 9. The diffusion time τ_D of the molecules is determined as fit parameter from the decay of the auto-correlation function $G(\tau)$. The interaction of the GAD 65 molecule with its antibody can be determined from the increase of the diffusion time.

2.1.4. Experiments

The sensitivity of the FCS method for the detection of GAD 65 was determined in clean and spiking experiments. Alexa 647 and Alexa 488 were used as dyes. In order to avoid disturbing auto-fluorescence for standardization, the detection of GAD 65 was carried out in bi-distillate water. By step-wise dilution, a minimal precisely detectable amount of 2.65 microgram/ml of GAD 65 was measured in such clean systems. To verify the minimal precisely detectable amount in sera, normal healthy controls were used, where the same amount of GAD 65 as to the clean systems was added (spiking experiment). Sera from 27 juvenile patients were investigated. All the children between 5 and 12 years were diabetes mellitus type 1 patients in an early stage and already had auto-antibodies. 126 sera of adult persons from normal admissions to the clinic served as controls. The sera from the paediatric patients came from a serum bank (Department of Paediatrics of the Medical University of Graz), the adult sera were fresh.

2.2. Enzyme-Linked ImmunoSorbent Assay (ELISA)

The second assay for the detection of the antigen GAD 65 in sera is the enzyme-linked immunosorbent assay (ELISA). As a heterogeneous assay, ELISA separates specifically components in a mixture by adsorbing them onto a solid phase which is physically immobilized. Therefore, the linking and adsorption of proteins (for example antibodies and antigens) is necessary. The chemical linking of proteins was developed by S. Avrameas and G. B. Pierce. The adsorption of proteins at solid states was developed in 1966 by L Wide and J.Porath. Based on these results, ELISA was developed in 1971 independently by two working groups, namely by P. Perlmann and E. Engvall at Stockholm University in Sweden and A. Schuurs and B. van Weemen in the Netherlands [44,45]. There exist different types of

ELISA which differ in more or less steps: the 'indirect' ELISA, the 'sandwich' ELISA, the 'competitive' ELISA and the 'multiple' ELISA. One of the most useful and common of the immunoassays for the detection of antigens is the two antibodies 'sandwich' ELISA. This assay enables it to determine fast and accurately the antigen concentration in biological sera [46-48].

2.2.1. *Principle and experimental setup*

The sandwich ELISA requires two monoclonal antibodies, the capture and the detection antibody, that bind to different epitopes on the antigen. A microtiter plate (with a size of 127.76 mm×85.48 mm×14.35 mm) is a flat plate with multiple wells, arranged in a regular 8x12 matrix array, which serve as small test tubes. Each well holds tens of nanolitres to several millilitres of liquid. The capture antibodies are fixed to the wells of the microtiter plate (Figure 10). In a first step, the serum is added to the capture antibodies and the corresponding antigen is picked up (Figure 10). The unbounded substances are washed away. In the next step, the detection antibodies are added and bind to the antigen. The detection antibodies are labelled with an enzyme. Again the enzyme-linked antibodies that do not bind are washed away. The remaining molecules form a "sandwich" consisting of layers of antibody/antigen/enzyme-linked antibody (Figure 10). In the last step, a colorimetric substrate is added, which is digested by the enzyme. This reaction results in a change of colour in the substrate, producing a visible signal, which indicates the quantity of antigen in the sample. Then, as result, the antigen is present in the sera if the substrate changes colour. The substrate concentration is measured by a photometer, whereby the concentration of the substrate is proportional to the antigen concentration in the serum.

2.2.2. *Evaluation of the results, calculation of the calibration curve*

For the evaluation of the ELISA output, the extinction is measured as a function of the concentration c of the coloured substrate inside the wells. The extinction E_λ is a measure for the diminishing of the intensity of light, with a wavelength λ, after passing a medium:

$$E_\lambda = -ln\left(\frac{I}{I_0}\right) \tag{18}$$

I_0 is the intensity of the incident light, I is the light intensity after passing the medium. If the extinction values are applied on the y-axis and the logarithm of the concentration $ln(c)$ on the x-axis, there results a sigmoid curve (mathematical function with an S-shape curve, including one turning-point and two asymptotes). Prior to the calculation of the calibration curve by a linear regression, the sigmoid curve must be transformed into a linear curve. The logit-function L is used for the linearization of sigmoid curves, which is of great importance for the evaluation of ELISA curves. From this operation results a linear curve. First, the measured extinction E_λ values are normalized so that the resulting values lie in the range between 0 and 1. The normalized extinction values are then expressed as:

$$N_E = \frac{E_\lambda - l_a}{u_a - l_a} \tag{19}$$

Whereby the upper (u_a) and lower (l_a) asymptotes of the sigmoid curve are used. The normalized extinction values are put into the logit-function L:

$$L = ln\left(\frac{N_E}{1 - N_E}\right) \tag{20}$$

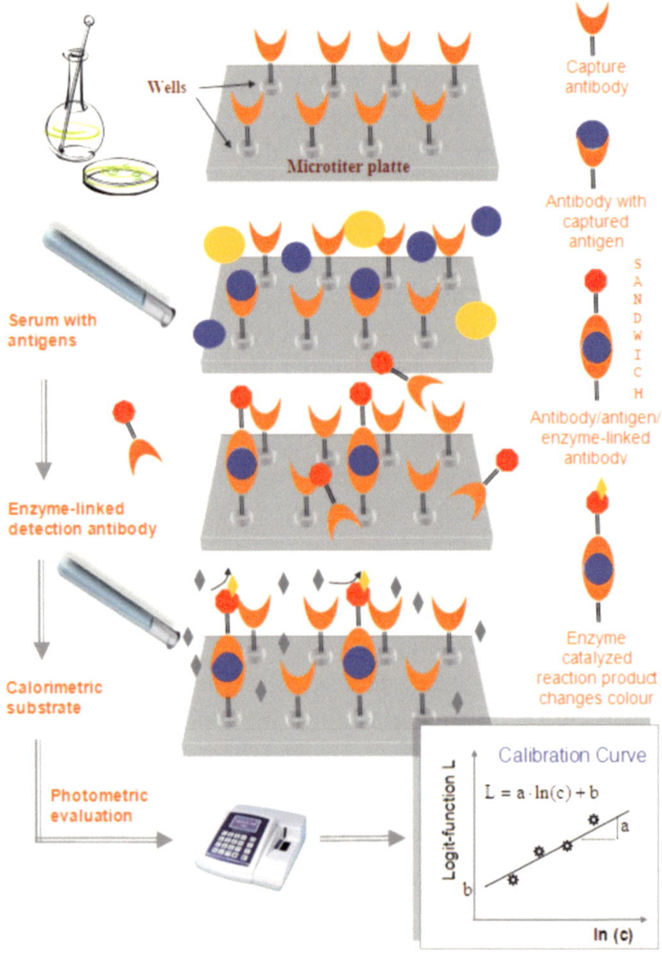

Figure 10. The capture antibodies are bound on a microtiter plate. The serum is added and the antigen GAD 65 is picked up. Then, the detection antibodies, labelled with an enzyme, are added and bind to the antigen. The enzyme catalyses a substrate reaction, whereby results a change of colour which is measured quantitatively by a photometer.

The value pairs of the logit-log-plot (x-value is the logarithm of the substrate concentration and the y-value is the logit of the normalized extinction values) are used for the linear regression. From the linear regression results the high (b) and ascent (a) of the linear calibration curve:

$$L = a ln(c) + b \tag{21}$$

Where: $ln(c)$ is the x-value and L is the y-value (Figure 10). Then, the concentration c of the substrate is calculated out of the measured extinction values. The best accuracy is obtained in the neighborhood of the turning-point of the sigmoid curve, because in this range the ascent has a maximum value.

2.2.3. *Experiments*

In order to evaluate the stability of the GAD 65 molecule in sera, the concentration measurements in the samples were repeated after a time delay. Additionally the correlation between the GAD 65 concentrations from samples stored at different temperatures was determined. The correlation between the GAD 65 concentrations at different time steps is calculated by linear regression. Given a series of *N* measurements of the variables y_n and x_n (*n*=1,2,…,*N*), then the correlation coefficient *R* is applied to quantify the strength of their linear dependence:

$$R = \frac{\sum_{n=1}^{N}(x_n - \overline{x})(y_n - \overline{y})}{(N-1)\sigma_x\sigma_y} \tag{22}$$

The quantities $\overline{x}$ and $\overline{y}$ are the mean values of x and y and σ_x and σ_y are the respective standard deviations. If the coefficient equals 1, then the concentrations are completely linearly correlated. If the coefficient equals 0, then the variables are completely independent. Serum samples from 64 persons representing a cross-section of the samples in a blood bank (in Freiburg, Germany) were used. The specimens were randomly selected. Each sample was stored at room temperature and additionally in a refrigerator cooled at -80°C.

2.3. Surface Enhanced Laser Desorption Ionisation – Time Of Flight (SELDI-TOF)

Mass spectrometry is an analytical technique that measures the mass-to-charge ratio of charged particles. Based on preceding works of B. Goldstein and W. Wien, J.J. Thomson developed the first mass spectrograph [49]. End of the 1950's the mass spectrometry was applied to the analysis of amino acids and peptides. K. Tanaka developed the laser desorption which was applied for the ionization of biological macromolecules, especially proteins [50]. In this study mass spectrometry was carried out according to the surface enhanced laser desorption ionisation – time of flight (SELDI-TOF) system. SELDI-TOF has been proven as suitable tool in the clinical laboratory for the profiling of biomarkers in complex biological specimens such as: serum, plasma, intestinal fluid and urine [51-56].

SELDI–TOF consists of an aluminium carrier, called the array, a laser unit and a system which measures the time of flight (TOF) of the molecules (Figure 11). The TOF system includes an electric field, induced by the acceleration potential, and a detector. Photomultipliers, avalanche diodes etc. are used as detectors.

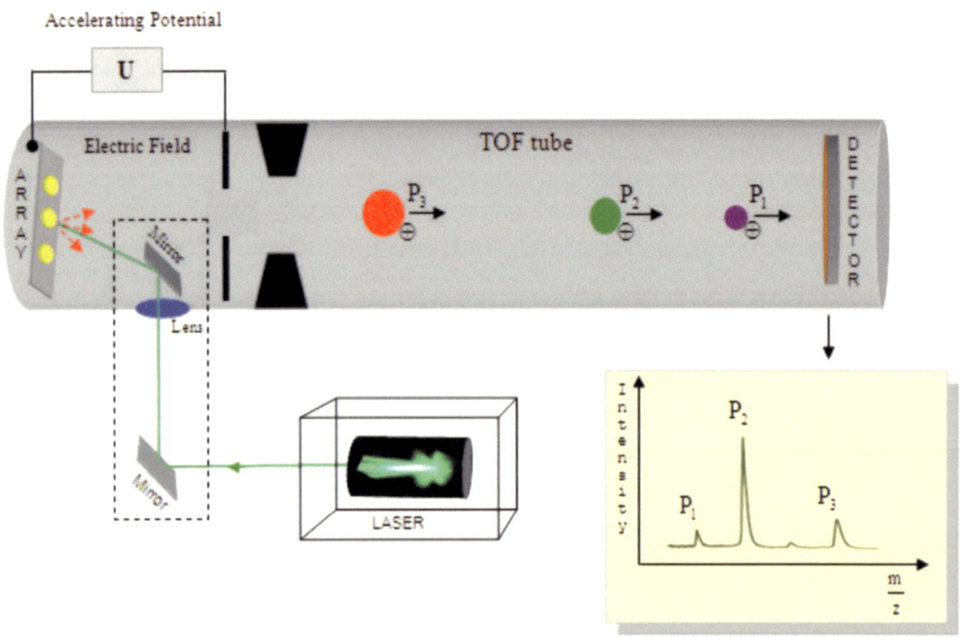

Figure 11. Surface enhanced laser desorption ionisation– time of flight (SELDI-TOF). The proteins are "eluted" from the matrix array by laser desorption and ionization. The ionized proteins are accelerated in the electric field and enter the TOF tube, according to their mass to charge ratio, with different velocities and each detection signal is represented by a peak in the mass spectrum.

2.3.1. Chip array

Proteins are captured by adsorption, electrostatic interaction, or affinity chromatography on the solid-phase protein chip array. The different chip types have either: surfaces that bind many different proteins or surfaces with a specific biomolecular affinity. The chips of the fist type are composed of chemical surfaces, which have: hydrophobic, hydrophilic, anionic, cationic or metal affinity properties. The chips of the second type are composed of biochemically active surfaces, such as: immobilized antibodies, receptor proteins, DNA fragments or enzymes. The first type of surface binds many different proteins, whereas the second type binds only specific molecules, such as: antibodies, factors, DNA binding proteins and substrates. Therefore, the biochemically active surfaces are used to exploit specific molecular recognition mechanisms.

After putting the sample on the chosen chip type, the weakly bound molecules are washed away. The remaining sample molecules are mixed with small photosensitive molecules. These molecules cause the sample to crystallize and form the matrix as it dries. (The matrix is composed of the molecules in the sample mix which are not analyzed). The photosensitive molecules facilitate desorption and ionization of the proteins in the mixture.

2.3.2. *Laser desorption and ionization*

The chip with the samples is put into a vacuum chamber, the flight tube of the mass spectrometer (Figure 11). The laser pulse excites the photosensitive matrix molecules. The energy of the excited molecules is converted into thermal energy which heats up the sample spot. The overheated part of the sample mix explodes into a plume and the molecules are liberated from the array (Figure 12). The protein molecules in the plume collide with the excited matrix molecules, whereby the matrix molecules transfer protons to the proteins and create charged proteins. Due to repeated processes, the proteins can get multiple charges.

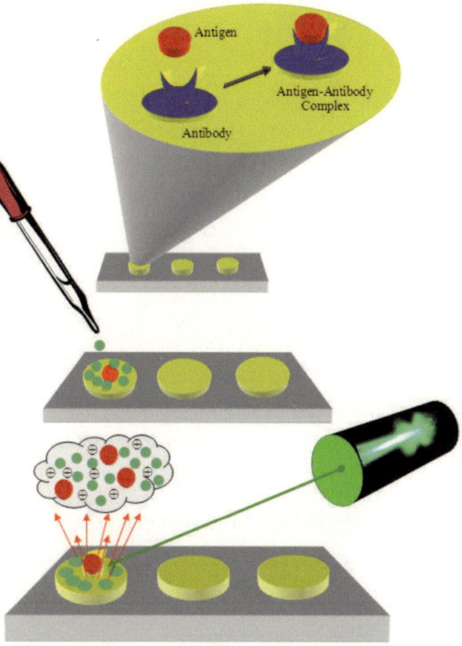

Figure 12. The chip array (aluminium carrier) contains immobilized GAD 65 antibodies, enabling it to focus specially on the GAD 65 antigen. The sample molecules are mixed with small matrix molecules, facilitating desorption and ionization of the proteins in the mixture. The laser pulse excites the matrix molecules; the serum molecules are liberated from the array and protonized.

2.3.3. *TOF-measurement*

Inside the vacuum chamber, an electric field (along the direction *r*) is generated by an electrostatic accelerating potential U :

$$\vec{E} = -\frac{\partial}{\partial r}U \tag{23}$$

The electric field is switched on synchronously with the end of the laser pulse. The protonated molecules are then accelerated in the electrical field by a force:

$$\vec{F} = ze\vec{E} \tag{24}$$

Where z is the net charge of the ionized molecule and e is the elementary electron charge ($1.602 \cdot 10^{-19}$ C). The molecules are accelerated into a field-free region, the TOF tube (Figure 11). Inside the TOF tube, the ionized molecules move toward the ion detector. The physical principle of the TOF analyser is that proteins, which have a different mass over charge ratio $\left({}^{m}\!/_{z}\right)$ are accelerated differently and enter the TOF tube with different velocities. The ratio of each protein molecule is recorded on the basis of the time required to pass through the tube. A protein with a net charge z, which passes through a potential difference of U, acquires an energy of:

$$E_{Pot} = zeU \tag{25}$$

The net charge is always a multiple whole number of the elementary electron charge e. The potential energy is converted, during the acceleration of the charged protein, into kinetic energy:

$$\frac{m}{2}v^2 = zeU \tag{26}$$

Where m is the protein mass and v is its velocity. Then the velocity of the protein inside the TOF tube equals:

$$v = \sqrt{\frac{2zeU}{m}} \tag{27}$$

Because the molecules gain the same kinetic energy in the electric field, the velocity of the molecules with a small mass is bigger than the velocity of molecules with greater masses. If the TOF tube has a length of d, the time of flight to the detector is given by:

$$t_{TOF} = \frac{d}{v} \tag{28}$$

The introduction of the molecule velocity (formula 27) into the equation yields:

$$t_{TOF} = \sqrt{\frac{m}{2zeU}}\, d \tag{29}$$

Then, the mass over charge ratio can be expressed as a function of the time of flight of the molecule:

$$\left(\frac{m}{z}\right) = \left(\frac{2eU}{d^2}\right)\left(t_{TOF}\right)^2 \tag{30}$$

The detector measures the time interval between the switch on of the electric field and the moment a charged molecule hits the detector. When the molecules strike the detector plates, the plates release a certain multiple of electrons. The release of electrons is generally amplified by a cascade of successive releases (avalanche effect). The detector signal is then defined by the ratio of released electrons and the number of molecules striking the detector plate.

2.3.4. *Mass spectrum and calibration*

The counted totals per time interval are displayed in the spectrum (Figure 11). The detection of molecules with the same molecular weight and the same electric charge produce a signal which is called a singleton peak. A peak in the spectrum is then the signal induced by neighbouring singleton peaks. The peak area is proportional to the number of detected molecules. The baseline of the spectrum is formed by the dark current inside the detector and the detected air molecules. In practice, linear deviations from the expected (theoretical) relation are observed. Therefore a calibration must be performed before the measurement. The calibration equation is given by:

$$\left(\frac{m}{z}\right) = \alpha U\left(t_{TOF} - t_0\right)^2 + \beta \tag{31}$$

The calibration equation considers the linear deviation in the spectrum by inserting the extraction delay t_0 and the calibration parameters α and β. The parameter α is given by:

$$\alpha = a\left(\frac{2e}{d^2}\right) \tag{32}$$

The factor a is a temporary dummy variable. By measuring the time of flight t_{TOF} of molecules with well known masses, the calibration parameters α and β are determined.

2.3.5. *Experiments*

The sera were tested on a PS20 slide provided by Phadia, Sweden-Diagnostic, Freiburg/Breisgau, Germany. PS20 Protein chip arrays are 8 spot chips with 2 mm diameter spots, spatially compatible with one column of a standard 96-well microplate. The investigations were made with the Ciphergen system (Ciphergen Protein Chip Software 3.0) and the calibrations of the spectra were realized in point of view of the GAD 65. The serum was applied on the array and covered with the matrix from the laboratory of the Pasteur Institute in Paris. In a first experiment, sera without dilution were used and in a second experiment, the sera were diluted. To realize a diagnostic procedure, every serum was tested in duplicate with different successive dilutions (1:5, 1:10, 1:20.). Within the latter of "marker molecules" with known molecular weight such as Albumin and the analytical GAD 65 molecule purisimum and in spiking experiments, the existence of GAD 65 can be estimated. The concentration of albumin in sera is of course tremendously higher than the concentration of the expected GAD 65. By use of the protein chip PS20 with fixation by covalent bonds of the GAD 65 antibodies, the contamination of the exuberant albumin is less disturbing. The sera from 2 paediatric patients (also contained in the sample set of the FCS measurements) with early onset of diabetes mellitus type 1 were kindly provided from the serum bank of the Department of Paediatrics of the Medical University of Graz.

3. Results

3.1. FCS

Clean and spiking experiments allowed a minimal precisely detectable amount of the GAD 65 at the concentration of 2.65 microgram/ml. The measured diffusion times are shown in figure 9. This enabled a sufficient serum dilution and avoids interference by auto fluorescence and other proteins in the FCS system. With diffusion times of 985 resp. 630 microseconds, GAD 65 could be found in 8 sera from patients with diabetes in an early onset. 4 of the patients were juvenile patients and 4 were adults, which were initially used as controls, who retrospectively showed signs of autoimmunity.

3.2. ELISA

GAD 65 was found in different concentrations, where the values range from 0.10-514.7 ng/ml (1 ng/ml = 10^{-9} g/ml), in all the samples (Figure 13). This leads to an average concentration of 58.00 ng/ml. The correlation between the GAD 65 concentrations from samples stored at room temperature and the same samples stored in a refrigerator cooled at -80°C are shown in Figure 14.

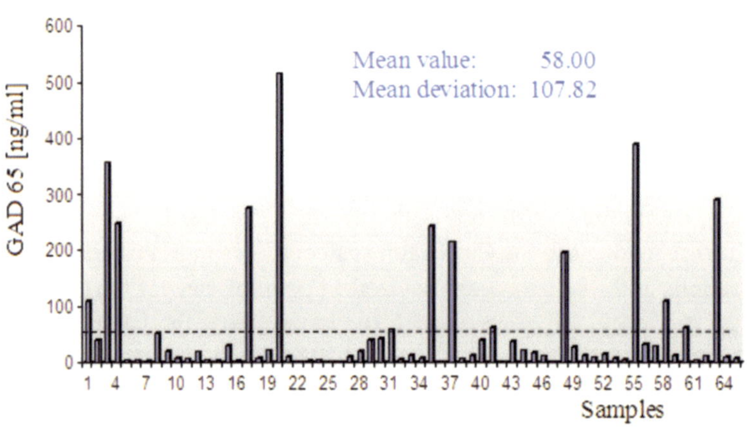

Figure 13. With the ELISA setup, GAD 65 was found in human sera from a blood bank, with values ranging from 0.10-514.7 ng/ml.

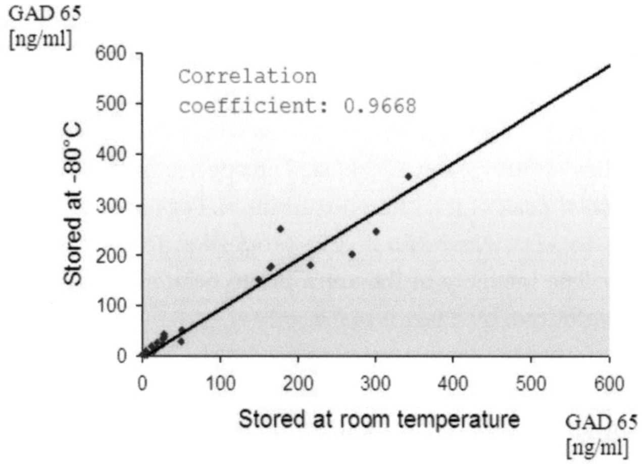

Figure 14. Correlation between the GAD 65 concentrations from samples stored at room temperature and cooled at -80°C.

The high value of the correlation coefficient (0.9668) shows that there is practically no difference in the concentrations between samples at room temperature and the same samples at -80°C. Additionally, the correlation between the GAD 65 concentrations taken from samples stored at room temperature and taken from the same samples after a time delay of one week was calculated. During this week, the samples were stored at room temperature (Figure 15). The value of the correlation coefficient (0.9897) demonstrates that the GAD 65 molecule remains highly stable over a time period of one week.

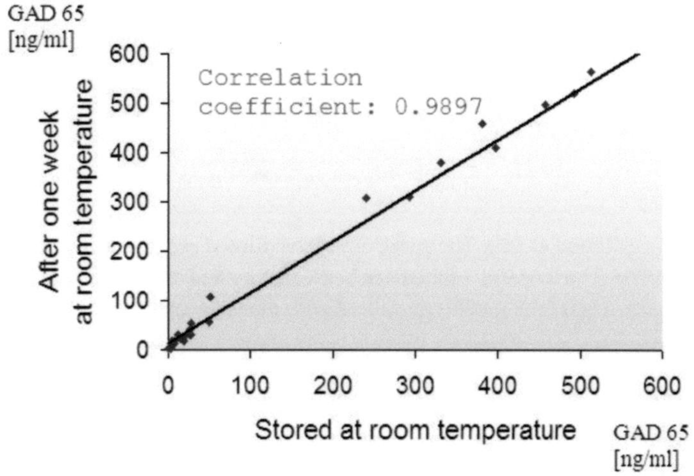

Figure 15. Correlation analysis between the GAD 65 concentrations taken from samples stored at room temperature and taken from the same samples after a time delay of one week.

3.3. SELDI-TOF

Evidence for GAD 65 in one serum sample in the mass spectrum was found, giving a peak very close to albumin with a molecular weight of 65 kDa. This serum was from a juvenile patient with an early onset of diabetes mellitus type 1. Peak evaluation after spiking experiments was done to have comparable results as with FCS. The spectra always show the peaks of the antibodies at 50, 75 and 150 kDa. The spectra of the diluted sera (Figure 16) show a much diminished peak of the reference albumin. For the interpretation of the results, the peak intensity at 65 kDa was calibrated in proportion to the intensity of the albumin peak in the reference. The intensity of the appropriate peak in the spectrum is greater than the peak obtained for albumin by a factor of 8.4.

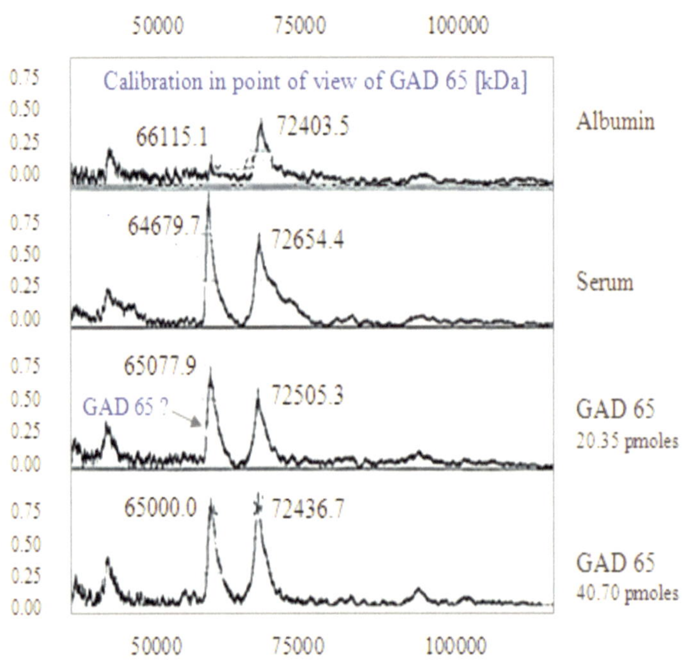

Figure 16. The sera are diluted at 1:20. The spectrum of the diluted serum shows a peak at 65kDa which may results from GAD65. The intensity of the peak is greater, by a factor of 8.4, than the corresponding albumin peak. This serum is from a paediatric patient with diabetes mellitus type 1 at an early stage.

4. Molecular analysis and visualization

Functional specificity and biological function of a protein are linked to its structure. Due to the 3-D folding structure, the residues, which are responsible for the protein function, are brought into a precise geometric arrangement. The rest of the protein structure is mainly necessary to enable and maintain the correct spatial position between the amino acids on the active site. Therefore, to understand a protein function, the 3-D structure of the protein reveals far more information than its sequence.

For an analysis and planning of neutralization of GAD 65 with antibodies in the sera, the locations and shapes of the epitopes on the GAD 65 molecule are important. The structural visualization of the GAD 65 molecule and its epitope locations is illustrative and may help the reader to speculate on the antigenic sites of the molecule, enabling an understanding of the interaction with the immune-receptor, which is the basis for the development of active or passive immunotherapy in the near future. The epitopes are well known in literature and were identified by homolog-scanning mutagenesis, where segments of sequences from a homologous molecule (GAD 67) known not to bind to the specific antibodies are systematically substituted throughout the GAD 65 gene [57,58]. A complete or partial loss of antibody reactivity by the resulting mutated molecules (chimeras) suggests that GAD65 specific sequences required for contact with the antibody has been exchanged by the point mutation. The quaternary structure of GAD 65 was determined experimentally by X-ray diffraction [59]. In this paper the visualization is done with the Swiss-Pdb Viewer (http://spdbv.vital-it.ch) [60].

4.1. Visualisation of macromolecules

Bioinformatics is an interdisciplinary discipline between computer science and molecular biology. On one side, bioinformatics is a science with interconnected data banks, connecting sequence information to structural, biomedical and clinical data. On the other side, bioinformatics is a science which provides mathematical algorithms and computational tools for: detecting sequence similarities and finding homologous sequences; prediction, analysis and visualization of protein 3-D structure etc.

Structural information about proteins is available in the PDB structure database, an international repository for 3-D structure files [61]. Once a protein structure has been determined experimentally, either with crystallographic methods or by nuclear magnetic resonance spectroscopy, the structural information is deposited into the PDB. The structural information is stored in the PDB as data files, which contain mainly the Cartesian coordinates of all atoms involved in the protein (Figure 17). The entry point to the structural protein data is the PDB web site: http://www.rcsb.org/pdb. The database is accessed via Internet and the selected PDB data files, containing the atomic coordinates, are downloaded. The data files are used as input for protein visualization and the viewer software transforms the information in the PDB data file into an appropriate representation of the protein 3-D structure. Usually the molecules are visualized by "balls-and-sticks" models or by ribbons showing their secondary structures (Figure 5). The step from a molecule (set of connected atoms) to geometric shape is done by space filling diagrams. The theory of space filling diagrams is part of topology: the area of mathematics concerned with spatial properties that are preserved under continuous deformations of objects.

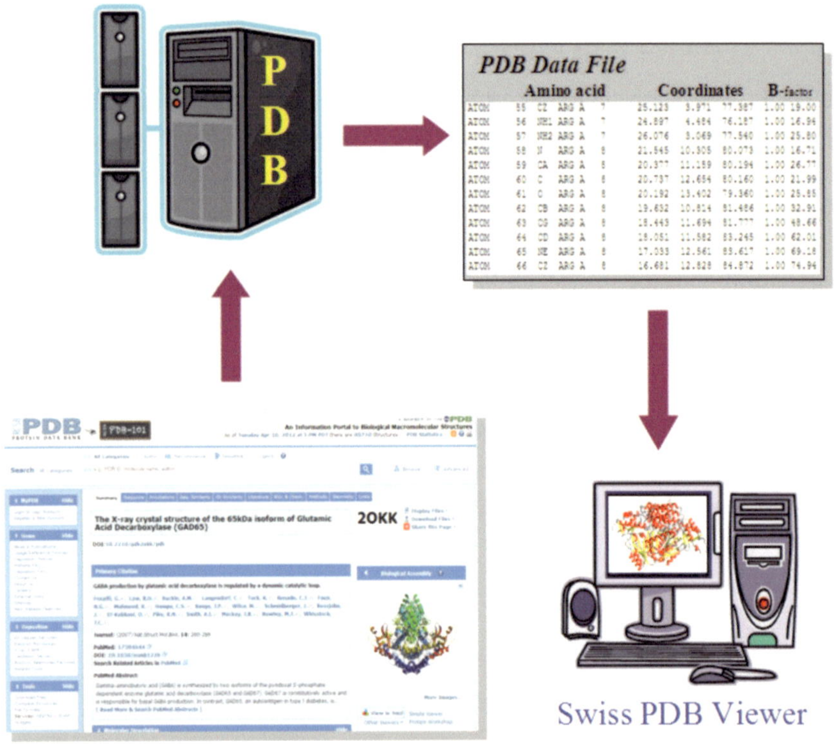

Figure 17. Protein structural information is available at the Protein Data Base (PDB). At the moment the database contains more than 80.700 experimentally determined structures. The PDB is contacted through the Internet. The structural information is stored in the PDB data files as atomic coordinates. The B-factor indicates the precision of each atom position. The requested PDB data files are downloaded and the protein structure visualized locally.

4.2. Space filling models and molecular shapes

Space filling diagrams are models that represent a molecule by the space it occupy [62-65]. They are embedded in the 3-D space ($\mathbb{R}^3$) and show properties that make them suitable for molecular analysis. Each atom in a space filling diagram is represented by its location in space and a quantitative expression of influence on its surrounding. Most commonly, the space-filling diagram of a molecule is defined as the union of overlapping balls A_i :

$$SFM = \bigcup_{i \in \mathbb{N}} A_i \tag{33}$$

The molecular boundary is defined as the envelope of the union of overlapping spheres. Three types are of special interest: the van der Waals model, the solvent accessible model and the molecular surface model.

Van der Waals model (VW): Due to the movement of the electrons around the atomic nucleus, an atom can be considered as an electric dipole. The dipole of an atom polarises the neighbour atom resulting in a transient attractive force between the atoms. Conversely, at short ranges a repulsive force between the electrons of both atoms arises. The radius at which the repulsive force begins to increase sharply is called the van der Waals radius. The van der Waals sphere A_i of the i -th atom of a molecule is specified by its atom type and has a location in space: $z_i \in \mathbb{R}^3$ and a radius $r_i \in \mathbb{R}_+$. This radius r_i is the same for all atoms of the same type i. The van der Waals model of a molecule is a union of balls:

$$VW = \left\{ x \in \mathbb{R}^3 \middle| \exists_i : \|x - z_i\| \le r_i; i = 1,...,N \in \mathbb{N} \right\} \tag{34}$$

N is the number of atoms in the molecule. That means: the van der Waals model is the set of points x which are located inside the distance r_i from the centre of the van der Waals sphere A_i. The van der Waals spheres of binding atoms overlap, whereas the spheres of non-binding atoms do not overlap (Figure 18). As the van der Waal model, the following space filling models depend on the atomic van der Waals radii and the coordinates of the atoms in the molecule.

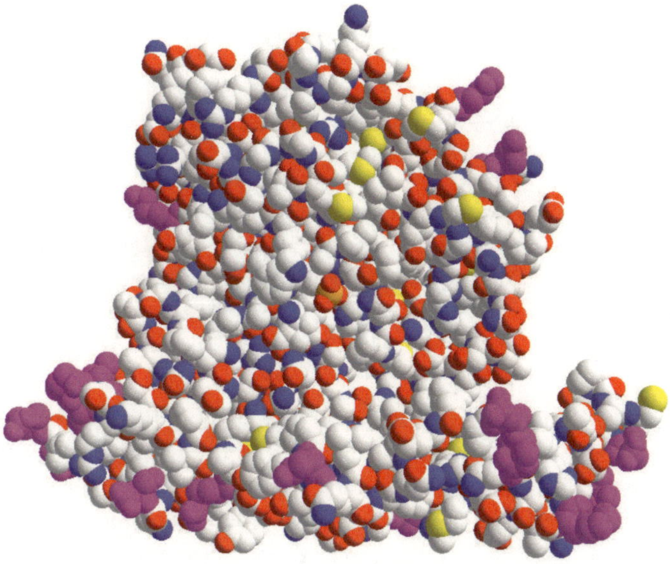

Figure 18. Van der Waals surface of GAD 65: The boundary of the space filling diagram is made up as envelope of the union of spheres with van der Waals radii.

Solvent accessible model (SA): The interaction of the Van der Waals model and a solvent molecule, represented as sphere of radius ρ, is studied by increasing the radius r_i of every van der Waals sphere, associated to an atom A_i, by ρ. That means: the radius of the van der Waals sphere is expanded by the radius of the solvent (Figure 19). The solvent accessible model is then defined (similar to the van der Waals model) as the union of the enlarged balls:

$$SA = \left\{ x \in \mathbb{R}^3 \middle| \exists_i : \|x - z_i\| \le r_i + \rho; i = 1,...,N \in \mathbb{N} \right\} \tag{35}$$

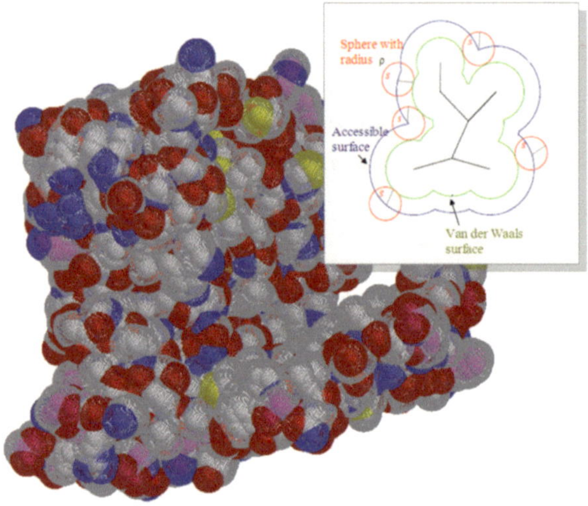

Figure 19. Solvent accessible model of GAD 65: The boundary of the space filling diagram is made up as union of spheres which are grown by the radius of the sphere of a single solvent molecule. The accessible surface is the surface generated by the centre of the solvent sphere rolling of the van der Waal surface.

The accessible surface is the surface generated by the centre of the solvent sphere rolling of the van der Waals surface. The radius ρ of the solvent sphere is usually set to 1.4 angstrom (the approximate radius of a water molecule).

Molecular surface model (MS): A model that resembles in size the van der Waals model and in connectivity the solvent accessible model is the molecular surface model. It consists of all points $x \in \mathbb{R}^3$ that lie outside all solvent spheres disjoint from van der Waal modell:

$$MS = \left\{ x \in \mathbb{R}^3 \middle| \forall_{y \notin SA} : \|x - y\| > \rho \right\} \tag{36}$$

The surface is generated by a sphere of radius ρ rolling about the van der Waals model. The molecular surface is the envelope generated by the rolling sphere. It differs from the van der Waal surface by covering portions of the volume inaccessible to the rolling sphere (Figure 20). It consists of sphere and torus patches connected in a tangent continuous manner. The shape of a molecule is described by the molecular surface, which is the boundary of the molecule volume within which no other molecule can enter. The molecular shape of the antigen and the corresponding antibody is of special importance for the understanding of their intermolecular interaction. The interaction is usually described in terms of locks and keys: The shape of the lock (the antigen) must be complimentary to the shape of the key (the antibody) to initiate an immune response. The body develops antibodies with the right shape to attack specific antigens. The docking places for the antibodies are the epitopes of the antigen. The locations of the sequence fragments, constituting the epitopes, are highlighted on the GAD 65 3D structure (Figure 21). Molecular surfaces are suitable for the visualization of the epitope shapes, which enables a pictorial analysis of the local docking sites and their fitting. For the quantification of the epitope accessibility to the paratopes of the antibodies, dual models of the space filling diagrams are used.

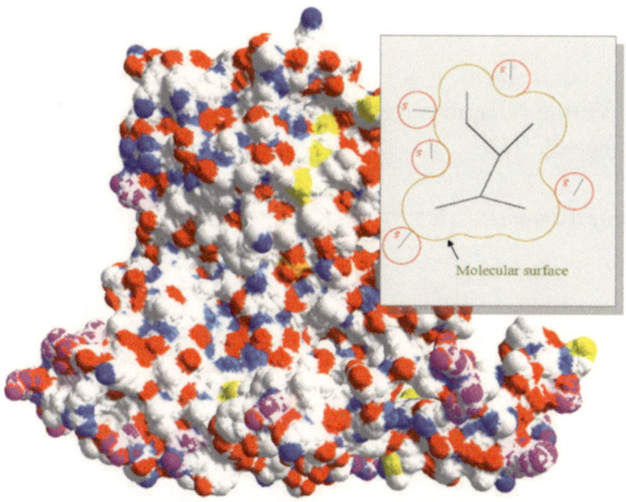

Figure 20. Molecular surface of GAD 65: Boundary that is obtained by rolling the solvent sphere over the van der Waals surface. The molecular surface is the envelope generated by the rolling sphere. It consists of sphere and torus patches connected in a tangent continuous manner and filling up the inaccessible crevices and cusps.

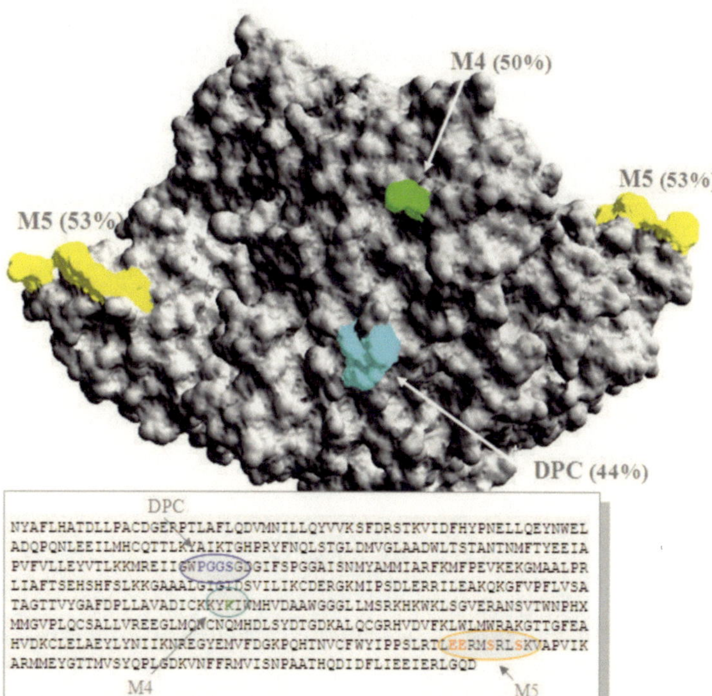

Figure 21. The GAD 65 molecule is represented by its molecular surface. The shapes of the GAD 65 epitopes, enable a pictorial analysis of the local docking sites. The exposure values of the residues, constituting the epitopes, were calculated by Voronoi tessellation. These values (in %) indicate how much the epitopes are exposed to the surrounding solvent, indicating the accessibility to potential antibodies.

4.3. Dual models and exposure values

The space filling models have a common dual counterpart. The dual counterpart is constructed by the Voronoi diagram that decomposes the union of balls (VW or SA model) into convex pieces [66-68].

Space-filling diagrams	⟷	*Dual structures*
Van der Waals model		Voronoi diagram
Solvent accessible model		Delaunay triangulation
Molecular surface		

The weighted distance of a point $x \in \mathbb{R}^3$ from A_i is defined as:

$$\pi_i(x) = \|x - z_i\|^2 - r_i^2 \tag{37}$$

The Voronoi cell V_i of A_i is the region of points whose weighted distance to A_i is as least as small as to any other ball:

$$V_i = \left\{ x \in \mathbb{R}^3 \middle| \forall_j : \pi_i(x) \le \pi_j(x) \right\} \tag{38}$$

Each Voronoi cell is an intersection of closed half-spaces and therefore a convex polyhedron. Any two Voronoi cells overlap at most along some piece of their boundary and together the collection of cells covers the entire $\mathbb{R}^3$. The common intersection of $k+1>1$ Voronoi cells is either empty or a common (3-k)-dimensional face. In Voronoi tessellation, the space, containing a set of discrete points P_l, is subdivided into the non overlapping Voronoi cells [68]. Each cell V_l is associated with an element of the set of points P_l in that way, that every region contains space points x, which have the shortest distance to the associated point:

$$V_l = \left\{ x \in \mathbb{R}^3 \mid \|P_l - x\| < \|P_k - x\|, l \ne k \right\} \tag{39}$$

This partition of the space is called Voronoi tessellation. In the definition, the Euclidean metric is used as measure:

$$\| P_k - x \| = \sqrt{\sum_{i=1}^{3} | P_k - x_i |^2} \tag{40}$$

For a given set of points the Voronoi decomposition is unique. The set of Voronoi cells is called a Voronoi diagram, which defines the topological relations of the set of discrete points (Figure 23A). The Voronoi tessellation describes the space filled by a packing of solid polyhedrons, connected by their faces, without empty space between them. The configuration of the cells provides information about the package of the associated set of points. Each cell in the diagram is characterized by its number of edges and faces (Figure 22). All the values concerning the individual cells, such as: cell volume, cell surface, number of sides, number of faces, area of contact faces and distances between the representative points, are derived from the geometry of the tessellation.

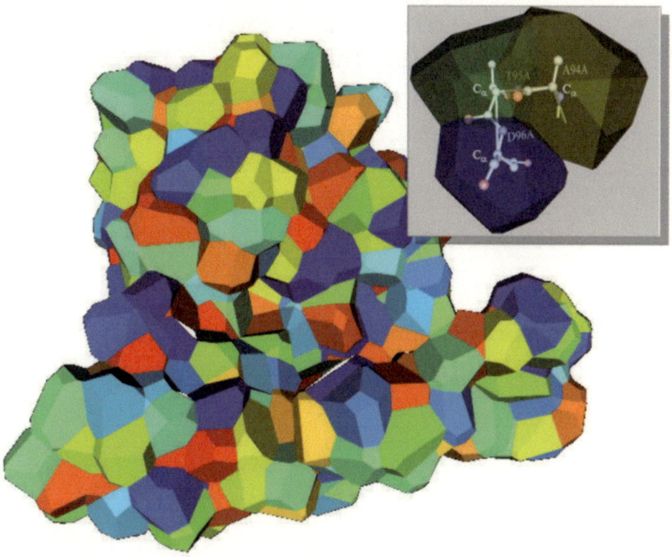

Figure 22. Voronoi tessellation of the GAD 65 molecule. Each Voronoi cell V_l is a polyhedron which is uniquely associated with one of the residues. The C_α atoms are used as centre points. Each cell in the Voronoi diagram is characterized by its number of edges and faces. The common faces of the cells define the contacts with nearest residues.

For completeness, let us shortly introduce the Delaunay triangulation. The Delaunay complex is a collection of simplices that records the overlap pattern among Voronoi cells. The complex contains the convex hull of $k+1$ ball centres if their corresponding Voronoi cells have a non-empty common intersection. Let B be a subset of $k+1$ atoms with $Z_B = \left\{ z_i \middle| A_i \in B \right\}$ and $V_B = \left\{ V_i \middle| A_i \in B \right\}$. Then the Delaunay complex is:

$$D = \left\{ \sigma = H_{conv}(Z_B) \middle| \bigcap V_B \neq \varnothing \right\} \tag{41}$$

Where ($H_{conv}(Z_B)$ denotes the convex hull of the points in Z_B. Figure 23A shows a Voronoi tessellation of a set of 4 points in the plane. In 2-D the Voronoi cell of a point is given by a polygon, where the intersection of the contact lines is build with aid of the lines joining the neighbour points. The set of segments joining the points two by two is called Delaunay triangulation, which is the dual of the Voronoi diagram (that means that it represents the same geometrical information about the set of points).

A Voronoi tessellation can be used to quantify the contact areas of individual residues in proteins. The tessellations are mostly performed on the alpha carbon atoms (as point P_l) of the structure. The tetrahedron set, sharing a particular alpha carbon C_α as a vertex, defines its closest neighbourhood. The circumscribed sphere of each tetrahedron does not contain any other alpha carbon (Figure 22). Two residues are in direct contact if their corresponding cells share a common face. To obtain quantitative values for the epitopes area, the exposure rate of the epitopes to the surrounding solvent was calculated. The contribution of an amino acid, at the epitope, to the exposure rate, is characterized by the number and size of the faces of its Voronoi cell exposed to the solvent. The total area of the Voronoi cell V_l of the l-te residue is denoted by F_l. The area of the i-te common face to the solvent is: a_i. N_a is the number of common faces. Thus a measure for the exposure of the l-te residue to the solvent is the relative exposure value:

$$E_l = \frac{1}{F_l}\sum_{i=1}^{N_a} a_i \tag{42}$$

The total area of the epitope can be quantified by summing up the areas for all the involved residues. Then, the contribution of the l-te residue of the epitope is given by the relative contribution:

$$I_l = \frac{E_l F_l}{\sum_j E_j F_j} \tag{43}$$

The relative exposure values (in %) of the epitope residues give hints about the accessibilities of the antibodies to the GAD 65 molecule and are shown in Figure 21. The Voro3D software was used for the Voronoi tessellations (http://www.lmcp.jussieu.fr/~mornon/voronoi.html) [69].

4.4. Molecular electronic states and molecular recognition

The structural visualization of the GAD 65 molecule and its epitopes, together with their electrostatic field, is illustrative and may help the clinical immunologist to better imagine the mechanisms of the GAD 65 antigenicity. The specific antigen-antibody recognition and the attraction of the two molecules are done by the electrostatic fields surrounding the molecules. The electrostatic potential can be studied locally at the epitopes or globally, surrounding the whole molecule at different distances. The local electrostatic potential generated by the epitope residues, at the epitope location play a role in the recognition and adjustment of the antibody at the docking place. The global electrostatic potential is extending in the surrounding solvent influencing other molecules.

The electron behaviour in molecules is treated by methods based on quantum theoretical calculations. The Hamiltonian operator for the electronic Schrödinger equation describes the dynamic of the involved electrons [70-72]. For a molecule with N electrons and K nuclei, the Hamiltonian operator is given by:

$$H = -\sum_{i=1}^{N}\frac{\hbar^2}{2m}\Delta_i - \sum_{i=1}^{N}\sum_{a=1}^{K}\frac{Z_a e^2}{r_{ai}} + \sum_{i=1}^{N}\sum_{\substack{j=1 \\ j>i}}^{N}\frac{e^2}{r_{ij}} \tag{44}$$

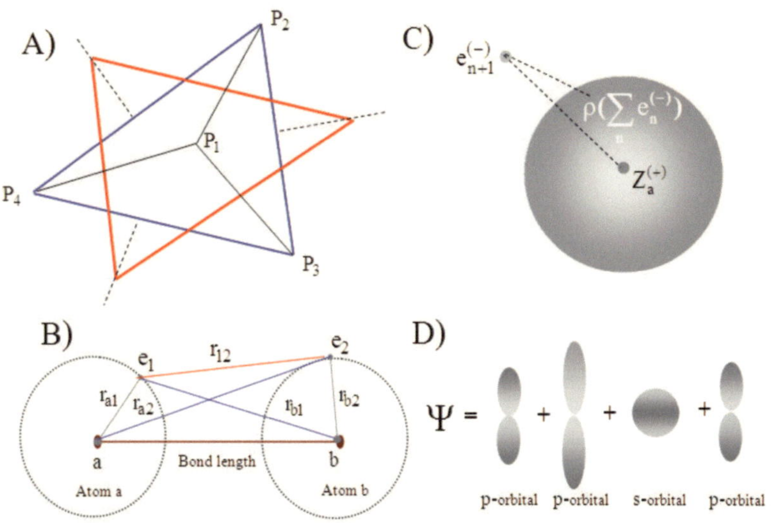

Figure 23. A) Voronoi tessellation (red) of a set of 4 points in the plane together with the dual Delaunay triangulation (blue). B) The interactions between the electrons e and nuclei a, b of a molecule. C) The independent electron moves in the electrostatic field of the nuclei and the averaged field of all other electrons. D) The molecular orbital Ψ is build as linear combination of atomic orbital.

The Hamiltonian operator involves the kinetic energy of the N electrons (first term: $\hbar = \frac{h}{2\pi}$, h is Planck's constant $6.626 \cdot 10^{-34}$ Js) the interaction of the electrons with the K nuclei (second term), the electron-electron interactions (third term). Z_a is the nuclear charge in atom a, r_{ai} is the distance between electron i and nucleus a, r_{ij} is the distance between electron i and electron j (Figure 23B). Then the electronic properties are calculated with the nuclei coordinates as parameters which are provided by the corresponding PDB data files. The resulting major part of the further calculation remains in solving the electronic Schrödinger equation:

$$H\Psi_n = E_n\Psi_n \tag{45}$$

The only possible values for the energy in quantum theory are the eigenvalues E_n of the Hamiltonian operator in the Schrödinger (eigenstate) equation with eigenfunctions Ψ_n. A significant simplification can be obtained by introducing an independent-particle model where the dynamic of an electron is considered to be independent of all other electrons and the interaction is taken into account in an average fashion. That means that the electron moves independently in the electric field of the nuclei and the field of all other electrons (Figure 23C). In the independent-particle model, the total state function Ψ of a molecule with N electrons is the product of the N single electron state functions Ψ_k ($k = 1,...,N$). In quantum theory, the values of an observable are the expectation values of the corresponding operator in pure (eigenstates) or mixed states (linear combination of eigenstates). The energy of a molecular system, described by an appropriate state function, is therefore calculated as the expectation value of the Hamiltonian operator (in Dirac bra-ket notation):

$$E = \langle \Psi | H | \Psi \rangle = \int \Psi^*(r_i) H \Psi(r_i) dV \tag{46}$$

The energy of the molecular system, in the independent-particle model, is then given by:

$$E = \sum_{k=1}^{N} \langle \Psi_k(i) | h_i | \Psi_k(i) \rangle + \sum_{k=1}^{N} \sum_{\substack{l=1 \\ l>k}}^{N} \left[\langle \Psi_k(i)\Psi_l(j) | h_{ij} | \Psi_k(i)\Psi_l(j) \rangle - \langle \Psi_k(i)\Psi_l(j) | h_{ij} | \Psi_l(i)\Psi_k(j) \rangle \right] \tag{47}$$

The first expression describes the mean kinetic energy of the electrons and the potential energy in the electrostatic field of the nuclei.

$$\langle \Psi_k(i) | h_i | \Psi_k(i) \rangle = \int \Psi_k^*(r_i) \left[-\frac{\hbar^2}{2m} \Delta_i - \sum_{a=1}^{K} \frac{Z_a e^2}{r_{ai}} \right] \Psi_k(r_i) dV_i \tag{48}$$

The second term describes the Coulomb interaction between 2 electrons, where one electron is located in the *k*-orbital and the second in the *l*-orbital (the charge is distributed inside the orbitals).

$$\langle \Psi_k(i)\Psi_l(j) | h_{ij} | \Psi_k(i)\Psi_l(j) \rangle = \iint \Psi_k^*(r_i)\Psi_k(r_i) \frac{e^2}{r_{ij}} \Psi_l^*(r_j)\Psi_l(r_j) dV_i dV_j \tag{49}$$

The third term describes the exchange interaction resulting from the indistinguishability of the electrons (this is a pure quantum effect and has no classical analogue).

$$\langle \Psi_k(i)\Psi_l(j) | h_{ij} | \Psi_l(i)\Psi_k(j) \rangle = \iint \Psi_k^*(r_i)\Psi_l^*(r_j) \frac{e^2}{r_{ij}} \Psi_l(r_i)\Psi_k(r_j) dV_i dV_j \tag{50}$$

Since molecular systems, involve the motions of a large number of electrons, their Schrödinger equations cannot be solved exactly and approximate solutions must be used. The molecular orbitals are expanded in terms of the basis functions, the atomic orbitals:

$$\Psi_n(r_i) = \sum_{\mu=1}^{M} c_{n\mu} \phi_\mu(r_i) \tag{51}$$

This expansion is called "Linear Combination of Atomic Orbitals" (LCAO). $\phi_\mu(r_i)$ are the well known atomic orbitals: s-orbital, p-orbital, d-orbital. The coefficients $c_{n\mu}$ define the contribution of the atomic orbital's to the molecular orbitals and are the weight of the μ-the atomic orbital in the *n*-te molecular orbital (Figure 23D). These coefficients have to be determined to find the molecular orbitals. Until now the molecules were considered as a system of electrons and nuclei, the expansion in atomic orbitals reflects the chemical view where molecules are building up of single atoms. The objective is now to find molecular orbitals that make the energy a minimum. This is done by determining a set of coefficients $c_{n\mu}$ that minimize the energy:

$$\delta E = \frac{\partial E}{\partial c^*_{n\mu}} = 0 \tag{52}$$

($c^*_{n\mu}$ is the complex conjugate of $c_{n\mu}$). The variation procedure yields the HF-LCAO (HF: Hartree-Fock) equation system (also called Roothan-Hall equations) for the coefficients:

$$\sum_{\beta=1}^{M} \left(H_{\alpha\beta} - \varepsilon_n S_{\alpha\beta} \right) c_{n\beta} = 0 \tag{53}$$

This is the most important equation in the quantum theory of molecules. $S_{\alpha\beta}$ is the overlap matrix:

$$S_{\alpha\beta} = \int \phi^*_\alpha(r_i)\phi_\beta(r_i)dV_i \tag{54}$$

The solutions of the HF-LCAO equation system are the energy $\varepsilon_n; (n = 1,...,M)$ and the coefficients $c_{n\beta}; (\beta = 1,...,M)$ for the molecular orbitals $\Psi_n; (n = 1,...,M)$. It is a linear equation system, of dimension MxM, where the solutions for larger molecules highly depend on computer power. The dimension of the equation system depends on the number of atoms and the involved atomic orbitals. In the simplest version only the p-orbital's contributing to the delocalized π-bonds are considered (Hückel molecular orbitals), in a higher version all the valence orbitals contributing to the chemical bonds are used (Extended Hückel). In more sophisticated versions, beside the valence orbitals also inner atomic orbitals are used. The complexity of the equation system and the computational power depend on the evaluation of the integrals. The matrix elements of the Hamiltonian are given by:

$$\begin{aligned} H_{\alpha\beta} &= \langle \phi_\alpha(i) | h_i | \phi_\beta(i) \rangle \\ &+ \sum_{\rho=1}^{M} \sum_{\sigma=1}^{M} P_{\rho\sigma} \left[\langle \phi_\alpha(i)\phi_\rho(j) | h_{ij} | \phi_\beta(i)\phi_\sigma(j) \rangle - \frac{1}{2} \langle \phi_\alpha(i)\phi_\rho(j) | h_{ij} | \phi_\sigma(i)\phi_\beta(j) \rangle \right] \end{aligned} \tag{55}$$

$P_{\alpha\beta}$ is the density matrix, which is defined by:

$$P_{\alpha\beta} = 2\sum_{n=1}^{N/2} c^*_{n\alpha} c_{n\beta} \tag{56}$$

A principal difficulty in solving the HF-LCAO equations is the large number ($\sim M^4$) of two-electron integrals. These integrals can involve up to four atomic centres. Therefore calculations for large molecules require enormous computer power. Semi-empirical methods reduce the computational cost by neglecting all three-centre and four-centre two-electron integrals and the use of empirical parameters.

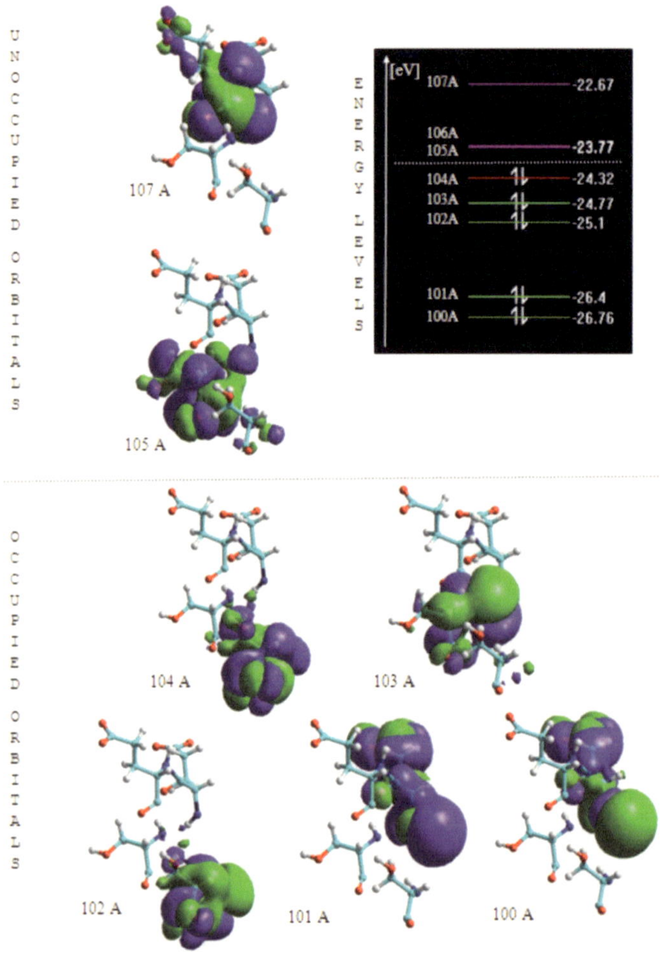

Figure 24. A subset of the molecular orbitals from the epitope M5 is shown together with their energy levels. Positive values of the molecular orbitals are green encoded, negative values violet. The most important orbitals in organic chemistry are the highest occupied molecular orbital (HOMO: 104 A) and the lowest unoccupied molecular orbital (LUMO: 105 A).

The molecular orbitals are arranged in order of increasing energy ε_n (Figure 24). Then the electrons are assigned to the orbitals beginning with the lowest energy. As a result, in a system with N electrons, the $N/2$ lowest molecular orbitals are occupied by respectively up to two electrons with opposite spins. The remaining M-$N/2$ (virtual) orbitals are unoccupied in the ground state and are occupied in excited electronic states (Figure 24). Physically, the square of the orbitals represents the electron spatial density distribution or in other words: the probability for finding the electron in a certain space volume element. Because of the protein size, a full treatment on the quantum level is beyond the realm of the available computers. Therefore mixed quantum/classical (QM/MM) methods are chosen, whereby the GAD 65 molecule is divided into the epitopes, where a quantum description is required, and the rest of the molecule which is treated classically by molecular force fields (Figure 25). Once the molecular orbitals are known, a number of molecular properties can be calculated out of the molecular orbitals. The electron density is given by:

$$\rho(r) = \sum_{n} \Psi_n^*(r)\Psi_n(r) \tag{57}$$

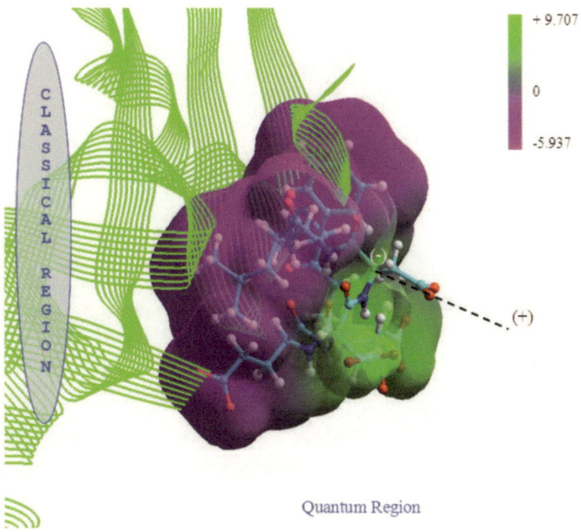

Figure 25. The electron density distribution at the residues of the epitope M5 is shown. The electron density in the visualisation is colour encoded according to its electrostatic potential. For large molecules, like GAD 65, the molecule is divided into a classical region and a quantum region. The epitope residues are treated by quantum mechanics and the rest of the molecule is treated classical by using molecular force fields. The spatial orientation of the dipole moment is shown (dotted lines). The surface shows electron density values of $8 \cdot 10^{-5} e / a_0^3$.

It describes the distribution of the electrons in the molecule (Figure 25). The values of the electron density are expressed in units of e / a_0^3, where *e* is the electron charge and a_0 is the Bohr radius (0.5 angstrom).

The electrostatic potential $V(r)$ is expressed as an electrostatic potential map, showing constant contouring values.

$$V(r) = \sum_{a=1}^{K} \frac{Z_a}{|R_a - r|} - \int \frac{\rho(r')}{|r' - r|} dr' \tag{58}$$

The first part of the equation results from the electrostatic potential of the atomic nuclei (point charge at position R_a) and the second part from the electron distribution (Figure 25). The values of the electrostatic field are expressed in units of e / a_0. The electrostatic field $\vec{E}$ acts perpendicular on the potential surfaces. It is a measure of the force exerted between molecules. The electrostatic potential at the epitope location plays an important role in the specific antigen-antibody recognition e.g. the specific interaction of the antigen GAD 65 with antibodies (Figure 26). At greater distances, the charge distribution of the whole molecule is taken into consideration and the electrostatic potential attracts molecules in more extended ranges (Figure 27). The quantum mechanical calculations were done with HyperChem (http://www.hyper.com).

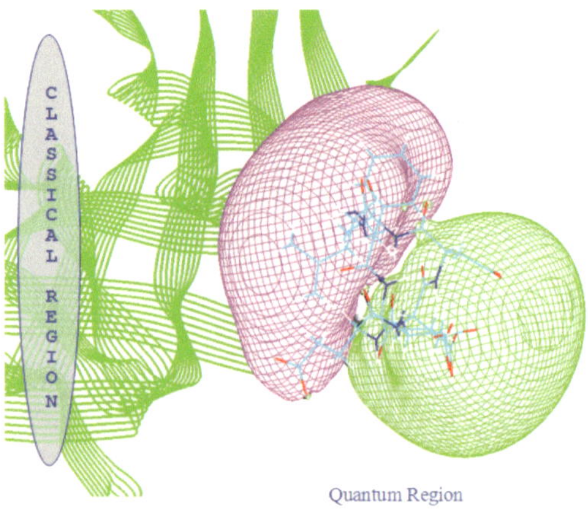

Figure 26. The spatial distribution of the electrostatic potential surrounding the residues of the M5 epitope. Negative values are red encode, positive values green. The surface shows where in 3D the electrostatic potential has a value of $3.8 e / a_0$.

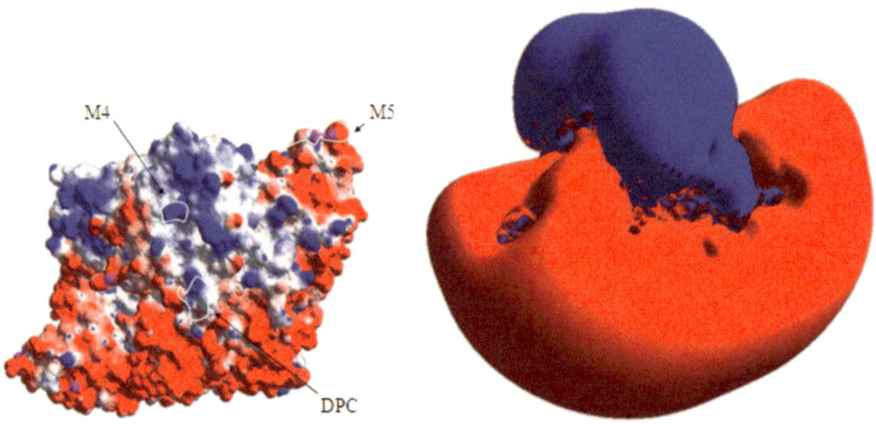

Figure 27. The electrostatic potential surrounding the GAD 65 molecule plays an important role in the specific antibody recognition. The electrostatic potential map shows contours of constant values. Positive potential values are drawn in blue, negative values in red. Different constant electrostatic potential values, ranging from the neighbourhood (left) to more extended ranges (right) are shown.

5. Discussion

The enzyme GAD 65 was generally considered to be strictly intracellular. But such a strictly intra-cytoplasmatic antigen would never have access to the immune system. With the ultrasensitive FCS technology, GAD 65 could be found to exist in peripheral blood of patients with diabetes mellitus type 1. It was measured with a sensitivity of 2.65 microgram/ml in the sera of adult and paediatric patients. The antigen was not found in all the patients' sera. The reason of the incidence is probably due to the complexed form (antigen-antibody complex) of GAD 65 at the time of investigation, hence hiding the antigen in the antibody excess. This could make it undetectable for FCS.

To understand the procedure and development of immunization and therefore the occurrence of GAD 65 antibodies in the blood, it was proposed that in an initial step the immune system is primed by the accessibility to GAD 65. The assumption was that the enzyme has to be in the human serum and should be found in higher concentrations before the onset of the disease. FCS is a very sensitive method, but the technique requires a labelling of the antibodies with dyes, which is very difficult to achieve and makes the measurements with FCS time consuming and expensive. Furthermore, the method is very sensitive to disturbance, resulting from other proteins (like albumin) and free dye contamination. Therefore and encouraged by the relative high concentration of GAD 65 in the blood of patients with diabetes mellitus type 1, we used in the following an ELISA setup. In the ELISA setup, the antigen GAD 65 was detected, in the peripheral blood of persons representing a cross-section of 64 samples in a blood bank. The result from the ELISA experiments demonstrates that GAD 65 exists, in mostly small amounts, in the sera of the blood-donors. The average concentration of GAD 65, by taking all these samples into consideration, is 58.00 ng/ml. By assuming that the most blood-donors are healthy, it can be expected that GAD 65 exists in at least small concentrations in the human peripheral blood. (For the diabetes mellitus type 1 patients the concentrations are by factors 40-50 higher). The correlation analysis of the samples stored at -80°C and additionally at room temperature showed that the GAD 65 molecule in the sera is stable at room temperature. By determining the correlation between the GAD 65 concentrations, taken from samples stored at room temperature and taken from the same samples after a time delay of one week, it was found that he molecule GAD 65 is sufficiently stable in sera.

By the use of SELDI-TOF and the study of some specimens used in the previous work with FCS we found some evidence for the diabetic antigen GAD 65 in a peak close to albumin. The albumin, produced in the liver, is the most abundant protein in human blood plasma. The reference range for albumin in blood is 35 to 53 mg/ml. Its concentration is therefore higher, by a factor above 10.000, than the expected value of GAD 65 (2.65 microgram/ml). The molecular weight of albumin is 66.47 kDa and therefore near the molecular weight of GAD (65 kDa). The weights differ only by 2.26%. Because of the tremendously higher concentration of albumin in the sera, a peak evaluation in regard of GAD 65 could not be achieved in a proper manner. Although an array with GAD 65 antibodies was used to pick out the antigen of the sera, it seems that the omnipresent albumin could not be completely washed out, but remained partially on the chip bounded by van der Waals interactions. This leads to a superposition of the GAD 65 peak and the albumin peak at $\approx 65\,\text{kD}$, which complicate the proper detection of the antigen. The results of these first trials show that the application of SELDI-TOF for the detection of GAD 65 in human sera, in the manner presented here is not reliable for a routine procedure. In conclusion, the development of new techniques for the separation of GAD 65 from albumin is necessary for an accurate and reliable diction of the diabetes type 1 antigen.

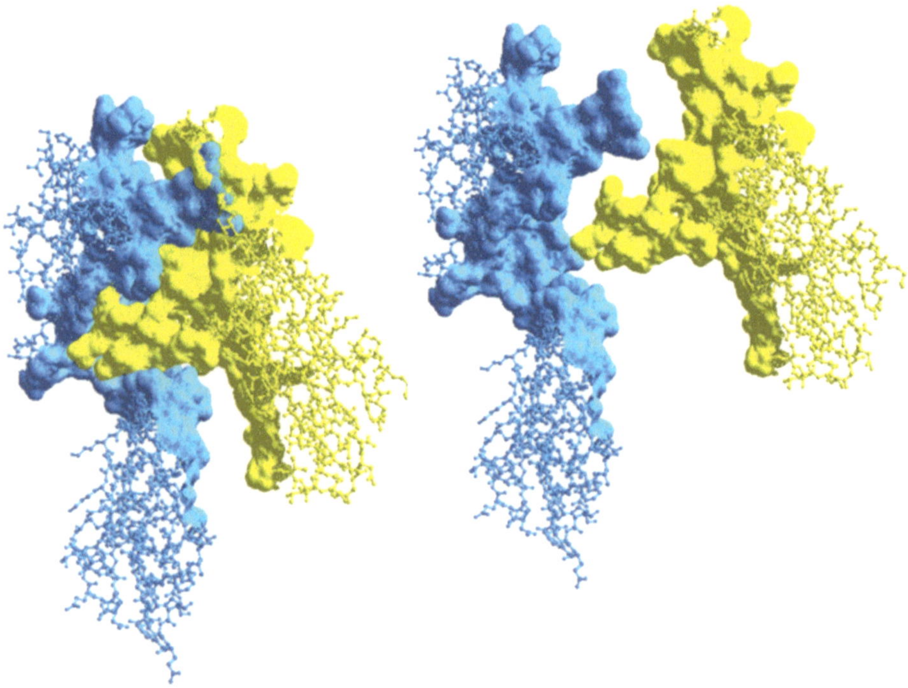

Figure 28. Interacting molecular surfaces. The major histocompatibility complex (MHC) protein (blue) I-Ag7 interacts with GAD 65.

The source of GAD 65 in serum of normal healthy human is unknown. Numerous hydrophobic parts at the protein surface enable a potential interaction with the hydrophobic membrane lipids, leading to a reversible anchoring of the molecule to the cell membrane. Another source may be the normal turn-over of beta cells. To explain the mechanism of autoimmunization, the visualization of the GAD 65 tertiary structure, together with its antigenic determinants and the associated electrostatic field, is essential. Molecular modelling enables an imagination of the GAD 65-antibody interaction and understanding of antigenicity and binding sites, which is the basis for the development of an active or passive immunotherapy [73]. The 3-D molecular surface, derived from space filling models, illustrates the fitting of the GAD 65 epitopes to the paratopes of the antibodies (GADA) and other associated molecules (Figure 28). It enables a pictorial understanding of the interaction with the antibody via complementary surfaces. Quantitative values for the GAD 65 antigenic properties were obtained with Voronoi tessellation (dual model) by calculating the exposure rate of its epitopes to the surrounding solvent and the GAD antibodies. The electrostatic potential and details of the electronic structure of the GAD 65 epitopes were calculated by quantum theoretical methods. The specific antigen-antibody recognition and the attraction of the two molecules are done by the electrostatic fields surrounding the molecules. The local electrostatic field at the epitope location plays a crucial role in the antibody-antigen recognition.

6. Conclusion

Biomarkers are molecules which are associated with a particular disease, whereby he identification of specific biomarkers in the early stage of disease, improves the success of the therapy. However, a single value is not expressive for interpretation. Only the time progression of the biomarkers is interpretable. Due to its stability and its frequent existence in the human blood, it might be that GAD 65 could be a suitable candidate as biomarker for diabetes mellitus type 1. The results from the GAD 65 studies could also be important for the therapy of diabetes mellitus type 1 by passive administration of GAD 65 antibodies or even the application of GAD 65 for vaccination. First trials of injections with the antigen GAD 65 has been shown to preserve some insulin production for 30 months in humans with diabetes mellitus type 1. To gain more insight into the role of GAD 65 for early diagnosis and therapy, an additional screening of further samples, with corresponding case history, is planned. To use GAD 65 as a biomarker of diabetes mellitus type 1, a big longitudinal study will be necessary to follow children of high risk category by monitoring their GAD 65 serum level over time. By comparing to normal healthy subjects, a potential differentiator may be indentified.

Author details

Wiltgen Marco* and Gernot P. Tilz
Institute for Medical Informatics, Statistics and Documentation,
Medical University of Graz, Graz, Austria

7. References

[1] Tierney LM, S J McPhee SJ, Papadakis MA (2002) Current medical Diagnosis & Treatment. International edition. New York: Lange Medical Books/McGraw-Hill.
[2] Rother KI (2007) Diabetes treatment—bridging the divide . The New England Journal of Medicine. 356(15): 1499–1501.
[3] Duckworth WC, Kitabchi AE (1981) Insulin metabolism and degradation. Endocr Rev. 2:210–233.

* Corresponding Author

[4] Duckworth WC (1988) Insulin degradation: mechanisms, products, and significance. Endocr Rev. 9:319–345.

[5] Capes SE, Hunt D, Malmberg K, Pathak P, Gerstein HC (2001) Stress hyperglycemia and prognosis of stroke in nondiabetic and diabetic patients: a systematic overview. Stroke. 32(10): 2426–2432.

[6] Hill NR, Thompson B, Bruce J, Matthews DR, Hindmarsh P (2009) Glycaemic risk assessment in children and young people with Type 1 diabetes mellitus. Diabet Med. 26(7):740-743.

[7] Huysman E, Mathieu C (2009) Diabetes and peripheral vascular disease. Acta Chir Belg. 109(5):587-594.

[8] Goyal BR, Solanki N, Goyal RK, Mehta AA (2009) Investigation into the cardiac effects of spironolactone in the experimental model of type 1 diabetes. J Cardiovasc Pharmacol. 54(6):502-509.

[9] Vergès B (2009) Lipid disorders in type 1 diabetes. Diabetes Metab. 35(5):353-560.

[10] Grauslund J, Hodgson L, Kawasaki R, Green A, Sjølie AK, Wong TY (2009) Retinal vessel calibre and micro- and macrovascular complications in type 1 diabetes. Diabetologia. 52(10):2213-2217.

[11] Wild S, Roglic G, Green A, Sicree R, King H (2004) Global prevalence of diabetes: estimates for 2000 and projections for 2030. Diabetes Care. 27(5):1047–1053.

[12] Craig ME, Hattersley A, Donaghue KC (2009) Definition, epidemiology and classification of diabetes in children and adolescents. Pediatr Diabetes. (10)12: 3-12.

[13] Karagianni P, Sampanis Ch, Katsoulis Ch, Miserlis G, Polyzos S, Zografou I, Stergiopoulos S, Douloumbakas I, Zamboulis Ch (2009) Continuous subcutaneous insulin infusion versus multiple daily injections. Hippokratia. 13(2):93-96.

[14] Grossi SA, Lottenberg SA, Lottenberg AM, Della Manna T, Kuperman H (2009) Home blood glucose monitoring in type 1 diabetes mellitus. Rev Lat Am Enfermagem. 17(2):194-200.

[15] Veleminsky Sr M, Buresova G (2008) Health Related Quality of Life of Children and Adolescents with Type 1 Diabetes. Neuro Endocrinol Lett. (5):29(6).

[16] Report of the Expert Committee on the Diagnosis and Classification of Diabetes Mellitus. Diabetes Care 25, 2002.

[17] Sabin MA, Cameron FJ, Werther GA (2009) Type 1 diabetes--still the commonest form of diabetes in children. Aust Fam Physician. 38(9):695-697.

[18] Patterson CC, Dahlquist GG, Gyürüs E, Green A, Gyula Soltész G (2009) The EURODIAB study group: Incidence trends for childhood diabetes mellitus type 1 in Europe during 1989-2003 and predicted new cases 2005-2020: a multicentre prospective registration study. The Lancet. 373(9680):2027-2033.

[19] Johnson JD, Luciani DS (2010) Mechanisms of Pancreatic beta-Cell Apoptosis in Diabetes and Its Therapies. Adv Exp Med Biol. 654:447-462.

[20] Harrison LC (1992) Islet cell antigens in insulin-dependent diabetes: Pandora's box revisited. Immunol Today. 13(9):348-352.

[21] Cooke DW, Plotnick L (2008) Type 1 diabetes mellitus in pediatrics. Pediatr Rev. 29(11):374–384.

[22] Van der Werf N, Kroese FG, Rozing J, Hillebrands JL (2007) Viral infections as potential triggers of type 1 diabetes. Diabetes Metab Res Rev. 23(3):169-183.

[23] Tirabassi RS, Guberski DL, Blankenhorn EP, Leif JH, Woda BA, Liu Z, Winans D, Greiner DL, Mordes JP (2010) Infection with viruses from several families triggers autoimmune diabetes in LEW*1WR1 rats: prevention of diabetes by maternal immunization. Diabetes. 59(1):110-118.

[24] Richer MJ, Horwitz MS (2009) Preventing viral-induced type 1 diabetes. Ann N Y Acad Sci. 1173:487-492.

[25] Burgess MA, Forrest JM (2009) Congenital rubella and diabetes mellitus. Diabetologia. 52(2):369-370.

[26] Shehadeh N, Shamir R, Berant M, Etzioni A (2001) Insulin in human milk and the prevention of type 1 diabetes. Pediatric Diabetes. 2(4):175–177.

[27] Virtanen SM, Knip M (2003) Nutritional risk predictors of beta cell autoimmunity and type 1 diabetes at a young age. The American Journal of Clinical Nutrition. 78(6):1053–1067.

[28] Bantle JP (2009) Dietary fructose and metabolic syndrome and diabetes. J Nutr. 139(6):1263-1268.

[29] Atkinson, M.A., Kaufman, D.L., Newman, D., Tobin, A.J. & Maclaren, N.K (1993) Islet cell cytoplasmic autoantibody reactivity to glutamate decarboxylase in insulin-dependent diabetes. J. Clin. Invest. 91:350–356.

[30] Franke B, Galloway TS, Wilkin TJ (2005) Developments in the prediction of type 1 diabetes mellitus, with special reference to insulin autoantibodies. Diabetes Metab Res Rev. 21(5):395-415.

[31] Tuomilehto J, Zimmet P, Mackay IR, Koskela P, Vidgren G, Toivanen L, Tuomilehto-Wolf E, Kohtamäki K, Stengård J, Rowley MJ (1994) Antibodies to glutamic acid decarboxylase as predictorsofinsulin-dependent diabetes mellitus before clinical onset of disease. Lancet. 343(8910):1383-1385.

[32] Solimena, M. et al (1988) Autoantibodies to glutamic acid decarboxylase in a patient with stiff-man syndrome, epilepsy and type-1 diabetes. N. Engl. J. Med. 318: 1012–1020.

[33] Solimena, M., Folli, F., Aparisi, R., Pozza, G. & De Camilli, P (1990) Autoantibodies to GABA-ergic neurons and pancreatic beta cells in stiff-man syndrome. N. Engl. J. Med. 322:1555–1560.

[34] Baekkeskov, S. et al (1982) Autoantibodies in newly diagnosed diabetic children with immunoprecipitate human pancreatic islet cell proteins. Nature. 298: 167–169.

[35] Jun HS, Khil LY, Yoon JW (2002) Role of glutamic acid decarboxylase in the pathogenesis of type 1 diabetes. Cell Mol Life Sci. 59:1892-1901.

[36] Tilz GP, Dausset J, Wiltgen M (2009) The Diabetic Antigen Glutamic Acid Decarboxylase (GAD 65) in the Human Peripheral Blood. Int Arch Allergy Immunol. 16;152(2):184-194.

[37] Tilz GP, Wiltgen M Borkenstein M (2011) On the occurrence of the diabetes-associated antigen GAD 65 in human sera. Int Arch Allergy Immunol. 155(2):167-179.

[38] Magde D, Elson EL, Webb WW (1974) Fluorescence correlation spectroscopy. II. An experimental realization. Biopolymers. 13(1):29-61.

[39] Eigen M, Rigler R (1994) Sorting single molecules: application to diagnostics and evolutionary biotechnology. Proc Natl Acad Sci USA. 91:5740-5747.

[40] Dittrich P, Malvezzi-Campeggi F, Jahnz M, Schwille P (2001) Accessing molecular dynamics in cells by fluorescence correlation spectroscopy. Biol Chem. 382(3):491-494.

[41] Schwille P (2001) Fluorescence correlation spectroscopy and its potential for intracellular applications. Cell Biochem Biophys. 34(3):383-408.

[42] Medina MA, Schwille P (2002) Fluorescence correlation spectroscopy for the detection and study of single molecules in biology. Bioessays. 24(8):758-764.

[43] Schlaman HR, Schmidt K, Ottenhof D, van Es MH, Oosterkamp TH, Spaink HP (2008) Analysis of interactions of signaling proteins with phage-displayed ligands by fluorescence correlation spectroscopy. J Biomol Screen. 13(8):766-776.

[44] Van Weemen BK, Schuurs AH (1971) Immunoassay using antigen-enzyme conjugates. FEBS Letters. 15(3):232–236.

[45] Engvall E, Perlman P (1971) Enzyme-linked immunosorbent assay (ELISA). Quantitative assay of immunoglobulin G. Immunochemistry. 8(9): 871–874.

[46] S. Leng, J. McElhaney, J. Walston, D. Xie, N. Fedarko, G. Kuchel (2008) Elisa and Multiplex Technologies for Cytokine Measurement in Inflammation and Aging Research. J Gerontol A Biol Sci Med Sci. 63:879-884.

[47] Bexley J, Hogg JE, Hammerberg B, Halliwell RE (2009) Levels of house dust mite-specific serum immunoglobulin E (IgE) in different cat populations using a monoclonal based anti-IgE enzyme-linked immunosorbent assay. Vet Dermatol. 20(5-6): 562-568.

[48] Nishifuji K, Tamura K, Konno H, Olivry T, Amagai M, Iwasaki T (2009) Development of an enzyme-linked immunosorbent assay for detection of circulating IgG autoantibodies against canine desmoglein 3 in dogs with pemphigus. Vet Dermatol. 20(5-6):331-337.

[49] Thomson G (1956) Centenary of J. J. Thomson. Science. 124(3233):1191-1195.

[50] Koomen J, Hawke D, Kobayashi R (2005) Developing an understanding of proteomics: an introduction to biological mass spectrometry. Cancer Invest. 23(1):47-59.

[51] Dijkstra M, Vonk RJ, Jansen RC (2007) SELDI-TOF mass spectra: A view on sources of variation. Journal of Chromatography B. (847): 12-23.

[52] Issaq HJ, Conrads TP, Prieto DA, Tirumalai R, Veenstra TD (2003) SELDI-TOF MS for diagnostic proteomics. Analytical Chemistry A. 149-155.

[53] Clarke CH, Buckley JA, Fung ET (2005) SELDI-TOF-MS proteomics of breast cancer. Clin Chem Lab Med. 43,12:1314-1320.

[54] Boyce EA, Kohn EC (2005) Ovarian cancer in the proteomics era: diagnosis, prognosis and therapeutics targets. Int J Gynecol cancer. 15: 266-373.

[55] Vorderwülbecke S, Cleverley S, Weinberger SR, Wiesner A (2005) Protein quantification by the SELDI-TOF-MS-based ProteinChip System. Nature Methods. 2,5:393-395.

[56] Gast MC, Van Gils CH, Wessels LF, Harris N, Bonfrer JM, Rutgers EJ, Schellens JH, Beijnen JH (2009) Serum protein profiling for diagnosis of breast cancer using SELDI-TOF. MS.Oncol Rep. 22(1):205-213.

[57] Myers MA, Fenalti G, Gray R, Scealty M, Tong JC, El-Kabbani O, Rowley MJ (2003) A diabetes-related epitope of GAD65: a major diabetes-related conformational epitope on GAD65. Ann NY Acad Sci. 1005: 250-252.

[58] Schwartz HL, Chandonia JM, Kash SF, Kanaani J, Tunnell E, Domingo A, Cohen FE, Banga JP, Madec AM, Richter W, Baekkeskov S (1999) High-resolution autoreactive epitope mapping and structural modelling of the 65 kDa form of glutamic acid Decarboxylase. J Mol Biol. 287: 983-999.

[59] Fenalti G, Law RH, Buckle AM, Langendorf C, Tuck Rosado CJ, Faux NG, Mahmood K, Hampe CS, Banga JP, Wilce M, Schmidberger J, Rossjohn J, El-Kabbani O, Pike RN, Smith AI, Mackay IR, Rowley MJ, Whisstock JC (2007) GABA production by glutamic acid decarboxylase is regulated by a dynamic catalytic loop. Struct. Mol. Biol. 14, 280-286.

[60] Guex N, Peitsch MC (1997) SWISS-MODEL and the Swiss-Pdb Viewer: An environment for comparative protein modelling. Electrophoresis. 18:2714-2723.

[61] Berman HM, Westbrook J, Feng Z, Gilliland G, Bhat TN, Weissig H, Shindyalov IN, Bourne PE (2000) The PDB data uniformity project. Nucleic Acids Research. 28:235-242.

[62] Edelsbrunner H, Harer JL (2010) Computational Topology. An Introduction. Amer. Math. Soc., Providence, Rhode Island.

[63] Liang J, Edelsbrunner H, Woodward C (1998) Anatomy of protein pockets and cavities: measurement of binding site geometry and implications for ligand design. Protein Science. 7:1884-1897.

[64] Edelsbrunner H, Facello MA, Liang J (1998) On the definition and the construction of pockets in macromolecules. Discrete Appl. Math. 88:83-102.

[65] Headd J,. Ban YHA, Brown P, Edelsbrunner H, Vaidya M, Rudolph J (2007) Protein-protein interfaces: properties, preferences, and projections. Proteome Research. 6:2576-2586.

[66] Voronoi G (1908) Recherche sur les paralleloedres primitifs. J. Reine Angw Math 134:198-287.

[67] Dupuis F, Sadoc JF, Mornon JP (2004) Protein Secondary Structure Assignment Through Voronoi Tessellation. Proteins: Structure, Function, and Bioinformatics. 55:519-528.

[68] Angelov B, Sadoc JF, Jullien R, Soyer A, Mornon JP, Chomilier J (2002) Nonatomic Solvent-Driven Voronoi Tessellation of Proteins: A Open Tool to Analyze Protein Folds. Proteins: Structure, Function, and Genetics. 49:446-456.

[69] Dupuis F, Sadoc JF, Jullien R, Angelov B, Mornon J (2005) Voro3D: 3D voronoi tessellations applied to protein structures. Bioinformatics. 21(8):1715-1716.

[70] Perruccio F, Ridder L, Mulholland AJ (2003) Quantum-mechanical/Molecular-mechanical Methods in Medicinal Chemistry, In: Carloni P, Alber F (Eds), Quantum Medicinal Chemistry. WILEY_VCH Verlag GmbH&Co. Weinheim.

[71] Jensen F (2007) Introduction to computational chemistry. John Wiley&Sons Ltd, UK.

[72] Szabo A, Ostlund NS (1996) Modern quantum chemistry. Dover Publications, INC, Mineola, New York.

[73] Corper AL, Stratmann T, Apostolopoulos V, Scott CA, Garcia KC, Kang AS, Wilson IA, Teyton L (2000) A structural framework for deciphering the link between I-Ag7 and autoimmune diabetes. Science. 21;288(5465):505-511.

Section 3

Stem Cell and Other Therapies for Autoimmune Disease

Chapter 11

New Therapeutic Challenges in Autoimmune Diseases

Eun Wha Choi

Additional information is available at the end of the chapter

http://dx.doi.org/10.5772/48207

1. Introduction

The immune system is the body's main line of defense against invasion by infectious organisms, such as bacteria, virus, and fungi. In normal immune systems, an immune response does not occur against the self-antigen, and is called self-tolerance. Autoimmune diseases occur when body tissues are attacked by the body's own immune system due to loss of tolerance to self-antigens (Dejaco et al., 2006). Under these conditions, body tissues are destroyed by antigen-specific cytotoxic T cells or auto-antibodies, and the accompanying inflammation can cause functional disability and morbidity. Autoimmune diseases are a heterogenous group of diseases with a wide spectrum of symptoms that affect approximately 6% of the population (Siatskas et al., 2006). They can be broadly classified as organ-specific or systemic depending on the location of the target antigen and clinical features (Sakaguchi, 2000). Common examples of systemic autoimmune diseases include systemic lupus erythematosus (SLE), rheumatoid arthritis, systemic sclerosis, ankylosing spondylitis, and polymyositis; examples of organ-specific autoimmune diseases include type 1 diabetes, Addison's disease, Hashimoto thyroiditis, Graves' disease, Sjögren's syndrome, vitiligo, pernicious anemia, glomerulonephritis, myasthenia gravis, Goodpasture's syndrome, autoimmune hemolytic anemia, idiopathic thrombocytopenia purpura, and pulmonary fibrosis. The clinical features of autoimmune diseases are very different, but immune-mediated mechanisms are associated with the generation of an adaptive immune response toward the target antigen (Kuby, 1994; Siatskas et al., 2006).

Conventional treatments, such as corticosteroids, cyclophosphamide, azathioprine, and methotrexate, are effective in some patients with autoimmune disease, but they are not uniformly effective and are associated with side effects and toxicity (Jantunen et al., 2000; Wiesik-Szewczyk et al., 2010).

With a better understanding of the pathophysiology of autoimmune diseases, many potential novel therapies focusing on cellular or molecular targets have been developed and evaluated (Nepom, 2002). This chapter provides a review of the pathophysiology and mechanisms underlying the induction of autoimmune diseases and the target sites and mechanisms of new therapies, and may help to understand the concept of new therapeutic trials that enhance or replace conventional therapies by reducing inflammatory immune responses and achieving immunological balance.

2. Pathophysiology and mechanisms for the induction of autoimmune diseases

The etiology of autoimmune diseases is unknown; however, autoimmune diseases may be caused by interplays between genetic factors, inappropriate immune regulation, and hormonal and environmental factors. Regarding immune regulation, lymphocytes and antigen-presenting cells play important roles in the generation of an effective immune response. Immune responses can be broadly divided into humoral and cell-mediated immune responses. The term "humoral" is derived from the Latin word "humor," which means body fluid. The humoral immune response involves the interaction of B cells with an antigen and subsequent B-cell proliferation and differentiation into antibody-secreting plasma cells (Kuby, 1994). Apart from mediating the humoral response via antibody production in adaptive immunity, B cells function as antigen-presenting cells and have the ability to activate T cells. Furthermore, activated B cells may produce pro-inflammatory cytokines, which aggravate local inflammation (Mok MY, 2010). T cells regulate B-cell responses, and inflammatory T cells infiltrate target tissues, which can lead to tissue damage. Cells expressing major histocompatibility complex (MHC) class II molecules that can present peptides to CD4+ T helper (Th) cells are called antigen-presenting cells. Cells that constitutively express MHC class II molecules, such as B cells, dendritic cells, monocytes, macrophages, thymic dendritic cells, thymic epithelial cells, and human vascular endothelial cells, function as antigen-presenting cells (Kuby, 1994). However, inducible expression of MHC class II molecules can occur in fibroblasts, glial cells, pancreatic beta cells, thyroid epithelial cells, and non-human vascular endothelial cells during an inflammatory response (Kuby, 1994).

In autoimmune disease, immune-mediated mechanisms are associated with the generation of an adaptive immune response against the target self-antigen (Siatskas et al., 2006). Many self-reactive lymphocytes are deleted during development or maturation, but not all self-reactive lymphocytes are eliminated. In normal healthy individuals, the activity of mature, recirculating self-reactive lymphocytes are regulated by clonal anergy or clonal suppression. A breakdown in this regulation results in the activation of self-reactive T- or B-cell clones, inducing humoral or cell-mediated responses against the self-antigen.

As described above, autoimmune diseases do not develop from a single event, but rather from many different events. Many mechanisms have been proposed for the induction of autoimmune diseases. Some of the well-known mechanisms include release of sequestered antigens, molecular mimicry, inappropriate expression of MHC class II molecules, cytokine imbalance, dysfunction of idiotype network regulatory pathways, general regulatory T-cell defects, and polyclonal B-cell activation (Kuby, 1994). An overview of the "pathophysiology and mechanisms for the induction of autoimmune disease" is presented in Figure 1.

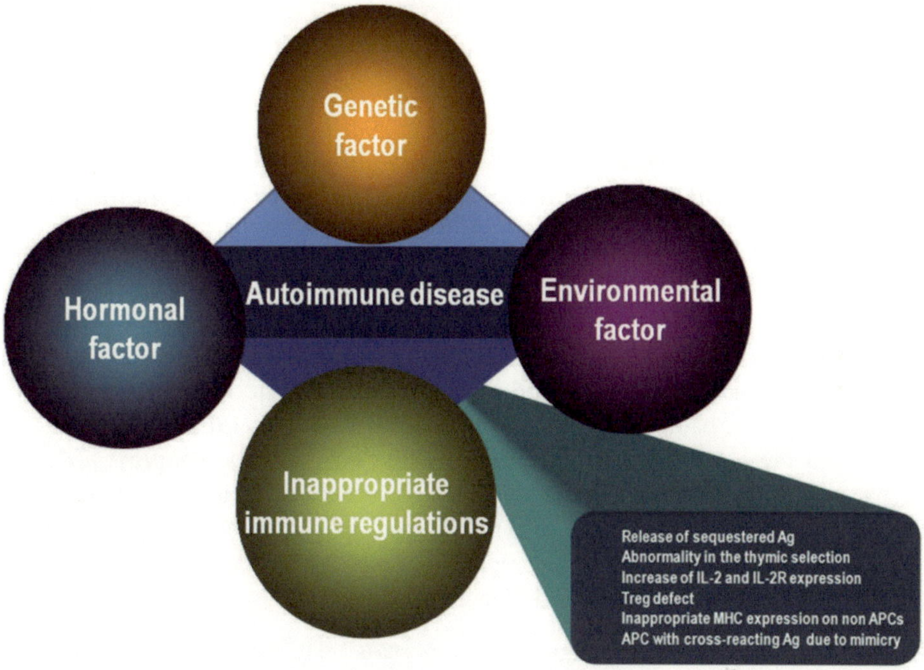

Autoimmune diseases may be caused by interplays between genetic factors, inappropriate immune regulation, and hormonal and environmental factors. Immune-mediated mechanisms underlie the development of autoimmune diseases. (Ag: antigen, IL-2R: IL-2 receptor, Treg: regulatory T cell, MHC: major histocompatibility complex, APC: antigen presenting cell)

Figure 1. Pathophysiology of autoimmune diseases

2.1. Sequestered antigens

Induction of tolerance in self-reactive T cells is thought to occur via exposure of immature lymphocytes to self-antigens during development. Thus, sequestered antigens not seen by the developing immune system will not induce self-tolerance. However, trauma to tissues following an accident or a viral or bacterial infection may release the sequestered self-antigens into circulation, leading to auto-antibody formation on occasion (Kuby, 1994). Multiple sclerosis is the most common autoimmune disorder of the central nervous system (CNS). A study on multiple sclerosis revealed that CD8 T cells specific for protein sequestered in oligodendrocytes can mount a spontaneous lethal demyelinating attack on the CNS without help from other T- or B-cell subsets or signals from the innate immune system (Na et al., 2008).

2.2. Molecular mimicry

A variety of bacteria and viruses possess antigenic determinants that are identical or similar to host cell components. This molecular mimicry between microbial antigens and host proteins can induce the production of activated T cells and antibodies that can cross-react with the host's own cells and lead to autoimmune disease. For example, a recent study using bioinformatics tools revealed that some of the identified antigens have been detected in established autoimmune diseases associated with mycobacterial infection (Chodisetti et al., 2012).

2.3. Inappropriate expression of MHC class II molecules on non-antigen-presenting cells & MHC molecules and susceptibility to autoimmune diseases

Inappropriate MHC class II expression was first observed on thyroid cells derived from patients with Graves' disease (Hanafusa et al., 1983) and led to the hypothesis that such expression can lead to the presentation of thyroid autoantigens to T cells, thereby initiating an autoimmune response. Normally, MHC class II molecules are expressed only on antigen-presenting cells. Healthy beta cells and thyroid acinar cells do not express MHC class II molecules. However, pancreatic beta cells in patients with type I diabetes mellitus (Bosi et al., 1987) and thyroid acinar cells in patients with Grave's disease express high levels of MHC class II (Hanafusa et al., 1983). This inappropriate expression of MHC class II molecules may serve to sensitize Th cells to peptides derived from cells that inappropriately express MHC class II molecules, allowing activation of B cells and cytotoxic T (Tc) cells, or sensitization of T_{DTH} cells against self-antigen.

Individuals susceptible to autoimmunity must possess MHC molecules and T-cell receptors capable of binding self-antigens. Expression of certain MHC alleles causes susceptibility to autoimmune diseases, and the presence of certain domains in T-cell receptors has also been linked to many autoimmune diseases (Kuby, 1994). Indeed, several autoimmune diseases, including type I diabetes and rheumatoid arthritis, exhibit a strong association and linkage with specific sequence polymorphisms in MHC class II molecules (Castaño et al., 1990).

Trauma or viral infection in an organ may induce localized inflammation. Increased levels of interferon (IFN)-γ can induce the expression of MHC class II molecules on a wide variety of non-antigen-presenting cells, thereby causing autoimmune disease (Todd et al., 1985). Further, the combination of IFN-γ with tumor necrosis factor (TNF)-α or interleukin (IL)-1β increases the expression of class I and II antigens in human thyroid follicular cells, compared with the effect of IFN-γ alone (Migita et al., 1990).

2.4. Cytokine imbalance

CD4+ Th cells can be subdivided into Th1, Th2, Th17, and regulatory T cells, on the basis of the cytokines they produce and the functions they perform (Cooke, 2006). Th1-type cytokines tend to produce the pro-inflammatory responses responsible for killing intracellular parasites such as viruses and certain bacteria, perpetuating autoimmune responses, and causing cell-mediated allergies. Preferential activation of Th1 cells plays a central role in the pathogenesis of many autoimmune diseases, including type 1 diabetes mellitus, multiple sclerosis, and rheumatoid arthritis (Emamaullee et al., 2009). The primary cytokines secreted from Th1 cells include IL-2, IFN-γ, and TNF-β. Overproduction of these cytokines from activated Th1 cells can induce excessive B-cell activation and autoantibody production (Kuby, 1994). In contrast, induction of Th2 populations results in a dominant protective effect against autoimmunity (Suarez-Pinzon and Rabinovitch, 2001; Sia, 2005). Th2-type cytokines include IL-4, IL-5, and IL-13, which are associated with the promotion of allergic responses, and IL-10, which produces anti-inflammatory responses. In fact, autoimmune diseases can be ameliorated by a reduced Th1 response or a shift toward Th2 responses in some cases, but there are exceptions.

Th17 occurs at the sites of interaction between the internal and external environments of the body. Important cytokines of Th17 include IL-17, IL-12, and IL-23. IL-17 is a potent pro-inflammatory cytokine that elicits the production of other inflammatory cytokines and chemokines such as TNF-α, IL-1ß, IL-6, IL-8, GM-CSF, and MCP-1 by endothelial cells, epithelial cells, and other cell types such as fibroblasts, keratinocytes, synoviocytes, and macrophages (Waite and Skokos, 2012). Thus, IL-17 can amplify ongoing inflammation. IL-17 levels were elevated in many inflammatory autoimmune diseases, including systemic sclerosis, psoriasis, and rheumatoid arthritis (Chabaud et al., 1999). Furthermore, several autoimmune conditions that were previously assumed to be mediated by Th1 have now been shown to involve Th17 cells (Cooke, 2006).

2.5. General regulatory T cell defects

The CD4+ regulatory T cell subsets include IL-10–producing T regulatory cell type 1 (Tr1), transforming growth factor (TGF)-β–secreting T helper cell type 3 (Th3), and a subpopulation of naturally occurring regulatory T cells that express high levels of CD25 and the forkhead box P3 (FoxP3) (Dejaco et al., 2005). Lack of regulatory T cells that express CD4, CD25, and FoxP3 induces severe autoimmunity in both mice and humans (Buckner, 2010). General regulatory T-cell defects cause hyperactivity of both B and T cells. Thus, restoration of regulatory T cells can reverse autoimmunity. Studies on the functional assays revealed that regulatory T cells play a crucial role in the modulation of local immune responses (de kleer et al., 2004). Altered generation of regulatory T cells and insufficient suppression of inflammation are considered pivotal for the initiation and perpetuation of autoimmune diseases because imbalance between pro-inflammatory and regulatory T cells can lead to the breakdown of self-tolerance (Dejaco et al., 2005). In fact, reduced levels of circulating CD4+CD25high T cells were observed in patients with juvenile idiopathic arthritis (de kleer et al., 2004). Further, lower levels of circulating CD4+CD25high T cells also correlate with higher disease activity or poorer prognosis (de kleer et al., 2004).

2.6. Dysfunction of the idiotype network regulatory pathways

Production of anti-idiotype antibodies against self-proteins can contribute to autoimmune disease. For example, in Grave's disease, antibodies produced against the thyroid-stimulating hormone (TSH) receptor bind to the receptor and inappropriately stimulate the thyroid. Antibodies against the "TSH-specific antibody" (anti-idiotype antibody) can stimulate the TSH receptor. Anti-idiotype antibodies were found in patients with myasthenia gravis (Dwyer et al., 1983) and a patient with Grave's disease (Kuby, 1994).

2.7. Polyclonal B-cell activation

Many bacteria and viruses, such as gram-negative bacteria, cytomegalovirus, and Epstein-Barr virus, can induce nonspecific polyclonal B-cell activation without the help of Th cells. Lipopolysaccharide from gram-negative bacteria is sufficient to induce autoimmune disease in an immunologically normal host, suggesting that polyclonal B-cell activation plays a central role in the pathogenesis of systemic autoimmune diseases (Granholm, 1992). Indeed, autoimmune diseases can be arrested by suppressing excessive polyclonal B-cell activation, and autoimmune diseases can be exacerbated by enhancing polyclonal B-cell activation.

3. Strategies to influence specific immune cells and molecules such as co-stimulatory molecules, cytokines, and chemokines

The immunity-related strategy for treating autoimmune diseases is to arrest ongoing inflammatory responses, prevent the adaptive memory response, and achieve antigen-specific immunomodulation (Nepom GT, 2002). During the past several decades, strategies using agents that influence cytokines, hyperactivity of B cells, and B cell-T cell interaction have proven to be effective and safe therapies for autoimmune disease (Lacki JK, 2000). Overviews of the "Generation of adaptive immune response against the target self-antigen" and "Target sites of new therapies influencing specific immune cells, molecules, cytokines, and chemokines" are presented in Figure 2.

3.1. B-cell-based therapy

Strategies targeting B cells include B-cell depletion therapies, anti-cytokine therapies, B-cell tolerogens, and inhibition of co-stimulatory molecules (Mok MY, 2010).

Potential targets for B-cell therapy include cell surface molecules and co-stimulatory molecules, such as CD20, CD22, B220, MHC class II molecules, CD35 (CR1), CD21 (CR2), CD32 (FcγRII), CD80 (B7-1), CD86 (B7-2), and CD40.

3.1.1. B-cell depletion therapies

CD20 is a B-cell-restricted surface molecule and an activated-glycosylated phosphoprotein that is expressed from pre-B to memory B cells (Mok MY, 2010). Anti-CD20 antibody (Ab) treatment results in B-cell depletion via antibody-dependent cell-mediated cytotoxicity, complement-mediated lysis, and stimulation of apoptosis (Pescovitz, 2006). Anti-CD20 Ab treatment was administered for B-cell depletion in human SLE (Anolik et al., 2007, Smith et al., 2006), autoimmune hemolytic anemia (Quartier et al., 2001; Perrotta et al., 2002), and rheumatoid arthritis (Furst et al., 2007). Clinical trials for SLE proved that anti-CD20 Ab treatment has beneficial effects only on B-cell-driven SLE because beneficial effects were seen only in the African American and Hispanic subgroups, which are refractory to standard treatment and are more B-cell dependent (Isenberg et al., 2008). The main complication relating to anti-CD20 Ab treatment is an increased rate of serious infection, which terminated the clinical trials (Hutas et al., 2008).

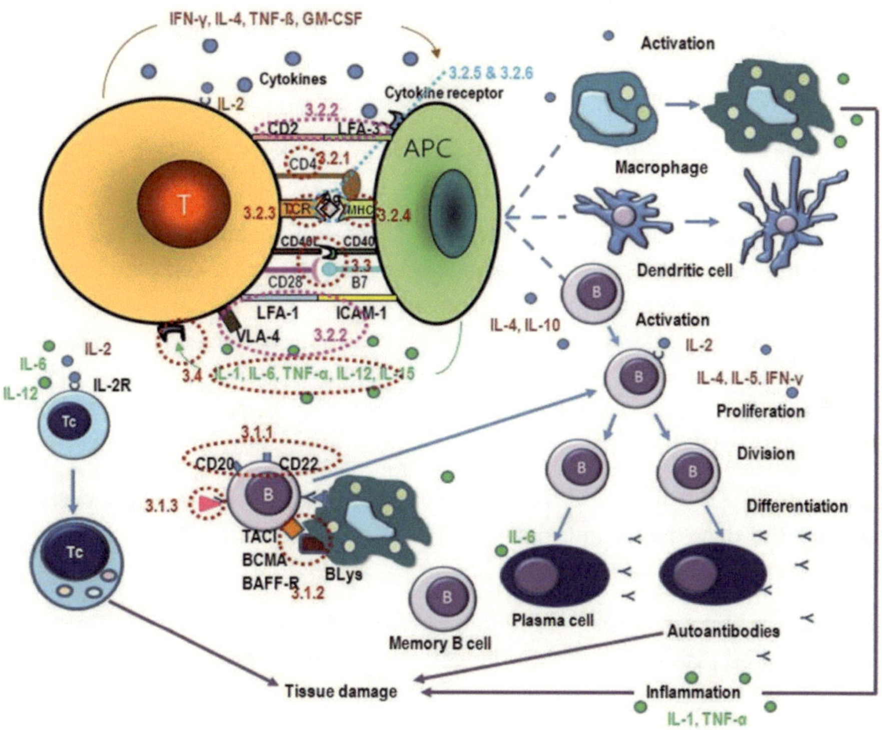

In autoimmune diseases, an adaptive immune response is mounted against the target self-antigen. The target sites of the new therapies are shown.
3.1.1 B-cell depletion therapies
3.1.2 B-cell-related anti-cytokine therapies
3.1.3 Therapy using B-cell tolerogens
3.2.1 Therapies targeting T-cell surface molecules
3.2.2 Therapies targeting T-cell pathways related to trafficking and co-stimulation
3.2.3 T-cell vaccination
3.2.4 Therapies targeting MHC molecules or antigen-presenting cells in the first signal
3.2.5 Therapies targeting antigens in the first signal
3.2.6 Therapy using T-cell tolerogens
3.3 Therapy targeting B cell-T cell interaction (inhibition of co-stimulatory molecules)
3.4 Anti-cytokine therapy (prevention of ongoing inflammatory responses)
(APC: antigen presenting cell, Tc: cytotoxic T cell, TCR: T cell receptor, MHC: major histocompatibility complex, Ag: antigen, LFA: lymphocyte function-associated antigen, CD: cluster of differentiation, VLA: very late antigen, ICAM: intercellular adhesion molecule, TACI: transmembrane activator and calcium modulator and cyclophilin ligand interactor, BCMA: B-cell maturation antigen, BAFF-R: B-cell-activating factor receptor, BLys: B-lymphocyte stimulator, IFN: interferon, IL: interleukin, GM-CSF: granulocyte-macrophage colony-stimulating factor, TNF: tumor necrosis factor)

Figure 2. Target sites of new therapies influencing specific immune cells, molecules, cytokines, and chemokines

CD22 is a B-cell surface glycoprotein and a specific adhesion molecule that regulates antigen receptor signaling, B-cell activation, and interaction with T cells (Tedder et al., 1997). Anti-CD22 Ab treatment was tested in 14 SLE patients in an open-labeled study. No reduction in ANA or anti-dsDNA antibodies (Abs) was observed, but induction of B-cell modulation and evidence of clinical improvement were seen (Dörner et al., 2006; Carnahan et al., 2007). The action of anti-CD22 Abs is achieved by antibody-dependent cell cytotoxicity and induction of signal transduction via downmodulation of B-cell receptor signaling (Carnahan et al., 2007).

3.1.2. B-cell-related anti-cytokine therapies

The B-lymphocyte stimulator (BLys), also called B-cell-activating factor (BAFF), is important in B-cell immunity (Moore et al., 1999). BLys is a TNF family ligand expressed on the cells of myeloid origin, such as monocytes, macrophages, and dendritic cells, and can bind to 3 membrane receptors on B cells, including transmembrane activator and calcium modulator and cyclophilin ligand interactor (TACI), B-cell maturation antigen (BCMA), and BAFF receptor (BAFF-R). Anti-BLys Ab treatment decreased CD20+ B cells, reduced anti-dsDNA Abs and disease flares, and stabilized SLE, in particular, in serologically active SLE patients (Wallace et al., 2009; Wiglesworth et al., 2010).

Treatment with BAFF-R linked to the Fc domain of human IgG1 ameliorated murine SLE, judging from the decrease in anti-dsDNA Abs and proteinuria and the improvement in glomerular lesions (Kayagaki et al., 2002).

TACI-IgG can inhibit BLys and a proliferation-inducing ligand (APRIL), and TACI-IgG treatment decreased proteinuria and prolonged survival in murine lupus (Gross et al., 2000).

3.1.3. Therapy using B-cell tolerogens

Abetimus sodium is a synthetic compound of 4 deoxynucleotide sequences bound to a triethylene glycol backbone that can bind to anti-dsDNA Abs and crosslink B-cell receptors that recognize dsDNA. Thus, treatment with abetimus sodium induces deletion or anergy of anti-dsDNA Ab-producing B cells. Abetimus sodium was used as a B-cell tolerogen in SLE patients with lupus nephritis and it exhibited potential efficacy in some SLE patients with elevated anti-dsDNA Abs. However, a phase IV trial was prematurely terminated because of lack of clinical efficacy (Wiesik-Szewczyk et al., 2010).

3.2. T-cell-based therapy and therapies targeting the first signal

3.2.1. Therapies targeting T-cell surface molecules

Monoclonal antibodies to T-cell surface molecules (CD3, CD4, and CD52) have been effectively used in clinical efficacy trials for autoimmune diseases, but all of them were associated with transient depression of circulating T cells. For example, treatment of New Zealand black × New Zealand white (NZB/W) F1 and the autoimmune disease-prone non-obese diabetic

(NOD) mice with anti-CD4 Abs blocked nonspecific overall immune responses (Phillips et al., 2000). A clinical trial using anti-CD52 Abs revealed that profound lymphopenia, with recovery B cells and CD8+ cells and longer lasting CD4 cytopenia can occur (Willis et al., 2001). A monoclonal antibody directed against the α subunit of the high-affinity IL-2 receptor can more specifically block autoreactive Th cells in autoimmunity, because only activated Th cells express the high affinity IL-2R α subunit, CD25. Therapy with a monoclonal antibody to the IL-2 receptor CD25 led to downregulation of the receptor without depleting T cells. Egan et al. (2001) and Haufs and Haneke's (2001) studies showed the efficacy of anti-CD25 Abs in epidermolysis bullosa acquista. In a study on multiple sclerosis, maintenance therapy with anti-CD25 Abs reduced the frequency of CD4+CD25+ regulatory T cells, but inflammatory activity in multiple sclerosis was substantially reduced with anti-CD25 Ab treatment despite reduction of circulating regulatory T cells (Oh et al., 2009).

3.2.2. Therapies targeting T-cell pathways related to trafficking and co-stimulation

Lymphocyte function-associated antigen-3 (LFA-3, CD58) is a cell-bound immunoglobulin superfamily receptor with only one known ligand, namely, CD2 (Springer et al., 1987). LFA-3 is widely expressed on human hematopoietic and non-hematopoietic tissues, leukocytes, erythrocytes, endothelial and epithelial cells, and fibroblasts. The engagement of LFA-3 with CD2 optimizes immune recognition and initiates T-cell expansion and activation. These contact activities can occur between helper T cells and antigen-presenting cells and cytolytic effectors and target cells. The soluble LFA3/IgG1 fusion protein binds CD2 on T cells and Fc receptor on natural killer cells, macrophages, neutrophils, and mast cells. Thus, the soluble LFA3/IgG1 fusion protein can inhibit immune recognition as well as T-cell expansion and activation.

LFA-1 is found on all T-cells and also on B-cells, macrophages and neutrophils and is involved in recruitment to the site of infection. It binds to ICAM-1 on antigen-presenting cells and functions as an adhesion molecule. Anti-LFA1 Ab treatment elicited an improvement in psoriasis (Papp et al., 2001; Tutrone et al., 2001).

Very late antigen-4 (VLA-4) is an integrin dimer composed of CD49d (alpha) and CD29 (beta). VCAM-1 (integrin receptor) binds to VLA-4 normally expressed on leukocyte plasma membrane, but does not adhere to the appropriate ligands until the leukocytes are activated by chemotactic agents or other stimuli. Treatment with the anti-α4 integrin Abs (VLA-4 Abs), which targets T-cell trafficking pathways, also showed clinical benefit in Crohn's disease and multiple sclerosis (Tubridy et al., 1999; Gordon et al., 2001).

3.2.3. T-cell vaccination

Cross-linked T cells apparently elicit regulatory T cells specific to T-cell receptor variable region determinants of the autoimmune clones, and it has been shown that a synthetic T-cell receptor variable region peptide can function as a vaccine and an effective therapy (Kuby, 1994). For example, treatment with the IR501 therapeutic vaccine, which consists of a combination of 3 peptides derived from T cell receptors (Vβ3, Vβ14, and Vβ17) in Freund's incomplete adjuvant, was safe and well tolerated, and showed clinical improvement in rheumatoid arthritis patients (Moreland et al., 1998).

3.2.4. Therapies targeting MHC molecules or antigen-presenting cells in the first signal

Expression of certain MHC alleles causes susceptibility to autoimmune diseases. Thus, selective inhibition of MHC molecules, which are associated with autoimmunity, by using monoclonal antibodies can delay and ameliorate autoimmune diseases (Kuby, 1994). For example, treatment with anti-MHC class II monoclonal Abs (monoclonal Abs to the murine I-E equivalent) prevented thyroidal and pancreatic autoimmunity in BioBreeding/Worcester (BB/W) rats (Boitard et al., 1985). Treatment of anti-I-A monoclonal Abs ameliorated many autoimmune diseases in animal models including lupus nephritis (NZB/W F1) (Adelman et al., 1983), experimental autoimmune uveoretinitis (Rao et al., 1989), and experimental autoimmune myasthenia gravis (Waldor et al., 1983). Engineered antigen-presenting cells have also been used for immunomodulation and tolerance induction. For example, FasL-expressing antigen-presenting cells that specifically interact with Fas molecules on the surface of lymphocytes induce lymphocyte apoptosis (Zhang et al., 1999).

3.2.5. Therapies targeting antigens in the first signal

Oral presentation of T-cell-dependent antigens can lead to immunity or tolerance depending on the form of the antigen, dose, and number of feedings (Tomasi, 1980, Titus and Chiller, 1981). Thus, parenteral administration of antigens or antigen analogs was evaluated as immunotherapy for autoimmune diseases. Myelin basic protein (MBP)-specific T cells and symptoms of multiple sclerosis were reduced in myelin-fed, HLA-DR2-negative patients (Weiner et al., 1993). Mice fed MBP do not develop experimental autoimmune encephalomyelitis (experimental allergic encephalomyelitis, EAE) following subsequent injection of MBP (Kuby, 1994). Type II collagen-induced arthritis is an animal model of polyarthritis induced in susceptible mice and rats by immunization with type II collagen, a major component of cartilage. Intragastric administration of soluble type II collagen, prior to immunization with type II collagen in adjuvant, suppressed the incidence of collagen-induced arthritis (Nagler-Anderson C, 1986; Trentham et al., 1993).

A synthetic polypeptide comprising a random mixture of alanine, glutamate, lysine, and tyrosine, which can bind MHC and elicit T-cell recognition, acts as an altered antigen ligand. Treatment using this synthetic polypeptide showed beneficial effects on multiple sclerosis (Fusco C, 2001).

3.2.6. Therapy using T-cell tolerogens

hCDR1 (TV-4710, Edratide) is a peptide derived from the immunoglobulin Vh region of human anti-dsDNA Abs. Treatment with hCDR1 as a T-cell tolerogen induced regulatory T cells and reduced proteinuria and immune complexes in the kidneys of SLE patients. In this study on gene expression in peripheral blood mononuclear cells from SLE patients, treatment using hCDR1 increased in vivo gene expression of TGF-β, FoxP3 and the anti apoptotic molecule Bcl-xL, but significantly decreased the gene expression of IL-1β, TNF-α, IFN-γ, IL-10, BLyS, caspase-3, and caspase-8. hCDR1 treatment also markedly decreased disease activity (Sthoeger et al., 2009).

3.3. Therapy targeting B cell-T cell interaction (inhibition of co-stimulatory molecules)

T-cell activation requires 2 signals and cytokines. The first signal is mediated via binding of the T-cell receptor to the antigen presented with MHC molecules on antigen-presenting cells. However, the first signal alone is not sufficient; a second co-stimulatory signal is also required. Thus, co-stimulation is important not only for normal immunity, but also for the pathogenesis of autoimmunity. Therapies targeting the 2 main co-stimulatory pathways B7-CD28 and CD40-CD40L have been evaluated. Anti-CD40L Ab treatment reduced inflammation, vasculitis, and fibrosis in the kidney and increased survival in a murine lupus model, the SNF1 mouse (Kalled et al, 1998). Anti-CD40L Ab treatment also elicited clinical improvements such as decrease in anti-dsDNA Abs and hematuria and increase in C3 in some SLE patients. However, thromboembolism complications prevented continuation of the phase II study (Mok et al., 2010). CTLA4Ig is a fusion protein comprising the extracellular domain of CTLA4 and the constant region of immunoglobulin. CTLA4Ig competes with CD28 for binding to B7 thereby inhibiting the B7-CD28 co-stimulatory signal. CTLA4Ig treatment elicited improvements in murine SLE, judging from the decrease in proteinuria and increase in survival (Finck et al., 1994). CTLA4Ig gene therapy also had beneficial effects on canine SLE (Choi et al., 2005) and canine experimental autoimmune thyroiditis (Choi et al., 2008). A phase III clinical trial using CTLA4Ig in human SLE is currently underway (Mok, 2010).

3.4. Anti-cytokine therapy (prevention of ongoing inflammatory responses)

Inhibitors of inflammatory cytokines, such as a decoy receptor for inflammatory cytokines, have produced promising results in animal models of autoimmune diseases.

TNF-α is an inflammatory cytokine produced by various cells such as monocytes, macrophages, T cells, and B cells. TNF-α stimulates the production of other cytokines such as IL-1, IL-6, IL-8, and GM-CSF. To prevent ongoing inflammatory responses, TNF-blocking agents were administered in patients with psoriasis, rheumatoid arthritis, or Crohn's disease, and were shown to be efficacious (Chaudhari et al., 2001; Keating and Perry, 2002). However, ANA and anti-dsDNA Abs were observed in some rheumatoid arthritis or Crohn's disease patients treated with TNF-blocking agents (De Bandt et al., 2005; Mohan et al., 2002). TNF-blocking agents were ineffective in multiple sclerosis (Skurkovish et al., 2001). The diseases frequently recurred after discontinuation of TNF-blocking agent therapy. Further, Furst et al. recommend that caution should be exercised when using TNF-blocking agents. According to them, TNF-blocking agents should not be initiated or should be discontinued when serious infections occur (Furst et al., 2001). Instances of demyelinating-like disorders, pancytopenia, and aplastic anemia have been reported in patients receiving TNF blockers (Furst et al., 2002). A recent study reported the association of TNF inhibitor treatment with the risk of elevated liver enzymes, such as ALT and AST in patients with rheumatoid arthritis (Sokolove et al., 2010). A TNF-blocking agent in conjunction with baseline immunosuppressive therapy significantly decreased proteinuria and attenuated arthritis in SLE patients (Aringer et al., 2004). A trial evaluating a TNF-blocking agent in membranous nephritis is currently underway (Wiesik-Szewczyk et al., 2010).

IFN-γ is also a pleiotropic cytokine that is a key effector in the pathogenesis of various autoimmune diseases. Intramuscular injections of plasmids with cDNA encoding IFN-γR/Fc can retard lupus development and progression in MRL-Fas(lpr) mice. The therapy significantly reduced serum levels of IFN-γ and autoantibodies, lymphoid hyperplasia, and glomerulonephritis, and increased survival (Lawson et al., 2000).

IL-12 is an inflammatory cytokine that plays a pivotal role in the development of autoimmune diseases, such as those in the NOD mouse. Gene transfer using a modified form of IL-12 into pancreatic beta islet cells decreased the activity of natural IL-12 and prevented the onset of diabetes in NOD mice (Yasuda et al., 1998).

IL-6 is produced by monocytes, T cells, B cells, and mesangial cells. IL-6 stimulates B-cell maturation and immunoglobulin production. Combined with other cytokines, IL-6 also induces neutrophil activation, T-cell proliferation, and differentiation to cytotoxic T cells (Tackey et al., 2004). A monoclonal antibody against the IL-6 receptor α chain inhibits the binding of IL-6 to its receptor. Some SLE patients treated with this monoclonal antibody exhibited a significant decrease in acute phase reactant, activated B cells and memory B cells (Lacki et al., 1997). Furthermore, IL-6 receptor Ab treatment has been shown to be rapidly efficacious in patients with severe rheumatoid arthritis (Jones and Ding, 2010). However, complications relating to abnormalities in CBC and serum chemistry, such as neutropenia, increased concentrations of liver enzymes, cholesterol, and triglycerides, were observed in rheumatoid arthritis patients treated with anti-IL-6 receptor α chain monoclonal Abs (Iebba et al., 2012). The US Food and Drug Administration (FDA) approved the intravenous infusion of a monoclonal antibody against the IL-6 receptor α chain (tocilizumab) in adult patients with severely active rheumatoid arthritis who had an inadequate response to TNF antagonist therapies (http://www.fda.gov/NewsEvents/Newsroom/PressAnnouncements/ucm251572.htm).

An IL-1-blocking agent (IL-1 receptor antagonist) has been approved for use in rheumatoid arthritis. However, its use also increased the incidence of serious bacterial infections. A recent meta-analysis study revealed that the IL-1 receptor antagonist is less effective than TNF-α inhibitors for the treatment of rheumatoid arthritis (Furst et al., 2010).

As described in the previous section, IL-17 plays a central role in early inflammation and eosinophil recruitment. Therapeutic agents that target Th17, such as anti-IL-17 Ab and IL-25, showed promising results in animal models of autoimmunity. Anti-IL-17 Ab treatment reduced Th17 population, and prevented inflammation and bone erosion in experimental rheumatoid arthritis by decreasing RANKL and IL-1 (Koenders et al., 2005). Multiple treatments with anti-IL-17 Abs dramatically reduced inflammatory lesions and neurological signs in experimental autoimmune encephalomyelitis (Hofsttter et al., 2005). IL-25 has shown to inhibit Th17 cells and promote the development of Th2 responses (Angkasekwinai et al., 2007). Further, a recent study showed that IL-25 regulates Th17 function in autoimmune inflammation (Kleinschek et al., 2007). Treatment with anti-IL-17 Abs or IL-25 prevented progression to diabetes in pre-diabetic NOD mice, reduced islet inflammation, and prevented glutamic acid decarboxylase (GAD) 65 autoantibody formation (Emamaulle et al., 2009). Clinical trials of anti-IL-17 Abs in autoimmune diseases, including rheumatoid arthritis, psoriasis, and Crohn's disease, are currently underway (www. clinicaltrials.gov). A recent study revealed that a small molecule, halofuginone (HF), selectively inhibits mouse and human Th17 differentiation by activating a cytoprotective signaling pathway, the amino acid starvation response (AAR) (Sundrud et al., 2009). Further, this study showed that HF prevented experimental autoimmune encephalomyelitis by inducing AAR.

3.5. Protective cytokine gene therapy and induction or replacement of regulatory T cells

Studies on cytokine gene therapy using viral or nonviral vectors have been conducted in animal models of autoimmune diseases, including type 1 diabetes mellitus, EAE, SLE, colitis, thyroiditis, and various forms of arthritis. The purpose of this therapy is to modify the inappropriate inflammatory immune responses in autoimmune disease. Genes encoding TGF-β, IL-4, and IL-10 are most frequently protective. For example, IL-10 gene therapy using replication-deficient adenovirus administered directly into the CNS prevented disease progression in murine EAE, whereas systemic administration of IL-10 gene therapy using adenovirus had little effect on EAE (Cua et al., 2001). Intramuscular injection of IL-10 gene therapy prevented diabetes induced by streptozotocin injections in mice (Zhang et al., 2003). IL-4 gene therapy using adenovirus administered directly into limb joints decreased inflammation and improved pathology in a rat model of adjuvant-induced arthritis (Woods et al., 2001). Monthly intramuscular injections of cDNA expression vectors encoding TGF-β1 significantly elevated the serum levels of TGF-β, prolonged survival, and elicited beneficial effects in the MRL/lpr murine model of SLE (Raz et al., 1995). Systemic TGF-β1 gene therapy using an adenoviral system followed by syngeneic islet transplantation induced Foxp3+ regulatory cells, restored self-tolerance, and facilitated the survival of islet grafts and recovery of β-cell function in overtly diabetic NOD mice (Luo et al., 2005). Chen et al. reported that TGF-β-induced Foxp3 gene expression has the ability to convert CD4+CD25- naive T cells to regulatory T cells with potent immunosuppressive potential (Chen et al., 2003).

The transfer of CD4+CD25+ regulatory T cells conferred significant protection against clinical EAE in a mouse model of multiple sclerosis (Kohm et al, 2002). Treatment with in vitro-expanded antigen-specific regulatory T cells from autoimmune-prone NOD mice also reversed diabetes after disease onset (Tang et al., 2004). Further, antigen-specific T cells transduced with FoxP3 using a retroviral system prevented diabetes in NOD mice (Jaeckel et al., 2005). These studies suggested that regulatory T cells act as main regulators of the immune system and provide a novel approach to cellular immunotherapy for autoimmune diseases.

4. Stem cell therapy for autoimmune diseases

4.1. Hematopoietic stem cell transplantation

Non-disease prone animals that received bone marrow derived from diseased hosts developed autoimmune diseases (Berisso et al., 1999) and vice versa. This suggested that the hematopoietic compartment plays an important role in autoimmune disease susceptibility, and transplantation of autologous or allogeneic non-autoimmune disease-prone hematopoietic cells can attenuate autoimmune disease. Autologous, syngeneic, and allogeneic bone marrow (or hematopoietic stem cell) transplantations have been performed in animal models of human autoimmune diseases, including EAE (Burt et al., 1998; Karussis et al., 1993), experimental autoimmune myasthenia gravis (Pestronk et al., 1983), adjuvant-induced arthritis (van Bekkum, 1989), collagen-induced arthritis (Kamiya et al., 1993), type 1 diabetes (NOD mice) (Beilhack et al., 2003), and SLE-like autoimmune diseases (MLR/lpr mice and NZB/W F1 mice) (Ikehara, 2001; Smith-Berdan et al., 2007). The results from these animal studies suggested that myelo-ablative therapy supported by stem cell transplantation can result in remission of disease or induction of immune tolerance. The bone marrow was the initial source of hematopoietic stem cells, but peripheral blood is currently used following mobilization procedures comprising a combination of cyclophosphamide and G-CSF (Saccardi and Gualandi, 2008).

The therapeutic concept of hematopoietic stem cell transplantation is to reset the immune system. Thus, patients receive aggressive immunosuppression to eliminate autoreactive lymphocytes (to ablate the immune system), and disease remission occurs via de novo regeneration of immunocytes from hematopoietic stem cells. Two mechanisms have been proposed. The first is re-education of the defective immune system by restoring diverse antigen-specific clones via reactivation of the thymic output and regenerating the adaptive immune system that had became apparently tolerant to self-antigens (Abrahamsson and Muraro, 2008). The second mechanism is reconstitution of the regulatory T-cell pool after stem cell transplantation. Regulatory T cells are important for preventing autoreactivity and control autoimmunity throughout life (Zhang et al., 2009). The rationale of allogeneic stem cell transplantation is substitution of the faulty immune system with a normal healthy one. However, the burden of higher mortality and morbidity due to graft versus host disease prevents its use in autoimmune disease except immune cytopenia. Allogeneic transplantation may be an option for selective patients who are not suitable for or have previously undergone autologous hematopoietic stem cell transplantation.

Autologous BM transplantation for autoimmune diseases has no risk of graft-versus-host disease, but relapses are common (Chan et al., 2008). For example, a case report on autologous hematopoietic stem cell transplantation in non-Hodgkin's lymphoma concurrent with Crohn's disease discussed that autologous hematopoietic stem cell transplantation will not provide a long-term cure for Crohn's disease (Anumakonda et al., 2007). In this case report, the authors postulated that autologous hematopoietic stem transplantation led to ablation of activated T cells for a prolonged period (8 years), but the genetic predisposition (positive family history) concurrent with other environmental factors such as smoking subsequently led to disease relapse. In case of genetically determined autoimmunity, an allogeneic source of stem cells is necessary to prevent a relapse of autoimmunity (Jorgensen et al., 2003). Patients with a refractory autoimmune disease that does not respond to current conventional treatments may be considered for stem cell transplantation. Pilot studies were conducted in systemic sclerosis (Tyndall et al., 1997; Martini et al., 1999), rheumatoid arthritis (Durez et al., 1998), SLE (Burt et al., 1997; Marmont et al., 1997), multiple sclerosis (Burt et al., 1998), and hematological autoimmune diseases, such as idiopathic thrombocytopenia (Lim et al., 1997), autoimmune hemolytic anemia, and Evans syndrome. Some promising results have been reported from phase I/II trial studies, and phase III randomized controlled trials are currently underway (http://clinicaltrials.gov/). Over one-third of patients achieved durable remission and transplant-related mortality reached 12% in the initial "European group for Blood and Marrow Transplants" (EBMT) registry, which decreased to around 5% in a recent EBMT study (Farge et al., 2010). Susceptibility to bacterial, viral, and fungal infections increases until the immune system is reconstituted, which makes the hematopoietic stem cell transplantation a high-risk therapy. The major complications of hematopoietic stem cell transplantation include septicemia, pneumonia, increased risk of late infection, infertility, and secondary malignancies, such as acute leukemia and myelodysplastic syndrome.

4.2. Mesenchymal stem cell transplantation

Mesenchymal stem cells (MSCs) are multipotent adult stem cells that are the progenitors of multiple mesenchymal lineages (Pittenger et al., 1999). The therapeutic mechanisms of MSC transplantation include capacity for differentiation and transdifferentiation, paracrine effects, immunomodulatory properties, and capacity for directional migration. MSCs have immunoprivileges. MSCs can escape the immune system because they lack MHC class II or co-stimulatory molecules, such as B7, CD40, and CD40L, which leads to poor recognition by T cells (Deans et al., 2000). Moreover, a number of in vitro studies have revealed that MSCs exert immunosuppressive and immunomodulatory effects on MHC-mismatched lymphocyte proliferation by inhibiting naïve, memory, and activated T cells, B cells, NK cells, and dendritic cells (Bartholomew et al., 2002; Di Nicola et al., 2002). MSCs release paracrine factors, including trophic, chemoattractant, and immunomodulatory factors. Immunomodulatory factors secreted by human MSCs include TGF-β, HGF, PGE2, hemoxygenase-1, human leukocyte antigen-G5, and IL-10 (Wang et al., 2011). They are constitutively produced by MSCs or after cross-talk with target cells, and their production is also enhanced by cytokines secreted by target cells after cross-talk (Wang et al., 2011). MSCs exhibit immunomodulatory properties by direct cell-to-cell contact and/or release of soluble immunosuppressive factors (Uccelli et al., 2008). MSCs possess the capacity to home to mesenchymal tissues, and injured sites in particular, which may also contribute to autoimmune disease treatment. According to the study by Ponte et al., human bone marrow MSCs (BMMSCs) express the following tyrosine kinase receptors: platelet-derived growth factor receptor (PDGF-R)α; PDGF-Rβ; and insulin-like growth factor receptor (IGF-R). MSCs also express 'regulated upon activation, normal T-cell expressed, and secreted (RANTES) and macrophage-derived chemokine (MDC) receptors (CCR2, CCR3, and CCR4)' and 'stromal-derived factor (SDF)-1 receptor (CXCR4)' (Ponte et al., 2007).

Survival results from an animal study comparing whole bone marrow cell transplantation with adherent cell (MSC)-removed bone marrow cell transplantation revealed that MSCs play a critical role in the treatment of lupus in the MLR/lpr mouse model. All mice treated with whole bone marrow cells survived more than 1 year, but 75% of mice treated with MSC-removed bone marrow cells died within 3 months (Ishida et al., 1994). Total bone marrow transplants consist of both hematopoietic stem cells and stromal cells, and MSCs play a pivotal role in tolerance induction (Jorgensen et al., 2003).

Initially, MSCs were isolated from the bone marrow and later from various other tissues, including placenta, muscle, cartilage, and fat (da Silva Meirelles L et al., 2006).

Recently, syngeneic, allogeneic, and xenogeneic MSC transplantations have been performed for autoimmune diseases in various animal models, including autoimmune encephalomyelitis (Zappia et al., 2005; Rafei et al., 2009; Constantin et al., 2009), type I diabetes (Fiorina et al., 2009), inflammatory bowel disease (Gonzalez-Rey et al., 2009), rheumatoid arthritis (González et al., 2009), and SLE (Zhou et al., 2008; Sun et al., 2009; Choi et al., 2012). These studies yielded some promising results. For example, long-term serial administration of human adipose tissue-derived MSCs increased survival rates, improved serologic, immunologic, and histologic abnormalities, and decreased the incidence of severe proteinuria in NZB/W F1 mice, a murine SLE model. The levels of IL-4 and IL-10 in the serum and the proportion of CD4+FoxP3+ regulatory T cells in the spleen were increased in NZB/W F1 mice treated with MSCs, compared to control NZB/W F1 mice treated with saline (Choi et al., 2012). Clinical studies using allogeneic MSC transplantation in refractory SLE patients revealed improvements in serologic parameters and renal function (Sun et al., 2009; Liang J et al., 2010). Furthermore, pilot studies using autologous BMMSC transplantation in patients with refractory Crohn's disease also yielded promising results (Duijvestein et al., 2010; Ciccocioppo R et al., 2011). Clinical trials using MSCs for diabetes and lupus nephritis are underway (http://clinicaltrials.gov/).

4.3. Genetically modified stem cell therapy (Stem cell-based gene therapy)

Gene therapy-assisted stem cell transplantation has become one of the most attractive therapies in clinical immunology (Marmont, 2011). The use of genetically selected or genetically engineered cell types can further control the possibility of disease progression or relapse. Hematopoietic stem cells engineered to express autoantigens in resting antigen-presenting cells can be used to prevent autoimmune diseases. For example, syngeneic transplantation of hematopoietic stem cells encoding proinsulin transgenically targeted to antigen-presenting cells completely prevents the development of spontaneous autoimmune diabetes in NOD mice (Steptoe et al., 2003). Transplantation of BM genetically engineered to express myelin oligodendrocyte glycoprotein (MOG) led to the deletion of MOG-specific thymocytes and prevented the induction and progression of EAE (Chan et al., 2008).

Transplantation of genetically engineered autologous BM cells expressing diabetes-resistant MHC class II molecules (I-A^b) into NOD mice prevented the development of autoreactive T cells via negative selection and prevented the progression of diabetes (Tian et al., 2004).

Genetic modification of stem cells or differentiated tissue cells with a decoy receptor for inflammatory cytokines can be used to treat autoimmune diseases. For example, NOD/SCID mice administered with MSCs genetically modified to secrete the soluble TNF receptor II exhibit decreased concentration of serum TNF-α.

My previous study revealed that transplantation of adipose tissue-derived MSCs transduced with the CTLA4Ig gene by using a lentiviral vector reduces the inflammatory immune response and improves Th1/Th2 balance in experimental autoimmune thyroiditis (Choi EW et al., 2011). This study showed that MSCs can be efficiently transduced using lentiviral vectors to express therapeutic proteins and can retain their immunophenotype even after genetic manipulation. Moreover, the concentration of murine CTLA4Ig in the culture supernatants of CTLA4Ig-transduced MSCs was sustained at higher passages, indicating that MSCs genetically modified using the lentiviral system provide durable expression of therapeutic genes. Similarly, insertion of inducible regulatory genes into the stem cell compartment is expected to alter disease activity. Genetically modified stem cells that secrete immunomodulatory factors (e.g., IL-10, IDO, PGE2, TGF-β) and home to injured targets have great potential for treating various diseases, including autoimmune diseases.

5. Conclusion

During the past several decades, strategies using agents that influence cytokines, hyperactivity of B cells, and B cell-T cell interaction have been developed and some of these agents have proven to be effective and well tolerated therapies for autoimmune diseases. Although some of these treatments have yielded encouraging and promising results, prospective well-planned studies and international cooperation are required to collect experiences and clarify further details on safety and clinical efficacy depending on the disease states and the condition of patients.

Hematopoietic stem cell therapy removes misguided inappropriate immune cells, restores immune cells, and resets or re-educates the immune system. Promising results have been reported from clinical trial studies. Some patients achieved durable remission, and transplant-related mortality has decreased. MSCs are easily available, possess extensive capacity for in vitro expansion, and exhibit homing effects and immunomodulatory functions. Thus, MSCs have been targeted by researchers as an alternative source of treatment for autoimmune diseases. Stem cell therapy may be integrated with other therapeutic agents, including biologics and new intelligent molecules, for greater immunomodulation.

Stem cell-based gene therapy has great potential as a novel method for immunomodulation in autoimmune diseases. By identifying the correct gene for autoimmune disease treatment, stem cell-based gene therapy will be able to produce a synergic effect of gene therapy and stem cell therapy. Before they are put to clinical use, genetically engineered cells should be carefully tested at the genetic, molecular, and cellular levels.

Selection and application of the appropriate therapy from among the various new therapeutic agents should be based on the risk-benefit analysis for each patient, because patients with autoimmune diseases exhibit different symptoms and severities and different responses to each treatment. Further studies are warranted to identify new specific targets and determine regimens to optimize the clinical response depending on the disease states. The development of non-toxic and effective novel gene transfer systems and clinical trials to evaluate combination therapies using agents that achieve immunomodulation or induce immune tolerance via different targets are also needed.

Author details

Eun Wha Choi

Laboratory Animal Research Center, Samsung Biomedical Research Institute, Republic of Korea

School of Medicine, Sungkyunkwan University, Republic of Korea

6. References

Abrahamsson S, Muraro PA. Immune re-education following autologous hematopoietic stem cell transplantation. Autoimmunity. 2008;41(8):577-84.

Adelman NE, Watling DL, McDevitt HO. Treatment of (NZB x NZW)F1 disease with anti-I-A monoclonal antibodies. J Exp Med. 1983;158(4):1350-5.

Angkasekwinai P, Park H, Wang YH, Wang YH, Chang SH, Corry DB, Liu YJ, Zhu Z, Dong C. Interleukin 25 promotes the initiation of proallergic type 2 responses. J Exp Med. 2007;204(7):1509-17.

Anolik JH, Barnard J, Owen T, Zheng B, Kemshetti S, Looney RJ, Sanz I. Delayed memory B cell recovery in peripheral blood and lymphoid tissue in systemic lupus erythematosus after B cell depletion therapy. Arthritis Rheum. 2007;56(9):3044-56.

Anumakonda V, Hayee B, Chung-Faye G. Remission and relapse of Crohn's disease following autologous haematopoietic stem cell transplantation for non-Hodgkin's lymphoma. Gut. 2007; 56(9): 1325.

Aringer M, Graninger WB, Steiner G, Smolen JS. Safety and efficacy of tumor necrosis factor alpha blockade in systemic lupus erythematosus: an open-label study. Arthritis Rheum. 2004;50(10):3161-9.

Bartholomew A, Sturgeon C, Siatskas M, Ferrer K, McIntosh K, Patil S, Hardy W, Devine S, Ucker D, Deans R, Moseley A, Hoffman R. Mesenchymal stem cells suppress lymphocyte proliferation in vitro and prolong skin graft survival in vivo. Exp Hematol. 2002;30(1):42-8.

Beilhack GF, Scheffold YC, Weissman IL, Taylor C, Jerabek L, Burge MJ, Masek MA, Shizuru JA. Purified allogeneic hematopoietic stem cell transplantation blocks diabetes pathogenesis in NOD mice. Diabetes. 2003;52(1):59-68.

Berisso GA, van Lint MT, Bacigalupo A, Marmont AM. Adoptive autoimmune hyperthyroidism following allogeneic stem cell transplantation from an HLA-identical sibling with Graves' disease. Bone Marrow Transplant. 1999;23(10):1091-2.

Boitard C, Michie S, Serrurier P, Butcher GW, Larkins AP, McDevitt HO. In vivo prevention of thyroid and pancreatic autoimmunity in the BB rat by antibody to class II major histocompatibility complex gene products. Proc Natl Acad Sci U S A. 1985;82(19):6627-31.

Bosi E, Todd I, Pujol-Borrell R, Bottazzo GF. Mechanisms of autoimmunity: relevance to the pathogenesis of type I (insulin-dependent) diabetes mellitus. Diabetes Metab Rev. 1987;3(4):893-923.

Buckner JH. Mechanisms of impaired regulation by CD4+CD25+FOXP3+ regulatory T cells in human autoimmune diseases. Nat Rev Immunol. 2010;10:849-59.

Burt RK, Padilla J, Begolka WS, Canto MC, Miller SD. Effect of disease stage on clinical outcome after syngeneic bone marrow transplantation for relapsing experimental autoimmune encephalomyelitis. Blood. 1998 ;91(7):2609-16.

Burt RK, Traynor AE, Cohen B, Karlin KH, Davis FA, Stefoski D, Terry C, Lobeck L, Russell EJ, Goolsby C, Rosen S, Gordon LI, Keever-Taylor C, Brush M, Fishman M, Burns WH. T cell-depleted autologous hematopoietic stem cell transplantation for multiple sclerosis: report on the first three patients. Bone Marrow Transplant. 1998;21(6):537-41.

Burt RK, Traynor A, Ramsey-Goldman R. Hematopoietic stem-cell transplantation for systemic lupus erythematosus. N Engl J Med. 1997;337(24):1777-8.

Carnahan J, Stein R, Qu Z, Hess K, Cesano A, Hansen HJ, Goldenberg DM. Epratuzumab, a CD22-targeting recombinant humanized antibody with a different mode of action from rituximab. Mol Immunol. 2007;44(6):1331-41.

Castaño L, Eisenbarth GS. Type-I diabetes: a chronic autoimmune disease of human, mouse, and rat. Annu Rev Immunol. 1990;8:647-79.

Chabaud M, Durand JM, Buchs N, Fossiez F, Page G, Frappart L, Miossec P. Human interleukin-17: A T cell-derived proinflammatory cytokine produced by the rheumatoid synovium. Arthritis Rheum. 1999;42(5):963-70.

Chan J, Ban EJ, Chun KH, Wang S, Bäckström BT, Bernard CC, Toh BH, Alderuccio F. Transplantation of bone marrow transduced to express self-antigen establishes deletional tolerance and permanently remits autoimmune disease. J Immunol. 2008;181: 7571–7580.

Chaudhari U, Romano P, Mulcahy LD, Dooley LT, Baker DG, Gottlieb AB. Efficacy and safety of infliximab monotherapy for plaque-type psoriasis: a randomised trial. Lancet. 2001;357(9271):1842-7.

Chen W, Jin W, Hardegen N, Lei KJ, Li L, Marinos N, McGrady G, Wahl SM. Conversion of peripheral CD4+CD25- naive T cells to CD4+CD25+ regulatory T cells by TGF-beta induction of transcription factor Foxp3. J Exp Med. 2003;198(12):1875-86.

Chodisetti SB, Rai PK, Gowthaman U, Pahari S, Agrewala JN. Potential T cell epitopes of Mycobacterium tuberculosis that can instigate molecular mimicry against host: implications in autoimmune pathogenesis. BMC Immunol. 2012;13(1):13. [Epub ahead of print]

Choi EW, Shin IS, Lee HW, Park SY, Park JH, Nam MH, Kim JS, Woo SK, Yoon EJ, Kang SK, Ra JC, Youn HY, Hong SH. Transplantation of CTLA4Ig gene-transduced adipose tissue-derived mesenchymal stem cells reduces inflammatory immune response and improves Th1/Th2 balance in experimental autoimmune thyroiditis. J Gene Med. 2011 Jan;13(1):3-16.

Choi EW, Shin IS, Lee CW, Youn HY. The effect of gene therapy using CTLA4Ig/silica-nanoparticles on canine experimental autoimmune thyroiditis. J Gene Med. 2008;10(7):795-804.

Choi EW, Shin IS, Park SY, Park JH, Kim JS, Yoon EJ, Kang SK, Ra JC, Hong SH. Reversal of serologic, immunologic, and histologic dysfunction in mice with systemic lupus erythematosus by long-term serial adipose tissue-derived mesenchymal stem cell transplantation. Arthritis Rheum. 2012;64(1):243-53.

Choi EW, Shin IS, Youn HY, Kim DY, Lee H, Chae YJ, Lee CW. Gene therapy using non-viral peptide vector in a canine systemic lupus erythematosus model. Vet Immunol Immunopathol. 2005;103(3-4):223-33.

Ciccocioppo R, Bernardo ME, Sgarella A, Maccario R, Avanzini MA, Ubezio C, Minelli A, Alvisi C, Vanoli A, Calliada F, Dionigi P, Perotti C, Locatelli F, Corazza GR. Autologous bone marrow-derived mesenchymal stromal cells in the treatment of fistulising Crohn's disease. Gut. 201;60(6):788-98.

Constantin G, Marconi S, Rossi B, Angiari S, Calderan L, Anghileri E, Gini B, Bach SD, Martinello M, Bifari F, Galiè M, Turano E, Budui S, Sbarbati A, Krampera M, Bonetti B. Adipose-Derived Mesenchymal Stem Cells Ameliorate Chronic Experimental Autoimmune Encephalomyelitis. Stem Cells. 2009;27(10):2624-35.

Cooke A. Th17 cells in inflammatory conditions. Rev Diabet Stud. 2006;3(2):72-5.

Cua DJ, Hutchins B, LaFace DM, Stohlman SA, Coffman RL. Central nervous system expression of IL-10 inhibits autoimmune encephalomyelitis. J Immunol. 2001;166(1):602-8.

da Silva Meirelles L, Chagastelles PC, Nardi NB. Mesenchymal stem cells reside in virtually all post-natal organs and tissues. J Cell Sci. 2006;119(Pt 11):2204-13.

Deans RJ, Moseley AB. Mesenchymal stem cells: biology and potential clinical uses. Exp Hematol. 2000;28(8):875-84.

De Bandt M, Sibilia J, Le Loët X, Prouzeau S, Fautrel B, Marcelli C, Boucquillard E, Siame JL, Mariette X and the Club Rhumatismes et Inflammation. Systemic lupus erythematosus induced by anti-tumour necrosis factor alpha therapy: a French national survey. Arthritis Res Ther. 2005;7(3):R545-51.

de Kleer IM, Wedderburn LR, Taams LS, Patel A, Varsani H, Klein M, de Jager W, Pugayung G, Giannoni F, Rijkers G, Albani S, Kuis W, Prakken B. CD4+CD25bright regulatory T cells actively regulate inflammation in the joints of patients with the remitting form of juvenile idiopathic arthritis. J Immunol. 2004;172(10):6435-43.

Dejaco C, Duftner C, Grubeck-Loebenstein B, Schirmer M. Imbalance of regulatory T cells in human autoimmune diseases. Immunology. 2006;117(3):289-300.

Di Nicola M, Carlo-Stella C, Magni M, Milanesi M, Longoni PD, Matteucci P, Grisanti S, Gianni AM. Human bone marrow stromal cells suppress T-lymphocyte proliferation induced by cellular or nonspecific mitogenic stimuli. Blood. 2002;99(10):3838-43.

Dörner T, Kaufmann J, Wegener WA, Teoh N, Goldenberg DM, Burmester GR. Initial clinical trial of epratuzumab (humanized anti-CD22 antibody) for immunotherapy of systemic lupus erythematosus. Arthritis Res Ther. 2006;8(3):R74.

Duijvestein M, Vos AC, Roelofs H, Wildenberg ME, Wendrich BB, Verspaget HW, Kooy-Winkelaar EM, Koning F, Zwaginga JJ, Fidder HH, Verhaar AP, Fibbe WE, van den Brink GR, Hommes DW. Autologous bone marrow-derived mesenchymal stromal cell treatment for refractory luminal Crohn's disease: results of a phase I study. Gut. 2010;59(12):1662-9.

Durez P, Toungouz M, Schandené L, Lambermont M, Goldman M.

Remission and immune reconstitution after T-cell-depleted stem-cell transplantation for rheumatoid arthritis. Lancet. 1998;352(9131):881.

Dwyer, Donard S.; Bradley, Ronald J.; Urquhart, C. Kendrick; Kearney, John F. Naturally occurring anti-idiotypic antibodies in myasthenia gravis patients Nature. 1983;301 (5901):611-4.

Egan CA, Brown M, White JD, Yancey KB. Treatment of epidermolysis bullosa acquisita with the humanized anti-Tac mAb daclizumab. Clin Immunol. 2001;101(2):146-51.

Emamaullee JA, Davis J, Merani S, Toso C, Elliott JF, Thiesen A, Shapiro AM. Inhibition of Th17 cells regulates autoimmune diabetes in NOD mice. Diabetes. 2009;58(6):1302-11.

Farge D, Labopin M, Tyndall A, Fassas A, Mancardi GL, Van Laar J, Ouyang J, Kozak T, Moore J, Kötter I, Chesnel V, Marmont A, Gratwohl A, Saccardi R. Autologous hematopoietic stem cell transplantation for autoimmune diseases: an observational study on 12 years' experience from the European Group for Blood and Marrow Transplantation Working Party on Autoimmune Diseases. Haematologica. 2010;95(2):284-92.

Finck BK, Linsley PS, Wofsy D. Treatment of murine lupus with CTLA4Ig. Science 1994;265, 1225–7.

Fiorina P, Jurewicz M, Augello A, Vergani A, Dada S, La Rosa S, Selig M, Godwin J, Law K, Placidi C, Smith RN, Capella C, Rodig S, Adra CN, Atkinson M, Sayegh MH, Abdi R. Immunomodulatory function of bone marrow-derived mesenchymal stem cells in experimental autoimmune type 1 diabetes. J Immunol. 2009;183(2):993-1004.

Furst DE, Breedveld FC, Kalden JR, Smolen JS, Antoni CE, Bijlsma JW, Burmester GR, Cronstein B, Keystone EC, Kavanaugh A, Klareskog L. Updated consensus statement on biological agents for the treatment of rheumatoid arthritis and other rheumatic diseases (May 2002). Ann Rheum Dis. 2002 Nov;61 Suppl 2:ii2-7.

Furst DE, Breedveld FC, Kalden JR, Smolen JS, Burmester GR, Sieper J, Emery P, Keystone EC, Schiff MH, Mease P, van Riel PL, Fleischmann R, Weisman MH, Weinblatt ME. Updated consensus statement on biological agents for the treatment of rheumatic diseases, 2007. Ann Rheum Dis. 2007;66 Suppl 3:iii2-22.

Furst DE, Keystone EC, Breedveld FC, Kalden JR, Smolen JS, Antoni CE, Burmester GR, Crofford LJ, Kavanaugh A. Updated consensus statement on tumour necrosis factor blocking agents for the treatment of rheumatoid arthritis and other rheumatic diseases. Ann Rheum Dis. 2001;60 Suppl 3:iii2-5.

Fusco C, Andreone V, Coppola G, Luongo V, Guerini F, Pace E, Florio C, Pirozzi G, Lanzillo R, Ferrante P, Vivo P, Mini M, Macrì M, Orefice G, Lombardi ML. HLA-DRB1*1501 and response to copolymer-1 therapy in relapsing-remitting multiple sclerosis. Neurology. 2001;57(11):1976-9.

González MA, Gonzalez-Rey E, Rico L, Büscher D, Delgado M. Treatment of experimental arthritis by inducing immune tolerance with human adipose-derived mesenchymal stem cells. Arthritis Rheum. 2009;60(4):1006-1019.

Gonzalez-Rey E, Anderson P, González MA, Rico L, Büscher D, Delgado M. Human adult stem cells derived from adipose tissue protect against experimental colitis and sepsis. Gut. 2009;58(7):929-939.

Gordon FH, Lai CW, Hamilton MI, Allison MC, Srivastava ED, Fouweather MG, Donoghue S, Greenlees C, Subhani J, Amlot PL, Pounder RE. A randomized placebo-controlled trial of a humanized monoclonal antibody to alpha4 integrin in active Crohn's disease. Gastroenterology. 2001;121(2):268-74.

Granholm NA. Autoimmunity, Polyclonal B-Cell Activation and Infection. Lupus. 1992;1(2):63-74.

Gross JA, Johnston J, Mudri S, Enselman R, Dillon SR, Madden K, Xu W, Parrish-Novak J, Foster D, Lofton-Day C, Moore M, Littau A, Grossman A, Haugen H, Foley K, Blumberg H, Harrison K, Kindsvogel W, Clegg CH. TACI and BCMA are receptors for a TNF homologue implicated in B-cell autoimmune disease. Nature. 2000;404(6781):995-9.

Hanafusa T, Pujol-Borrell R, Chiovato L, Russell RC, Doniach D, Bottazzo GF. Aberrant expression of HLA-DR antigen on thyrocytes in Graves' disease: relevance for autoimmunity. Lancet. 1983;2(8359):1111-5.

Haufs MG, Haneke E. Epidermolysis bullosa acquisita treated with basiliximab, an interleukin-2 receptor antibody. Acta Derm Venereol. 2001;81(1):72.

Hofstetter HH, Ibrahim SM, Koczan D, Kruse N, Weishaupt A, Toyka KV, Gold R. Therapeutic efficacy of IL-17 neutralization in murine experimental autoimmune encephalomyelitis. Cell Immunol. 2005;237(2):123-30.

Hutas G. Ocrelizumab, a humanized monoclonal antibody against CD20 for inflammatory disorders and B-cell malignancies. Curr Opin Investig Drugs. 2008;9(11):1206-15.

Iebba F, Di Sora F, Tarasi A, Leti W, Montella T, Montella F. Case report: safety and efficacy of tocilizumab in a patient with rheumatoid arthritis and chronic hepatitis C. Case Report Med. 2012;2012:212381. Epub 2012 Feb 16.

Ikehara S. Treatment of autoimmune diseases by hematopoietic stem cell transplantation. Exp Hematol. 2001;29(6):661-9.

Isenberg D, Gordon C, Merrill J, Urowitz M. New therapies in systemic lupus erythematosus - trials, troubles and tribulations.... working towards a solution. Lupus. 2008;17(11):967-70.

Ishida T, Inaba M, Hisha H, Sugiura K, Adachi Y, Nagata N, Ogawa R, Good RA, Ikehara S. Requirement of donor-derived stromal cells in the bone marrow for successful allogeneic bone marrow transplantation. Complete prevention of recurrence of autoimmune diseases in MRL/MP-Ipr/Ipr mice by transplantation of bone marrow plus bones (stromal cells) from the same donor. J Immunol. 1994;152(6):3119-27.

Jaeckel E, von Boehmer H, Manns MP. Antigen-specific FoxP3-transduced T-cells can control established type 1 diabetes. Diabetes. 2005;54(2):306-10.

Jantunen E, Myllykangas-Luosujärvi R. Stem cell transplantation for treatment of severe autoimmune diseases: current status and future perspectives. Bone Marrow Transplant. 2000;25(4):351-6.

Jones G, Ding C. Tocilizumab: a review of its safety and efficacy in rheumatoid arthritis. Clin Med Insights Arthritis Musculoskelet Disord. 2010;3:81-9.

Jorgensen C, Djouad F, Apparailly F, Noël D. Engineering mesenchymal stem cells for immunotherapy. Gene Ther. 2003;10(10):928-31.

Kalled SL, Cutler AH, Datta SK, Thomas DW.Anti-CD40 ligand antibody treatment of SNF1 mice with established nephritis: preservation of kidney function. J Immunol. 1998;160(5):2158-65.

Kamiya M, Sohen S, Yamane T, Tanaka S. Effective treatment of mice with type II collagen induced arthritis with lethal irradiation and bone marrow transplantation. J Rheumatol. 1993;20(2):225-30.

Karussis DM, Vourka-Karussis U, Lehmann D, Ovadia H, Mizrachi-Koll R, Ben-Nun A, Abramsky O, Slavin S. Prevention and reversal of adoptively transferred, chronic relapsing experimental autoimmune encephalomyelitis with a single high dose cytoreductive treatment followed by syngeneic bone marrow transplantation. J Clin Invest. 1993;92(2):765-72.

Kayagaki N, Yan M, Seshasayee D, Wang H, Lee W, French DM, Grewal IS, Cochran AG, Gordon NC, Yin J, Starovasnik MA, Dixit VM. BAFF/BLyS receptor 3 binds the B cell survival factor BAFF ligand through a discrete surface loop and promotes processing of NF-kappaB2. Immunity. 2002;17(4):515-24.

Keating GM, Perry CM. Infliximab: an updated review of its use in Crohn's disease and rheumatoid arthritis. BioDrugs. 2002;16(2):111-48.

Kleinschek MA, Owyang AM, Joyce-Shaikh B, Langrish CL, Chen Y, Gorman DM, Blumenschein WM, McClanahan T, Brombacher F, Hurst SD, Kastelein RA, Cua DJ. IL-25 regulates Th17 function in autoimmune inflammation. J Exp Med. 2007;204(1):161-70.

Koenders MI, Lubberts E, Oppers-Walgreen B, van den Bersselaar L, Helsen MM, Di Padova FE, Boots AM, Gram H, Joosten LA, van den Berg WB. Blocking of interleukin-17 during reactivation of experimental arthritis prevents joint inflammation and bone erosion by decreasing RANKL and interleukin-1. Am J Pathol. 2005;167(1):141-9.

Kohm AP, Carpentier PA, Anger HA, Miller SD. Cutting edge: CD4+CD25+ regulatory T cells suppress antigen-specific autoreactive immune responses and central nervous system inflammation during active experimental autoimmune encephalomyelitis. J Immunol. 2002;169(9):4712-6.

Kuby J. 1994: Autoimmunity. In: Kuby J (ed), Immunology, 2nd edn, pp. 445-467. WH Freeman and Company, New York.

Lacki JK. Management of the patient with severe refractory rheumatoid arthritis: are the newer treatment options worth considering? BioDrugs. 2000;13(6):425-35.

Lacki JK, Samborski W, Mackiewicz SH. Interleukin-10 and interleukin-6 in lupus erythematosus and rheumatoid arthritis, correlations with acute phase proteins. Clin Rheumatol. 1997;16(3):275-8.

Lawson BR, Prud'homme GJ, Chang Y, Gardner HA, Kuan J, Kono DH, Theofilopoulos AN. Treatment of murine lupus with cDNA encoding IFN-gammaR/Fc. J Clin Invest. 2000;106(2):207-15.

Liang J, Zhang H, Hua B, Wang H, Lu L, Shi S, Hou Y, Zeng X, Gilkeson GS, Sun L. Allogenic mesenchymal stem cells transplantation in refractory systemic lupus erythematosus: a pilot clinical study. Ann Rheum Dis. 2010;69(8):1423-9.

Lim SH, Kell J, al-Sabah A, Bashi W, Bailey-Wood R. Peripheral blood stem-cell transplantation for refractory autoimmune thrombocytopenic purpura. Lancet. 1997;349(9050):475.

Luo X, Yang H, Kim IS, Saint-Hilaire F, Thomas DA, De BP, Ozkaynak E, Muthukumar T, Hancock WW, Crystal RG, Suthanthiran M. Systemic transforming growth factor-beta1 gene therapy induces Foxp3+ regulatory cells, restores self-tolerance, and facilitates regeneration of beta cell function in overtly diabetic nonobese diabetic mice. Transplantation. 2005;79(9):1091-6.

Marmont AM. Hematopoietic stem cell transplantation for severe autoimmune disease: Progress and perspectives. Cellular Therapy and Transplantation. 2011;2(6): 1-8.

Marmont AM, van Lint MT, Gualandi F, Bacigalupo A. Autologous marrow stem cell transplantation for severe systemic lupus erythematosus of long duration. Lupus. 1997;6(6):545-8.

Martini A, Maccario R, Ravelli A, Montagna D, De Benedetti F, Bonetti F, Viola S, Zecca M, Perotti C, Locatelli F. Marked and sustained improvement 2 years after autologous stem cell transplantation in a girl with systemic sclerosis. Rheumatology (Oxford). 1999;38(8):773.

Migita K, Eguchi K, Otsubo T, Kawakami A, Nakao H, Ueki Y, Shimomura C, Kurata A, Fukuda T, Matsunaga M, Ishikawa N, Ito K, Nagataki S. Cytokine regulation of HLA on thyroid epithelial cells. Clin Exp Immunol. 1990;82(3):548-52.

Mohan AK, Edwards ET, Coté TR, Siegel JN, Braun MM. Drug-induced systemic lupus erythematosus and TNF-alpha blockers. Lancet. 2002;360(9333):646.

Mok MY. The immunological basis of B-cell therapy in systemic lupus erythematosus.
Int J Rheum Dis. 2010;13(1):3-11.

Moore PA, Belvedere O, Orr A, Pieri K, LaFleur DW, Feng P, Soppet D, Charters M, Gentz R, Parmelee D, Li Y, Galperina O, Giri J, Roschke V, Nardelli B, Carrell J, Sosnovtseva S, Greenfield W, Ruben SM, Olsen HS, Fikes J, Hilbert DM. BLyS: member of the tumor necrosis factor family and B lymphocyte stimulator. Science. 1999;285(5425):260-3.

Moreland LW, Morgan EE, Adamson TC 3rd, Fronek Z, Calabrese LH, Cash JM, Markenson JA, Matsumoto AK, Bathon J, Matteson EL, Uramoto KM, Weyand CM, Koopman WJ,

Heck LW, Strand V, Diveley JP, Carlo DJ, Nardo CJ, Richieri SP, Brostoff SW. T cell receptor peptide vaccination in rheumatoid arthritis: a placebo-controlled trial using a combination of Vbeta3, Vbeta14, and Vbeta17 peptides. Arthritis Rheum. 1998;41(11):1919-29.

Na SY, Cao Y, Toben C, Nitschke L, Stadelmann C, Gold R, Schimpl A, Hünig T. Naive CD8 T-cells initiate spontaneous autoimmunity to a sequestered model antigen of the central nervous system. Brain. 2008;131(Pt 9):2353-65.

Nagler-Anderson C, Bober LA, Robinson ME, Siskind GW, Thorbecke GJ. Suppression of type II collagen-induced arthritis by intragastric administration of soluble type II collagen. Proc Natl Acad Sci U S A. 1986;83(19):7443-6.

Nepom GT. Therapy of autoimmune diseases: clinical trials and new biologics. Curr Opin Immunol. 2002;14(6):812-5.

Oh U, Blevins G, Griffith C, Richert N, Maric D, Lee CR, McFarland H, Jacobson S. Regulatory T cells are reduced during anti-CD25 antibody treatment of multiple sclerosis. Arch Neurol. 2009;66(4):471-9.

Papp K, Bissonnette R, Krueger JG, Carey W, Gratton D, Gulliver WP, Lui H, Lynde CW, Magee A, Minier D, Ouellet JP, Patel P, Shapiro J, Shear NH, Kramer S, Walicke P, Bauer R, Dedrick RL, Kim SS, White M, Garovoy MR. The treatment of moderate to severe psoriasis with a new anti-CD11a monoclonal antibody. J Am Acad Dermatol. 2001;45(5):665-74.

Perrotta S, Locatelli F, La Manna A, Cennamo L, De Stefano P, Nobili B. Anti-CD20 monoclonal antibody (Rituximab) for life-threatening autoimmune haemolytic anaemia in a patient with systemic lupus erythematosus. Br J Haematol. 2002;116(2):465-7.

Pescovitz MD. Rituximab, an anti-cd20 monoclonal antibody: history and mechanism of action. Am J Transplant. 2006;6(5 Pt 1):859-66.

Pestronk A, Drachman DB, Teoh R, Adams RN. Combined short-term immunotherapy for experimental autoimmune myasthenia gravis. Ann Neurol. 1983;14(2):235-41.

Phillips JM, Harach SZ, Parish NM, Fehervari Z, Haskins K, Cooke A. Nondepleting anti-CD4 has an immediate action on diabetogenic effector cells, halting their destruction of pancreatic beta cells. J Immunol. 2000;165(4):1949-55.

Pittenger MF, Mackay AM, Beck SC, Jaiswal RK, Douglas R, Mosca JD, Moorman MA, Simonetti DW, Craig S, Marshak DR. Multilineage potential of adult human mesenchymal stem cells. Science. 1999;284(5411):143-7.

Ponte AL, Marais E, Gallay N, Langonné A, Delorme B, Hérault O, Charbord P, Domenech J. The in vitro migration capacity of human bone marrow mesenchymal stem cells: comparison of chemokine and growth factor chemotactic activities. Stem Cells. 2007;25(7):1737-45.

Quartier P, Brethon B, Philippet P, Landman-Parker J, Le Deist F, Fischer A. Treatment of childhood autoimmune haemolytic anaemia with rituximab. Lancet. 2001;358(9292):1511-3.

Rafei M, Campeau PM, Aguilar-Mahecha A, Buchanan M, Williams P, Birman E, Yuan S, Young YK, Boivin MN, Forner K, Basik M, Galipeau J. Mesenchymal stromal cells ameliorate experimental autoimmune encephalomyelitis by inhibiting CD4 Th17 T cells in a CC chemokine ligand 2-dependent manner. J Immunol. 2009;182(10):5994-6002.

Rao NA, Atalla L, Linker-Israeli M, Chen FY, George FW 4th, Martin WJ, Steinman L. Suppression of experimental uveitis in rats by anti-I-A antibodies. Invest Ophthalmol Vis Sci. 1989;30(11):2348-55.

Raz E, Dudler J, Lotz M, Baird SM, Berry CC, Eisenberg RA, Carson DA. Modulation of disease activity in murine systemic lupus erythematosus by cytokine gene delivery. Lupus. 1995;4(4):286-92.

Saccardi R, Gualandi F. Hematopoietic stem cell transplantation procedures. Autoimmunity. 2008;41(8):570-6.

Sakaguchi S. Animal models of autoimmunity and their relevance to human diseases. Curr Opin Immunol. 2000;12(6):684-90.

Sia C. Imbalance in Th cell polarization and its relevance in type 1 diabetes mellitus. Rev Diabet Stud. 2005;2(4):182-6.

Siatskas C, Chan J, Field J, Murphy K, Nasa Z, Toh BH, Alderuccio F. Gene therapy strategies towards immune tolerance to treat the autoimmune diseases. Curr Gene Ther. 2006;6(1):45-58.

Skurkovich S, Boiko A, Beliaeva I, Buglak A, Alekseeva T, Smirnova N, Kulakova O, Tchechonin V, Gurova O, Deomina T, Favorova OO, Skurkovic B, Gusev E. Randomized study of antibodies to IFN-gamma and TNF-alpha in secondary progressive multiple sclerosis. Mult Scler. 2001;7(5):277-84.

Smith-Berdan S, Gille D, Weissman IL, Christensen JL. Reversal of autoimmune disease in lupus-prone New Zealand black/New Zealand white mice by nonmyeloablative transplantation of purified allogeneic hematopoietic stem cells. Blood. 2007;110(4):1370-8.

Smith KG, Jones RB, Burns SM, Jayne DR. Long-term comparison of rituximab treatment for refractory systemic lupus erythematosus and vasculitis: Remission, relapse, and re-treatment. Arthritis Rheum. 2006;54(9):2970-82.

Sokolove J, Strand V, Greenberg JD, Curtis JR, Kavanaugh A, Kremer JM, Anofrei A, Reed G, Calabrese L, Hooper M, Baumgartner S, Furst DE. Risk of elevated liver enzymes associated with TNF inhibitor utilisation in patients with rheumatoid arthritis. Ann Rheum Dis. 2010;69(9):1612-7.

Springer TA, Dustin ML, Kishimoto TK, Marlin SD. The Lymphocyte Function Associated LFA-1, CD2, and LFA-3 Molecules: Cell Adhesion Receptors of the Immune System. Ann Rev Immunol. 1987;5:223-252.

Steptoe RJ, Ritchie JM, Harrison LC. Transfer of hematopoietic stem cells encoding autoantigen prevents autoimmune diabetes. J Clin Invest. 2003;111(9):1357-63.

Sthoeger ZM, Sharabi A, Molad Y, Asher I, Zinger H, Dayan M, Mozes E. Treatment of lupus patients with a tolerogenic peptide, hCDR1 (Edratide): immunomodulation of gene expression. J Autoimmun. 2009;33(1):77-82.

Suarez-Pinzon WL, Rabinovitch A. Approaches to type 1 diabetes prevention by intervention in cytokine immunoregulatory circuits. Int J Exp Diabetes Res. 2001;2(1):3-17.

Sun L, Akiyama K, Zhang H, Yamaza T, Hou Y, Zhao S, Xu T, Le A, Shi S. Mesenchymal stem cell transplantation reverses multiorgan dysfunction in systemic lupus erythematosus mice and humans. Stem cells. 2009; 27(6):1421-1432.

Sundrud MS, Koralov SB, Feuerer M, Calado DP, Kozhaya AE, Rhule-Smith A, Lefebvre RE, Unutmaz D, Mazitschek R, Waldner H, Whitman M, Keller T, Rao A. Halofuginone inhibits TH17 cell differentiation by activating the amino acid starvation response. Science. 2009;324(5932):1334-8.

Tackey E, Lipsky PE, Illei GG. Rationale for interleukin-6 blockade in systemic lupus erythematosus. Lupus. 2004;13(5):339-43.

Tang Q, Henriksen KJ, Bi M, Finger EB, Szot G, Ye J, Masteller EL, McDevitt H, Bonyhadi M, Bluestone JA. In vitro-expanded antigen-specific regulatory T cells suppress autoimmune diabetes. J Exp Med. 2004;199(11):1455-65.

Tedder TF, Tuscano J, Sato S, Kehrl JH. CD22, a B lymphocyte-specific adhesion molecule that regulates antigen receptor signaling. Annu Rev Immunol. 1997;15:481-504.

Tian C, Bagley J, Cretin N, Seth N, Wucherpfennig KW, Iacomini J. Prevention of type 1 diabetes by gene therapy. J Clin Invest. 2004;114(7):969-78.

Titus RG, Chiller JM. Orally induced tolerance. Definition at the cellular level. Int Arch Allergy Appl Immunol. 1981;65(3):323-38.

Todd I, Pujol-Borrell R, Hammond LJ, Bottazzo GF, Feldmann M. Interferon-gamma induces HLA-DR expression by thyroid epithelium. Clin Exp Immunol. 1985;61(2):265-73.

Tomasi TB Jr. Oral tolerance. Transplantation. 1980;29(5):353-6.

Trentham DE, Dynesius-Trentham RA, Orav EJ, Combitchi D, Lorenzo C, Sewell KL, Hafler DA, Weiner HL. Effects of oral administration of type II collagen on rheumatoid arthritis. Science. 1993;261(5129):1727-30.

Tubridy N, Behan PO, Capildeo R, Chaudhuri A, Forbes R, Hawkins CP, Hughes RA, Palace J, Sharrack B, Swingler R, Young C, Moseley IF, MacManus DG, Donoghue S, Miller DH. The effect of anti-alpha4 integrin antibody on brain lesion activity in MS. The UK Antegren Study Group. Neurology. 1999;53(3):466-72.

Tutrone WD, Kagen MH, Barbagallo J, Weinberg JM. Biologic therapy for psoriasis: a brief history, II. Cutis. 2001;68(6):367-72.

Tyndall A, Black C, Finke J, Winkler J, Mertlesmann R, Peter HH, Gratwohl A. Treatment of systemic sclerosis with autologous haemopoietic stem cell transplantation. Lancet. 1997;349(9047):254.

Uccelli A, Moretta L, Pistoia V. Mesenchymal stem cells in health and disease.

Nat Rev Immunol. 2008;8(9):726-36.

van Bekkum DW, Bohre EP, Houben PF, Knaan-Shanzer S. Regression of adjuvant-induced arthritis in rats following bone marrow transplantation. Proc Natl Acad Sci U S A. 1989;86(24):10090-4.

Waite JC, Skokos D. Th17 response and inflammatory autoimmune diseases. Int J Inflam. 2012;2012:819467.

Waldor MK, Sriram S, McDevitt HO, Steinman L. In vivo therapy with monoclonal anti-I-A antibody suppresses immune responses to acetylcholine receptor. Proc Natl Acad Sci U S A. 1983;80(9):2713-7.

Wallace DJ, Stohl W, Furie RA, Lisse JR, McKay JD, Merrill JT, Petri MA, Ginzler EM, Chatham WW, McCune WJ, Fernandez V, Chevrier MR, Zhong ZJ, Freimuth WW. A phase II, randomized, double-blind, placebo-controlled, dose-ranging study of belimumab in patients with active systemic lupus erythematosus. Arthritis Rheum. 2009;61(9):1168-78.

Wang J, Liao L, Tan J. Mesenchymal-stem-cell-based experimental and clinical trials: current status and open questions. Expert Opin Biol Ther. 2011;11(7):893-909.

Weiner HL, Mackin GA, Matsui M, Orav EJ, Khoury SJ, Dawson DM, Hafler DA. Double-blind pilot trial of oral tolerization with myelin antigens in multiple sclerosis. Science. 1993;259(5099):1321-4.

Wiesik-Szewczyk E, Lacki JK, Feleszko W, Olesinska M. Target therapies in systemic lupus erythematosus: current state of the art. Mini Rev Med Chem. 2010;10(10):956-65.

Wiglesworth AK, Ennis KM, Kockler DR. Belimumab: a BLyS-specific inhibitor for systemic lupus erythematosus. Ann Pharmacother. 2010;44(12):1955-61.

Willis F, Marsh JC, Bevan DH, Killick SB, Lucas G, Griffiths R, Ouwehand W, Hale G, Waldmann H, Gordon-Smith EC. The effect of treatment with Campath-1H in patients with autoimmune cytopenias. Br J Haematol. 2001;114(4):891-8.

Woods JM, Katschke KJ, Volin MV, Ruth JH, Woodruff DC, Amin MA, Connors MA, Kurata H, Arai K, Haines GK, Kumar P, Koch AE. IL-4 adenoviral gene therapy reduces inflammation, proinflammatory cytokines, vascularization, and bony destruction in rat adjuvant-induced arthritis. J Immunol. 2001;166(2):1214-22.

Yasuda H, Nagata M, Arisawa K, Yoshida R, Fujihira K, Okamoto N, Moriyama H, Miki M, Saito I, Hamada H, Yokono K, Kasuga M. Local expression of immunoregulatory IL-12p40 gene prolonged syngeneic islet graft survival in diabetic NOD mice. J Clin Invest. 1998;102(10):1807-14.

Zappia E, Casazza S, Pedemonte E, Benvenuto F, Bonanni I, Gerdoni E, Giunti D, Ceravolo A, Cazzanti F, Frassoni F, Mancardi G, Uccelli A. Mesenchymal stem cells ameliorate experimental autoimmune encephalomyelitis inducing T-cell anergy. Blood. 2005;106(5):1755-1761.

Zhang L, Bertucci AM, Ramsey-Goldman R, Burt RK, Datta SK. Regulatory T cell (Treg) subsets return in patients with refractory lupus following stem cell transplantation, and TGF-beta-producing CD8+ Treg cells are associated with immunological remission of lupus. J Immunol. 2009;183(10):6346-58.

Zhang ZL, Shen SX, Lin B, Yu LY, Zhu LH, Wang WP, Luo FH, Guo LH. Intramuscular injection of interleukin-10 plasmid DNA prevented autoimmune diabetes in mice. Acta Pharmacol Sin. 2003;24(8):751-6.

Zhang HG, Su X, Liu D, Liu W, Yang P, Wang Z, Edwards CK, Bluethmann H, Mountz JD, Zhou T. Induction of specific T cell tolerance by Fas ligand-expressing antigen-presenting cells. J Immunol. 1999;162(3):1423-30.

Zhou K, Zhang H, Jin O, Feng X, Yao G, Hou Y, Sun L. Transplantation of human bone marrow mesenchymal stem cell ameliorates the autoimmune pathogenesis in MRL/lpr mice. Cell Mol Immunol. 2008;5(6):417-24.

Chapter 12

Stem Cell Therapies for Type I Diabetes

Jesus Ciriza and Jennifer O. Manilay

Additional information is available at the end of the chapter

http://dx.doi.org/10.5772/47803

1. Introduction

Diabetes mellitus is a chronic metabolic disease that results in high levels of glucose in the blood. Normally, glucose is transported into cells from the blood for energy, and this transport is initiated in response to the hormone, insulin. In diabetic patients, cellular glucose uptake is defective, in part due to the inability of cells to respond to insulin, or the inability of the body to produce the insulin itself. According to the International Diabetes Foundation, 366 million people worldwide had been diagnosed with diabetes in 2011, and this number is continuing to increase in every country (http://www.idf.org/). It is an especially challenging health problem, as treatments to both control hyperglycemia as well as the debilitating side effects of diabetes, such as injury to the blood vessels and nerves, must be addressed. Amongst the three types of diabetes (Type I - autoimmune, gestational and Type II – adult onset), Type II diabetes is the most prevalent, in which hyperglycemia is uncontrolled due to the body's inability to produce enough insulin or due to the body's inability to respond appropriately to lower the blood glucose level. In contrast, in patients with Type I diabetes (TID), insulin-producing beta (β) cells are destroyed by the immune system. Studies of TID by many groups have provided extensive insight to the fields of immunological tolerance and pancreatic developmental biology. In this chapter, we will briefly describe TID, provide a synopsis of pancreatic β cell development in mice as compared to humans, review of some of the medical treatments currently available for TID, and discuss current studies that have explored the use of stem cells as alternative possible therapies for TID.

2. Type I diabetes in humans and mice

2.1. TID in humans

A fully comprehensive comparison of TID in humans and mice has recently been published, so we will only highlight certain areas (van Belle, Coppieters et al. 2011). TID is a multigenic disease, and several candidates have been discovered that implicate disruptions in the normal process of negative selection of autoreactive T cells during thymic development, genetic association with specific major histocompatibility complex (MHC) genes in the human leukocyte antigen (HLA) locus, as well as dysregulation of mature T lymphocyte responses. For example, patients with mutations in the *FoxP3* or *Aire* genes, which are important for the development and function of regulatory T cells (T_{regs}) and expression of "self-antigens" by medullary thymic epithelial cells, often present with autoimmune diabetes, as well as other autoimmune disorders (Michels and Gottlieb 2010). On the other end of the spectrum, the inability to downregulate or prevent mature T cell responses due to mutations in cytokine receptor expression (Garg, Tyler et al. 2012) or low surface expression of CTLA-4 (Haseda, Imagawa et al. 2011) can also result in sustained T cell cytotoxicity or lack of T_{reg} response towards diabetes-related antigens. Environmental insults, such as viral infections, molecular mimicry between some viral proteins and diabetes-related autoantigens, changes in gut flora and the intestinal microenvironment, have also been linked with the onset of TID in humans.

2.2. TID in mice

The identification of the mechanisms underlying the autoimmunity of TID in humans has been facilitated by the use of rodent models of the disease (Van Belle, Taylor et al. 2009; von Herrath and Nepom 2009). Despite the fact that TID is a multigenic disease with heterogeneous etiologies, there is overall consensus that TID is caused by the destruction of pancreatic β cells by sets of immune cells that recognize many potential autoantigens (such as insulin, glutamate decarboxylase (GAD), islet antigens, and heat shock proteins-60 and -70) and that the disease can be transferred by the transplantation of autoreactive T lymphocytes that are specific for these antigens (Mallone, Brezar et al. 2011). Several spontaneous, induced and transgenic mouse models currently exist, which have provided important insights into the genetics, cellular mechanisms and immunological aspects of TID. However, the non-obese diabetic (NOD) mouse strain remains the primary animal strain for studies of TID. The utility of the NOD mouse and comparison of the TID in the NOD mouse with human TID have been extensively reviewed and debated, and we direct the reader to these excellent reviews for further reference (Anderson and Bluestone 2005; Roep and Peakman 2011). The NOD mouse strain, when housed in specific-pathogen free conditions, displays the onset of diabetes after 12 weeks of age in both sexes. Insulitis is observed as mononuclear infiltration in the islets before full blown diabetes is evident, and this cellular infiltrate is comprised of primary T lymphocytes, but other lymphoid and myeloid cells are also present. The insulitis results in the destruction of the pancreatic islets and the insulin-producing β cells. The NOD mouse also displays defects in functional macrophages and natural killer cells, NKT cells and regulatory T cells and complement. The NOD mouse, therefore, has allowed for the investigation of numerous immune mechanisms that contribute to the development of TID. The peripheral neuropathy that accompanies TID in humans is also evident in the NOD mouse, which has allowed for analysis and management of the side effects of TID (Anderson and Bluestone 2005; Roep and Peakman 2011). Similar to human diabetes, the MHC of the NOD mouse contains several loci that are linked to increased susceptibility to TID. The NOD mouse background has also been used to derive the NOD/*scid*/$\gamma_c^{-/-}$ (NSG) immunocompromised strain, into which human cells can be transplanted (Shultz, Saito et al. 2010).

Many studies in mice have focused on mechanisms to control the aberrant autoimmune response in TID, as well as strategies to replace dysfunctional β cells, using simple insulin replacement or rescue/regeneration of the β cells. Despite the similarities between TID in humans and in the NOD mouse, clear differences have been noted. TID in the NOD mouse appears to be a more aggressive disease compared than that in humans, so the NOD mouse may be more beneficial for studies of therapies for long-term TID than for discovery of pre-susceptibility markers of TID. β cells in the NOD mouse may also be more proliferative and could possibly regenerate better than other strains (Sherry, Kushner et al. 2006), and evidence that pancreatic development is altered in the NOD mouse also exists (Homo-Delarche 2001). Therefore, in addition to its clear autoimmune etiology, TID may also result from defects in pancreatic development.

2.3. Pancreatic development in the mouse and human

The adult pancreas organ is comprised of many cell types, including exocrine and endocrine cells, and is highly vascularized. Although TID is a disease that occurs in the fully formed pancreas, strategies to treat or cure TID via β cell regeneration or β cell differentiation from embryonic stem cells (ESCs) or induced pluripotent cells (iPSCs) have relied on the current knowledge of pancreatic development during the fetal period. Here, we briefly review the development of pancreas in the mouse and human, and then move to a description of development of β cells only.

In the mouse, pancreas formation occurs in three phases (Jorgenson, Ahnfelt-Ronne et al. 2007). In the first phase, pancreatic formation from the endodermal gut tube begins at embryonic day (e) 8.5. Patterning of the gut tube in the pancreatic region is reliant on retinoic acid (RA) signaling from the mesoderm. The dorsal and ventral pancreas buds form from the pancreatic epithelium in the primitive gut tube. Recently, the critical role of the Wnt signaling in the pancreatic mesenchyme in the differentiation of pancreatic epithelial cells was shown *in vivo* (Landsman, Nijagal et al. 2011). Eventually, the ventral pancreas rotates toward the dorsal pancreas, and they fuse into one organ by e12.5. At this stage, the pancreas organ undergoes significant cell proliferation and branching. In the second phase (e13.5), the cells within the immature pancreas begin to differentiate into exocrine cells that are required for the production of digestive enzymes, and endocrine cells that secrete hormones into the blood, such as glucagon, insulin, somatostatin, pancreatic polypeptide and ghrelin. Each of these hormones is produced by a distinct endocrine cell type (with insulin produced by the β cells) (**Figure 1**). The third phase of pancreatic development occurs after birth, and is associated with the ability of the pancreas to respond to dietary intake and maintain glucose homeostasis.

Islet development in humans occurs at a slower rate compared to what is observed in mice, but the reasons for this are not understood. The size of the human islet is comparable to that of the mouse, but in the mouse, the mean area ratio of β cells is higher than observed in the human (Kim, Miller et al. 2009). Fetal antigen-1 is a protein expressed exclusively in human endodermal tissue and pancreatic epithelial cells before islet formation (Tornehave, Jansen et al. 1993). Islets can be located in the human fetus as early as 12-13 weeks post coitus (Piper, Brickwood et al. 2004), although functional β cells that are insulin-positive can be detected as early as 8 weeks.

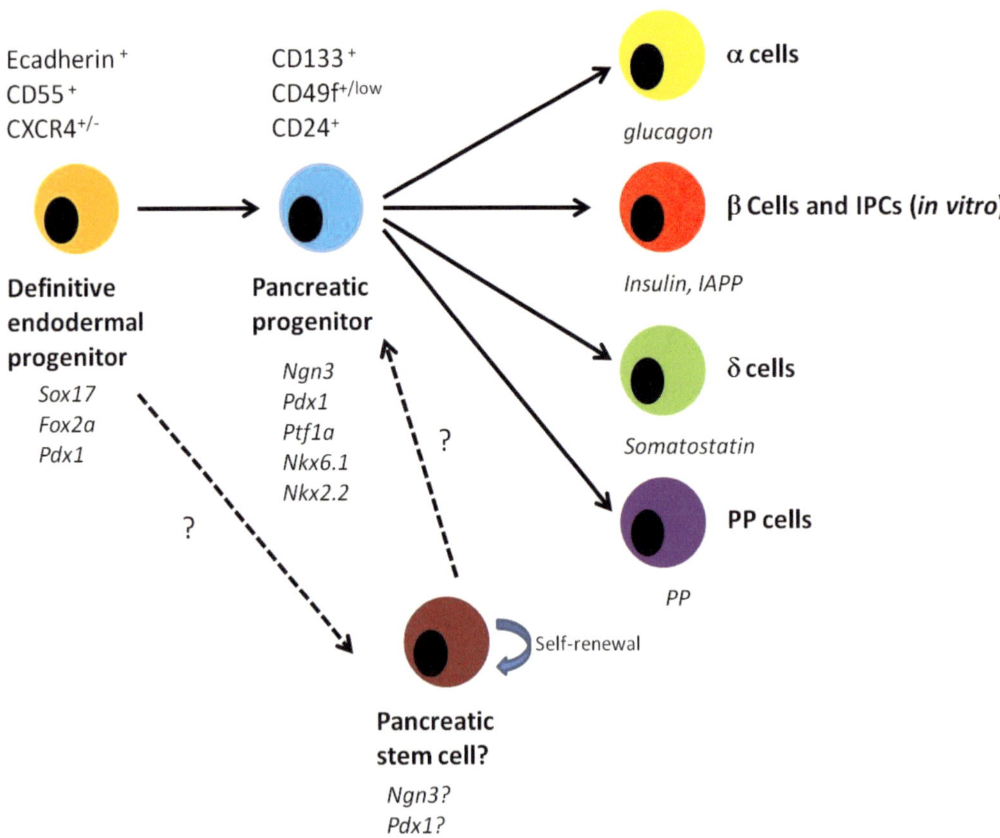

Figure 1. *An overview of pancreatic endocrine cell development*. The development of pancreatic endocrine cells starts with an early endocrine progenitor and ends with mature hormone-producing islet cell types. Cell surface markers (noted above the cell types) and gene expression (in italics) in distinct pancreatic cell lineages are shown. The existence of the self-renewing pancreatic stem cell is still controversial.

An overview of pancreatic endocrine cell development is shown in **Figure 1**. **Definitive endodermal progenitor cells** can differentiate into pancreatic progenitor cells, which have been identified by the expression of two critical transcriptional factors: *Pdx1* and *neurogenin 3* (*Ngn3*). Experiments with conditional *Pdx1* transgenic reporter mice (inducible Cre-ER™-LoxP system to mark the progeny of cells that express *Pdx1*) demonstrated that *Pdx1*$^{+}$ cells give rise to all three types of pancreatic tissue: exocrine, endocrine and duct (Gu, Dubauskaite et al. 2002). In line with this, *Pdx1* deficiency in mouse and humans leads to a complete pancreas agenesis at birth (Ahlgren, Jonsson et al. 1996). *Pdx1* is also a critical transcriptional activator of insulin and somatostatin in adult islet cells (Ohlsson, Thor et al. 1991; Leonard, Peers et al. 1993). Similar to *Pdx1*, *Ngn3*$^{+}$ cells give rise to all islet lineage cells during embryogenesis (Gradwohl, Dierich et al. 2000), with peak Ngn3 expression at 15.5 days post-coitus. Although some have reported that *Ngn3* is undetectable in adult pancreas (Gradwohl, Dierich et al. 2000; Johansson, Dursun et al. 2007), *Ngn3*$^{+}$ cells in duct-ligated adult pancreas were detected and observed to differentiate into islet cells (Gu, Dubauskaite et al. 2002; Xu, D'Hoker et al. 2008). Beta cells in the human, like in the mouse, are derived from a heterogeneous population of **pancreatic progenitor cells** (Scharfmann, Xiao et al. 2008). Whether or not the pancreatic progenitors are derived from a self-renewing **pancreatic stem cell** is still under debate (Jiang and Morahan 2011), and is discussed further in Section 3.1.

For β cell development, the essential role of three key transcription factors, Pax4, Nkx6.1, Nkx2.2, in the mouse and their relationships to the human β cell development is clear. Pax4 (paired box 4) is required for the commitment to the pancreatic lineages (Wang, Elghazi et al. 2004), as well as for the regulation of β cell mass size, proliferation and survival in mice (Brun and Gauthier 2008), and mutations in the *Pax4* gene have been linked to susceptibility to both Type I and Type II diabetes in humans (Yokoi, Kanamori et al. 2006; Chavali, Mahajan et al. 2011). In addition, both human and mice insulinoma cells overexpress Pax4 in comparison to mature β cells, suggesting that Pax4 may also play a role in β cell proliferation and resistance to apoptosis. *Nkx2.2* is expressed early during embryonic pancreatic development (Doyle, Loomis et al. 2007), whereas *Nkx6.1* is expressed later and restricted to the β cells. *Nkx2.2* and *Nkx6.1* knockout mice die in the neonatal period due to the lack of IPCs (Sussel, Kalamaras et al. 1998). Nkx2.2 has both activator and repressor functions; the repressor function is important for regulation of β cell function postnatally (Doyle and Sussel 2007). Nkx6.1 functions exclusively in β cells and is required for β cell development and specification, control of insulin secretion after glucose challenge, and can also induce human and rat β cell proliferation (Schisler, Fueger et al. 2008). However, *in vivo* overexpression of Nkx6.1 does not have any effect on β cells in the mouse (Schaffer, Yang et al. 2011).

2.4. Current therapies for TID

A fully mature, functional β cell produces and appropriately secretes the mature form of insulin (i.e. proteolytic processing of pro-insulin to form C-peptide is evident), in response to glucose to maintain normal glycemic levels in the blood. The current treatment for TID is long-term insulin replacement therapy that is delivered via injection, insulin pens or pumps, and has been quite successful for control of hyperglycemia. However, insulin replacement therapy is not considered a cure for TID, as patients receiving insulin long-term still manifest abnormalities in metabolism, as measured by above-normal levels of glycated hemoglobin (HbA1c). Furthermore, for children, the daily requirement for insulin replacement can limit their day-to-day activities, and TID-related complications, such as vascular disease, retinopathy and neuropathy, still persist even with insulin therapy.

Pancreatic transplantation has been performed for TID patients with success, but the main limitations of this strategy are the low number of suitable donors required for transplant and the decision if the risks of surgery and transplantation outweigh the benefits (Jahansouz, Kumer et al. 2011). Furthermore, even with insulin replacement therapy or pancreatic transplantation, autoreactive immune cells that can attack and destroy any residual β cells in the patient can still remain. For this reason, therapies that modulate the immune response to β cells and β cell antigens also exist, and their safety and efficacy have been or are currently being tested in clinical trials (Bluestone, Herold et al. 2010; Waldron-Lynch and Herold 2011). GAD65 specific-antigen-based immunotherapy with alum adjuvant demonstrated preservation of C-peptide fasting levels in younger new-onset patients four years after treatment (Ludvigsson, Hjorth et al. 2011), but this was not supported in the larger Phase III trial (Ludvigsson, Krisky et al. 2012). Humanized anti-CD3 antibody (in which human Fc immunoglobulin domains are engineered to mouse CD3-binding portions of the antibody) therapy given in a single dose reduced the decline of insulin production and the amount of exogenous insulin required in the patients (Herold, Gitelman et al. 2009). Interestingly, the anti-CD3 antibodies reduced the numbers of circulating T lymphocytes, but whether or not autoreactive T cells are specifically depleted is unclear. There is evidence that the anti-CD3 antibody acts as a weak TCR agonist and stimulates the production of regulatory T cells (T_{regs}) in humans. B lymphocytes in TID have been postulated to act as antigen-presenting cells and also to produce autoantibodies that can result in β cell destruction (Bluestone, Herold et al. 2010). Anti-CD20 antibodies target and deplete B lymphocytes, and lead to a preservation of β cell function in patients, as measured by C-peptide production and reduction of HbA1c levels compared to controls. However, the level of autoantibodies in these TID patients was not determined, so the mechanism by which anti-CD20 therapy works in TID patients is still uncertain. As we will explain further below, these immune modulation therapies may also be important for the future success of β cell regeneration and transplantation.

3. Experimental alternative treatments for TID: Stem cells

Pancreas transplantation has succeeded as a replacement for insulin-secreting β cells for TID patients, but this relies on a limited source of cadaveric pancreatic tissue (Danovitch, Cohen et al. 2005). Early studies demonstrated that isolated human islets did not proliferate in suspension culture, and that adherent islet cells showed limited replication of β cells (Nielsen, Brunstedt et al. 1979; Nielsen, Galsgaard et al. 2001). Therefore, alternative sources of IPCs are needed, and stem cells have been suggested as this source. Stem cells are undifferentiated cells that are capable of self-renewal and differentiation into any cell type. They can be classified depending on their origin. Embryonic stem cells (ESCs) are derived from the inner cell mass of implanted embryos (Evans and Kaufman 1981), induced pluripotent stem cells (iPSCs) are adult or fetal cells that have been "reprogrammed" to an ESC-like state (Takahashi and Yamanaka 2006), adult stem cells are isolated from adult tissues (Becker, Mc et al. 1963) and germline-derived stem cells are generated from embryonic or adult gonads (Shamblott, Axelman et al. 1998). In this section, we will discuss the state-of-the-art technologies in which the different types of stem cells are generated and differentiated and their possible clinical applications as cellular replacement therapies for TID.

3.1. Tissue-specific pancreatic stem cells

The existence of pancreatic stem cells was proposed in the last decade (Ramiya, Maraist et al. 2000), and is still a topic of debate (Dor, Brown et al. 2004; Smukler, Arntfield et al. 2011) (**Figure 1**). When defining a "stem cell" by function, the standard tests are to examine the ability of a putative stem cell to **self-renew,** often using proliferation assays; and **differentiate**, measured by changes in function, cell surface marker and/or gene expression.

Evidence from fetal and adult pancreas biology in physiological as well as pathological conditions support the hypothesis of the existence of **pancreatic adult stem cells** based on proliferation assays. For example, pancreas from pregnant rats and mice displayed an uptake of bromodeoxyuridine (BrdU) during pregnancy, suggesting the proliferation of islets (Parsons, Brelje et al. 1992; Karnik, Chen et al. 2007). This proliferation was stimulated by prolactin (Nielsen, Svensson et al. 1999; Rieck and Kaestner) that reduced expression of *multiple endocrine neoplasia type 1* (*MEN1*), a tumor suppressor (Karnik, Chen et al. 2007), and enhanced expression of *tryptophan hydroxylase 1* (*Tph1*), which allows for incorporation of BrdU in the cell (Kim, Toyofuku et al. 2010). In addition, expression of Ki-67 (a marker associated with proliferation) and β-cell mass increase has been described in the pancreas of obese mice, perhaps as a response to insulin resistance (Butler, Janson et al. 2003; Butler, Janson et al. 2003). Other authors have shown that mature β cells are capable of self-replication (**Figure 2**), and that this is the mechanism by which new beta cells in the adult are generated. Young diabetic rats are able to regenerate β cells after streptozotocin (STZ)-induced β cell destruction, but this capacity for regeneration declines rapidly during the first days of life (Wang, Bouwens et al. 1996). β cell regeneration is also detected after pancreatectomies, but the regeneration response is different between species, with a higher rate of regeneration in rodents than in larger mammals (Stagner and Samols 1991; Bonner-Weir and Sharma 2002; Robertson, Lanz et al. 2002; Matveyenko, Veldhuis et al. 2006). More recently, human islet precursor cells were identified from IPCs that underwent an epithelial-to-mesenchymal transition, demonstrating that, *in vitro*, human IPCs from the islets of cadaveric pancreas donors could spontaneously produce highly proliferative "de-differentiated" fibroblast-like cells that could then possibly be expanded and later re-induced into insulin-producing, β-like cells (Gershengorn, Hardikar et al. 2004; Russ, Bar et al. 2008; Russ, Sintov et al. 2011).

As mentioned previously, *Pdx1* and *Ngn3* are two transcription factors which are essential for endocrine cell differentiation during pancreas development, and have been targets in the search of pancreatic stem cells. However, it has not been demonstrated if *Pdx1*$^{+}$ cells can self-renew (Jiang and Morahan 2011), a requirement for stem cell definition. *Ngn3*$^{+}$ cells from duct-ligated adult pancreas can develop into islet cells (Xu, D'Hoker et al. 2008), satisfying the stem cell differentiation requirement. However, *Ngn3* expression in the embryo inhibits proliferation by inducing *cyclin-dependent kinase inhibitor 1a* (*Cdkn1a*) (Miyatsuka, Kosaka et al. 2011), resulting in limited mitotic potential of *Ngn3*⁺ cells (Gradwohl, Dierich et al. 2000; Johansson, Dursun et al. 2007), which is evidence against self-renewal.

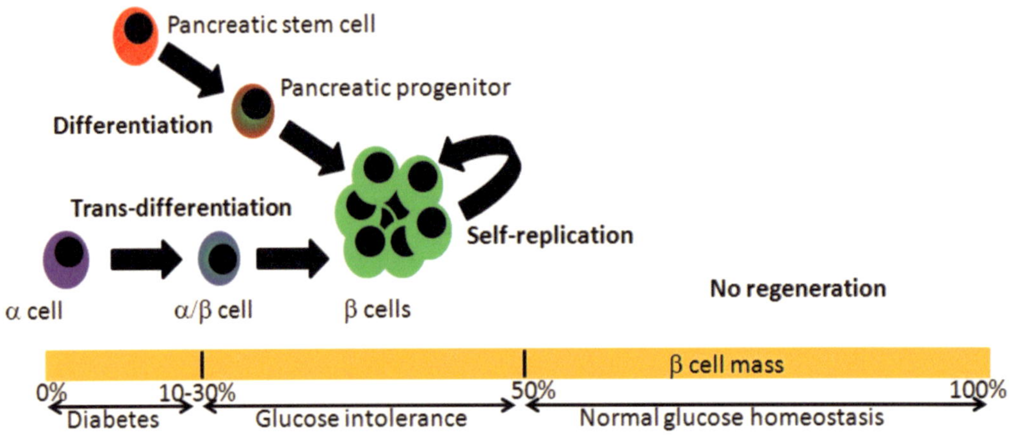

Figure 2. *Different mechanisms for β cell regeneration based on β cell mass.* Differentiation from pancreatic stem cells and transdifferentiation from β cells would occur when less than 30% of the normal β cell mass is present, whereas self-replication of residual β cells would occur if 30-50% of the normal β cell mass is present.

To test whether β cells can self-replicate in the adult, transgenic mice in which pre-existing β cells were specifically labeled were utilized (Dor, Brown et al. 2004). In the absence of pancreatic injury, these labeled cells were not replaced by new IPCs, arguing against the existence of an adult pancreatic stem cell. However, the labeled IPCs were able to uptake BrdU after pancreatectomy, indicating that adult β cells contain regenerative ability (Dor, Brown et al. 2004). A different model in which apoptosis was induced specifically in β cells using a diphtheria toxin receptor (DTR) transgenic mouse model showed β cell recovery, restoration to euglycemia, and that the surviving β cells were involved in their own regeneration (Nir, Melton et al. 2007). These studies assumed that insulin expression was limited exclusively to cells, but it has been shown that in certain circumstances, other cells and tissues can express insulin (Kojima, Fujimiya et al. 2004). In support of this, rare multipotent stem cells which express insulin have been described in both embryonic and adult mouse and human pancreas that are distinct from mature β cells (Smukler, Arntfield et al. 2011). Importantly, these cells were shown to self-renew, expressed *Pdx1*, *Nkx6.1*, *Ngn3* and *insulin*, and differentiate into IPCs that could alleviate diabetes in mice. Therefore, it appears that adult pancreatic stem cells do indeed exist, and the assumption that insulin is not expressed in β cell progenitors is incorrect. These findings can now be used to model additional cellular alternatives for β cell replacement in TID.

Questions regarding the existence and location of pancreatic stem cells and progenitors outside of the pancreas are still an area of investigation. Hepatic and pancreatic cells are derived from a common endodermal progenitor during embryogenesis, and this has led to the hypothesis that cells from fetal liver tissue could be used as an alternative β cell source.

Pancreatic duct cells and liver cells can be induced to express certain β cell gene products in culture (Heremans, Van De Casteele et al. 2002; Sapir, Shternhall et al. 2005). In support of this, $CD45^-$ $Ter119^-$ c-kit^- hepatic stem cells were isolated from mouse fetal liver and differentiated into IPCs in vitro. These differentiated cells were then transplanted into drug-induced diabetic mice, which showed a significant reduction of their blood glucose levels (Feng, Du et al. 2005). Bone marrow has also been proposed as another possible source of IPCs. For example, human fetal bone marrow-derived $CD45^-$ Glycophorin A^- mesodermal progenitor cells generated insulin secreting islet-like clusters when injected into human fetal pancreatic tissues that were implanted in STZ-treated NOD/severe combined immunodeficiency (SCID) mice (Ai, Todorov et al. 2007). In the mouse, progeny of Mac-1^- Sca^+ bone marrow cells cultured with cytokines such as IL-3, IL-6, IL-11 and stem cell factor (SCF) migrate into the pancreas islets and have been reported to convert into $CD45^-$ $CD34^+$ insulin-expressing cells (Luo, Luo et al. 2009). The mechanisms involved in the conversion of these bone marrow cells into IPCs were not investigated.

3.2. Transdifferentiated cells as heterologous sources of β cells

Transdifferentiation is defined as a process by which a "terminally" differentiated cell changes into another type of differentiated cell. Transdifferentiation of pancreatic α cells into β cells has been suggested as a source of β cell replacement for TID. Transdifferentiation of α cells into β cells has been observed *in vivo* (Thorel, Nepote et al. 2010). Mice in which more than 99% of β cells were ablated eventually recovered β cell mass, due to transdifferentiated α cells. The rates of recovery from α cells ranged between 32 to 81% among individuals. These data have led to a model in which several β cell regenerative mechanisms can occur, but each mechanism is used under different pathological conditions (**Figure 2**). For example, in this model, pancreatic stem cells and progenitors, as well as transdifferentiated cells, naturally replace β cells when β cell mass is extremely depleted (less than 30% of normal), but β cell mass is regenerated by self-replication of β cells when the loss is 30 - 50% of normal (Thorel, Nepote et al. 2010). Interestingly, during transdifferentiation from the α to β phenotype, cells that express both insulin and glucagon can be temporally detected (Thorel, Nepote et al. 2010). These "bi-hormonal" cells have been described during pancreas development by immunohistochemistry or single cell gene expression analysis (Chiang and Melton 2003). Their existence is controversial and more studies are required before they can be accepted to be true endocrine progenitor cells, such as clear isolation of the population and definitive evidence that they can give rise to α or β cells *in vitro* or *in vivo* (Alpert, Hanahan et al. 1988; Teitelman, Alpert et al. 1993; Herrera, Huarte et al. 1994; Herrera 2000; Jensen, Heller et al. 2000).

One important question that has not yet been answered pertains to the location of the cells that can undergo transdifferentiation into β cells *in vivo*. Two major pancreas compartments contain cells with the potential of generating new β cells via transdifferentiation *in vivo*: ductal epithelium and acinar tissue. Islet-like clusters of human ductal epithelium cells reverse diabetes after transplantation (Bonner-Weir, Taneja et al. 2000; Ramiya, Maraist et al. 2000). After pancreatic duct ligation, ductal cells that express *Ngn3* (a marker of pancreatic progenitors, see Section 2.3*)* differentiate into β cells if transplanted into fetal pancreas (Xu, D'Hoker et al. 2008). Experiments using ductal cell lineage tracing with the carbonic anydrase II (*CA2,* an enzyme specific for ductal cells) promoter showed *CA2* expression in islet cells under normal conditions or after pancreatic duct ligation, adding more evidence of ductal epithelial cells' ability to differentiate into islet cells. Some authors have suggested that these pancreatic ductal cells are mesenchymal stem cells (MSC) (Seeberger, Dufour et al. 2006). Whether these MSC differentiate directly into pancreatic stem cells or transdifferentiate from epithelial cells to pancreatic stem cells still remains unclear (Bonner-Weir, Inada et al. 2008; Inada, Nienaber et al. 2008). The exocrine tissue, in particular acinar cells, could provide a new alternative β cell replacement source for the treatment of diabetes. Acinar cells are usually discarded after islet purification from donated pancreas for transplantation, but could be reprogrammed *in vivo* to β cells by introducing a combination of the transcription factors *Ngn3, Pdx1* and *Mafa* by means of adenovirus. These transcription factors are required only transiently and they are not detectable after two months of transfection (Zhou, Martin et al. 2008). Epithelial cells that were purified from non-endocrine islet cells were co-transplanted with fetal pancreatic cells and differentiated into endocrine cells (Hao, Tyrberg et al. 2006). Moreover, cells which express *amylase/elastase*, specific markers of acinar cells, differentiated into insulin expressing cells, as measured by cell tracing (Minami, Okuno et al. 2005).

Taken together, the studies cited in this section demonstrate that there are many possible pluripotent and even terminally differentiated cells *in vivo* that could be used to derive new IPCs that can alleviate hyperglycemia in diabetic mouse models. However, the alternative source that been most exhaustively researched is the totipotent **embryonic stem cell** (ESC). In the next section, we review studies of ESC differentiation into IPCs.

3.3. Differentiation of embryonic stem cells into insulin producing cells

The use of ESCs for cell replacement therapies has great promise, due to the potentially unlimited self-renewal of ESC in their undifferentiated state, and the potential of ESC to differentiate into any type of cellular derivatives. Many groups have used diverse methodologies to differentiate human or murine ESCs into IPCs for β cell replacement in diabetes (**Figure 3**). The most common obstacles amongst the different protocols are the inability of ESC-derived IPCs (ESC-IPCs) to secrete insulin after glucose-stimulation, the risk of teratoma formation due to undifferentiated ESC that remain in the ESC-IPC culture, and immune rejection of the ESC-IPC after transplantation *in vivo*. Moreover, murine and human ESC lines do not behave similarly when they are differentiated into IPCs, which has led to species-distinct protocols (**Figure 3**).

The efficiency of ESC-IPC differentiation *in vitro* between murine and human ESC cells is clearly different. One reason for this appears to be the manner by which the endodermal germ layer is initiated in ESC culture. The embryoid body (EB) is a three-dimensional cluster of ESC that induces the differentiation of the endoderm, mesoderm, and ectoderm germ layers. In contrast to the EB method, ESCs can also differentiate in two-dimensional monolayers. For ESC-IPC differentiation, murine ESCs have been observed to differentiate very efficiently to endodermal cells via EB formation, with approximately 50% of the cells expressing *Foxa2*. In contrast, production of definitive endoderm cells in human EBs is less efficient, ranging from 5% to 19% of cells expressing *Foxa2* or *Sox17* (Shim, Kim et al. 2007). Instead, when cultured in monolayers, human ESCs show an efficiency of definitive endoderm differentiation over 80%, as measured by co-expression of *Foxa2* and *Sox17* (D'Amour, Agulnick et al. 2005; McLean, D'Amour et al. 2007), but murine ESCs are not efficiently differentiated into endoderm with this method (Kim, Hoffman et al. 2010). Consequently, most methods described for murine ESCs utilize EB formation, whereas human ESC methods use monolayers. Finding a common consensus protocol is one future challenge to the improvement of ESC-IPC differentiation and function. A summary of some murine and human IPC differentiation studies that includes a comparison of the IPC functional tests performed is presented in **Table 1 and Table 2,** respectively.

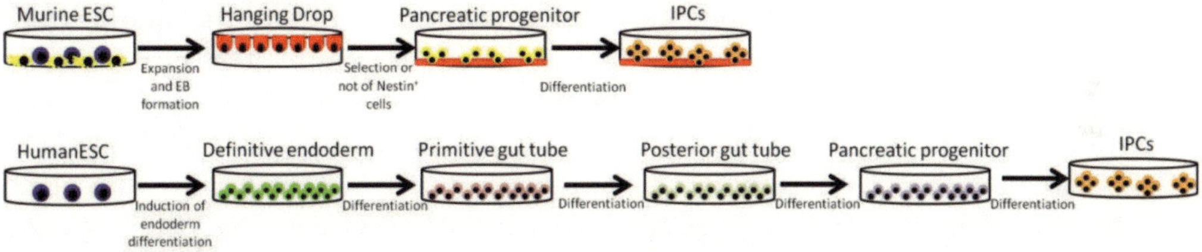

Figure 3. *Comparison of murine versus human ESC differentiation protocols to insulin-producing cells*. The schematic shows the differences in culture methods to produce IPCs from murine ESC (top) and human ESC (bottom). Please see the main text for more details.

ES cell lines used	Insulin mRNA	c-peptide protein expression	*In vitro* glucose response	Rescue of diabetic mice	Differentiation protocol reference
R1	Not done	Not done	Yes	Yes	(Soria, Roche et al. 2000)
B5, E14.1 and ESF122	Yes	Yes (controversial)	Yes	Failed (Fujikawa, Oh et al. 2005)	(Lumelsky, Blondel et al. 2001)
JM1, ROSA, and ESF122	Yes	Yes	Yes	Yes	(Hori, Rulifson et al. 2002)
R1 and ESF122	Yes	Yes	Yes	Yes with *Pax4* transfection	(Blyszczuk, Asbrand et al. 2004)
D3	Yes	Not done	Not done	Not done	(McKiernan, O'Driscoll et al. 2007)
D3	Yes	Not done	Yes	Not done	(Wang and Ye 2009)
B6	Yes	Yes	Yes	Not done	(Kim, Hoffman et al. 2010)
EB3	Yes	Yes	Yes	Not done	(Miyazaki, Yamato et al. 2004)
R1	Yes	Yes	Yes	Not done	(Banerjee, Sharma et al.)

Table 1. Murine ESC-IPC differentiation protocols

ES cell lines used	Insulin mRNA	c-peptide protein expression	*In vitro* glucose response	Rescue of diabetic mice	Differentiation protocol reference
CyT25, CyT49 CyT203	Yes	Yes	Yes	Yes	(D'Amour, Bang et al. 2006; Kroon, Martinson et al. 2008)
H1and H9	Yes	Yes	Yes	Yes	(Jiang, Shi et al. 2007)
H1, H7 and H9	Yes	Yes	Yes	Not done	(Jiang, Au et al. 2007)
Hes3	Yes	Yes	Yes	No	(Phillips, Hentze et al. 2007)

Table 2. Human ESC-IPC differentiation protocols

The first successful approach differentiating ESCs into functional IPCs utilized murine ESCs that were transfected with a neomycin selection gene under the control of the human *insulin* promoter (Soria, Roche et al. 2000). IPCs from EBs were selected with neomycin and nicotinamide, and no teratoma formation was described after transplantation. These ESC-IPCs normalized blood glycemia in diabetic mice during the first 4 weeks after transplant; however, 40% of the mice became hyperglycemic 12 weeks after implantation, suggesting that the ESC-IPCs function or lifespan was diminished (Soria, Roche et al. 2000). Since this initial report, numerous other approaches for differentiating ES cells into IPCs have been described, but three protocols by Lumelsky et al., Hori et al., and Blyszczuk et al. appear to be the most referenced (Lumelsky, Blondel et al. 2001; Hori, Rulifson et al. 2002; Blyszczuk, Asbrand et al. 2004). Non-transgenic ESCs were differentiated into IPCs by means of a five-step protocol: 1) expansion of ES cells, 2) formation of EBs, 3) selection of *nestin*-expressing cells with a serum-free medium containing insulin, transferrin, selenium and fibronectin (ITSFn), 4) expansion of pancreatic endocrine progenitor cells with a N2 medium containing B27 and the mitogenic basic fibroblast growth factor (bFGF) and 5) induction of differentiation of IPCs by withdrawal of bFGF in presence of nicotinamide (Lumelsky, Blondel et al. 2001). ESC-IPCs expressed insulin-1 and insulin-2 (murine isoforms) as detected by immunohistochemistry and PCR, and secreted insulin after glucose challenge (Lumelsky, Blondel et al. 2001). However, two years later, ESC-IPCs produced by this method became controversial, as it was reported that they were incapable of *de novo* insulin synthesis, and instead acquired insulin from the culture medium (Rajagopal, Anderson et al. 2003). This controversy currently is still unresolved, as some groups suggest that the insulin released by the ESC-IPCs is a mixture of insulin produced *de novo,* as well as insulin uptake from the medium (Paek, Morgan et al. 2005), and other groups state that the insulin expression by ESC-IPCs is an artifact due to apoptotic or necrotic cells (Hansson, Tonning et al. 2004).

To settle this controversy, the detection of C-peptide, a by-product of endogenous insulin synthesis, will be needed in order to prove that ESC-IPCs produce insulin *de novo*. ESC-IPCs produced with the Lumelsky protocol have been shown to express C-peptide, but they failed to alleviate diabetes in mice, due to teratoma formation (indicating that not all of the ESCs were completely differentiated) (Fujikawa, Oh et al. 2005). Hori et al. provided an alternative methodology, using the selection of *nestin*$^{+}$ cells, a marker for mitotically active cells. Nestin is a neuronal marker, and it is not surprising that the Lumelsky and the Hori protocols would also generate neuronal cells when differentiating ES cells into IPCs (Lumelsky, Blondel et al. 2001; Hori, Rulifson et al. 2002). Moreover, Hori et al. added LY294002, an inhibitor of phosphoinositide 3-kinase, an essential intracellular signaling regulator, to the culture media at the IPC induction step (Hori, Rulifson et al. 2002). ESC-IPCs produced via the Hori protocol were smaller, with a reduced cytoplasmic volume compared to pancreatic β cells, probably due to the ability of LY294002 to reduce cell size (Vanhaesebroeck, Leevers et al. 2001). Compared to the Lumelsky protocol, IPCs produced by the Hori protocol were able to release more insulin and rescue glycemic blood levels after 3 weeks of transplantation in diabetic mice (Hori, Rulifson et al. 2002). However, these results could not been reproduced by other authors (Boyd, Wu et al. 2008).

Blyszczuk et al. described a third ESC-IPC differentiation protocol (Blyszczuk, Asbrand et al. 2004). This protocol consisted of three steps: 1) formation of EBs, 2) spontaneous differentiation of EBs into cells of ectodermal, mesodermal and endodermal lineages by transferring EBs into gelatin-coated plates, and 3) induction of differentiation into IPCs by culturing the gelatin-plated EB cell suspension with culture media containing progesterone, laminin, putrescine, selenium, nicotinamide, insulin, transferrin and B27 (Blyszczuk, Asbrand et al. 2004; Schroeder, Kania et al. 2006; Schroeder, Rolletschek et al. 2006). ESC-IPCs generated by the Blyszczuk protocol released insulin *in vitro* after glucose challenge, but they did not succeed in rescuing diabetic mice *in vivo*. The generation of ESC-IPC via the activation of differentiation genes such as *Pax4* was also studied. When *Pax4*-transduced ESCs differentiated into IPCs and transplanted to diabetic mice, blood glucose levels were reduced for at least 4 weeks. Similar reduced blood glucose levels were detected in diabetic mice transplanted with IPCs transfected with *Pax4* by nucleofection (Lin, Kao et al. 2007). However, mice treated either with unmodified or *Pax4*-modified ESC-IPCs developed teratomas (Blyszczuk, Asbrand et al. 2004). Exhaustive microarray studies have compared gene expression in ESC-IPC derived from wild type and *Pax4*$^{+}$ ESC at different stages of *in vitro* differentiation in order to attempt understand the mechanisms and factors required to produce fully functional ESC-IPC. The authors conclude that murine ESC-derived pancreatic cells are unable to complete pancreatic differentiation *in vitro*, as they appear to be blocked at the embryonic/fetal stage of development, as deduced by their gene expression profiles (Rolletschek, Schroeder et al. 2010). To date, murine ESC-IPCs are only able to acquire full functional β cell characteristics *in vivo*, but not *in vitro*, so the challenge to identify the missing factors to induce complete maturation of ESC-IPC *in vitro* remains.

Solving the ESC-IPC differentiation problem is complicated, as individual ESC lines do not behave similarly before and after differentiation, which also makes direct cross-comparison of the published ESC-IPC differentiation protocols difficult (Osafune, Caron et al. 2008). The three ESC-IPC differentiation protocols described above were compared using three different ESC cell lines, with the ES122 ESC line providing the best results (Boyd, Wu et al.

2008). When the ES122 ESC line was differentiated using the Lumelsky, Hori or Blyszczuk protocols, the Blyszczuk protocol proved to be superior: higher insulin-1 and insulin-2 gene and protein expression, greater increase in insulin secretion after glucose challenge *in vitro* and longer duration of normoglycemic blood level in diabetic mice after transplantation were achieved. However, consistent with previous reports, IPCs formed teratomas after three weeks of transplantation (Boyd, Wu et al. 2008). Therefore, in order for ESC-IPCs to be used in the clinic, it is clear that additional measures must included in the ESC-IPC protocols before transplantation, such as: the depletion of undifferentiated cells, using markers like stage-specific embryonic antigen 1 (SSEA-1) in order to avoid teratoma formation, methods to efficiently scale-up cell numbers before transplantation in order to reach similar blood glycemia levels as with healthy β cells, and/or the identification and addition of factors that can induce ESC-IPC to more mature, functional status when cultured *in vitro*.

More differentiation protocols to generate ESC-IPCs from murine ESCs have been described, but all of the known assays to test function of ESC-IPC have not been performed (**Table 1**). A comparative analysis in which the murine ESC D3 line was differentiated through the formation of EBs in the presence of retinoic acid showed how the subsequent exposure to sodium butyrate produced IPCs that expressed insulin-1 and insulin-2. However, C-peptide was not expressed and *in vitro* glucose response assays or transplantation in diabetic mice were not performed (McKiernan, O'Driscoll et al. 2007). Another approach, using a three-dimensional (3D) system with a Type I rat tail collagen solution, generated IPCs from the murine ESC D3 line that secreted more insulin after *in vitro* glucose challenge than IPCs generated in a two-dimensional (2D) system (Wang and Ye 2009); however, no *in vivo* functional analysis of these IPCs was performed. Comparing the 3D system with the differentiation protocols described by Blyszczuk et al., Lumelsky et al. or Hori et al. using the same cell line would be interesting. In another protocol that omitted EB formation, ESC-IPCs were generated by following a four step protocol: 1) treatment of ES cells with all-*trans*-retinoic acid (ATRA) and fibroblast growth factor (bFGF), 2) withdrawal of ATRA, 3) induction of formation of cell cluster by growth in presence of N2 and B27 supplements and 4) culture of clusters in dibutyryl cAMP and nicotinamide (Kim, Hoffman et al. 2010). These ESC-IPCs expressed insulin and responded to glucose challenge, but transplantation into diabetic mice was not performed, so the functionality of these cells *in vivo* is unknown. As transgenesis of ESCs with *Pax4* seemed to influence ESC-IPC differentiation, other groups have attempted to control the expression of pancreatic genes during ESC-IPC differentiation. For instance, regulation of *Pdx1* expression via the "Tet-off" system generated IPCs that increased *insulin-2* and *Ngn3* expression and secreted more insulin after glucose challenge *in vitro* (Miyazaki, Yamato et al. 2004). The co-culture of ESCs with other cell types has also successfully generated IPCs that express insulin and C-peptide, and respond to glucose. Banerjee et al. used 3 co-culture steps: 1) induction toward endoderm-like cells by co-culturing with primary hepatocytes, 2) inhibition of Sonic hedgehog by culturing in presence of KAAD-cyclopamine on Matrigel and retinoid induction, and 3) maturation to islet cells by co-culture with endothelial cells in medium containing nicotinamide, insulin, selenium, transferring and B27 (Banerjee, Sharma et al.). These studies are all examples of the diverse approaches that have been explored to produce ESC-IPCs; however, none of the ESC-IPCs generated by these protocols have shown regulation of blood glucose levels after transplantation, as has been shown by Lumelsky et al., Hori et al. and Blyszczuk et al.

For human ESCs, differentiation into IPCs through monolayers, without EB formation, is the methodology most commonly followed. The protocol by D'Amour *et al.*, in which the *in vivo* differentiation steps from the definitive endoderm to endocrine pancreatic islets are mimicked *in vitro,* is currently considered the reference protocol for differentiating human ESC to IPC (D'Amour, Bang et al. 2006; Kroon, Martinson et al. 2008). Endodermal intermediates can be identified at each step: 1) definitive endoderm markers (*Sox17, FoxA2* and *Cxcr4*) are detected after the addition of activin A and Wnt3a in a medium with low serum concentration, 2) primitive gut tube markers (*Hnf1b* and *Hnf4a*) are induced by addition of FGF1- and KAAD-cyclopamine , 3) posterior foregut markers (*Pdx1, Hnf6* or *Sox9*) are observed by induction with ATRA, KAAD-cyclopamine, FGF10 and B27, 4) pancreatic endoderm and endocrine precursor gene and protein expression (*Nkx6-1, Ngn3, Pax4* or *Nkx2-2*) can be detected by induction with exendin-4, and 5) hormone-expressing endocrine cell markers (*insulin, glucagon, somatostatin* or *poly-peptide Y*) are induced by exposure of cells to IGF1 and HGF. Human ESC-IPCs generated via this protocol release C-peptide at levels similar to β cells from islets in response to multiple secretory stimuli, but unfortunately, not to glucose (D'Amour, Bang et al. 2006). Interestingly, cells that co-express insulin and glucagon are observed, indicating that IPCs generated by the D'Amour protocol may still be immature β cell progenitors. A slight modification of the D'Amour protocol generated pancreatic endodermal cells from human ESCs, which protected diabetic immunocompromised SCID-Bg mice from hyperglycemia after transplant (Kroon, Martinson et al. 2008).

Further modifications to the D'Amour protocol have shown some improvements in IPC properties. For example, human ESC-IPC that secrete insulin and respond to glucose were generated by combining activin A and ATRA in a chemically defined medium, and other maturation factors, such as bFGF and nicotinamide in DMEM/F12. ESC-IPCs differentiated by this system were able to rescue 30% of diabetic *nu/nu* mice from hyperglycemia for at least 6 weeks, with no teratoma formation observed for three months post-transplantation (Jiang, Shi et al. 2007). Other modifications, such as increasing the time of suspension cultures and different growth factor combinations have succeeded in producing ESC-IPCs. Those suspension cultures contained ductal, exocrine and endocrine-like cells and secreted insulin in response to glucose challenge, but their therapeutic potential for diabetes was not tested *in vivo* (Jiang, Au et al. 2007).

Human ESC-IPCs have been also generated through the formation of EBs. Human EBs in a 3D matrix were induced to differentiate into definitive endoderm by the presence of activin A and Bmp4, and then into IPCs via the addition of growth factors such as FGF18, EGF, TGF-α, IGF-1, IGF-1 and VEGF. In contrast with other reports, these ESC-IPCs expressed only insulin and no other pancreatic hormones; however, they did not rescue diabetic mice and formed teratomas instead. When *Pdx1* gene expression was quantified among six human ESC lines following this protocol, different levels of expression were detected (Phillips, Hentze et al. 2007). This result is not surprising, since distinct cell behaviors and differentiation potentials have been observed amongst independent stem cell lines (Osafune, Caron et al. 2008).

Therefore, for human and murine ESC-IPC differentiation, no "standard" protocol currently exists, as the results appear to be dependent on the ESC line utilized. In addition, there is no consensus on the composition of the differentiation culture mediums to guide cells from definitive endoderm to the IPC fate. However, some compounds appear to be key factors for the success of ESC-IPC differentiation. Activin A, a member of the transforming growth factor-beta (TGF-β) family, is involved in cellular proliferation and differentiation, and seems to be essential at the first steps of differentiation of human ESC into definitive endodermal cells (D'Amour, Bang et al. 2006; Kroon, Martinson et al. 2008). Nicotinamide, the amide of vitamin B3, is a well-known inducer of endocrine differentiation (Otonkoski, Beattie et al. 1993), and has been used in the differentiation of human and murine ESCs into IPCs (Jiang, Shi et al. 2007; Boyd, Wu et al. 2008). Epidermal Growth Factor (EGF) and Basic Fibroblast Growth Factor (bFGF) have been also applied in human and murine ESC-IPC differentiation, as both factors induce cell proliferation and differentiation (Lumelsky, Blondel et al. 2001; Jiang, Au et al. 2007). However, EGF, but not bFGF, needs to be removed from the cultures during the last stages of the differentiation protocols in order to allow the formation of islet-like cell aggregates (Cras-Meneur, Elghazi et al. 2001; Hardikar, Marcus-Samuels et al. 2003). Hepatocyte Growth Factor (HGF) is an inducer of cell proliferation that is secreted by mesenchymal cells, and has been used for human ESC-IPC differentiation (Otonkoski, Cirulli et al. 1996; D'Amour, Bang et al. 2006; Phillips, Hentze et al. 2007) as well as murine fetal liver differentiation into IPCs (Feng, Du et al. 2005). Exendin-4 stimulates β cell proliferation (Xu, Stoffers et al. 1999) and it has been used for murine and human ESC-IPC differentiation (Tang, Cao et al. 2004; Wu, Liu et al. 2007; Gabr, Sobh et al. 2008; Gao, Wu et al. 2008; Li, Lam et al.). A combination of insulin, transferrin, selenium and fibronectin (ITSFn) has been a common cocktail in murine ESC-IPC differentiation, although the presence of insulin in the medium brought some controversy about the endogenous insulin production of IPCs (Lumelsky, Blondel et al. 2001; Hori, Rulifson et al. 2002; Blyszczuk, Asbrand et al. 2004; Hansson, Tonning et al. 2004). The concentration of glucose in the culture media can also influence ESC-IPC differentiation and their properties. Low glucose concentrations (5mM) increase the content of insulin in islet-like clusters, whereas higher concentrations (20-30 mM) induce their replication (Bonner-Weir, Deery et al. 1989; Guillemain, Filhoulaud et al. 2007). Importantly, the presence or absence of serum has a clear effect on ESC-IPC differentiation. It is widely accepted by all cell culture professionals that lot-to-lot variation of serum sources can affect the success of *in vitro* cell culture and assays. The most referenced protocols for murine or human ESC-IPC use serum-free medium, as they claim serum inhibits differentiation; however, the specific component in the serum has not been identified (Blyszczuk, Asbrand et al. 2004; Jiang, Au et al. 2007; Jiang, Shi et al. 2007). The inhibitory role of serum is somewhat controversial, as other reports have described how reduced serum concentrations (0-10%) are permissive for murine ESC-IPC differentiation (Vincent and Odorico 2009), yet other authors produced

ESC-IPC successfully with relatively high 15% serum concentrations (Ibii, Shimada et al. 2007). Inherent variability in the behavior of individual ESC lines, in conjunction with these responses in the absence or presence of serum, could explain these results. Studies that identify the molecules released by developing pancreas could help to determine the main factors needed in ESC-IPC differentiation *in vitro* (Vaca, Martin et al. 2006). These studies could also be applied in the development of synthetic molecules, such as indolactam V, IDE1 or IDE2, for easier production and control of murine and human ESC-IPC differentiation (Borowiak, Maehr et al. 2009; Chen, Borowiak et al. 2009).

In summary, despite the progress made to date, investigation must continue to optimize ESC-IPC differentiation before their clinical use is possible. ESC-IPC cultures contain heterogeneous cell populations, and have not been well-identified. Moreover, the ESC-IPCs do not always respond to glucose challenge and do not release insulin, limiting their use as a pancreatic β cell replacement in TID. Identification of novel factors to induce maturation of ESC-IPC phenotypes may help to achieve full functional status. However, perhaps a better strategy would be to identify and transplant the immature pancreatic progenitor cells within the ESC-IPC cultures, as they may mature and respond more appropriately *in vivo*.

3.4. Identifying markers of endoderm and pancreatic progenitor cells in ESC-IPC cultures

ESC-IPCs to date have not recapitulated pancreatic mature β cell phenotypes. Pancreatic progenitors that are generated within the heterogeneous ESC-IPCs may be suitable for cellular replacement therapy in TID. The pancreatic progenitors may not self-renew as stem cells do, but could differentiate into endocrine cells after transplantation, including β cells. The identification of specific cell surface markers on pancreatic progenitors would allow for their isolation and for the transplantation of a homogenous population of ESC-derived pancreatic progenitors. We will discuss some current advances in the identification of pancreatic progenitors *in vivo* that could be applied to the detection and isolation of ESC-derived pancreatic progenitors from ESC-IPC cultures.

3.4.1. Definitive endoderm progenitors

In mice, putative definitive endodermal cells that co-express E-cadherin and Decay Accelerating Factor (DAF1/CD55) cell surface markers also express *Pdx1* (Shiraki, Harada et al. 2010). Discoidin domain receptor tyrosine kinase 1 (DDR1) and delta/notch-like EGF related receptor (DNER) have been also indicated as possible murine pancreatic progenitor surface markers with bioinformatics studies confirmed by immunohistochemistry (Hald, Galbo et al. 2011). Murine ESCs bearing the GFP reporter gene and human IL2Rα (CD25) marker genes in the *goosecoid* (GSc) and *Soc17* loci have allowed for the identification of seven surface markers that are differentially expressed between definitive and visceral endoderm cells: Amn (Amnionless), Sdc4 (Syndecan-4), Pthr1 (Parathyroid hormone receptor 1), Tmprss2 (Transmembrane protease, serine 2), Tm4sf2 (Transmembrane 4 superfamily 2), Cxcr4 and Gpc1 (Glypican 1). Cxcr4, in combination with E-cadherin, proved to be appropriate extracellular markers for the identification and isolation of definitive endoderm cells (E-cadherin^{+} Cxcr4^{+}) from unmanipulated ES-derived cells (Yasunaga, Tada et al. 2005). Thus, Cxcr4 permits the isolation of definitive endoderm cells from human ES cells after 5 days of differentiation to nearly 100% purity, eliminating undifferentiated ESCs (D'Amour, Agulnick et al. 2005). However, Cxcr4 expression decreases during development, making the isolation of late definitive endoderm cells difficult. The combination of E-cadherin with CD55 has circumvented this problem by identifying early and late definitive endoderm cells in the embryo, and in ESC-derived cell cultures where GFP is expressed under the promoter of *Pdx1* (Shiraki, Harada et al. 2010). Our group has also observed the presence of E-cadherin^{+} CD55^{+} cells in our ESC-IPC cultures (**Figure 4B**). *Pdx1*$^{+}$Cxcr4^{+} ESC-derived cells spontaneously undergo differentiation into IPCs *in vivo*, and lead to a sustained correction of hyperglycemia in diabetic mice (Raikwar and Zavazava 2011).

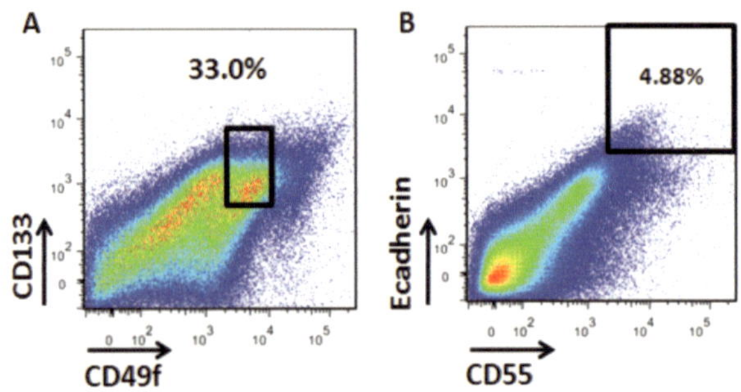

Figure 4. *Identification of putative pancreatic progenitor from murine ESC-IPC cultures.* ESC-IPCs were stained for markers of pancreatic progenitors found in the mouse embryo. A) CD133^{+}CD49f$^{low/+}$ cells. B) E-cadherin^{+}CD55^{+} cells. The differentiation potential and properties of these in vitro-derived putative pancreatic progenitors requires further study.

3.4.2. Pancreatic progenitors

First isolated using *Ngn3*-fluorescent reporter mice (Gu, Wells et al. 2004; Mellitzer, Martin et al. 2004), *Ngn3*$^{+}$ cells have been suggested as possible pancreatic progenitors. In later studies, CD133 (prominin 1) was described as an extracellular marker that identified cells which expressed *Ngn3* in fetal and adult pancreas (Oshima, Suzuki et al. 2007; Sugiyama, Rodriguez et al. 2007). Mouse ductal cells with the phenotype CD133^{+}CD34^{-}CD45^{-}Ter119^{-} CD49f$^{low/+}$ were isolated from fetal and adult murine tissues by flow cytometry. CD133^{+}CD49f$^{low/+}$ cells expressed *Ngn3*, increasing their isolation purity 1.4 fold when co-stained for CD24. Moreover, CD133^{+}CD49f$^{low/+}$ cells expressed *insulin-1, glucagon, somatostatin* and *pancreatic polypeptide* after culturing them with mitomycin C-treated mouse embryonic fibroblast (MEFs) for 2 days (Sugiyama, Rodriguez et al. 2007). Pancreatic progenitors isolated from neonatal, but not from adult, pancreases were able to differentiate into endocrine cells when cultured *in vitro* with HGF and EGF (Oshima, Suzuki et al. 2007). A newer study confirmed CD133 as well as platelet-derived growth factor receptor β (PDFGRβ) as markers of pancreatic progenitors in murine fetal pancreas (Hori, Fukumoto et al. 2008). CD133$^+$ PDFGRβ $^-$ cells were CD49f$^{low/+}$ and expressed *Ngn3* and *Pdx1*. *In vitro* co-culture of CD133$^+$ PDFGRβ $^-$ cells with MEFs or their *in vivo* transplantation induced the formation of IPCs that expressed C-peptide in 7 days. Moreover, serial transplantation of these CD133$^+$ PDFGRβ $^-$ cells demonstrated self-renewal properties and suggested they might be true pancreatic stem cells (Hori, Fukumoto et al. 2008). Inclusion of CD24 as a positive marker with CD133 and CD49f during cell isolation increases the yield of *Ngn3*$^+$ cells after sorting from mouse embryos (Sugiyama, Rodriguez et al. 2007).

Murine *Ngn3*-GFP ESC lines have been differentiated and *Ngn3*$^+$ cells were detected and isolated from EBs. *Ngn3*$^+$ cells were then sorted and differentiated *in vitro* into cells that expressed *insulin, glucagon* and *Pdx1*, among other pancreatic markers (Ku, Chai et al. 2007). Inducible *Ngn*3 expression in ESCs enhances expression of glucagon, somatostatin and insulin when they are differentiated into endocrine lineages, which reinforces the idea that *Ngn3* is an intermediate gene during IPCs differentiation (Serafimidis, Rakatzi et al. 2008). However, the description of non-transgenic *Ngn3*-expressing-pancreatic progenitor cells identified by cell surface markers in ESC-differentiation cultures has not been reported in the primary literature. Our group has analyzed the percentage of CD133$^+$CD49f$^{low/+}$ cells during ESC-IPC differentiation following the Blyszczuk protocol, and we have detected an increase in the number of CD133$^+$CD49f$^{low/+}$ cells in our cultures (**Figure 4A**). CD24 has been cited as a marker of murine pancreatic progenitors, and CD24$^+$ cells isolated from human ESC-IPC express *Pdx1,* and express insulin after 1 week *in vitro* (Jiang, Sui et al. 2011). Studies *in vivo* will confirm the differentiation potential of CD24$^+$ cells in ESC-IPC cultures. The CD142 protein is expressed in the human fetal pancreatic epithelium at 8 weeks of gestation, and has been implicated in human ESC-IPC differentiation. Isolation of CD142$^+$ cells allowed for the enrichment of pancreatic endoderm cells, and after transplantation into SCID/Bg mice, CD142$^+$ cells differentiated to all pancreatic cell lineages, including IPCs that responded to glucose stimulation *in vivo* and did not form teratomas (Kelly, Chan et al. 2011). However, these recipients were not diabetic, so future studies are required to demonstrate if they can rescue hyperglycemia in diabetic mice.

The establishment of intermediate lineage-restricted progenitor cell lines (similar to the pancreatic progenitor cells) that generate homogeneous IPCs could be useful for scalable IPC production. Several clones were isolated from differentiation protocols into IPCs with the E-RoSH cell line (an endothelial lineage-restricted clonal murine ES cell derived line). The eight clones that were isolated could be frozen and thawed for months, and when cultured, they displayed properties of pancreatic β cells, such as expression of *insulin-1, insulin-2, Pdx1, Nkx2.2, Nkx6.1, Isl1, and Foxa2,* no expression of *Ngn3*, and expression of C-peptide. Moreover, the clones were able to rescue diabetic mice and did not form teratomas, demonstrating the absence of undifferentiated ESC. However, these cells continued proliferating after transplantation and showed an abnormal karyotype, suggesting an insulinoma phenotype, that may be responsible for the hyperinsulinemia and hypoglycemia observed in the animals (Li, Luo et al. 2009).

In summary, isolation and characterization of pancreatic progenitors from embryonic development and ESC-IPCs could provide another possible β cell replacement source for the treatment of diabetes. These multipotent cells are not teratoma-forming, and can differentiate into IPCs and other hormone expressing cells, and have been shown to reverse hyperglycemic blood levels after transplantation. However, the isolation of pure or enriched pancreatic progenitors using cell-specific surface markers from ESC-IPCs cell differentiation cultures that are able to cure diabetic mice still has not been demonstrated. More studies to assess the efficiency of human ESC-IPC differentiation and optimization of sorting methods to remove any undifferentiated teratoma-forming cells are necessary before clinical translation. Nevertheless, even if fully functional, teratoma-free ESC-IPCs are derived, they must circumvent another possible barrier after transplantation: the host immune system (see Section 3.6). For this reason, induced pluripotent stem cells have been proposed as an autologous alternative to ESCs.

3.5. Differentiation of induced pluripotent stem cells into insulin-producing cells

Induced pluripotent stem cells (iPSCs) are reprogrammed somatic cells that behave like ESCs and can be re-differentiated into all three germ layers and potentially, any terminally differentiated cell type (Takahashi and Yamanaka 2006). The generation of iPSCs was firstly achieved by the viral delivery of reprogramming factors (Takahashi and Yamanaka 2006) in murine cells, and later by non-viral methods (Yu, Hu et al. 2009). Human iPSCs have also been generated (Yu, Hu et al. 2009). iPSC are envisioned as the future of "personalized" medicine since they could be used to generate autologous therapies that will not require pharmacologic immune suppression after transplantation (Okita, Ichisaka et al. 2007). However, the immunogenicity of syngeneic iPSC, which was unexpected by the stem cell biology field, demonstrated that this is not the case (Zhao, Zhang et al. 2011). Moreover, autologous iPSC generated from patients with genetic diseases likely will retain the propensity to develop disease following re-differentiation, unless they are modified (Raya, Rodriguez-Piza et al. 2009). The use of allogeneic iPSC could alleviate this possibility, but would have the disadvantage of possible immune rejection. iPSCs differ from ESCs in gene expression profiles (Chin, Mason et al. 2009), persistence of donor-cell gene expression (Marchetto, Yeo et al. 2009; Ghosh, Wilson et al. 2010), differentiation abilities (Feng, Lu et al. 2010; Hu, Weick et al. 2010) and genetic stability (Mayshar, Ben-David et al. 2010; Laurent, Ulitsky et al. 2011).

Currently, there is no standard iPSC to IPC differentiation protocol, but scientists have followed strategies similar to ESC to IPC differentiation (**Table 3**). Murine skin fibroblasts reprogrammed into iPSCs were differentiated into IPCs that were glucose responsive *in vitro* and normalized hyperglycemia in syngeneic mice with Type I and Type II diabetes. Teratoma formation was prevented by sorting out SSEA1$^+$ IPCs before transplantation, and no immune rejection was detected (Alipio, Liao et al. 2010). Human iPSC to IPC differentiation has been performed using a four-stage protocol: 1) endoderm induction by activin A and wortmannin, 2) pancreatic differentiation with retinoic acid, Noggin and FGF7, 3) expansion of pancreatic endoderm cells with EGF and 4) maturation of IPCs with nicotinamide, bFGF, exendin-4 and BMP4 (Zhang, Jiang et al. 2009), and another method following a human ESC-IPC protocol (Maehr, Chen et al. 2009; Thatava, Nelson et al. 2010). These IPCs expressed and released C-peptide after glucose challenge *in vitro*. Differentiation of distinct human iPSC lines also produced IPC that expressed C-peptide and insulin, but at lower levels than ESC-IPCs (Zhang, Jiang et al. 2009). Interestingly, iPSC-IPC generated from TID patients also appear to be responsive to glucose challenge *in vitro* (Maehr, Chen et al. 2009). iPSC generated from human β-cells (BiPSCs) appear to be predisposed to re-differentiation into IPCs, as shown by the epigenetics of *Pdx1* and *insulin* promoters. BiPSC express more insulin and C-peptide than ESC-IPCs after transplantation into SCID mice (Bar-Nur, Russ et al. 2011; Russ, Sintov et al. 2011). Human iPSC-IPCs have not yet been transplanted into diabetic humanized mouse models, so their therapeutic potential to normalize blood glucose levels and their safety *in vivo* still requires further investigation.

Source	Insulin mRNA	c-peptide protein expression	*In vitro* glucose response	Rescue of diabetic mice	Differentiation protocol reference
Murine skin fibroblast	Yes	Not done	Yes	Yes	(Alipio, Liao et al. 2010)
Human fibroblast	Yes	Yes	Not done	Not done	(Zhang, Jiang et al. 2009)
Skin human TID adult and healthy neonatal fibroblast	Yes	Yes	Yes	Not done	(Maehr, Chen et al. 2009; Thatava, Nelson et al. 2010)

Table 3. iPS to IPC differentiation protocols

3.6. Addressing the immunogenicity of ESC-IPCs and iPSC-IPCs

Inflammation, due to local tissue damage, is a regular occurrence during transplantation of cells or organs, even in a syngeneic setting (Turvey, Gonzalez-Nicolini et al. 2000; Carvalho-Gaspar, Billing et al. 2005). For instance, cellular infiltrates are evident in rat islet β cell allografts within one week post-transplant, and are completely destroyed within 2 weeks. Depletion of major histocompatibility complex class II (MHC II)-positive islet cells (which presumably are antigen-presenting cells) delays β cell rejection up to 5 weeks, while re-aggregation of islet β cells after islet dissociation and β cell purification promotes allograft survival up to 20 weeks (Pipeleers, Pipeleers-Marichal et al. 1991). Embryonic tissue has not been considered to be highly immunogenic, mainly based on the "immune privileged" status of the fetus during gestation, which protects it from the maternal immune system. However, this immune privileged status is not generally observed outside the womb. For example, transplanted human β cells from fetal pancreas, which have a greater proliferative capacity than adult tissue (Hayek and Beattie 1997; Castaing, Peault et al. 2001), normalize blood glucose levels in diabetic immunoincompetent rodents (Hullett, Falany et al. 1987; Tuch, Osgerby et al. 1988; Tuch and Monk 1991; Castaing, Peault et al. 2001), but are rejected when transplanted into humanized SCID mice (immune reconstituted with human fetal liver and thymus tissue) (Rouleau, Namikawa et al. 1996). Human pancreas obtained from first trimester fetus are less immunogenic that pancreas from the second trimester of gestation, as indicated by cellular infiltrates that contain high levels of host $CD45^+$ cells. This is consistent with an upregulation of T cell activating molecules, such as MHC II, the chemokine ligand 19 (CCL19), complement component 3 (C3) and tumour necrosis factor superfamily 10 (TNFSF10, also known as TNF-related apoptosis-inducing ligand, TRAIL), in second trimester human fetal pancreas compared to first trimester tissue (Brands, Colvin et al. 2008).

ESCs and iPSCs were also considered to be non-immunogenic, until recently. Murine ESCs do not express MHC I or MHC II, but increase MHC I expression when they differentiate spontaneously (Wu, Boyd et al. 2008). Despite of the lack of MHC I expression, ESCs are not deleted by natural killer (NK) cells (Koch, Geraldes et al. 2008). Interestingly, MHC I-positive murine ESCs are not recognized by cytotoxic $CD8^+$ T cells, even when antigen presenting cells (APCs) are used to prime T cells, suggesting that ES cells have some immune privilege. Nevertheless, this immune privilege is fragile and the addition of $CD4^+$ helper T cells can induce ESC rejection *in vivo* (Wu, Boyd et al. 2008). In immunocompetent mice, ESC allografts contain infiltrates of $CD11b^+$ macrophages, $CD4^+$ and $CD8^+$ T cells as early as 10 days post-transplantation (Wu, Boyd et al. 2008). In line with this, allogeneic EBs are not rejected if the CD4 and CD8 co-receptors are blocked, suggesting that ESC-derived tissues could be tolerated in allogeneic host (Lui, Boyd et al. 2010). In the absence of blocking, rejection of allogeneic EBs is mediated by $CD8^+$ T cells and active $F4/80^+$ $MHC\ II^+$ mannose receptor-negative macrophages. IL-10, a cytokine that downregulates immune responses, is expressed in syngeneic and allogeneic EBs grafts that are not rejected (Lui, Boyd et al. 2010). This tolerance is completely eliminated when host $CD4^+$ $FoxP3^+$ regulatory T cells (T_{reg}) are ablated. T_{regs} seem to protect EBs by keeping $F4/80^+$ macrophages in a low activation state by preventing their upregulation of MHC II, as well as by suppressing cytotoxic $CD8^+$ T cell responses by downregulating their expression of granzyme B (Lui, Boyd et al. 2010). It remains to be seen whether or not these mechanisms will apply universally to all ESC-derived tissues.

To date, there have been few descriptions of the immunogenicity of ESC-IPCs, but the existing data indicate that both innate and adaptive arms of the host immune system could be activated after ESC-IPC transplantation. ESC-IPCs can normalize blood glucose levels of diabetic immune compromised mice short-term, but when transplanted into immunocompetent hosts, their functionality is impaired, even under syngeneic conditions (Wu, Boyd et al. 2008). One explanation for the immune rejection of ESC-IPCs is that they express higher levels of MHC I than ES cells, and express higher levels of both MHC I and MHC II after exposure with IFNγ *in vitro*. Incidentally, IFNγ is up-regulated within both syngeneic and allogeneic ESC-IPC grafts three days after transplantation (Boyd and Wood 2009). However, the level of cellular infiltration differs between syngeneic and allogeneic ESC-IPC grafts. For example, $Gr1^+$ leukocytes can be observed in allogeneic, but not syngeneic, ESC-IPC grafts, within the first 24 hours post-transplantation. $CD11b^+$ macrophages can be detected in both syngeneic and allogeneic grafts by three days after transplantation, indicating a general response to local injury (Boyd and Wood 2010). In addition, early inflammatory molecules that activate macrophages and granulocytes, such as IL-6, Gro-β (CXCL2 or macrophage inflammatory protein 2), Lix (CXCL5 or epithelial-derived neutrophil-activating peptide 78), MIP-1α (CCL3 or macrophage inflammatory protein 1-alpha) and MIP-1β (CCL4 or macrophage inflammatory protein 1-beta, IP-10 (Interferon gamma-induced protein 10 or CXCL10) and Mig (monokine induced by gamma interferon or CXCL9), are induced within both syngeneic and allogeneic ESC-IPC grafts within three days post-transplantation. Of these cytokines, IP-10, and Mig are associated with acute graft rejection (Burns, Wang et al. 2005). The adaptive immune system, as expected, is slower to respond, and infiltrates of reactive $CD8^+$ T cells are observed in allogeneic ESC-IPCs 10 days post-transplantation. In all cases, the immune response to allogeneic ESC-IPC observed was lower than the response to transplanted allogeneic pancreatic islets (Boyd and Wood 2010). These studies suggest that IPCs are suitable for transplantation, but some immune response by macrophages and T cells should be expected, so it is likely that immunosuppressive drugs to prevent graft rejection will have to be administered with ESC-IPC grafts.

Strategies to circumvent the immune system barrier to ESC-IPCs will be needed if they will be used for the treatment of diabetic patients. For instance, a short term immunosuppression approach blocking cytotoxic T-lymphocyte-associated antigen 4 (CTLA-4), CD40 ligand (CD40L) or lymphocyte function-associated antigen 1(LFA-1) for 6 days, has shown to allow for the engraftment of murine and human ESCs (Pearl, Lee et al. 2011). Since CTLA4Ig treatment has previously induced long-term survival of xenogeneic pancreatic islet grafts (Lenschow, Zeng et al. 1992; Eventov-Friedman, Tchorsh et al. 2006), it is possible that similar pre-conditioning treatments in recipients will allow for the acceptance of ESC-IPC grafts. An alternative strategy is the co-culture of ESC-IPC with bone marrow-derived mesenchymal stem cells, since co-culture of β cells with bone marrow-derived mesenchymal stem cells induces the expression of protective molecules such as IL6 (in a paradoxically anti-inflammatory role) and TGFβ1, an immunosuppressive cytokine, and anti-apoptotic genes like *Mapkapk2, Tnip1* or *Bcl3* (Karaoz, Genc et al. 2010). Another interesting strategy to prevent immune rejection of pancreatic progenitors is their encapsulation in alginate capsules with pores that allow for the passage of nutrients and insulin, but not immune cells (Tuch, Hughes et al. 2011). The use of autologous iPSC, instead of ESCs, was thought to avoid these immune rejection issues, but new evidence has demonstrated that syngeneic iPS-derived tissues can in fact, be rejected, as shown by T cell infiltration in the grafts (Zhao, Zhang et al. 2011). This rejection appears to involve minor histocompatibility antigens. Candidate genes, such as *Hormad1* (Horma Domain-Containing 1) or *Zg16* (zymogen granule protein 16), were shown to be directly involved in the activation of antigen-specific T cells, as shown by IFN-γ release. Based on this evidence, it is clear that the potential of immune rejection of both ESC- and iPSC-derived tissues will be an obstacle to be overcome before they can be applied in the clinic. Moreover, a detailed understanding of the immunogenicity profiles of ESC- and iPSC-derived tissues of any type (i.e. not only IPCs) could provide important information about the type of potential immune response(s) to expect and prevent before transplantation and helping to identify alternative strategies to facilitate their acceptance.

3.7. Hematopoietic stem cell transplantation to induce immune tolerance for type I diabetes

The autoimmune nature of TID provides two main targets in which hematopoietic stem cell transplantation (HSCT) could be used to ameliorate disease: the replacement of autoimmune T cells to prevent the onset of TID, and the induction of immunological tolerance to islet replacements via a previous HSCT or HSC co-transplantation. In both cases, induction of immunological tolerance to donor antigens is required for long-term survival of a transplanted organ. This is more easily achieved with autologous bone marrow transplantation, but can also occur when allogeneic bone marrow donors are used. In allogeneic bone marrow transplantation, induction of central and peripheral tolerance to donor antigens has been accomplished by creating mixed hematopoietic chimerism using non-myeloablative conditioning regimens (Sykes 2007; Sykes 2009). An important component to the induction of this tolerance is the education of donor and host T cells to recognize each other as "self" to avoid graft-versus-host disease (GVHD) and well as host-versus-graft reactions.

HSCT has been used to induce immune tolerance to TID antigens. Gene therapy approaches in which transplantation of syngeneic HSCs that were engineered to express pro-insulin under the MHC-II promoter transferred protection against insulitis and the development of spontaneous autoimmune diabetes (Steptoe, Ritchie et al. 2003; Chan, Clements et al. 2006). Transplant of fully allogeneic purified adult hematopoietic stem cells into lethally irradiated NOD mice (Beilhack, Scheffold et al. 2003) and the induction of mixed allogeneic hematopoietic chimerism using a non-myeloablative conditioning regimen cured diabetes in NOD mice and established clear immunological tolerance to both host and donor MHC as well as to insulin (Nikolic, Takeuchi et al. 2004). Recently, it has been shown that mixed chimerism across MHC mismatches is superior than mixed chimerism amongst MHC matched hematopoietic cells for prevention of insulitis in TID (Racine, Wang et al. 2011). Moreover, mesenchymal stem cells (MSC) co-transplanted with hematopoietic stem cells without islets prevented the onset of TID in allogeneic recipients, and co-transplantation of MSC with allogeneic hematopoietic stem cells and islets have been used to prevent the onset of TID in rodent models (Itakura, Asari et al. 2007; Asari, Itakura et al. 2011).

The results of the first human clinical trial of the use of autologous HSC transplant to treat early-stage TID patients were excellent (Voltarelli, Couri et al. 2007). Importantly, in these studies TID was alleviated using hematopoietic grafts alone (i.e. without co-transplantation of islets). However, patients with late-stage TID can only currently be cured by islet transplantation protocols which require islets from multiple matched donors, exceeding donor availability (Shapiro, Ricordi et al. 2006), or other insulin producing cell sources (such as ESC-IPC and iPS-IPC), which will also require induction of immune tolerance. Combined islet and HSC allotransplantation using an 'Edmonton-like' immunosuppression, (i.e. without ablative conditioning) in which high doses of donor HSCs ($4.3 \pm 1.9 \times 10^6$ HSCs/kg) were transplanted after 5 and 11days of islet transplantation, has not resulted in stable hematopoietic chimerism or graft tolerance after 1 year post-transplantation (Mineo, Ricordi et al. 2008). Whether prior transplantation of HSCs could improve the engraftment of later islet transplantation is not clear, and is not easily tested in the clinic.

The induction of immunological tolerance to ESC-derived tissues is an active and emerging area of investigation. Recent studies have provided proof-of-principle that the induction of immunological tolerance to ESC-derived tissues can be achieved, but the mechanisms of tolerance induction to ESC-derived hematopoietic-progenitors (ES-HP), as well as the ability of ES-HP themselves to induce immunological tolerance across allogeneic barriers, are still not well understood (reviewed in (Thompson and Manilay 2011)). Transplantation of HoxB4-transduced ES-HP resulted in mixed hematopoietic chimersm and the induction of specific transplantation tolerance to allogeneic cardiac grafts (Bonde and Zavazava 2006; Bonde, Chan et al. 2008). It appears that HoxB4-ES-HP-derived T cells are actively "tolerized" to donor antigens in the thymus, and that if not, they can cause lethal GVHD (Kim, Stultz et al. 2011). In line with this, recipients of allogeneic ES-HP lacked evidence of GVHD (Burt, Verda et al. 2004; Bonde and Zavazava 2006; Bonde, Chan et al. 2008). Finally, another study has shown that non-HoxB4 transduced ES-HP can prevent onset of TID in mice (Verda, Kim et al. 2008), but the method of ES-HP production in this study is quite different from the other more recent protocols. Therefore, it appears that ES-HP are similar to bone-marrow derived hematopoietic progenitors, and that they could be used to induce tolerance of allogeneic tissues that are derived from the same ESC line, or that share MHC antigens. The same theory could apply to hematopoietic progenitors that are derived from iPSC (Niwa, Umeda et al. 2009).

4. Conclusion

The replacement of β cells is a promising therapy for diabetic patients, but the process depends on the discovery and detailed study of sources other than cadaveric pancreas. Pancreatic stem cells would be an ideal source for β cell replacement, since they are committed to differentiate into pancreatic cells. However, their cellular marker phenotype, as well as their anatomic location, has not yet been identified. If these questions are resolved, the conditions for their expansion and differentiation will require further optimization, such as emulating the properties of the pancreatic stem cell niche, improving their expansion, and perfecting the composition of culture media to induce their differentiation into endocrine cells. In addition, as pancreatic stem cells will likely be isolated from healthy patients, the immune system barrier to allogeneic transplants will also need to be addressed.

Another alternative to pancreatic stem cells is the differentiation of IPCs from ESC or iPSC, but this first requires the development and acceptance of a standard methodology to generate them. IPCs differentiated by this standard methodology will have to be completely mature and functional (i.e. respond appropriately when blood glucose level are altered, and have absolutely no teratoma-forming potential). The generation of a well-defined homogenous population of transplantable pancreatic progenitors that can be identified with extracellular markers would be an alternative to IPCs. Although they are not completely mature, pancreatic progenitors could perhaps differentiate more readily into mature endocrine cells in response to the signals in their *in vivo* microenvironment. Studies to demonstrate that pancreatic progenitors can be isolated and differentiated from human ESCs, and can normalize blood glucose levels in humanized diabetic animal models still have not been reported. Perhaps a more complete comprehension of normal pancreas development can shed light into the processes that lead to the complete maturation of β-cells *in vivo*, which can be translated to differentiation protocols from ESC and iPSC. iPSC that are reprogrammed from human β cells can be more efficiently differentiated into IPCs than ESCs, and would avoid the ethical issues related to the use of ESCs. However, optimization of non-viral strategies for reprogramming iPS cells would be preferable before clinical translation (Yu, Hu et al. 2009). Finally, independently of the type of cell transplanted (ESC-IPC, iPSC-IPC, or pancreatic progenitors), the immunogenicity of these cells will have to be considered and determined to predict the potential and type of immune response to block before and after transplantation. The data collected from such analyses will aid in the establishment of strategies that can promote immune tolerance of these IPC grafts.

Author details

Jesus Ciriza
Department of Molecular and Cell Biology, School of Natural Sciences, University of California, Merced, Merced, CA, USA

Jennifer O. Manilay*
Department of Molecular and Cell Biology and Quantitative and Systems Biology Graduate Group, School of Natural Sciences, University of California, Merced, Merced, CA, USA

Acknowledgement

This manuscript is supported by funding from the University of California and the California Institute for Regenerative Medicine (RN1-00554-1).

5. References

Ahlgren, U., J. Jonsson, et al. (1996). "The morphogenesis of the pancreatic mesenchyme is uncoupled from that of the pancreatic epithelium in IPF1/PDX1-deficient mice." *Development* 122(5): 1409-16.

Ai, C., I. Todorov, et al. (2007). "Human marrow-derived mesodermal progenitor cells generate insulin-secreting islet-like clusters in vivo." *Stem Cells Dev* 16(5): 757-70.

Alipio, Z., W. Liao, et al. (2010). "Reversal of hyperglycemia in diabetic mouse models using induced-pluripotent stem (iPS)-derived pancreatic beta-like cells." *Proc Natl Acad Sci U S A* 107(30): 13426-31.

* Corresponding Author

Alpert, S., D. Hanahan, et al. (1988). "Hybrid insulin genes reveal a developmental lineage for pancreatic endocrine cells and imply a relationship with neurons." *Cell* 53(2): 295-308.

Anderson, M. S. and J. A. Bluestone (2005). "The NOD mouse: a model of immune dysregulation." *Annu Rev Immunol* 23: 447-85.

Asari, S., S. Itakura, et al. (2011). "Mesenchymal stem cells facilitate mixed hematopoietic chimerism induction and prevent onset of diabetes in nonobese diabetic mice." *Pancreas* 40(6): 846-54.

Banerjee, I., N. Sharma, et al. (2010). "Impact of co-culture on pancreatic differentiation of embryonic stem cells." *J Tissue Eng Regen Med* 5(4): 313-23.

Bar-Nur, O., H. A. Russ, et al. (2011). "Epigenetic memory and preferential lineage-specific differentiation in induced pluripotent stem cells derived from human pancreatic islet beta cells." *Cell Stem Cell* 9(1): 17-23.

Becker, A. J., C. E. Mc, et al. (1963). "Cytological demonstration of the clonal nature of spleen colonies derived from transplanted mouse marrow cells." *Nature* 197: 452-4.

Beilhack, G. F., Y. C. Scheffold, et al. (2003). "Purified allogeneic hematopoietic stem cell transplantation blocks diabetes pathogenesis in NOD mice." *Diabetes* 52(1): 59-68.

Bluestone, J. A., K. Herold, et al. (2010). "Genetics, pathogenesis and clinical interventions in type 1 diabetes." *Nature* 464(7293): 1293-300.

Blyszczuk, P., C. Asbrand, et al. (2004). "Embryonic stem cells differentiate into insulin-producing cells without selection of nestin-expressing cells." *Int J Dev Biol* 48(10): 1095-104.

Bonde, S., K. M. Chan, et al. (2008). "ES-cell derived hematopoietic cells induce transplantation tolerance." *PLoS One* 3(9): e3212.

Bonde, S. and N. Zavazava (2006). "Immunogenicity and engraftment of mouse embryonic stem cells in allogeneic recipients." *Stem Cells* 24(10): 2192-201.

Bonner-Weir, S., D. Deery, et al. (1989). "Compensatory growth of pancreatic beta-cells in adult rats after short-term glucose infusion." *Diabetes* 38(1): 49-53.

Bonner-Weir, S., A. Inada, et al. (2008). "Transdifferentiation of pancreatic ductal cells to endocrine beta-cells." *Biochem Soc Trans* 36(Pt 3): 353-6.

Bonner-Weir, S. and A. Sharma (2002). "Pancreatic stem cells." *J Pathol* 197(4): 519-26.

Bonner-Weir, S., M. Taneja, et al. (2000). "In vitro cultivation of human islets from expanded ductal tissue." *Proc Natl Acad Sci U S A* 97(14): 7999-8004.

Borowiak, M., R. Maehr, et al. (2009). "Small molecules efficiently direct endodermal differentiation of mouse and human embryonic stem cells." *Cell Stem Cell* 4(4): 348-58.

Boyd, A. S. and K. J. Wood (2009). "Variation in MHC expression between undifferentiated mouse ES cells and ES cell-derived insulin-producing cell clusters." *Transplantation* 87(9): 1300-4.

Boyd, A. S. and K. J. Wood (2010). "Characteristics of the early immune response following transplantation of mouse ES cell derived insulin-producing cell clusters." *PLoS One* 5(6): e10965.

Boyd, A. S., D. C. Wu, et al. (2008). "A comparison of protocols used to generate insulin-producing cell clusters from mouse embryonic stem cells." *Stem Cells* 26(5): 1128-37.

Brands, K., E. Colvin, et al. (2008). "Reduced immunogenicity of first-trimester human fetal pancreas." *Diabetes* 57(3): 627-34.

Brun, T. and B. R. Gauthier (2008). "A focus on the role of Pax4 in mature pancreatic islet beta-cell expansion and survival in health and disease." *J Mol Endocrinol* 40(2): 37-45.

Burns, W. R., Y. Wang, et al. (2005). "Recruitment of CXCR3+ and CCR5+ T cells and production of interferon-gamma-inducible chemokines in rejecting human arteries." *Am J Transplant* 5(6): 1226-36.

Burt, R. K., L. Verda, et al. (2004). "Embryonic stem cells as an alternate marrow donor source: engraftment without graft-versus-host disease." *J Exp Med* 199(7): 895-904.

Butler, A. E., J. Janson, et al. (2003). "Beta-cell deficit and increased beta-cell apoptosis in humans with type 2 diabetes." *Diabetes* 52(1): 102-10.

Butler, A. E., J. Janson, et al. (2003). "Increased beta-cell apoptosis prevents adaptive increase in beta-cell mass in mouse model of type 2 diabetes: evidence for role of islet amyloid formation rather than direct action of amyloid." *Diabetes* 52(9): 2304-14.

Carvalho-Gaspar, M., J. S. Billing, et al. (2005). "Chemokine gene expression during allograft rejection: comparison of two quantitative PCR techniques." *J Immunol Methods* 301(1-2): 41-52.

Castaing, M., B. Peault, et al. (2001). "Blood glucose normalization upon transplantation of human embryonic pancreas into beta-cell-deficient SCID mice." *Diabetologia* 44(11): 2066-76.

Chan, J., W. Clements, et al. (2006). "Transplantation of bone marrow genetically engineered to express proinsulin II protects against autoimmune insulitis in NOD mice." *J Gene Med* 8(11): 1281-90.

Chavali, S., A. Mahajan, et al. (2011). "Association of variants in genes involved in pancreatic beta-cell development and function with type 2 diabetes in North Indians." *J Hum Genet* 56(10): 695-700.

Chen, S., M. Borowiak, et al. (2009). "A small molecule that directs differentiation of human ESCs into the pancreatic lineage." *Nat Chem Biol* 5(4): 258-65.

Chiang, M. K. and D. A. Melton (2003). "Single-cell transcript analysis of pancreas development." *Dev Cell* 4(3): 383-93.

Chin, M. H., M. J. Mason, et al. (2009). "Induced pluripotent stem cells and embryonic stem cells are distinguished by gene expression signatures." *Cell Stem Cell* 5(1): 111-23.

Cras-Meneur, C., L. Elghazi, et al. (2001). "Epidermal growth factor increases undifferentiated pancreatic embryonic cells in vitro: a balance between proliferation and differentiation." *Diabetes* 50(7): 1571-9.

D'Amour, K. A., A. D. Agulnick, et al. (2005). "Efficient differentiation of human embryonic stem cells to definitive endoderm." *Nat Biotechnol* 23(12): 1534-41.

D'Amour, K. A., A. G. Bang, et al. (2006). "Production of pancreatic hormone-expressing endocrine cells from human embryonic stem cells." *Nat Biotechnol* 24(11): 1392-401.

Danovitch, G. M., D. J. Cohen, et al. (2005). "Current status of kidney and pancreas transplantation in the United States, 1994-2003." *Am J Transplant* 5(4 Pt 2): 904-15.

Dor, Y., J. Brown, et al. (2004). "Adult pancreatic beta-cells are formed by self-duplication rather than stem-cell differentiation." *Nature* 429(6987): 41-6.

Doyle, M. J., Z. L. Loomis, et al. (2007). "Nkx2.2-repressor activity is sufficient to specify alpha-cells and a small number of beta-cells in the pancreatic islet." *Development* 134(3): 515-23.

Doyle, M. J. and L. Sussel (2007). "Nkx2.2 regulates beta-cell function in the mature islet." *Diabetes* 56(8): 1999-2007.

Evans, M. J. and M. H. Kaufman (1981). "Establishment in culture of pluripotential cells from mouse embryos." *Nature* 292(5819): 154-6.

Eventov-Friedman, S., D. Tchorsh, et al. (2006). "Embryonic pig pancreatic tissue transplantation for the treatment of diabetes." *PLoS Med* 3(7): e215.

Fabricius, D., S. Bonde, et al. (2005). "Induction of stable mixed chimerism by embryonic stem cells requires functional Fas/FasL engagement." *Transplantation* 79(9): 1040-4.

Feng, Q., S. J. Lu, et al. (2010). "Hemangioblastic derivatives from human induced pluripotent stem cells exhibit limited expansion and early senescence." *Stem Cells* 28(4): 704-12.

Feng, R. Q., L. Y. Du, et al. (2005). "In vitro cultivation and differentiation of fetal liver stem cells from mice." *Cell Res* 15(5): 401-5.

Fujikawa, T., S. H. Oh, et al. (2005). "Teratoma formation leads to failure of treatment for type I diabetes using embryonic stem cell-derived insulin-producing cells." *Am J Pathol* 166(6): 1781-91.

Gabr, M. M., M. M. Sobh, et al. (2008). "Transplantation of insulin-producing clusters derived from adult bone marrow stem cells to treat diabetes in rats." *Exp Clin Transplant* 6(3): 236-43.

Gao, F., D. Q. Wu, et al. (2008). "Extracellular matrix gel is necessary for in vitro cultivation of insulin producing cells from human umbilical cord blood derived mesenchymal stem cells." *Chin Med J (Engl)* 121(9): 811-8.

Garg, G., J. R. Tyler, et al. (2012). "Type 1 Diabetes-Associated IL2RA Variation Lowers IL-2 Signaling and Contributes to Diminished CD4+CD25+ Regulatory T Cell Function." *J Immunol.*

Gershengorn, M. C., A. A. Hardikar, et al. (2004). "Epithelial-to-mesenchymal transition generates proliferative human islet precursor cells." *Science* 306(5705): 2261-4.

Ghosh, Z., K. D. Wilson, et al. (2010). "Persistent donor cell gene expression among human induced pluripotent stem cells contributes to differences with human embryonic stem cells." *PLoS One* 5(2): e8975.

Gradwohl, G., A. Dierich, et al. (2000). "neurogenin3 is required for the development of the four endocrine cell lineages of the pancreas." *Proc Natl Acad Sci U S A* 97(4): 1607-11.

Gu, G., J. Dubauskaite, et al. (2002). "Direct evidence for the pancreatic lineage: NGN3+ cells are islet progenitors and are distinct from duct progenitors." *Development* 129(10): 2447-57.

Gu, G., J. M. Wells, et al. (2004). "Global expression analysis of gene regulatory pathways during endocrine pancreatic development." *Development* 131(1): 165-79.

Guillemain, G., G. Filhoulaud, et al. (2007). "Glucose is necessary for embryonic pancreatic endocrine cell differentiation." *J Biol Chem* 282(20): 15228-37.

Hald, J., T. Galbo, et al. (2011). "Pancreatic islet and progenitor cell surface markers with cell sorting potential." *Diabetologia* 55(1): 154-65.

Hansson, M., A. Tonning, et al. (2004). "Artifactual insulin release from differentiated embryonic stem cells." *Diabetes* 53(10): 2603-9.

Hao, E., B. Tyrberg, et al. (2006). "Beta-cell differentiation from nonendocrine epithelial cells of the adult human pancreas." *Nat Med* 12(3): 310-6.

Hardikar, A. A., B. Marcus-Samuels, et al. (2003). "Human pancreatic precursor cells secrete FGF2 to stimulate clustering into hormone-expressing islet-like cell aggregates." *Proc Natl Acad Sci U S A* 100(12): 7117-22.

Haseda, F., A. Imagawa, et al. (2011). "Low CTLA-4 expression in CD4+ helper T-cells in patients with fulminant type 1 diabetes." *Immunol Lett* 139(1-2): 80-6.

Hayek, A. and G. M. Beattie (1997). "Experimental transplantation of human fetal and adult pancreatic islets." *J Clin Endocrinol Metab* 82(8): 2471-5.

Heremans, Y., M. Van De Casteele, et al. (2002). "Recapitulation of embryonic neuroendocrine differentiation in adult human pancreatic duct cells expressing neurogenin 3." *J Cell Biol* 159(2): 303-12.

Herold, K. C., S. Gitelman, et al. (2009). "Treatment of patients with new onset Type 1 diabetes with a single course of anti-CD3 mAb Teplizumab preserves insulin production for up to 5 years." *Clin Immunol* 132(2): 166-73.

Herrera, P. L. (2000). "Adult insulin- and glucagon-producing cells differentiate from two independent cell lineages." *Development* 127(11): 2317-22.

Herrera, P. L., J. Huarte, et al. (1994). "Ablation of islet endocrine cells by targeted expression of hormone-promoter-driven toxigenes." *Proc Natl Acad Sci U S A* 91(26): 12999-3003.

Homo-Delarche, F. (2001). "Is pancreas development abnormal in the non-obese diabetic mouse, a spontaneous model of type I diabetes?" *Braz J Med Biol Res* 34(4): 437-47.

Hori, Y., M. Fukumoto, et al. (2008). "Enrichment of putative pancreatic progenitor cells from mice by sorting for prominin1 (CD133) and platelet-derived growth factor receptor beta." *Stem Cells* 26(11): 2912-20.

Hori, Y., I. C. Rulifson, et al. (2002). "Growth inhibitors promote differentiation of insulin-producing tissue from embryonic stem cells." *Proc Natl Acad Sci U S A* 99(25): 16105-10.

Hu, B. Y., J. P. Weick, et al. (2010). "Neural differentiation of human induced pluripotent stem cells follows developmental principles but with variable potency." *Proc Natl Acad Sci U S A* 107(9): 4335-40.

Hullett, D. A., J. L. Falany, et al. (1987). "Human fetal pancreas--a potential source for transplantation." *Transplantation* 43(1): 18-22.

Ibii, T., H. Shimada, et al. (2007). "Possibility of insulin-producing cells derived from mouse embryonic stem cells for diabetes treatment." *J Biosci Bioeng* 103(2): 140-6.

Inada, A., C. Nienaber, et al. (2008). "Carbonic anhydrase II-positive pancreatic cells are progenitors for both endocrine and exocrine pancreas after birth." *Proc Natl Acad Sci U S A* 105(50): 19915-9.

Itakura, S., S. Asari, et al. (2007). "Mesenchymal stem cells facilitate the induction of mixed hematopoietic chimerism and islet allograft tolerance without GVHD in the rat." *Am J Transplant* 7(2): 336-46.

Jahansouz, C., S. C. Kumer, et al. (2011). "Evolution of beta-Cell Replacement Therapy in Diabetes Mellitus: Pancreas Transplantation." *Diabetes Technol Ther* 13(3): 395-418.

Jensen, J., R. S. Heller, et al. (2000). "Independent development of pancreatic alpha- and beta-cells from neurogenin3-expressing precursors: a role for the notch pathway in repression of premature differentiation." *Diabetes* 49(2): 163-76.

Jiang, F. X. and G. Morahan (2011). "Pancreatic Stem Cells: From Possible to Probable." *Stem Cell Rev.*

Jiang, J., M. Au, et al. (2007). "Generation of insulin-producing islet-like clusters from human embryonic stem cells." *Stem Cells* 25(8): 1940-53.

Jiang, W., Y. Shi, et al. (2007). "In vitro derivation of functional insulin-producing cells from human embryonic stem cells." *Cell Res* 17(4): 333-44.

Jiang, W., X. Sui, et al. (2011). "CD24: a novel surface marker for PDX1-positive pancreatic progenitors derived from human embryonic stem cells." *Stem Cells* 29(4): 609-17.

Johansson, K. A., U. Dursun, et al. (2007). "Temporal control of neurogenin3 activity in pancreas progenitors reveals competence windows for the generation of different endocrine cell types." *Dev Cell* 12(3): 457-65.

Jorgenson, M. C., J. Ahnfelt-Ronne, et al. (2007). "An illustrated review of early pancreas development in the mouse." *Endocrine Reviews* 28(6): 685-705.

Karaoz, E., Z. S. Genc, et al. (2010). "Protection of rat pancreatic islet function and viability by coculture with rat bone marrow-derived mesenchymal stem cells." *Cell Death Dis* 1: e36.

Karnik, S. K., H. Chen, et al. (2007). "Menin controls growth of pancreatic beta-cells in pregnant mice and promotes gestational diabetes mellitus." *Science* 318(5851): 806-9.

Kelly, O. G., M. Y. Chan, et al. (2011). "Cell-surface markers for the isolation of pancreatic cell types derived from human embryonic stem cells." *Nat Biotechnol* 29(8): 750-6.

Kim, A., K. Miller, et al. (2009). "Islet architecture: A comparative study." *Islets* 1(2): 129-36.

Kim, E. M., R. Stultz, et al. (2011). "Embryonic stem cell-derived T cells induce lethal graft-versus-host disease and reject allogenic skin grafts upon thymic selection." *Am J Transplant* 12(3): 600-9.

Kim, H., Y. Toyofuku, et al. (2010). "Serotonin regulates pancreatic beta cell mass during pregnancy." *Nat Med* 16(7): 804-8.

Kim, P. T., B. G. Hoffman, et al. (2010). "Differentiation of mouse embryonic stem cells into endoderm without embryoid body formation." *PLoS One* 5(11): e14146.

Koch, C. A., P. Geraldes, et al. (2008). "Immunosuppression by embryonic stem cells." *Stem Cells* 26(1): 89-98.

Kojima, H., M. Fujimiya, et al. (2004). "Extrapancreatic insulin-producing cells in multiple organs in diabetes." *Proc Natl Acad Sci U S A* 101(8): 2458-63.

Kroon, E., L. A. Martinson, et al. (2008). "Pancreatic endoderm derived from human embryonic stem cells generates glucose-responsive insulin-secreting cells in vivo." *Nat Biotechnol* 26(4): 443-52.

Ku, H. T., J. Chai, et al. (2007). "Insulin-expressing colonies developed from murine embryonic stem cell-derived progenitors." *Diabetes* 56(4): 921-9.

Landsman, L., A. Nijagal, et al. (2011). "Pancreatic mesenchyme regulates epithelial organogenesis throughout development." *PLoS Biol* 9(9): e1001143.

Laurent, L. C., I. Ulitsky, et al. (2011). "Dynamic changes in the copy number of pluripotency and cell proliferation genes in human ESCs and iPSCs during reprogramming and time in culture." *Cell Stem Cell* 8(1): 106-18.

Lenschow, D. J., Y. Zeng, et al. (1992). "Long-term survival of xenogeneic pancreatic islet grafts induced by CTLA4lg." *Science* 257(5071): 789-92.

Leonard, J., B. Peers, et al. (1993). "Characterization of somatostatin transactivating factor-1, a novel homeobox factor that stimulates somatostatin expression in pancreatic islet cells." *Mol Endocrinol* 7(10): 1275-83.

Li, G., R. Luo, et al. (2009). "Generating mESC-derived insulin-producing cell lines through an intermediate lineage-restricted progenitor line." *Stem Cell Res* 2(1): 41-55.

Li, H., A. Lam, et al. (2010). "High dosage of Exendin-4 increased early insulin secretion in differentiated beta cells from mouse embryonic stem cells." *Acta Pharmacol Sin* 31(5): 570-7.

Lin, H. T., C. L. Kao, et al. (2007). "Enhancement of insulin-producing cell differentiation from embryonic stem cells using pax4-nucleofection method." *World J Gastroenterol* 13(11): 1672-9.

Ludvigsson, J., M. Hjorth, et al. (2011). "Extended evaluation of the safety and efficacy of GAD treatment of children and adolescents with recent-onset type 1 diabetes: a randomised controlled trial." *Diabetologia* 54(3): 634-40.

Ludvigsson, J., D. Krisky, et al. (2012). "GAD65 antigen therapy in recently diagnosed type 1 diabetes mellitus." *N Engl J Med* 366(5): 433-42.

Lui, K. O., A. S. Boyd, et al. (2010). "A role for regulatory T cells in acceptance of ESC-derived tissues transplanted across an major histocompatibility complex barrier." *Stem Cells* 28(10): 1905-14.

Lumelsky, N., O. Blondel, et al. (2001). "Differentiation of embryonic stem cells to insulin-secreting structures similar to pancreatic islets." *Science* 292(5520): 1389-94.

Luo, L., J. Z. Luo, et al. (2009). "Cytokines inducing bone marrow SCA+ cells migration into pancreatic islet and conversion into insulin-positive cells in vivo." *PLoS One* 4(2): e4504.

Maehr, R., S. Chen, et al. (2009). "Generation of pluripotent stem cells from patients with type 1 diabetes." *Proc Natl Acad Sci U S A* 106(37): 15768-73.

Mallone, R., V. Brezar, et al. (2011). "T cell recognition of autoantigens in human type 1 diabetes: clinical perspectives." *Clin Dev Immunol* 2011: 513210.

Marchetto, M. C., G. W. Yeo, et al. (2009). "Transcriptional signature and memory retention of human-induced pluripotent stem cells." *PLoS One* 4(9): e7076.

Matveyenko, A. V., J. D. Veldhuis, et al. (2006). "Mechanisms of impaired fasting glucose and glucose intolerance induced by an approximate 50% pancreatectomy." *Diabetes* 55(8): 2347-56.

Mayshar, Y., U. Ben-David, et al. (2010). "Identification and classification of chromosomal aberrations in human induced pluripotent stem cells." *Cell Stem Cell* 7(4): 521-31.

McKiernan, E., L. O'Driscoll, et al. (2007). "Directed differentiation of mouse embryonic stem cells into pancreatic-like or neuronal- and glial-like phenotypes." *Tissue Eng* 13(10): 2419-30.

McLean, A. B., K. A. D'Amour, et al. (2007). "Activin a efficiently specifies definitive endoderm from human embryonic stem cells only when phosphatidylinositol 3-kinase signaling is suppressed." *Stem Cells* 25(1): 29-38.

Mellitzer, G., M. Martin, et al. (2004). "Pancreatic islet progenitor cells in neurogenin 3-yellow fluorescent protein knock-add-on mice." *Mol Endocrinol* 18(11): 2765-76.

Michels, A. W. and P. A. Gottlieb (2010). "Autoimmune polyglandular syndromes." *Nat Rev Endocrinol* 6(5): 270-7.

Minami, K., M. Okuno, et al. (2005). "Lineage tracing and characterization of insulin-secreting cells generated from adult pancreatic acinar cells." *Proc Natl Acad Sci U S A* 102(42): 15116-21.

Mineo, D., C. Ricordi, et al. (2008). "Combined islet and hematopoietic stem cell allotransplantation: a clinical pilot trial to induce chimerism and graft tolerance." *Am J Transplant* 8(6): 1262-74.

Miyatsuka, T., Y. Kosaka, et al. (2011). "Neurogenin3 inhibits proliferation in endocrine progenitors by inducing Cdkn1a." *Proc Natl Acad Sci U S A* 108(1): 185-90.

Miyazaki, S., E. Yamato, et al. (2004). "Regulated expression of pdx-1 promotes in vitro differentiation of insulin-producing cells from embryonic stem cells." *Diabetes* 53(4): 1030-7.

Nielsen, J. H., J. Brunstedt, et al. (1979). "Preservation of beta cell function in adult human pancreatic islets for several months in vitro." *Diabetologia* 16(2): 97-100.

Nielsen, J. H., E. D. Galsgaard, et al. (2001). "Regulation of beta-cell mass by hormones and growth factors." *Diabetes* 50 Suppl 1: S25-9.

Nielsen, J. H., C. Svensson, et al. (1999). "Beta cell proliferation and growth factors." *J Mol Med (Berl)* 77(1): 62-6.

Nikolic, B., Y. Takeuchi, et al. (2004). "Mixed hematopoietic chimerism allows cure of autoimmune diabetes through allogeneic tolerance and reversal of autoimmunity." *Diabetes* 53(2): 376-83.

Nir, T., D. A. Melton, et al. (2007). "Recovery from diabetes in mice by beta cell regeneration." *J Clin Invest* 117(9): 2553-61.

Niwa, A., K. Umeda, et al. (2009). "Orderly hematopoietic development of induced pluripotent stem cells via Flk-1(+) hemoangiogenic progenitors." *J Cell Physiol* 221(2): 367-77.

Ohlsson, H., S. Thor, et al. (1991). "Novel insulin promoter- and enhancer-binding proteins that discriminate between pancreatic alpha- and beta-cells." *Mol Endocrinol* 5(7): 897-904.

Okita, K., T. Ichisaka, et al. (2007). "Generation of germline-competent induced pluripotent stem cells." *Nature* 448(7151): 313-7.

Osafune, K., L. Caron, et al. (2008). "Marked differences in differentiation propensity among human embryonic stem cell lines." *Nat Biotechnol* 26(3): 313-5.

Oshima, Y., A. Suzuki, et al. (2007). "Isolation of mouse pancreatic ductal progenitor cells expressing CD133 and c-Met by flow cytometric cell sorting." *Gastroenterology* 132(2): 720-32.

Otonkoski, T., G. M. Beattie, et al. (1993). "Nicotinamide is a potent inducer of endocrine differentiation in cultured human fetal pancreatic cells." *J Clin Invest* 92(3): 1459-66.

Otonkoski, T., V. Cirulli, et al. (1996). "A role for hepatocyte growth factor/scatter factor in fetal mesenchyme-induced pancreatic beta-cell growth." *Endocrinology* 137(7): 3131-9.

Paek, H. J., J. R. Morgan, et al. (2005). "Sequestration and synthesis: the source of insulin in cell clusters differentiated from murine embryonic stem cells." *Stem Cells* 23(7): 862-7.

Parsons, J. A., T. C. Brelje, et al. (1992). "Adaptation of islets of Langerhans to pregnancy: increased islet cell proliferation and insulin secretion correlates with the onset of placental lactogen secretion." *Endocrinology* 130(3): 1459-66.

Pearl, J. I., A. S. Lee, et al. (2011). "Short-term immunosuppression promotes engraftment of embryonic and induced pluripotent stem cells." *Cell Stem Cell* 8(3): 309-17.

Phillips, B. W., H. Hentze, et al. (2007). "Directed differentiation of human embryonic stem cells into the pancreatic endocrine lineage." *Stem Cells Dev* 16(4): 561-78.

Pipeleers, D. G., M. Pipeleers-Marichal, et al. (1991). "Transplantation of purified islet cells in diabetic rats. II. Immunogenicity of allografted islet beta-cells." *Diabetes* 40(7): 920-30.

Piper, K., S. Brickwood, et al. (2004). "Beta cell differentiation during early human pancreas development." *J Endocrinol* 181(1): 11-23.

Racine, J., M. Wang, et al. (2011). "Induction of mixed chimerism with MHC-mismatched but not matched bone marrow transplants results in thymic deletion of host-type autoreactive T-cells in NOD mice." *Diabetes* 60(2): 555-64.

Raikwar, S. P. and N. Zavazava (2011). "Spontaneous in vivo differentiation of embryonic stem cell-derived pancreatic endoderm-like cells corrects hyperglycemia in diabetic mice." *Transplantation* 91(1): 11-20.

Rajagopal, J., W. J. Anderson, et al. (2003). "Insulin staining of ES cell progeny from insulin uptake." *Science* 299(5605): 363.

Ramiya, V. K., M. Maraist, et al. (2000). "Reversal of insulin-dependent diabetes using islets generated in vitro from pancreatic stem cells." *Nat Med* 6(3): 278-82.

Raya, A., I. Rodriguez-Piza, et al. (2009). "Disease-corrected haematopoietic progenitors from Fanconi anaemia induced pluripotent stem cells." *Nature* 460(7251): 53-9.

Rieck, S. and K. H. Kaestner (2010). "Expansion of beta-cell mass in response to pregnancy." *Trends Endocrinol Metab* 21(3): 151-8.

Robertson, R. P., K. J. Lanz, et al. (2002). "Relationship between diabetes and obesity 9 to 18 years after hemipancreatectomy and transplantation in donors and recipients." *Transplantation* 73(5): 736-41.

Roep, B. O. and M. Peakman (2011). "Diabetogenic T lymphocytes in human Type 1 diabetes." *Curr Opin Immunol* 23(6): 746-53.

Rolletschek, A., I. S. Schroeder, et al. (2010). "Characterization of mouse embryonic stem cell differentiation into the pancreatic lineage in vitro by transcriptional profiling, quantitative RT-PCR and immunocytochemistry." *Int J Dev Biol* 54(1): 41-54.

Rouleau, M., R. Namikawa, et al. (1996). "Antigen-specific cytotoxic T cells mediate human fetal pancreas allograft rejection in SCID-hu mice." *J Immunol* 157(12): 5710-20.

Russ, H. A., Y. Bar, et al. (2008). "In vitro proliferation of cells derived from adult human beta-cells revealed by cell-lineage tracing." *Diabetes* 57(6): 1575-83.

Russ, H. A., E. Sintov, et al. (2011). "Insulin-producing cells generated from dedifferentiated human pancreatic beta cells expanded in vitro." *PLoS One* 6(9): e25566.

Sapir, T., K. Shternhall, et al. (2005). "Cell-replacement therapy for diabetes: Generating functional insulin-producing tissue from adult human liver cells." *Proc Natl Acad Sci U S A* 102(22): 7964-9.

Schaffer, A. E., A. J. Yang, et al. (2011). "Transgenic overexpression of the transcription factor Nkx6.1 in beta-cells of mice does not increase beta-cell proliferation, beta-cell mass, or improve glucose clearance." *Mol Endocrinol* 25(11): 1904-14.

Scharfmann, R., X. Xiao, et al. (2008). "Beta cells within single human islets originate from multiple progenitors." *PLoS One* 3(10): e3559.

Schisler, J. C., P. T. Fueger, et al. (2008). "Stimulation of human and rat islet beta-cell proliferation with retention of function by the homeodomain transcription factor Nkx6.1." *Mol Cell Biol* 28(10): 3465-76.

Schroeder, I. S., G. Kania, et al. (2006). "Insulin-producing cells." *Methods Enzymol* 418: 315-33.

Schroeder, I. S., A. Rolletschek, et al. (2006). "Differentiation of mouse embryonic stem cells to insulin-producing cells." *Nat Protoc* 1(2): 495-507.

Seeberger, K. L., J. M. Dufour, et al. (2006). "Expansion of mesenchymal stem cells from human pancreatic ductal epithelium." *Lab Invest* 86(2): 141-53.

Serafimidis, I., I. Rakatzi, et al. (2008). "Novel effectors of directed and Ngn3-mediated differentiation of mouse embryonic stem cells into endocrine pancreas progenitors." *Stem Cells* 26(1): 3-16.

Shamblott, M. J., J. Axelman, et al. (1998). "Derivation of pluripotent stem cells from cultured human primordial germ cells." *Proc Natl Acad Sci U S A* 95(23): 13726-31.

Shapiro, A. M., C. Ricordi, et al. (2006). "International trial of the Edmonton protocol for islet transplantation." *N Engl J Med* 355(13): 1318-30.

Sherry, N. A., J. A. Kushner, et al. (2006). "Effects of autoimmunity and immune therapy on beta-cell turnover in type 1 diabetes." *Diabetes* 55(12): 3238-45.

Shim, J. H., S. E. Kim, et al. (2007). "Directed differentiation of human embryonic stem cells towards a pancreatic cell fate." *Diabetologia* 50(6): 1228-38.

Shiraki, N., S. Harada, et al. (2010). "Identification of DAF1/CD55, a novel definitive endoderm marker." *Cell Struct Funct* 35(2): 73-80.

Shultz, L. D., Y. Saito, et al. (2010). "Generation of functional human T-cell subsets with HLA-restricted immune responses in HLA class I expressing NOD/SCID/IL2r gamma(null) humanized mice." *Proc Natl Acad Sci U S A* 107(29): 13022-7.

Smukler, S. R., M. E. Arntfield, et al. (2011). "The adult mouse and human pancreas contain rare multipotent stem cells that express insulin." *Cell Stem Cell* 8(3): 281-93.

Soria, B., E. Roche, et al. (2000). "Insulin-secreting cells derived from embryonic stem cells normalize glycemia in streptozotocin-induced diabetic mice." *Diabetes* 49(2): 157-62.

Stagner, J. I. and E. Samols (1991). "Deterioration of islet beta-cell function after hemipancreatectomy in dogs." *Diabetes* 40(11): 1472-9.

Steptoe, R. J., J. M. Ritchie, et al. (2003). "Transfer of hematopoietic stem cells encoding autoantigen prevents autoimmune diabetes." *J Clin Invest* 111(9): 1357-63.

Sugiyama, T., R. T. Rodriguez, et al. (2007). "Conserved markers of fetal pancreatic epithelium permit prospective isolation of islet progenitor cells by FACS." *Proc Natl Acad Sci U S A* 104(1): 175-80.

Sussel, L., J. Kalamaras, et al. (1998). "Mice lacking the homeodomain transcription factor Nkx2.2 have diabetes due to arrested differentiation of pancreatic beta cells." *Development* 125(12): 2213-21.

Sykes, M. (2007). "Mechanisms of tolerance induced via mixed chimerism." *Front Biosci* 12: 2922-34.

Sykes, M. (2009). "Hematopoietic cell transplantation for tolerance induction: animal models to clinical trials." *Transplantation* 87(3): 309-16.

Takahashi, K. and S. Yamanaka (2006). "Induction of pluripotent stem cells from mouse embryonic and adult fibroblast cultures by defined factors." *Cell* 126(4): 663-76.

Tang, D. Q., L. Z. Cao, et al. (2004). "In vivo and in vitro characterization of insulin-producing cells obtained from murine bone marrow." *Diabetes* 53(7): 1721-32.

Teitelman, G., S. Alpert, et al. (1993). "Precursor cells of mouse endocrine pancreas coexpress insulin, glucagon and the neuronal proteins tyrosine hydroxylase and neuropeptide Y, but not pancreatic polypeptide." *Development* 118(4): 1031-9.

Thatava, T., T. J. Nelson, et al. (2010). "Indolactam V/GLP-1-mediated differentiation of human iPS cells into glucose-responsive insulin-secreting progeny." *Gene Ther* 18(3): 283-93.

Thompson, H. L. and J. O. Manilay (2011). "Embryonic stem cell-derived hematopoietic stem cells: challenges in development, differentiation, and immunogenicity." *Curr Top Med Chem* 11(13): 1621-37.

Thorel, F., V. Nepote, et al. (2010). "Conversion of adult pancreatic alpha-cells to beta-cells after extreme beta-cell loss." *Nature* 464(7292): 1149-54.

Tornehave, D., P. Jansen, et al. (1993). "Fetal antigen 1 (FA1) in the human pancreas: cell type expression, topological and quantitative variations during development." *Anat Embryol (Berl)* 187(4): 335-41.

Tuch, B. E., T. C. Hughes, et al. (2011). "Encapsulated pancreatic progenitors derived from human embryonic stem cells as a therapy for insulin-dependent diabetes." *Diabetes Metab Res Rev* 27(8): 928-32.

Tuch, B. E. and R. S. Monk (1991). "Regulation of blood glucose to human levels by human fetal pancreatic xenografts." *Transplantation* 51(6): 1156-60.

Tuch, B. E., K. J. Osgerby, et al. (1988). "Normalization of blood glucose levels in nondiabetic nude mice by human fetal pancreas after induction of diabetes." *Transplantation* 46(4): 608-11.

Turvey, S. E., V. Gonzalez-Nicolini, et al. (2000). "Fas ligand-transfected myoblasts and islet cell transplantation." *Transplantation* 69(9): 1972-6.

Vaca, P., F. Martin, et al. (2006). "Induction of differentiation of embryonic stem cells into insulin-secreting cells by fetal soluble factors." *Stem Cells* 24(2): 258-65.

van Belle, T. L., K. T. Coppieters, et al. (2011). "Type 1 diabetes: etiology, immunology, and therapeutic strategies." *Physiol Rev* 91(1): 79-118.

Van Belle, T. L., P. Taylor, et al. (2009). "Mouse Models for Type 1 Diabetes." *Drug Discov Today Dis Models* 6(2): 41-45.

Vanhaesebroeck, B., S. J. Leevers, et al. (2001). "Synthesis and function of 3-phosphorylated inositol lipids." *Annu Rev Biochem* 70: 535-602.

Verda, L., D. A. Kim, et al. (2008). "Hematopoietic mixed chimerism derived from allogeneic embryonic stem cells prevents autoimmune diabetes mellitus in NOD mice." *Stem Cells* 26(2): 381-6.

Vincent, R. K. and J. S. Odorico (2009). "Reduced serum concentration is permissive for increased in vitro endocrine differentiation from murine embryonic stem cells." *Differentiation* 78(1): 24-34.

Voltarelli, J. C., C. E. Couri, et al. (2007). "Autologous nonmyeloablative hematopoietic stem cell transplantation in newly diagnosed type 1 diabetes mellitus." *Jama* 297(14): 1568-76.

von Herrath, M. and G. T. Nepom (2009). "Remodeling rodent models to mimic human type 1 diabetes." *Eur J Immunol* 39(8): 2049-54.

Waldron-Lynch, F. and K. C. Herold (2011). "Immunomodulatory therapy to preserve pancreatic beta-cell function in type 1 diabetes." *Nat Rev Drug Discov* 10(6): 439-52.

Wang, J., L. Elghazi, et al. (2004). "The concerted activities of Pax4 and Nkx2.2 are essential to initiate pancreatic beta-cell differentiation." *Dev Biol* 266(1): 178-89.

Wang, R. N., L. Bouwens, et al. (1996). "Beta-cell growth in adolescent and adult rats treated with streptozotocin during the neonatal period." *Diabetologia* 39(5): 548-57.

Wang, X. and K. Ye (2009). "Three-dimensional differentiation of embryonic stem cells into islet-like insulin-producing clusters." *Tissue Eng Part A* 15(8): 1941-52.

Wu, D. C., A. S. Boyd, et al. (2008). "Embryonic stem cells and their differentiated derivatives have a fragile immune privilege but still represent novel targets of immune attack." *Stem Cells* 26(8): 1939-50.

Wu, X. H., C. P. Liu, et al. (2007). "Reversal of hyperglycemia in diabetic rats by portal vein transplantation of islet-like cells generated from bone marrow mesenchymal stem cells." *World J Gastroenterol* 13(24): 3342-9.

Xu, G., D. A. Stoffers, et al. (1999). "Exendin-4 stimulates both beta-cell replication and neogenesis, resulting in increased beta-cell mass and improved glucose tolerance in diabetic rats." *Diabetes* 48(12): 2270-6.

Xu, X., J. D'Hoker, et al. (2008). "Beta cells can be generated from endogenous progenitors in injured adult mouse pancreas." *Cell* 132(2): 197-207.

Yasunaga, M., S. Tada, et al. (2005). "Induction and monitoring of definitive and visceral endoderm differentiation of mouse ES cells." *Nat Biotechnol* 23(12): 1542-50.

Yokoi, N., M. Kanamori, et al. (2006). "Association studies of variants in the genes involved in pancreatic beta-cell function in type 2 diabetes in Japanese subjects." *Diabetes* 55(8): 2379-86.

Yu, J., K. Hu, et al. (2009). "Human induced pluripotent stem cells free of vector and transgene sequences." *Science* 324(5928): 797-801.

Zhang, D., W. Jiang, et al. (2009). "Highly efficient differentiation of human ES cells and iPS cells into mature pancreatic insulin-producing cells." *Cell Res* 19(4): 429-38.

Zhao, T., Z. N. Zhang, et al. (2011). "Immunogenicity of induced pluripotent stem cells." *Nature* 474(7350): 212-5.

Zhou, B., G. J. Martin, et al. (2008). "Increased phenotypic stability and ethanol tolerance of recombinant Escherichia coli KO11 when immobilized in continuous fluidized bed culture." *Biotechnol Bioeng* 100(4): 627-33.

Chapter 13

Stem Cell-Based Cellular Therapy in Rheumatoid Arthritis

Rizwanul Haque, Fengyang Lei, Xiaofang Xiong and Jianxun Song

Additional information is available at the end of the chapter

http://dx.doi.org/10.5772/47804

1. Introduction

1.1. Potential mechanisms of pathogenesis of RA

Rheumatoid arthritis (RA) is a chronically systemic inflammatory disorder that ultimately leads to the destruction of joint architecture. RA affects more than two million people in America and about 1% of the world's population, women are three times more prone to RA than men (1, 2). About 58 million people suffer from RA all over the world. The disease has a variable course, from a mild, occasionally symptomatic illness requiring only symptomatic therapy to a fully onset requiring aggressive immunosuppressive therapy, surgery or both. The hallmarks of RA is the systemic loss of regulation of immune system characterized by either acute or chronic inflammation, in which the immune system primarily attacks the joints of the body leading to tissue pathology and clinical disease. The etiological factor causes the immune reaction is still unknown. The pathological insult starts with inflammation of the synovium (sinovita), which then takes the form of proliferative nature (pannus) with the damage of cartilage and bones. Plasmatic cells of joint produce antibody that form aggregates of IgG. In turn, IgG aggregates have been recognized by the immune system as foreign antigens and plasmatic cells (B cells, dendritic cells, T cells, and macrophages formed lymphoid follicle-like structures within the synovial membrane) begin to produce autoantibodies against those structures known as rheumatoid factors (RF). Autoantibodies directed against the Fc fragment of IgG. (3, 4). The most important type of RF is the IgM class, which appears in 70-80% of patients with RA. In the course of the disease, the normal, relatively avascular synovium then becomes heavily infiltrated by a wide variety of cells, including B cells, macrophages, fibroblasts, neutrophil granulocytes, dendritic cells, and many other cells (5). Because of the autoimmune inflammatory process, which leads to formation of pannus - granulation tissue that occurs from in the inflamed synovium, which is consists of actively proliferating fibroblasts, lymphocytes, macrophages and rich with vessels. The synovial lining increases to a thickness of up to 30 cell layers, presumably through influx of macrophages, and by expansion of synovial fibroblasts. Pannus grows intensively, percolates from the synovial tissue to the cartilage and destroys it by the influence of enzymes, which are induced by the production of high amount of proinflammatory cytokines mainly tumor necrosis factor (TNF), interleukin (IL)-1, and IL-6 within the pannus. Furthermore, many other cytokines such as IL-17, IL-18, IL-15, chemokines, and angiogenic molecules are present in the inflamed synovial membrane and drive the development of the disease. Subsequently, these proinflammatory cytokines activate signal transduction pathways and transcription factors, which, in turn, control the production of cytokines (6). Gradually, intrasynovial cartilage disappears, it is replaced by granulation tissue and ankylosis develops. Chronic inflammation of periarthric tissues, joint capsule, ligaments and tendons lead to deformation of joints, semiluxations, and contractures. Currently, there is a large body of literature which suggests that autoimmune processes play a central role in the early stages of RA, and in later stages non-immune mechanisms (*i.e.*, the ability of pannus for growth, invasion and destruction of joint cartilage) are more important. However, the crucial triggers for the onset of diseases that lead to pathogenic events in RA are still not fully understood. It is generally believed that RA is the result of interactions amongst genetic, environmental, biomechanical factors, neuroimmunological interactions and altered articular microvascular function (7). Several genetic loci have been proposed based on the genome wide association studies to have an association with the susceptibility and severity of RA (8-12). A disease association with HLA-DR4 alleles (which contain the shared epitope) is well established (13). However, apart from the major histocompatibility complex, genetic factors associated with RA severity have not yet been convincingly proved. However, other loci, including PTPN22 (protein tyrosine phosphatase, non-receptor type 22), PADI4 (peptidyl arginine deiminase, type IV), CTLA4 (cytotoxic T-lymphocyte antigen 4), Fc◎Rs (Fc receptors for IgG), CD40 and CDK6 were identified that involved in susceptibility and higher rate of joint destruction (14-17). Various cytokines and cytokine-receptor loci, such as those encoding TNF, IL-1, IL-10, and IL-18, have been implicated in disease association to various degrees in distinct populations (12). The area of identification of susceptible gene loci in RA is currently under intense investigation. The frequencies of bone marrow and circulating $CD34^{+}$ HPC (hematopoietic progenitor cells) in RA patient are reduced (18-20), the median apoptotic index of early bone marrow myeloid precursors is significantly higher than in controls (21, 22) and their proliferative activity is impaired (18, 19). Reduced colony formation by highly purified RA $CD34^{+}$ cells may be linked to an intrinsic defect in the clonogenic potential of RA progenitors. However, the molecular pathways responsible for this abnormality remain undetermined. HPC isolated from RA patients are hyporesponsive to hematopoietic growth factors and fail to expand appropriately. This defect appears specifically connected to the extracellular signal-regulated protein kinase (ERK) signaling pathway, a signaling cascade critically involved in cell cycle entry and progression of progenitor cells (23). The molecular defect causing RA has not been fully characterized although it is reported that many cell population have aberrant function, including monocytes, macrophages, B cells, T cells, endothelial cells, and fibroblasts, participate in the ongoing inflammatory process. Multiple inflammatory pathways contribute to the persistent chronic inflammation in RA (24). Recent advances in our understanding of the key cells (*i.e.*, T cells, B cells) and inflammatory cytokines (TNF and IL-6) have provided therapeutic opportunities, which are now directly targeted by biologic agents approved by the US Food and Drug Administration (FDA) for the treatment of RA.

2. Current biological therapies for RA

Biologic therapies have brought improved efficacy in the treatment of RA. However, these therapies sometimes fail or produce only partial responses, because of the lack of reliable predictive biomarkers of prognosis, therapeutic response, and toxicity data. Sustained remission is rarely achieved and requires ongoing pharmacological intervention. Although RA often responds to immunosuppressive medication including corticosteroids, methotrexate, azathioprine and cyclophosphamide, or non-steroidal anti-inflammatory drugs, none of these drugs showed a curative effect (25). Synthetic disease-modifying antirheumatic drugs (DMARDs), such as methotrexate, leflunomide, and sulfasalazine, have evidently improved clinical symptoms and reduced joint damage in RA patients. However, despite the effectiveness of synthetic DMARDs, many patients who have been taking those drugs continue to have clinical symptoms of inflammation and progressive joint destruction. Recently, FDA approved many TNF-α inhibitors including infliximab, etanercept, adalimumab, golimumab, and certolizumab pegol in the RA treatment. In randomized clinical trials, all of these agents have been shown effective in reducing clinical symptom of inflammation in RA patients who have failed synthetic DMARDs (26). Multiple studies have demonstrated significant benefits of early treatment with TNF-α inhibitors combined with methotrexate (27-29). Other FDA-approved biologic agents for treating moderate-to- severe RA include abatacept, rituximab, and tocilizumab (30-33). However, all biologic agents carry an increased risk of infections.

3. Current concept of stem cell therapy in RA

The natural healing process for RA requires a combination of stem cells, growth factors, and matrix to optimize tissue repair and regeneration. The use of these bioactive cells to supplement and hasten the natural healing process is considered by many to be a new era of clinical treatment. This ideal cell population for the treatment of RA should have a series of properties, namely a high osteogenic and chondrogenic potential, and at the same time, it should be easily expanded, *i.e.*, capable of self replicating and can be maintained in cultures for a long period of time. Due to their natural and intrinsic properties, stem cells are one of the best available cell types. There are mainly four types of stem cells undergoing current study. They are embryonic stem cells (ESCs), allogeneic (donor) stem cells (SCs), induced pluripotential adult stem cells (iPSCs), and last but not least autologous stem cells. Of these four, only two, donor SCs and autologous SCs have been used to treat arthritis in human at present. The multipotent autologous stem cells also know as mesenchyme stem cell (MSC) are sufficient to be used to treat disorders involving connective tissue, such as blood, tendon, ligament, cartilage, bone, nerve, muscle, and liver. During the last 1-2 decades, the scientific community witnessed and reported the appearance of several sources of stem cells with both osteogenic and chondrogenic potential. There are many different sources of adult stem cells (*e.g.*, bone marrow, periosteum, adipose tissue, skeletal muscle and umbilical cord) for bone and cartilage regenerative medicine, namely those focusing on the differentiation potential of the latter, as well as *in vivo* proof of concept of their applicability.

4. MSC based stem cell therapy in RA

MSCs are the non-hematopoietic progenitor cells found in various adult tissues. MSCs have been characterized by the ease of isolation and rapid growth *in vitro* while maintaining their differentiation potential, allowing for extensive culture expansion to obtain large quantities suitable for therapeutic use. MSCs are characterized by the capacity to adhere to plastic surface, the phenotype ($CD90^+$, $CD73^+$, $CD105^+$ and absence of hematopoietic markers including $CD45^-$, CD34, $CD11b^-$, $CD14^-$ CD79α or CD19 and HLA-DR^-), the ability to differentiate into at least three distinct lineages including adipocytes, chondrocytes, osteoblasts, and the capacity for self-renewal (34, 35). MSCs are hypoimmunogenic and are able to evade the host immune surveillance. MSCs express low (fetal) to intermediate (adult) level of major histocompatibility complex (MHC) class I molecules and do not express MHC class II molecules on the cell surface, although an intracellular pool of MHC class II molecules can be stimulated to express on the cell surface by interferon-gamma (IFN-γ) (36). However, because MSC do not express any costimulatory molecules, including B7-1 (CD80), B7-2 (CD86), or CD40, MSCs do not activate alloreative T cells (37). After differentiation into adipocytes, osteoblasts, and chondrocytes, MSCs continue to express MHC class I but not class II molecules on the cell surface, even under stimulation, and continue to be non-immunogenic (36, 38). However, the immune privilege of MSCs seem to be limited. A few studies in mouse system have reported that allogeneic mismatched MSCs were rejected by the host and could not form ectopic bone *in vivo*, while syngeneic recipient allowed ectopic bone formation despite the fact that, the MSCs showed immunosuppressive activity *in vitro* (39, 40). Recently, MSCs have been shown to possess several immunomodulatory properties. These include suppression of T cell proliferation, influencing dendritic cell maturation and function, suppression of B cell proliferation and terminal differentiation, and immune modulation of other immune cells such as NK cells and macrophages (41-44). Meanwhile, MSCs also express the Toll-like receptors (TLR)-2 -8. The addition of polyI:C (TLR3 ligand), Pam3Cys (TLR2 ligand) or LPS (TLR4 ligand) inhibited the differentiation potential of MSCs, but spared their immunosuppressive function (45). MSCs also inhibit the maturation and decrease the expression of antigen presentation molecules and costimulatory molecules on the surface of antigen-presenting cells (APCs) (42). Furthermore, MSCs not only have a direct inhibitory effect on T cells but also affect the first critical step of immune response in which they can inhibit the differentiation and maturation of the APCs and cause the dendritic cells to switch cytokine secretion profile to decrease the secretion of proinflammatory cytokines such as TNF-α, IFN-γ, and IL-12, and importantly, increase the production of IL-10, which is a suppressive, tolerogenic and potent inducer of regulatory T cells (Tregs) (42, 46, 47). An additional study, however, reported that TLR3 or -4 ligation resulted in a strong down-regulation of the Notch ligand Jagged-1, leading to the down-regulation of suppressive capacities (48). Thus, in the context of an inflammatory process, MSCs may lose the immunosuppressive function. MSCs have been shown in recent studies to have significant effects on a variety of conditions including both RA and osteoarthritis (49). MSCs are shown to have significant effects on a variety of autoimmune type of problems such as rheumatoid arthritis, osteoarthritis, lupus, colitis, mixed connective tissue disease, and scleroderma. The mechanism of the immunomodulatory effects of MSCs is not completely understood, although both direct and indirect actions have been suggested through either cell-cell interaction or soluble factors that create a local immunosuppressive environment. MSCs also alter the cytokine secretion profiles of dendritic cells, naive and effector T cells, and NK cells to induce a more profound anti-inflammatory or tolerant phenotype. Secretion of the proinflammatory cytokines, TNF-α and IFN-γ, is decreased whereas that of the suppressive IL-4 and IL-10 is strongly stimulated (46). Other factors involved in the immunosuppression have been shown to include hepatocyte growth factor, TGF-β1, IL-10, IL-6, prostaglandin E_2, nitric oxide, and possibly indoleamine 2,3-dioxygnease. Although the precise mechanism has yet to be clarified (38, 50), a large body of evidences suggests that MSCs are immunosuppressive and anti-inflammatory and can be transplanted between MHC-incompatible individuals. Single injection of primary murine MSCs could prevent the occurrence of severe arthritis, associated with a decreased pro-inflammatory cytokines in serum (51). Recently, the systemic injection of MSCs engineered to overexpress IL-10 significantly reduces the arthritic symptoms contrary to the injection of naïve MSCs (52). Several other studies have indicated the limitation of MSC based therapy due to its limited regeneration potentials, unidentified homing mechanism as well as long-term culture may leads to unstable culture and the possibility of malignancy. The first study on the use of MSCs in CIA (collagen induced arthritis) showed that the allogeneic C3H10T1/2 cells were unable to decrease the clinical signs of arthritis and even worsen the disease in a murine model (53). One of the groups suggested that the systemic injection of allogeneic, as well as autologous BM-derived primary MSCs could prevent the disease, but did not have any curative effects (54). Overall, the effect of MSCs on the immune cells is to tip off the immune response toward a tolerant and anti-inflammatory phenotype. These immunomodulatory effects appear not to be limited to MSCs themselves but also are shared by other mesenchymal cells. MSC- differentiated cells as well as various stromal cells from different tissues, including chondrocytes and fibroblasts, have also been shown to have immunosuppressive effects under certain conditions (36, 55). MSCs have been shown to decrease the severity of CIA, but so far very few clinical trials is going on despite the convincing evidence that primary MSCs could inhibit human T-cell proliferation by *in vitro* (56). Similar results have been recently obtained with human adipose-derived stem cells (ADSCs), which share similar properties with MSCs. The authors concluded that ADSCs suppressed T-cell response through the generation/activation of antigen-specific Tregs (57). The immunomodulatory role of MSCs is dose dependent, and two injections of bone marrow (BM)-MSCs on days 18 and 24 significantly improved arthritic symptoms (58). The mechanisms involved are suggested as to be through $CD4^{+}CD25^{+}Foxp3^{+}$ Treg cell induction as well as T-cell anergy or Treg activation (59, 60). MSCs treatment in immunized mice induced the proliferation of antigen-specific clones of Tregs with a CD4+CD25+CD27+Foxp3+ phenotype, suggesting that the immunosuppressive activity of MSCs could be prolonged by the action of Treg clones that is activated by an antigen-specific stimulus (51). A recent result showed that ADSCs both prevented and treated CIA by significantly reducing the incidence and severity of experimental arthritis (61). In this study, treatment with ADSCs inhibited the production of various inflammatory mediators, decreased the expansion of antigen-specific Th1/Th17 cell, and induced the production of anti-inflammatory cytokine interleukin-10. Moreover, ADSCs could induce the generation of antigen-specific Tregs with the capacity to suppress collagen-specific T cell responses. Currently, a clinical trial based on MSC transplantation has been initiated to treat RA; clinicians are trying to asses the safety and efficacy of umbilical cord-derived MSCs for RA at phase I/II levels (NCT01547091, www.Clinical.Trials.gov).

5. HSC (hematopoietic stem cell)-based therapy in RA

Out of several advantages of HSC-based therapy, one potential of using HSC lines for transplantation in patients with autoimmune diseases is that these cells can be recovered from unaffected individuals. Thus, genetic makeup is defined and will not be affected by genetic influence whereas ESCs will be affected by genetic influences (62). In addition, by using genetically selected or engineered cell types may further limit the possibility of disease progression or re-emergence. There are several studies in the past that used cell-based approaches to treat active, destructive, refractory and inflammatory arthritis that involved HSC transplantation (HSCT) (62-65) and juvenile idiopathic arthritis (66, 67). Although this treatment was curative for some patients, prolonged immunosuppression after HSCT was associated with a significant risk of infection, which limited the potential of this therapy (68, 69). One other potential problem of using non-self HSCs is the possible immune rejection of the transplanted cells. Under these circumstances, ESC-derived HSCs or other blood cells may offer distinct advantages over cord blood and BM-derived HSC lines in avoiding rejection of the transplant. In future, there is a hope for the development of deposit banks of ESCs expressing various combinations of the three most critical MHC molecules that can be utilized to allow close matching to the recipient's MHC composition. However, data from these trials implicated that Tregs, as a critical component of the regulatory state, will be functioning in the newly reconstituted immune system after transplant. In patients with juvenile idiopathic arthritis treated with HSCT, post-transplant reconstitution of $CD4^{+}CD25^{high}$ Treg was more rapid than that of $CD4^{+}CD25^{-}$ cells. This preferential recovery of Tregs could result from the relative resistance of Tregs to apoptosis after genotoxic stress (70). These results imply that there are other approaches to shift the balance of the immune system away from inflammation and toward regulation, *e.g.*, those that selectively bolster Treg numbers or function, may prove to be successful and less risky than HSCT.

6. Regulatory T cell-based therapy in RA

Tregs play an important role in the prevention of autoimmunity, and have ability to modulate the severity of CIA (71, 72). Deficiencies in Treg function have been identified in a wide variety of human autoimmune disorders, including RA (73-76). The majority of the reports suggested that biological or stem cells therapy will induce a potent population of Tregs in patients with RA (57, 59, 60), but the natural Treg defect will persist in responding patients after anti-TNF treatment (77). A few studies suggested that Tregs isolated from patients with active RA were competent at suppressing conventional T cell proliferation but not cytokine production (73). A recent report suggested that reduced expression and functional abnormalities in Tregs associated with cytotoxic T lymphocyte-associated antigen 4 (CTLA-4) could account for the Treg defect in patients with RA (78).

Tregs comprise about 5-10% of the mature CD4+ T helper cell subpopulation in mice and about 1-2% of CD4+ T cells in human. Tregs are composed of thymus-derived, naturally occurring $CD4^+CD25^+Foxp3^+$ Tregs (nTregs) as well as adaptive (also called 'induced') Tregs (iTregs) that are generated from $CD4^+CD25^-Foxp3^-$ naive T cells in the periphery. Unlike other cell-surface markers used to identify Tregs, Foxp3 is not up-regulated upon activation, and discriminates Tregs from activated effectors T cells. On the other hand, Foxp3 is also expressed in T cells without conferring any regulatory functions. nTregs are characterized by the expression of CD25, CD45RB, CD62L, CD103, CD95 (Fas), MHC class II, CD127, neuropiln-1 lymphocyt activation gene-3 (LAG-3), CTLA-4, glucocorticoid-induced TNFR family related gene (GITR), and Foxp3. iTreg cells are also characterized as expressing the same markers as nTreg cells but arise from $CD4^+D25^+FoxP3^-$ precursor cells. iTreg cells are further classified into two subgroups on the basis of TGF-β or IL-10 production. Recently, it was reported that human $CD4^+FoxP3^+$ T cells have three distinct populations with precise phenotypes and fates which includes, $CD25^{++}$ $CD45RA^+$ ($Foxp3^{lo}$) resting Tregs (rTreg cells), $CD25^{+++}$ $CD45RA^-$ ($Foxp3^{hi}$) activated Tregs (aTregs), and $CD25^{++}$ $CD45RA^-$ ($Foxp3^{hi}$) cytokines-secreting T cells which lack suppressive activity (79). The first two groups of phenotypes represent different stages of Treg cell differentiation and are both playing suppressive function *in vitro*. However, the new and exclusive cell surface marker of Tregs is still an area of intense research.

One critical factor in Treg cell-based therapy is the survival of Tregs. Tregs are highly susceptible to apoptosis in the absence of common gamma chain (γc) cytokines (*i.e.*, IL-2, IL-4, IL-7, IL-9, IL-15, and IL-21) because Tregs do not produce these cytokines and depend on other cells (80, 81). Tregs are also susceptible to apoptosis due to the low expression of the anti-apoptotic bcl-2 family members (82). Bcl-xL is an anti-apoptotic factor that is able to prolong the life span of apoptosis-prone lymphocytes. ß-catenin enhances the survival of $CD4^+CD25^+$ Tregs *in vitro* without altering their anergic state or suppressive function by modulating the antiapoptotic bcl-xl gene expression in Tregs (83). Recent reports (84) suggest that bcl-xL is involved in the development and function of Tregs by inducing the expression of Foxp3, CTLA-4, TGF-β, and repressing the programmed death receptor-1 (PD-I) expression. Additionally, Foxp3 and bcl-xL could cooperatively promote Treg cell survival and prevention of arthritis development due to the increased life span of Tregs (85). These approaches promote Treg cell differentiation and long-term survival thus results in the long-lasting Treg cell persistence.

Several studies have shown improvement of inflammation, *e.g.*, that seen in murine antigen-induced arthritis, by transfusion of functional Tregs (86-89). It has ignited some debates regarding the potential use in cellular therapy for RA. One approach to boost number of Tregs without myeloablative conditioning is to isolate Tregs from patients, expand them in culture, and then re-infuse the cells (90). Expansion of pre-existing Treg cell subsets *ex vivo* and transfuse back into patients in carefully controlled conditions to ensure the preservation of the regulatory capacity may be helpful, but could require large numbers of Tregs to be effective (91, 92). *Ex vivo* Treg cell expansion and re-infusion has successfully prevented or reversed a number of autoimmune diseases in mouse models, including models of inflammatory arthritis (93-97). There are several limitations and pitfalls in the treatment of patients with Tregs. Incomplete lineage commitment enables some human Tregs to express nuclear factor ROR-γt and to develop into IL-17-producing effector cells (98-100). It is also possible that cells become unstable after transfusion, particularly in an inflammatory environment, pathogenic responses might be exacerbated. Contamination of therapeutic Tregs with these unstable Tregs, or even with true autoreactive effector T cells, could lead to deterioration rather than attenuation of the autoimmune process. Tregs may be less effective in suppressing effector T cells in an autoimmune setting, and may even augment IL-17 production *in vitro (100-102)*. The ability to generate iTreg cells *in vitro* by culturing $CD4^+$ T cells in the presence of TGF-β provides a mechanism by which large numbers of functional iTreg cells could be generated for adoptive transfer into patients with RA, however, TGF-β-induced Tregs are potentially unstable and would pose a risk of converting into pathogenic responder T cells (103, 104). There are also several other disadvantages of the *in vitro* expansion or generation of Tregs for transfer back to patients, which include the risk of contamination from pathogenic responder T cells that could exacerbate the disease, and the generation of polyclonal Tregs that could initiate a generalized immunosuppression. In spite of these potential concerns, however, clinical trials are underway to test the therapeutic potential of Tregs in graft-versus-host diseases. Ectopic expression of the regulatory transcription factor, Foxp3, has been used to convert conventional $CD4^+$ T cells into Tregs with regulatory function (87, 105). A powerful approach to generating large numbers of antigen-specific Tregs has been demontrated by the introduction of T cell receptor (TCR) gene into purified CD4+CD25+ T cells as well as co-transfer of Foxp3 and TCR genes to convert conventional $CD4^+$ T cells into antigen-specific Tregs (88). However, important safety concerns remained for the application of this approach. TCR-transduced Tregs as well as Foxp3+TCR-transduced $CD4^+$ T cells selectively accumulated in the draining lymph nodes of the antigen-challenged knee, indicating that both were able to respond to the antigen stimulation in *vivo* compared to PBS-treated control mice. There was no increase in Th17 cells in the T cell-treated mice, indicating that in the *in vivo* environment of inflammatory arthritis neither the engineered Tregs nor the engineered $CD4^+$ T cells converted into Th17 cells. In a series of studies, both populations displayed characteristic markers of nTregs (CD25, CTLA-4, and GITR) and demonstrated suppressive activity. These studies open the possibility to target Tregs to tissue-specific antigens for the treatment of autoimmune tissue damage. Recent strategies have used the foot-and-mouth disease virus 2A or 2A-like elements to create multicistronic vectors capable of generating multiple proteins from the same transcript. A single 2A peptide-linked retroviral vector has been used successfully to generate reliable and versatile gene therapy vectors that can be used in biomedical research (106). In addition, co-expression of Foxp3 and bcl-xL linked by a 2A sequence in CD4$^+$ cells is critical for augmenting the differentiation and persistence of Tregs. Most significantly, the co-introduction of these molecules into CD4$^+$ T cells resulted in their ability to significantly block the development of arthritis in a murine model (87). These data provide new insights toward the generation of highly reactive Tregs for adoptive immunotherapy of autoimmune disease. However, adoptive cell transfer did not cure established arthritis, which could be explained by the absence of specificity that directs the movement of Tregs to the inflamed paw. Thus, generation of antigen-specific highly reactive Tregs may be a promising approach for the treatment of established autoimmune diseases.

7. Concept of stem cell-derived Treg-based therapy in RA

Because of the intrinsic resistance of Tregs to exogenous expansion and a high number of Tregs are required to perform the Treg-based immunotherapy, it becomes imminent to isolate a larger Treg cell subset for exogenous expansion and adoptive transfer, as discussed above, there are number problem and limitations to generate a large number of Tregs regardless of an increasing number of protocols for isolating subsets of Tregs, no approach to date has been confirmed the capacity to isolate the entire Treg cell population with 100 percent specificity. ESCs or iPSCs have the remarkable potential to develop into many different cell types in the body during early life and growth. ES or iPSC can give rise to all the blood cell types including myeloide (*e.g.*, monocytes and macrophages, neutrophiles, basophiles, eosinophiles, erythrocytes, megakaryocytes/platelets, dendritic cells) and lymphiode lineage (*e.g.*, T cells, B cells, NK cells). Whether ESCs or iPSCs will provide advantages over cord blood or adult BM-derived HSC remains to be determined. However, HSCs or MSCs, have limited potentials for self-renewal and the differentiation decline in response to differentiation signals with with each cycle compared to pluripotent ESCs or iPSCs (107). HSCs are present in differentiated cultures from human ESCs and from human fetal-derived embryonic germ stem cells (108-112). In contrast, iPSCs could be generated from mouse and human somatic cells by introducing Oct3/4 and Sox2 with either Klf4 and c-Myc or Nanog and Lin28 by using retroviruses or lentiviruses-mediated transduction (113-116). In addition, iPSCs are similar to natural pluripotent stem cells (*e.g.*, ESCs) in many respects, such as the expression of certain stem cell genes and proteins, chromatin methylation patterns, doubling time, embryoid body formation, teratoma formation, viable chimera formation, and potency and differentiability, but the full extent of the relations to natural pluripotent stem cells are still being assessed (117, 118). The use of iPSCs can bypass ethical and feasibility issues related to the use of ESCs and HSCs. The iPS technology continues to progress rapidly, and clinically applicable iPSCs can be generated from patients with noninvasive medical procedures. Collectively, iPSCs have a greater potential to be used in adoptive cell transfer (ACT)-based immunotherapy for autoimmune diseases compared to ESCs and HSCs.

Previously, pluripotent stem cells (*e.g.*, ESCs, HSCs) have been shown to differentiate into T cells *in vitro*, and recently iPSCs have been demonstrated to have the ability to differentiate into T cells (123) and antigen-specific CD8+ cytotoxic T lymphocytes (CTLs) (124). In these studies, murine iPSCs were genetically modified with ovalbumin (OVA)-specific MHC I-restricted TCR (OT-I) by retrovirus-mediated transduction. These iPSCs differentiated into functional antigen-specific CTLs *in vivo* and significantly protected the hosts from a tumor challenge (124). Thus, a new approach to generate a high number of functional Tregs from ESCs or iPSCs may be used for the treatment of autoimmune diseases (Figures 1-3). ESCs and iPSCs can be induced to differentiate into antigen specific or naïve Tregs *in vitro* through a Notch-mediated signaling. Genetic modification of iPSCs or ESCs with the Foxp3 gene and antigen specific TCR as well as stimulation with an *in vitro* Notch ligand will direct iPSC differentiation into Tregs, which are able to produce suppressive cytokines and inhibit

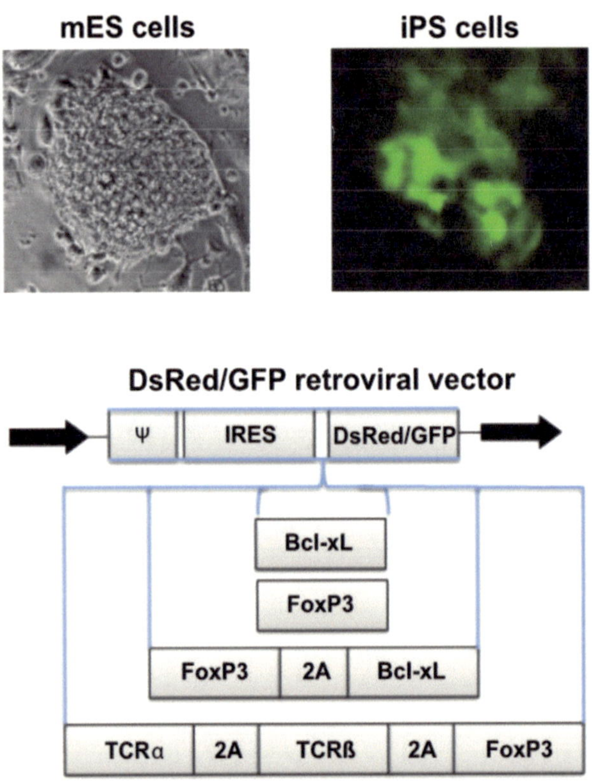

Figure 1. Generation of muticistronic construct for antigen-specific Tregs. (A) Mouse ES cells & iPS cells were maintained on feeder layers of irradiated SNL76/7 cells in 6-well culture plates and were passaged every 3 days. In brief, iPSCs were maintained in DMEM culture medium supplemented with 15% fetal calf serum (FCS), 0.1 mmol/L nonessential amino acids, 1 mmol/L l-glutamine, and 0.1 mmol/L β-mercaptoethanol. (B) Schematic representation of the retrovirus construct based on MiDR vector contain bcl-xL, or Foxp3, or Foxp3 + bcl-xL or TCRα + TCRβ + FoxP3, ψ, packaging signal; 2A, picornavirus self-cleaving 2A sequence; LTR, long terminal repeats; DsRed and IRES bidirectional promoter.

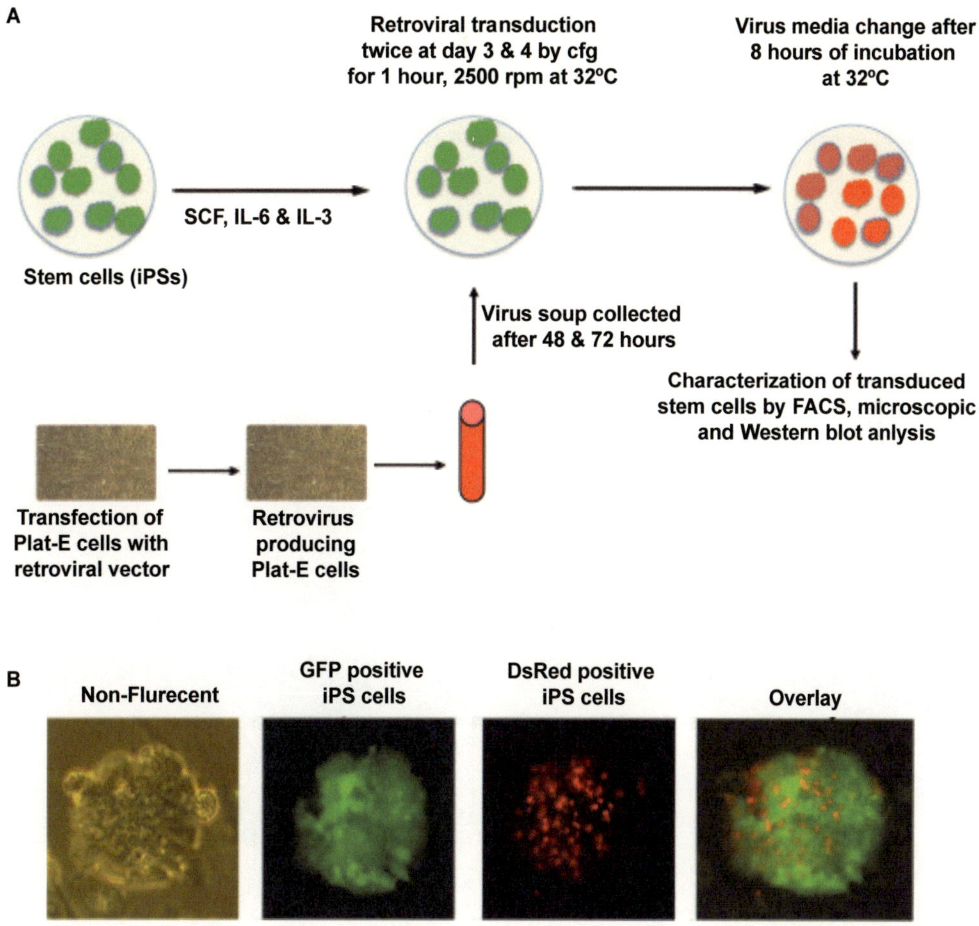

Figure 2. Retroviral transduction of stem cells. (A) Schematic representation of retroviral transduction. Retroviral transduction was performed as described before (124). 5×10^4 iPSCs were cultured in the presence of stem cell factor (SCF), IL-6 and IL-3 for 48 hours in 24 well plate coated with 1% gelatin. At the same time virus producing packaging cells line were transfected with retroviral construct containing gene of interests. After 2 days, the supernatant was replaced with 1 ml viral supernatant containing 10 µg/ml Polybrene, and the cells were spun for 1 h at 32°C and incubated at 32°C for 8 h. This was repeated the following day. Viral supernatant was removed and replaced with fresh medium, and iPSCs were re-cultured on fresh feeder layer. Expression of DsRed was determined by flow cytometry by gating on double positive (GFP + DsRed) iPSCs. DsRed-expressing iPSCs can be enriched and purified by cell sorting using a high-speed cell sorter and can be further use for differentiation and characterization. (B) Gene-transduced iPSCs were visualized by fluorescence microscopy.

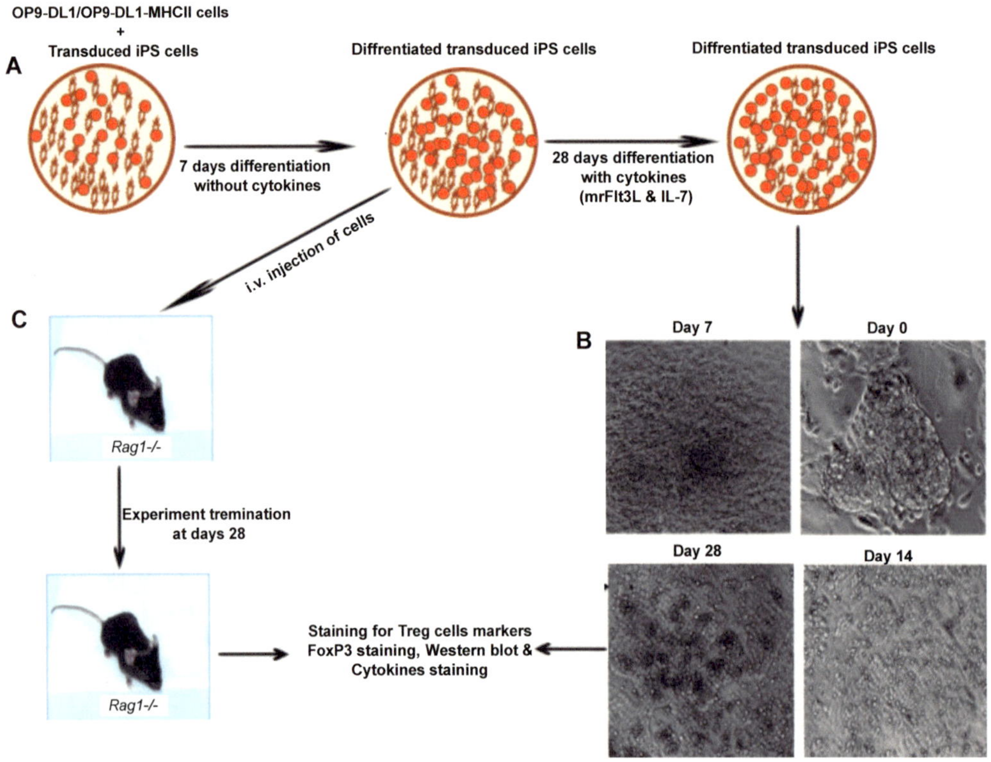

Figure 3. *In vivo* & *in vitro* differentiations of transduced iPSCs. (A) Schematic representation of *in vitro* stem cells differentiation. Monolayers of OP9-DL1/OP9DL-1-MHC-II cells were cultured in α-MEM medium supplemented with 20% FCS and 2.2 g/L sodium bicarbonate. Gene-transduced, sorted and purified iPSCs were washed once in OP9-DL1 medium before plating onto subconfluent OP9-DL1 monolayers for Treg lineage differentiation in the presence of murine recombinant 5 ng/ml Flt-3 ligand and 1 ng/ml murine rIL-7 after day 7. (B). Morphology of Treg cell differentiation on days 0, 7, 14, and 28. (C) Foxp3-transduced iPSCs were co-cultured on OP9-DL1 cells for 7 days, and adoptively transferred into *Rag1-/-* mice that had no mature T cells or B cells. After 6 weeks, antigen-specific Treg cell development can be determined (*e.g.*, we observed CD4+ CD25+ Foxp3+ Tregs in the lymph nodes (LN) and spleen and the cells had the ability to produce TGF-β and IL-10). Thus, Foxp3-tranduced iPSCs are capable of differentiating into functional Tregs both *in vitro* and *in vivo*.

other immune cell activities. In addition, gene transduction of antigen-specific TCR will result in iPSC or ESC-derived Tregs exhibiting a uniform expression of antigen-specific TCR following *in vitro* or *in vivo* development. This approach will help generate large numbers of functional antigen-specific Tregs. Therefore, gene transduction of iPSC or ESCs followed by T lineage differentiation through an *in vitro* Notch signaling or an *in vivo* approach will generate large numbers of monoclonal antigen-specific Tregs, which can be used for Treg-based immunotherapy. These cells could be able to persist *in vivo*, unlike cells generated via the current therapeutic regimen, and will likely contribute toward the treatment of autoimmune diseases (such as type I diabetes, RA, and system lupus erythematosus). The use of iPSCs as a mean to develop disease-specific immune cells for immunotherapy has a great potential in the prevention of many diseases. Collectively, iPSCs have a greater potential to be used in Treg-based immunotherapy for autoimmune diseases compared to ESCs and HSCs.

8. Conclusion

Biologic agents have revolutionized the treatment of RA by reducing the signs and symptoms and improving physical function and quality of life in affected patients, and also showed promising data to treat many diseases. However, question remains for their side effects. Improved knowledge of the pathophysiology will lead to the recognition of more reliable and practical predictors of the disease course and treatment response. Stem cell-based therapies offer many exciting opportunities for the development of novel treatment and cure for autoimmune diseases. The multipotent autologous stem cells have potential to treat disorders involving connective tissue because of their differentiation potential. In addition, the multipotent autologous stem cells have significant effects on a variety of autoimmune diseases because of their immunomodulatory immune response. Despite of the great potential and convincing evidence that primary MSCs inhibit human T-cell proliferation *in vitro* and decrease the severity of CIA in mouse models, there are very few clinical trials are going on worldwide and recent trials have produced mixed results. The results of clinical trails question the efficacy of MSCs in disease conditions in part due to incomplete understanding of the fate of MSC after infusion despite of the positive safety aspects. Because of the plasticity and potentially unlimited capacity for self-renewal, iPSC-derived Tregs may be applied for Treg cell adoptive immunotherapy, such as cancer, autoimmune disorders, and infectious or aging-related diseases. A challenging research effort remains to fully examine this potential and to address several remaining questions, which include how to direct the differentiation of specific cell types, generate large number of differentiated cells in the best possible ways and determine which particular type of stem cell will be optimal for each therapeutic approach. However, stem cells or their progeny may provide one of several better roads for future delivery of immune cell-based therapies. The approaches for generation of antigen-specific Tregs from iPSCs provide an important foundation for the ultimate generation of patient- and/or disease-specific Treg-based therapies. However, to explore the potential to alleviate these devastating chronic diseases with the use of stem cell-based technologies is still enormous.

Author details

Rizwanul Haque, Fengyang Lei, Xiaofang Xiong and Jianxun Song
Department of Microbiology and Immunology,
The Pennsylvania State University College of Medicine, Hershey, PA, USA

Acknowledgement

This project was funded, in part, under grants with the Grant Number K18CA151798 from the National Cancer Institute (NCI) and the Melanoma Research Foundation to J.S.

9. References

[1] Firestein GS. Evolving concepts of rheumatoid arthritis. Nature. [Research Support, U.S. Gov't, P.H.S. Review]. 2003 May 15;423(6937):356-61.

[2] Akil M, Amos RS. ABC of rheumatology. Rheumatoid arthritis--I: Clinical features and diagnosis. Bmj. [Review]. 1995 Mar 4;310(6979):587-90.

[3] Steiner G, Smolen J. Autoantibodies in rheumatoid arthritis and their clinical significance. Arthritis Res. [Research Support, Non-U.S. Gov't Review]. 2002;4 Suppl 2:S1-5.

[4] Cooke TD, Hurd ER, Jasin HE, Bienenstock J, Ziff M. Identification of immunoglobulins and complement in rheumatoid articular collagenous tissues. Arthritis Rheum. [Research Support, U.S. Gov't, P.H.S.]. 1975 Nov-Dec;18(6):541-51.

[5] Haraoui B, Pelletier JP, Cloutier JM, Faure MP, Martel-Pelletier J. Synovial membrane histology and immunopathology in rheumatoid arthritis and osteoarthritis. In vivo effects of antirheumatic drugs. Arthritis Rheum. [Research Support, Non-U.S. Gov't]. 1991 Feb;34(2):153-63.

[6] Sweeney SE, Firestein GS. Signal transduction in rheumatoid arthritis. Curr Opin Rheumatol. [Review]. 2004 May;16(3):231-7.

[7] McInnes IB, Schett G. The pathogenesis of rheumatoid arthritis. N Engl J Med. [Review]. 2011 Dec 8;365(23):2205-19.

[8] Plenge RM, Cotsapas C, Davies L, Price AL, de Bakker PI, Maller J, et al. Two independent alleles at 6q23 associated with risk of rheumatoid arthritis. Nat Genet. [Research Support, N.I.H., Extramural Research Support, Non-U.S. Gov't]. 2007 Dec;39(12):1477-82.

[9] Raychaudhuri S, Remmers EF, Lee AT, Hackett R, Guiducci C, Burtt NP, et al. Common variants at CD40 and other loci confer risk of rheumatoid arthritis. Nat Genet. [Comparative Study Meta-Analysis Research Support, N.I.H., Extramural Research Support, N.I.H., Intramural Research Support, Non-U.S. Gov't]. 2008 Oct;40(10):1216-23.

[10] Barton A, Thomson W, Ke X, Eyre S, Hinks A, Bowes J, et al. Rheumatoid arthritis susceptibility loci at chromosomes 10p15, 12q13 and 22q13. Nat Genet. [Comparative Study Research Support, Non-U.S. Gov't]. 2008 Oct;40(10):1156-9.

[11] van der Helm-van Mil AH, Verpoort KN, Breedveld FC, Huizinga TW, Toes RE, de Vries RR. The HLA-DRB1 shared epitope alleles are primarily a risk factor for anti-cyclic citrullinated peptide antibodies and are not an independent risk factor for development of rheumatoid arthritis. Arthritis Rheum. [Research Support, Non-U.S. Gov't]. 2006 Apr;54(4):1117-21.
[12] van der Helm-van Mil AH, Wesoly JZ, Huizinga TW. Understanding the genetic contribution to rheumatoid arthritis. Curr Opin Rheumatol. [Review]. 2005 May;17(3):299-304.
[13] van der Helm-van Mil AH, Huizinga TW, Schreuder GM, Breedveld FC, de Vries RR, Toes RE. An independent role of protective HLA class II alleles in rheumatoid arthritis severity and susceptibility. Arthritis Rheum. [Research Support, Non-U.S. Gov't]. 2005 Sep;52(9):2637-44.
[14] Hinks A, Eyre S, Ke X, Barton A, Martin P, Flynn E, et al. Overlap of disease susceptibility loci for rheumatoid arthritis and juvenile idiopathic arthritis. Ann Rheum Dis. [Multicenter Study Research Support, Non-U.S. Gov't]. 2010 Jun;69(6):1049-53.
[15] Hinks A, Ke X, Barton A, Eyre S, Bowes J, Worthington J, et al. Association of the IL2RA/CD25 gene with juvenile idiopathic arthritis. Arthritis Rheum. [Research Support, N.I.H., Extramural Research Support, Non-U.S. Gov't]. 2009 Jan;60(1):251-7.
[16] Alenius GM, Friberg C, Nilsson S, Wahlstrom J, Dahlqvist SR, Samuelsson L. Analysis of 6 genetic loci for disease susceptibility in psoriatic arthritis. J Rheumatol. [Multicenter Study Research Support, Non-U.S. Gov't]. 2004 Nov;31(11):2230-5.
[17] Bridges SL, Jr. The genetics of rheumatoid arthritis: influences on susceptibility, severity, and treatment response. Curr Rheumatol Rep. [Review]. 1999 Dec;1(2):164-71.
[18] Colmegna I, Diaz-Borjon A, Fujii H, Schaefer L, Goronzy JJ, Weyand CM. Defective proliferative capacity and accelerated telomeric loss of hematopoietic progenitor cells in rheumatoid arthritis. Arthritis Rheum. [Research Support, N.I.H., Extramural]. 2008 Apr;58(4):990-1000.
[19] Porta C, Caporali R, Epis O, Ramaioli I, Invernizzi R, Rovati B, et al. Impaired bone marrow hematopoietic progenitor cell function in rheumatoid arthritis patients candidated to autologous hematopoietic stem cell transplantation. Bone Marrow Transplant. 2004 Apr;33(7):721-8.
[20] Snowden JA, Nink V, Cooley M, Zaunders J, Keir M, Wright L, et al. Composition and function of peripheral blood stem and progenitor cell harvests from patients with severe active rheumatoid arthritis. Br J Haematol. [Research Support, Non-U.S. Gov't]. 1998 Dec;103(3):601-9.
[21] Papadaki HA, Kritikos HD, Gemetzi C, Koutala H, Marsh JC, Boumpas DT, et al. Bone marrow progenitor cell reserve and function and stromal cell function are defective in rheumatoid arthritis: evidence for a tumor necrosis factor alpha-mediated effect. Blood. [Research Support, Non-U.S. Gov't]. 2002 Mar 1;99(5):1610-9.
[22] Snowden JA, Biggs JC, Milliken ST, Fuller A, Staniforth D, Passuello F, et al. A randomised, blinded, placebo-controlled, dose escalation study of the tolerability and efficacy of filgrastim for haemopoietic stem cell mobilisation in patients with severe

active rheumatoid arthritis. Bone Marrow Transplant. [Clinical Trial Randomized Controlled Trial Research Support, Non-U.S. Gov't]. 1998 Dec;22(11):1035-41.

[23] Colmegna I, Pryshchep S, Oishi H, Goronzy JJ, Weyand CM. Dampened ERK signaling in hematopoietic progenitor cells in rheumatoid arthritis. Clin Immunol. 2012 Apr;143(1):73-82.

[24] Zivojinovic SM, Pejnovic NN, Sefik-Bukilica MN, Kovacevic LV, Soldatovic, II, Damjanov NS. Tumor necrosis factor blockade differentially affects innate inflammatory and th17 cytokines in rheumatoid arthritis. J Rheumatol. [Research Support, Non-U.S. Gov't]. 2012 Jan;39(1):18-21.

[25] Jurgens MS, Jacobs JW, Bijlsma JW. The use of conventional disease-modifying anti-rheumatic drugs in established RA. Best Pract Res Clin Rheumatol. [Review]. 2011 Aug;25(4):523-33.

[26] Aravena O, Pesce B, Soto L, Orrego N, Sabugo F, Wurmann P, et al. Anti-TNF therapy in patients with rheumatoid arthritis decreases Th1 and Th17 cell populations and expands IFN-gamma-producing NK cell and regulatory T cell subsets. Immunobiology. [Research Support, Non-U.S. Gov't]. 2011 Dec;216(12):1256-63.

[27] Boyce EG, Halilovic J, Stan-Ugbene O. Golimumab: Review of the efficacy and tolerability of a recently approved tumor necrosis factor-alpha inhibitor. Clin Ther. [Review]. 2010 Sep;32(10):1681-703.

[28] De Stefano R, Frati E, Nargi F, Baldi C, Menza L, Hammoud M, et al. Comparison of combination therapies in the treatment of rheumatoid arthritis: leflunomide-anti-TNF-alpha versus methotrexate-anti-TNF-alpha. Clin Rheumatol. [Comparative Study Randomized Controlled Trial]. 2010 May;29(5):517-24.

[29] van Vollenhoven RF, Geborek P, Forslind K, Albertsson K, Ernestam S, Petersson IF, et al. Conventional combination treatment versus biological treatment in methotrexate-refractory early rheumatoid arthritis: 2 year follow-up of the randomised, non-blinded, parallel-group Swefot trial. Lancet. 2012 Mar 28.

[30] Jani M, Hyrich KL. Abatacept in the long-term treatment of rheumatoid arthritis. Expert Rev Clin Immunol. 2012 Mar;8(3):231-4.

[31] Mori S, Sugimoto M. Is continuation of anti-tumor necrosis factor-alpha therapy a safe option for patients who have developed pulmonary mycobacterial infection? : Case presentation and literature review. Clin Rheumatol. 2012 Feb;31(2):203-10.

[32] Soliman MM, Hyrich KL, Lunt M, Watson KD, Symmons DP, Ashcroft DM. Effectiveness of rituximab in patients with rheumatoid arthritis: observational study from the British Society for Rheumatology Biologics Register. J Rheumatol. [Research Support, Non-U.S. Gov't]. 2012 Feb;39(2):240-6.

[33] Nam JL, Winthrop KL, van Vollenhoven RF, Pavelka K, Valesini G, Hensor EM, et al. Current evidence for the management of rheumatoid arthritis with biological disease-modifying antirheumatic drugs: a systematic literature review informing the EULAR recommendations for the management of RA. Ann Rheum Dis. [Review]. 2010 Jun;69(6):976-86.

[34] Dominici M, Le Blanc K, Mueller I, Slaper-Cortenbach I, Marini F, Krause D, et al. Minimal criteria for defining multipotent mesenchymal stromal cells. The International Society for Cellular Therapy position statement. Cytotherapy. 2006;8(4):315-7.

[35] Jorgensen C, Djouad F, Bouffi C, Mrugala D, Noel D. Multipotent mesenchymal stromal cells in articular diseases. Best Pract Res Clin Rheumatol. [Review]. 2008 Apr;22(2):269-84.

[36] Le Blanc K, Tammik C, Rosendahl K, Zetterberg E, Ringden O. HLA expression and immunologic properties of differentiated and undifferentiated mesenchymal stem cells. Exp Hematol. [Research Support, Non-U.S. Gov't]. 2003 Oct;31(10):890-6.

[37] Tse WT, Pendleton JD, Beyer WM, Egalka MC, Guinan EC. Suppression of allogeneic T-cell proliferation by human marrow stromal cells: implications in transplantation. Transplantation. 2003 Feb 15;75(3):389-97.

[38] Le Blanc K, Ringden O. Immunomodulation by mesenchymal stem cells and clinical experience. J Intern Med. [Research Support, Non-U.S. Gov't Review]. 2007 Nov;262(5):509-25.

[39] Eliopoulos N, Stagg J, Lejeune L, Pommey S, Galipeau J. Allogeneic marrow stromal cells are immune rejected by MHC class I- and class II-mismatched recipient mice. Blood. [Research Support, Non-U.S. Gov't Research Support, U.S. Gov't, Non-P.H.S.]. 2005 Dec 15;106(13):4057-65.

[40] Prigozhina TB, Khitrin S, Elkin G, Eizik O, Morecki S, Slavin S. Mesenchymal stromal cells lose their immunosuppressive potential after allotransplantation. Exp Hematol. 2008 Oct;36(10):1370-6.

[41] Corcione A, Benvenuto F, Ferretti E, Giunti D, Cappiello V, Cazzanti F, et al. Human mesenchymal stem cells modulate B-cell functions. Blood. [Research Support, Non-U.S. Gov't]. 2006 Jan 1;107(1):367-72.

[42] Jiang XX, Zhang Y, Liu B, Zhang SX, Wu Y, Yu XD, et al. Human mesenchymal stem cells inhibit differentiation and function of monocyte-derived dendritic cells. Blood. [Research Support, Non-U.S. Gov't]. 2005 May 15;105(10):4120-6.

[43] Noel D, Djouad F, Bouffi C, Mrugala D, Jorgensen C. Multipotent mesenchymal stromal cells and immune tolerance. Leuk Lymphoma. [Review]. 2007 Jul;48(7):1283-9.

[44] Spaggiari GM, Capobianco A, Abdelrazik H, Becchetti F, Mingari MC, Moretta L. Mesenchymal stem cells inhibit natural killer-cell proliferation, cytotoxicity, and cytokine production: role of indoleamine 2,3-dioxygenase and prostaglandin E2. Blood. [Research Support, Non-U.S. Gov't]. 2008 Feb 1;111(3):1327-33.

[45] Pevsner-Fischer M, Morad V, Cohen-Sfady M, Rousso-Noori L, Zanin-Zhorov A, Cohen S, et al. Toll-like receptors and their ligands control mesenchymal stem cell functions. Blood. [Research Support, Non-U.S. Gov't]. 2007 Feb 15;109(4):1422-32.

[46] Aggarwal S, Pittenger MF. Human mesenchymal stem cells modulate allogeneic immune cell responses. Blood. [Comparative Study Research Support, U.S. Gov't, Non-P.H.S.]. 2005 Feb 15;105(4):1815-22.

[47] Beyth S, Borovsky Z, Mevorach D, Liebergall M, Gazit Z, Aslan H, et al. Human mesenchymal stem cells alter antigen-presenting cell maturation and induce T-cell unresponsiveness. Blood. 2005 Mar 1;105(5):2214-9.

[48] Liotta F, Angeli R, Cosmi L, Fili L, Manuelli C, Frosali F, et al. Toll-like receptors 3 and 4 are expressed by human bone marrow-derived mesenchymal stem cells and can inhibit their T-cell modulatory activity by impairing Notch signaling. Stem Cells. [Research Support, Non-U.S. Gov't]. 2008 Jan;26(1):279-89.
[49] Chen FH, Tuan RS. Mesenchymal stem cells in arthritic diseases. Arthritis Res Ther. [Research Support, N.I.H., Intramural Review]. 2008;10(5):223.
[50] Uccelli A, Pistoia V, Moretta L. Mesenchymal stem cells: a new strategy for immunosuppression? Trends Immunol. [Research Support, Non-U.S. Gov't Review]. 2007 May;28(5):219-26.
[51] Augello A, Tasso R, Negrini SM, Cancedda R, Pennesi G. Cell therapy using allogeneic bone marrow mesenchymal stem cells prevents tissue damage in collagen-induced arthritis. Arthritis Rheum. [Research Support, Non-U.S. Gov't]. 2007 Apr;56(4):1175-86.
[52] Choi JJ, Yoo SA, Park SJ, Kang YJ, Kim WU, Oh IH, et al. Mesenchymal stem cells overexpressing interleukin-10 attenuate collagen-induced arthritis in mice. Clin Exp Immunol. [Comparative Study Research Support, Non-U.S. Gov't]. 2008 Aug;153(2):269-76.
[53] Djouad F, Fritz V, Apparailly F, Louis-Plence P, Bony C, Sany J, et al. Reversal of the immunosuppressive properties of mesenchymal stem cells by tumor necrosis factor alpha in collagen-induced arthritis. Arthritis Rheum. [Research Support, Non-U.S. Gov't]. 2005 May;52(5):1595-603.
[54] Bouffi C, Djouad F, Mathieu M, Noel D, Jorgensen C. Multipotent mesenchymal stromal cells and rheumatoid arthritis: risk or benefit? Rheumatology (Oxford). [Research Support, Non-U.S. Gov't Review]. 2009 Oct;48(10):1185-9.
[55] Jones S, Horwood N, Cope A, Dazzi F. The antiproliferative effect of mesenchymal stem cells is a fundamental property shared by all stromal cells. J Immunol. 2007 Sep 1;179(5):2824-31.
[56] Zheng ZH, Li XY, Ding J, Jia JF, Zhu P. Allogeneic mesenchymal stem cell and mesenchymal stem cell-differentiated chondrocyte suppress the responses of type II collagen-reactive T cells in rheumatoid arthritis. Rheumatology (Oxford). [Research Support, Non-U.S. Gov't]. 2008 Jan;47(1):22-30.
[57] Gonzalez-Rey E, Gonzalez MA, Varela N, O'Valle F, Hernandez-Cortes P, Rico L, et al. Human adipose-derived mesenchymal stem cells reduce inflammatory and T cell responses and induce regulatory T cells in vitro in rheumatoid arthritis. Ann Rheum Dis. [Research Support, Non-U.S. Gov't]. 2010 Jan;69(1):241-8.
[58] Bouffi C, Bony C, Courties G, Jorgensen C, Noel D. IL-6-dependent PGE2 secretion by mesenchymal stem cells inhibits local inflammation in experimental arthritis. PLoS One. [Research Support, Non-U.S. Gov't]. 2010;5(12):e14247.
[59] Roord ST, de Jager W, Boon L, Wulffraat N, Martens A, Prakken B, et al. Autologous bone marrow transplantation in autoimmune arthritis restores immune homeostasis through CD4+CD25+Foxp3+ regulatory T cells. Blood. [Research Support, Non-U.S. Gov't]. 2008 May 15;111(10):5233-41.
[60] Zappia E, Casazza S, Pedemonte E, Benvenuto F, Bonanni I, Gerdoni E, et al. Mesenchymal stem cells ameliorate experimental autoimmune encephalomyelitis

inducing T-cell anergy. Blood. [Research Support, Non-U.S. Gov't]. 2005 Sep 1;106(5):1755-61.

[61] Zhou B, Yuan J, Zhou Y, Ghawji M, Jr., Deng YP, Lee AJ, et al. Administering human adipose-derived mesenchymal stem cells to prevent and treat experimental arthritis. Clin Immunol. [Research Support, Non-U.S. Gov't]. 2011 Dec;141(3):328-37.

[62] Tyndall A, LeBlanc K. Stem cells and rheumatology: update on adult stem cell therapy in autoimmune diseases. Arthritis Rheum. 2006 Aug 15;55(4):521-5.

[63] Snowden JA, Passweg J, Moore JJ, Milliken S, Cannell P, Van Laar J, et al. Autologous hemopoietic stem cell transplantation in severe rheumatoid arthritis: a report from the EBMT and ABMTR. J Rheumatol. [Meta-Analysis]. 2004 Mar;31(3):482-8.

[64] Teng YK, Verburg RJ, Sont JK, van den Hout WB, Breedveld FC, van Laar JM. Long-term followup of health status in patients with severe rheumatoid arthritis after high-dose chemotherapy followed by autologous hematopoietic stem cell transplantation. Arthritis Rheum. [Multicenter Study Research Support, Non-U.S. Gov't]. 2005 Aug;52(8):2272-6.

[65] Verburg RJ, Kruize AA, van den Hoogen FH, Fibbe WE, Petersen EJ, Preijers F, et al. High-dose chemotherapy and autologous hematopoietic stem cell transplantation in patients with rheumatoid arthritis: results of an open study to assess feasibility, safety, and efficacy. Arthritis Rheum. [Clinical Trial Clinical Trial, Phase I Clinical Trial, Phase II Multicenter Study Research Support, Non-U.S. Gov't]. 2001 Apr;44(4):754-60.

[66] Brinkman DM, de Kleer IM, ten Cate R, van Rossum MA, Bekkering WP, Fasth A, et al. Autologous stem cell transplantation in children with severe progressive systemic or polyarticular juvenile idiopathic arthritis: long-term follow-up of a prospective clinical trial. Arthritis Rheum. [Clinical Trial Research Support, Non-U.S. Gov't]. 2007 Jul;56(7):2410-21.

[67] De Kleer IM, Brinkman DM, Ferster A, Abinun M, Quartier P, Van Der Net J, et al. Autologous stem cell transplantation for refractory juvenile idiopathic arthritis: analysis of clinical effects, mortality, and transplant related morbidity. Ann Rheum Dis. [Evaluation Studies Research Support, Non-U.S. Gov't]. 2004 Oct;63(10):1318-26.

[68] Daikeler T, Tichelli A, Passweg J. Complications of autologous hematopoietic stem cell transplantation for patients with autoimmune diseases. Pediatr Res. 2012 Apr;71(4-2):439-44.

[69] Snowden JA, Kapoor S, Wilson AG. Stem cell transplantation in rheumatoid arthritis. Autoimmunity. [Research Support, Non-U.S. Gov't Review]. 2008 Dec;41(8):625-31.

[70] Komatsu N, Hori S. Full restoration of peripheral Foxp3+ regulatory T cell pool by radioresistant host cells in scurfy bone marrow chimeras. Proc Natl Acad Sci U S A. [Research Support, Non-U.S. Gov't]. 2007 May 22;104(21):8959-64.

[71] Morgan ME, Flierman R, van Duivenvoorde LM, Witteveen HJ, van Ewijk W, van Laar JM, et al. Effective treatment of collagen-induced arthritis by adoptive transfer of CD25+ regulatory T cells. Arthritis Rheum. [Research Support, Non-U.S. Gov't]. 2005 Jul;52(7):2212-21.

[72] Oh S, Rankin AL, Caton AJ. CD4+CD25+ regulatory T cells in autoimmune arthritis. Immunol Rev. [Research Support, N.I.H., Extramural Research Support, Non-U.S. Gov't Review]. 2010 Jan;233(1):97-111.

[73] Ehrenstein MR, Evans JG, Singh A, Moore S, Warnes G, Isenberg DA, et al. Compromised function of regulatory T cells in rheumatoid arthritis and reversal by anti-TNFalpha therapy. J Exp Med. [Research Support, Non-U.S. Gov't]. 2004 Aug 2;200(3):277-85.

[74] Esensten JH, Wofsy D, Bluestone JA. Regulatory T cells as therapeutic targets in rheumatoid arthritis. Nat Rev Rheumatol. [Review]. 2009 Oct;5(10):560-5.

[75] Valencia X, Stephens G, Goldbach-Mansky R, Wilson M, Shevach EM, Lipsky PE. TNF downmodulates the function of human CD4+CD25hi T-regulatory cells. Blood. [Research Support, N.I.H., Intramural]. 2006 Jul 1;108(1):253-61.

[76] Viglietta V, Baecher-Allan C, Weiner HL, Hafler DA. Loss of functional suppression by CD4+CD25+ regulatory T cells in patients with multiple sclerosis. J Exp Med. [In Vitro Research Support, Non-U.S. Gov't Research Support, U.S. Gov't, P.H.S.]. 2004 Apr 5;199(7):971-9.

[77] Nadkarni S, Mauri C, Ehrenstein MR. Anti-TNF-alpha therapy induces a distinct regulatory T cell population in patients with rheumatoid arthritis via TGF-beta. J Exp Med. [In Vitro Research Support, Non-U.S. Gov't]. 2007 Jan 22;204(1):33-9.

[78] Flores-Borja F, Jury EC, Mauri C, Ehrenstein MR. Defects in CTLA-4 are associated with abnormal regulatory T cell function in rheumatoid arthritis. Proc Natl Acad Sci U S A. [Research Support, Non-U.S. Gov't]. 2008 Dec 9;105(49):19396-401.

[79] Miyara M, Wing K, Sakaguchi S. Therapeutic approaches to allergy and autoimmunity based on FoxP3+ regulatory T-cell activation and expansion. J Allergy Clin Immunol. 2009 Apr;123(4):749-55; quiz 56-7.

[80] Pandiyan P, Lenardo MJ. The control of CD4+CD25+Foxp3+ regulatory T cell survival. Biol Direct. 2008;3:6.

[81] Pandiyan P, Zheng L, Ishihara S, Reed J, Lenardo MJ. CD4+CD25+Foxp3+ regulatory T cells induce cytokine deprivation-mediated apoptosis of effector CD4+ T cells. Nat Immunol. 2007 Dec;8(12):1353-62.

[82] Taams LS, Smith J, Rustin MH, Salmon M, Poulter LW, Akbar AN. Human anergic/suppressive CD4(+)CD25(+) T cells: a highly differentiated and apoptosis-prone population. Eur J Immunol. 2001 Apr;31(4):1122-31.

[83] Ding Y, Shen S, Lino AC, Curotto de Lafaille MA, Lafaille JJ. Beta-catenin stabilization extends regulatory T cell survival and induces anergy in nonregulatory T cells. Nat Med. 2008 Feb;14(2):162-9.

[84] Sharabi A, Lapter S, Mozes E. Bcl-xL is required for the development of functional regulatory CD4 cells in lupus-afflicted mice following treatment with a tolerogenic peptide. J Autoimmun. Mar;34(2):87-95.

[85] Haque R, Lei F, Xiong X, Wu Y, Song J. FoxP3 and Bcl-xL cooperatively promote regulatory T cell persistence and prevention of arthritis development. Arthritis Res Ther.12(2):R66.

[86] Frey O, Petrow PK, Gajda M, Siegmund K, Huehn J, Scheffold A, et al. The role of regulatory T cells in antigen-induced arthritis: aggravation of arthritis after depletion and amelioration after transfer of CD4+CD25+ T cells. Arthritis Res Ther. [Research Support, Non-U.S. Gov't]. 2005;7(2):R291-301.

[87] Haque R, Lei F, Xiong X, Wu Y, Song J. FoxP3 and Bcl-xL cooperatively promote regulatory T cell persistence and prevention of arthritis development. Arthritis research & therapy. [Research Support, Non-U.S. Gov't]. 2010;12(2):R66.

[88] Wright GP, Notley CA, Xue SA, Bendle GM, Holler A, Schumacher TN, et al. Adoptive therapy with redirected primary regulatory T cells results in antigen-specific suppression of arthritis. Proc Natl Acad Sci U S A. [Research Support, Non-U.S. Gov't]. 2009 Nov 10;106(45):19078-83.

[89] Zaiss MM, Frey B, Hess A, Zwerina J, Luther J, Nimmerjahn F, et al. Regulatory T cells protect from local and systemic bone destruction in arthritis. J Immunol. [Research Support, Non-U.S. Gov't]. 2010 Jun 15;184(12):7238-46.

[90] Brusko T, Bluestone J. Clinical application of regulatory T cells for treatment of type 1 diabetes and transplantation. Eur J Immunol. [Research Support, N.I.H., Extramural Research Support, Non-U.S. Gov't]. 2008 Apr;38(4):931-4.

[91] Peters JH, Hilbrands LB, Koenen HJ, Joosten I. Ex vivo generation of human alloantigen-specific regulatory T cells from CD4(pos)CD25(high) T cells for immunotherapy. PLoS One. [Research Support, Non-U.S. Gov't]. 2008;3(5):e2233.

[92] Putnam AL, Brusko TM, Lee MR, Liu W, Szot GL, Ghosh T, et al. Expansion of human regulatory T-cells from patients with type 1 diabetes. Diabetes. [Research Support, Non-U.S. Gov't]. 2009 Mar;58(3):652-62.

[93] Kohm AP, Carpentier PA, Anger HA, Miller SD. Cutting edge: CD4+CD25+ regulatory T cells suppress antigen-specific autoreactive immune responses and central nervous system inflammation during active experimental autoimmune encephalomyelitis. J Immunol. [Research Support, U.S. Gov't, P.H.S.]. 2002 Nov 1;169(9):4712-6.

[94] Masteller EL, Warner MR, Tang Q, Tarbell KV, McDevitt H, Bluestone JA. Expansion of functional endogenous antigen-specific CD4+CD25+ regulatory T cells from nonobese diabetic mice. J Immunol. [Research Support, N.I.H., Extramural Research Support, Non-U.S. Gov't Research Support, U.S. Gov't, P.H.S.]. 2005 Sep 1;175(5):3053-9.

[95] Mottet C, Uhlig HH, Powrie F. Cutting edge: cure of colitis by CD4+CD25+ regulatory T cells. J Immunol. [Research Support, Non-U.S. Gov't]. 2003 Apr 15;170(8):3939-43.

[96] Scalapino KJ, Tang Q, Bluestone JA, Bonyhadi ML, Daikh DI. Suppression of disease in New Zealand Black/New Zealand White lupus-prone mice by adoptive transfer of ex vivo expanded regulatory T cells. J Immunol. [Comparative Study Research Support, Non-U.S. Gov't Research Support, U.S. Gov't, Non-P.H.S.]. 2006 Aug 1;177(3):1451-9.

[97] Tang Q, Henriksen KJ, Bi M, Finger EB, Szot G, Ye J, et al. In vitro-expanded antigen-specific regulatory T cells suppress autoimmune diabetes. J Exp Med. [Research Support, Non-U.S. Gov't Research Support, U.S. Gov't, P.H.S.]. 2004 Jun 7;199(11):1455-65.

[98] Beriou G, Costantino CM, Ashley CW, Yang L, Kuchroo VK, Baecher-Allan C, et al. IL-17-producing human peripheral regulatory T cells retain suppressive function. Blood.

[Research Support, N.I.H., Extramural Research Support, Non-U.S. Gov't]. 2009 Apr 30;113(18):4240-9.

[99] Koenen HJ, Smeets RL, Vink PM, van Rijssen E, Boots AM, Joosten I. Human CD25highFoxp3pos regulatory T cells differentiate into IL-17-producing cells. Blood. 2008 Sep 15;112(6):2340-52.

[100] Voo KS, Wang YH, Santori FR, Boggiano C, Arima K, Bover L, et al. Identification of IL-17-producing FOXP3+ regulatory T cells in humans. Proc Natl Acad Sci U S A. [Research Support, N.I.H., Extramural Research Support, Non-U.S. Gov't]. 2009 Mar 24;106(12):4793-8.

[101] Annunziato F, Cosmi L, Liotta F, Maggi E, Romagnani S. The phenotype of human Th17 cells and their precursors, the cytokines that mediate their differentiation and the role of Th17 cells in inflammation. Int Immunol. [Research Support, Non-U.S. Gov't Review]. 2008 Nov;20(11):1361-8.

[102] Evans HG, Suddason T, Jackson I, Taams LS, Lord GM. Optimal induction of T helper 17 cells in humans requires T cell receptor ligation in the context of Toll-like receptor-activated monocytes. Proc Natl Acad Sci U S A. [Research Support, N.I.H., Extramural Research Support, Non-U.S. Gov't]. 2007 Oct 23;104(43):17034-9.

[103] Zhou X, Bailey-Bucktrout SL, Jeker LT, Penaranda C, Martinez-Llordella M, Ashby M, et al. Instability of the transcription factor Foxp3 leads to the generation of pathogenic memory T cells in vivo. Nat Immunol. [Research Support, N.I.H., Extramural Research Support, Non-U.S. Gov't]. 2009 Sep;10(9):1000-7.

[104] Zhou X, Kong N, Zou H, Brand D, Li X, Liu Z, et al. Therapeutic potential of TGF-beta-induced CD4(+) Foxp3(+) regulatory T cells in autoimmune diseases. Autoimmunity. [Research Support, N.I.H., Extramural Research Support, Non-U.S. Gov't Research Support, U.S. Gov't, Non-P.H.S. Review]. 2011 Feb;44(1):43-50.

[105] Hori S, Nomura T, Sakaguchi S. Control of regulatory T cell development by the transcription factor Foxp3. Science. 2003 Feb 14;299(5609):1057-61.

[106] Zhao B, Song A, Haque R, Lei F, Weiler L, Xiong X, et al. Cooperation between molecular targets of costimulation in promoting T cell persistence and tumor regression. J Immunol. [Research Support, N.I.H., Extramural Research Support, Non-U.S. Gov't]. 2009 Jun 1;182(11):6744-52.

[107] Himburg HA, Muramoto GG, Daher P, Meadows SK, Russell JL, Doan P, et al. Pleiotrophin regulates the expansion and regeneration of hematopoietic stem cells. Nature medicine. [Research Support, N.I.H., Extramural]. 2010 Apr;16(4):475-82.

[108] Itskovitz-Eldor J, Schuldiner M, Karsenti D, Eden A, Yanuka O, Amit M, et al. Differentiation of human embryonic stem cells into embryoid bodies compromising the three embryonic germ layers. Mol Med. [Research Support, Non-U.S. Gov't]. 2000 Feb;6(2):88-95.

[109] Ledran MH, Krassowska A, Armstrong L, Dimmick I, Renstrom J, Lang R, et al. Efficient hematopoietic differentiation of human embryonic stem cells on stromal cells derived from hematopoietic niches. Cell Stem Cell. [Research Support, Non-U.S. Gov't]. 2008 Jul 3;3(1):85-98.

[110] Lu SJ, Feng Q, Caballero S, Chen Y, Moore MA, Grant MB, et al. Generation of functional hemangioblasts from human embryonic stem cells. Nat Methods. [Research Support, N.I.H., Extramural Research Support, Non-U.S. Gov't]. 2007 Jun;4(6):501-9.
[111] Shamblott MJ, Axelman J, Littlefield JW, Blumenthal PD, Huggins GR, Cui Y, et al. Human embryonic germ cell derivatives express a broad range of developmentally distinct markers and proliferate extensively in vitro. Proc Natl Acad Sci U S A. 2001 Jan 2;98(1):113-8.
[112] Wang L, Menendez P, Cerdan C, Bhatia M. Hematopoietic development from human embryonic stem cell lines. Exp Hematol. [Research Support, Non-U.S. Gov't Review]. 2005 Sep;33(9):987-96.
[113] Park IH, Zhao R, West JA, Yabuuchi A, Huo H, Ince TA, et al. Reprogramming of human somatic cells to pluripotency with defined factors. Nature. [Research Support, N.I.H., Extramural Research Support, Non-U.S. Gov't]. 2008 Jan 10;451(7175):141-6.
[114] Takahashi K, Tanabe K, Ohnuki M, Narita M, Ichisaka T, Tomoda K, et al. Induction of pluripotent stem cells from adult human fibroblasts by defined factors. Cell. 2007 Nov 30;131(5):861-72.
[115] Takahashi K, Yamanaka S. Induction of pluripotent stem cells from mouse embryonic and adult fibroblast cultures by defined factors. Cell. [Research Support, Non-U.S. Gov't]. 2006 Aug 25;126(4):663-76.
[116] Yu J, Vodyanik MA, Smuga-Otto K, Antosiewicz-Bourget J, Frane JL, Tian S, et al. Induced pluripotent stem cell lines derived from human somatic cells. Science. [Research Support, N.I.H., Extramural Research Support, Non-U.S. Gov't]. 2007 Dec 21;318(5858):1917-20.
[117] Chin MH, Mason MJ, Xie W, Volinia S, Singer M, Peterson C, et al. Induced pluripotent stem cells and embryonic stem cells are distinguished by gene expression signatures. Cell Stem Cell. [Research Support, N.I.H., Extramural Research Support, Non-U.S. Gov't]. 2009 Jul 2;5(1):111-23.
[118] Kiskinis E, Eggan K. Progress toward the clinical application of patient-specific pluripotent stem cells. J Clin Invest. [Research Support, Non-U.S. Gov't Review]. 2010 Jan;120(1):51-9.
[119] La Motte-Mohs RN, Herer E, Zuniga-Pflucker JC. Induction of T-cell development from human cord blood hematopoietic stem cells by Delta-like 1 in vitro. Blood. 2005 Feb 15;105(4):1431-9.
[120] Schmitt TM, Ciofani M, Petrie HT, Zuniga-Pflucker JC. Maintenance of T cell specification and differentiation requires recurrent notch receptor-ligand interactions. J Exp Med. [Comparative Study Research Support, Non-U.S. Gov't]. 2004 Aug 16;200(4):469-79.
[121] Schmitt TM, de Pooter RF, Gronski MA, Cho SK, Ohashi PS, Zuniga-Pflucker JC. Induction of T cell development and establishment of T cell competence from embryonic stem cells differentiated in vitro. Nat Immunol. [Research Support, Non-U.S. Gov't]. 2004 Apr;5(4):410-7.

[122] Timmermans F, Velghe I, Vanwalleghem L, De Smedt M, Van Coppernolle S, Taghon T, et al. Generation of T cells from human embryonic stem cell-derived hematopoietic zones. J Immunol. [Research Support, Non-U.S. Gov't]. 2009 Jun 1;182(11):6879-88.

[123] Lei F, Haque R, Weiler L, Vrana KE, Song J. T lineage differentiation from induced pluripotent stem cells. Cell Immunol. [Research Support, Non-U.S. Gov't]. 2009;260(1):1-5.

[124] Lei F, Zhao B, Haque R, Xiong X, Budgeon L, Christensen ND, et al. In vivo programming of tumor antigen-specific T lymphocytes from pluripotent stem cells to promote cancer immunosurveillance. Cancer Res. 2011 Jul 15;71(14):4742-7.

Chapter 14

Biologic Treatment in Rheumatoid Arthritis

Katerina Chatzidionysiou

Additional information is available at the end of the chapter

http://dx.doi.org/10.5772/50745

1. Introduction

Rheumatoid arthritis (RA) is a common, chronic, inflammatory disease. It affects around 1% of the adult population in all age groups, although the incidence peaks during the fifth decade of life. The aetiology of RA is unknown, but it is considered to be autoimmune in nature. Inflammation in the synovial tissues of the joints is the hallmark of RA, causing pain, stiffness, loss of function and progressive destruction of the cartilage and bone in the inflamed joints in the majority of patients. Early diagnosis and appropriate treatment is crucial for the amelioration of symptoms, improvement of function and prevention of structural damage.

Traditionally, treatment of RA has been based on the use of a group of disease-modifying antirheumatic drugs (DMARDs), of which methotrexate (MTX) is the most widely used, often in combination with corticosteroids and/or NSAIDs (non-steroid anti-inflammatory drugs). Leflunomide, sulphasalazine, azathioprine, are examples of other synthetic DMARDs. The landscape of RA treatment has changed dramatically during the last decade due to the introduction of biologic DMARDs, small molecules that target small molecules (like cytokines) and cells of the immune system, important mediators of the immunological mechanisms in RA. To date, nine biologic agents have been approved for the treatment of RA and more molecules with distinct mechanisms of action are currently being tested in laboratories and in clinical trials. The good efficacy and general safety of these agents is well established from both clinical and epidemiological trials, but there are still several issues that remain unclear or need further study, such as long-term safety, more individualized treatment by finding predictors of response, cost-effectiveness, when to introduce biologic treatment and the feasibility of discontinuation after achieving low disease activity or remission.

Biologic (generic name)	Adalimumab	Certolizumab pegol	Etanercept	Golimumab	Infliximab
Brand name	Humira	Cimzia	Enbrel	Simponi	**Remicade**
Structure	monoclonal antibody, fully humanized	PEGylated Fab' fragment of humanized anti-TNF monoclonal antibody	Dimerized soluble TNF receptor	monoclonal antibody, fully humanized	Chimeric anti-TNF monoclonal antibody
Mechanism of action	TNF inhibition				
Approved dosage	40 mg	200 mg	50 mg	50 mg	**3 mg/kg**
Approved interval	every 2 weeks	every 2 weeks	once weekly	once monthly	**every 8 weeks**
Route of administration	Subcutaneous	Subcutaneous	Subcutaneous	Subcutaneous	**Intravenous**
Biologic (generic name)	**Abatacept**	**Anakinra**	**Rituximab**	**Tocilizumab**	
Brand name	Orencia	Kineret	MabThera (Rituxan)	RoActemra (Actemra)	
Structure	Dimerized CTLA4 molecule	Recombinant IL-1 receptor antagonist	Chimeric anti-CD20 monoclonal antibody	Humanized anti-IL-6 receptor antibody	
Mechanism of action	Inhibits T-cell activation	Binds IL-1 receptor	Binds and eliminates B cells	Binds IL-6 receptor	
Approved dosage	500–1000 mg	100 mg	1000 mg x 2 (with 2 weeks interval)	8 mg/kg	
Approved interval	once monthly	once daily	every 6–12 months	once monthly	
Route of administration	Intravenous	Subcutaneous	Intravenous	Intravenous	

Table 1. Biologic agents approved for the treatment of rheumatoid arthritis (RA).

2. Biologic agents

TNF (tumor necrosis factor) is a key cytokine of the immune response. Analysis of cytokine mRNA and protein in rheumatoid arthritis tissue revealed that many proinflammatory cytokines such as TNF alpha, IL-1 and IL-6 are abundant in all patients regardless of therapy[1]. These cytokines are of major importance in rheumatoid arthritis and are therapeutic targets. Five TNF inhibitors have been approved for the treatment of RA: the monoclonal antibodies infliximab (chimeric), adalimumab and golimumab (fully human), the TNF receptor etanercept, and the PEGylated Fab fragment of a fully human anti-TNF monoclonal antibody certolizumab pegol. There are several differences in pharmacodynamics and pharmacokinetics between these agents (table 1). Apart from the TNF inhibitors, biologics with different mechanism of action have been increasingly used in the clinical practice. Rituximab targets CD20 on the surface of B-cells and have been widely used in hematology for lymphoma treatment; Tocilizumab is an IL-6 (interleukin 6) inhibitor while anakinra blocks IL-1. Finally, abatacept inhibits costimulation of T-cell by binding B7 (table 1).

3. Efficacy of biological DMARDs

Numerous randomized clinical trials provide clear evidence on the efficacy of biologic agents in RA, both in early disease (short disease duration) in biologic-naïve population and in late RA (longer disease duration) after failure of traditional DMARDs. These trials show the superiority of combination treatment of a biologic agent with methotrexate versus methotrexate monotherapy in both early and late disease[2-18]. In figure 1 and 2 the ACR 20, 50 and 70 responses[*] of TNF inhibitors and other biologics from the largest clinical trials in methotrexate naïve patients and after inadequate response to methotrexate, are shown. The data demonstrate also clearly, especially in the MTX-naïve population, that a considerable proportion of patients respond to the simpler and less expensive monotherapy with methotrexate (MTX). Thus, one should keep in mind that in the combination groups, there are patients who would have responded to MTX monotherapy as well.

In figure 2, the clinical responses of other biologic agents plus MTX versus placebo plus MTX are summarized. Again efficacy in early and in late disease is evident. Superiority of rituximab over placebo was observed in the IMAGE and SERENE trials[9,10]. Abatacept demonstrated acceptable safety and clinically meaningful efficacy in methotrexate naïve patients and methotrexate non responders[7,11]. Additionally, in the TOWARD trial[17], tocilizumab-treated patients achieved significantly better results than those who received placebo during the first 6 months of therapy, after inadequate response to traditional

[*] ACR responses is a validate tool for the evaluation of efficacy of treatment in RA. ACR 20/50/70 response is defined as at least 20, 50 or 70%, respectively, improvement in both swollen joint count (SJC) and tender joint count (TJC), and at least 20, 50 and 70% improvement in 3 of the 5 following measures: pain VAS (visual analogue scale), Patient global assessment, Physician global assessment, ESR (erythrocyte sedimentation rate) or CRP (C-reactive protein) and functional questionnaire.

DMARDs. A large trial on the efficacy of tocilizumab in early RA is currently conducted. All these biologic agents seem to have comparable efficacy and significantly greater efficacy than placebo.

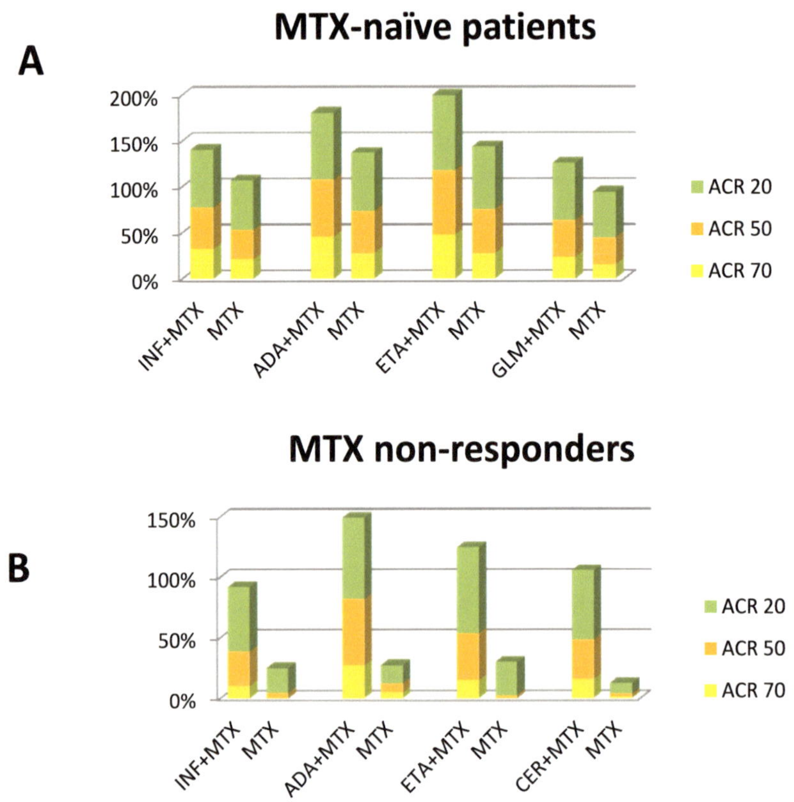

Figure 1. **A and B.** Efficacy of TNF inhibitors (infliximab INF, etanercept ETA, adalimumab ADA, golimumab GLM, certolizumab pegol (CER) in combination with methotrexate (MTX) versus MTX monotherapy in MTX-naïve RA patients (1A) and RA patients with an inadequate response to MTX (1B). Efficacy is assessed by ACR 20, 50 and 70 responses.

4. Safety of biological DMARDs

Extension phase of clinical trials as well as data from registry studies provide us with important information about the safety of biologic DMARDs. The safety profile is generally acceptable, with a small increase risk for infections being the most common adverse event[2-22]. Reactivation of latent tuberculosis is a well known risk during treatment with TNF inhibitors, therefore screening for tuberculosis is recommended before initiation of a TNF inhibitor. Infusion reaction is a common adverse event for rituximab and infliximab. Anti-TNF induced SLE and demyelinating disease are rare complications of TNF inhibitors. Regarding risk for malignancies, data so far have not shown any clear increase in risk for malignancies. A meta-analysis of clinical registries and prospective observational studies showed no increase in malignancies other than skin cancers, including lymphoma, associated with the use of TNF inhibitors[23]. However, longer follow up especially from large cohorts of patients, is needed.

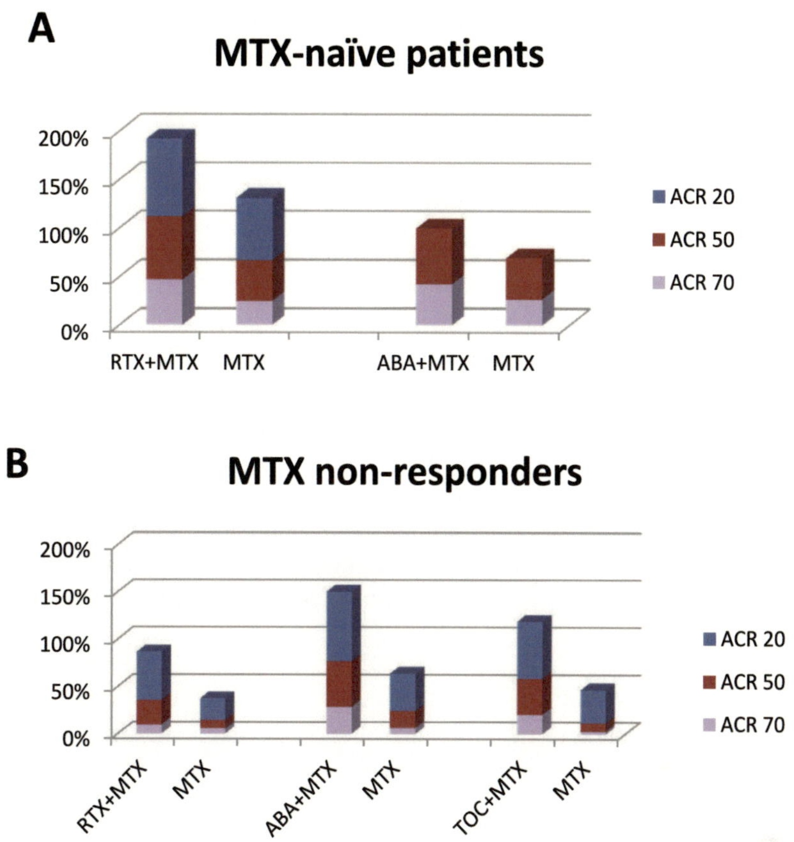

Figure 2. A and B. Efficacy of rituximab (RTX), abatacept (ABA) and tocilizumab (TOC) in combination with methotrexate (MTX) versus MTX monotherapy in MTX-naïve RA patients (2A) and RA patients with an inadequate response to MTX (2B). Efficacy is assessed by ACR 20, 50 and 70 responses.

5. When to start biologic agents

The effectiveness of biologic agents is well established in the above large, randomized clinical trials. These results do not, however, answer the question of when a biologic DMARD should be initiated. Traditional DMARDs, and most often methotrexate, unless contraindicated) is the first line treatment. However, about two third of patients who start treatment with methotrexate will discontinue treatment for reasons of either inefficacy or intolerance. The next step is either a combination of synthetic DMARDs (e.g. sulphasalazine and hydroxychloroquine) or introduction of a biologic agent. So far, only a few clinical trials have made a direct comparison of these two treatment options. In the SWEFOT trial, patients with early RA with an inadequate response to MTX after 3 months, defined as lack of achievement of low disease activity, were randomly allocated to addition of either sulphasalazine and hydroxychloroquine or infliximab. The latter group had significantly greater responses after 12 months of therapy, with 39% of patients achieving the primary endpoint (European League Against Rheumatism (EULAR) good response†, which is a widely used validated outcome) compared to 25% in the former group (p=0.016)[24]. However, at the 2-year follow-up assessment, the clinical difference was no longer present (EULAR Good response was 38% in infliximab group vs. 31% in the conventional DMARDs group (p=0.2), but radiological disease progression was significantly greater in the latter group than the former[25].

Similar results were established in the BeSt trial[26,27]. In the BeSt trial three treatment groups were formed: sequential DMARD monotherapy (group 1), step-up combination therapy (group 2), initial combination therapy with tapered high-dose prednisolone (group 3) and infliximab (group 4). It was shown that a more aggressive treatment strategy as in group 3 and 4 provided earlier clinical improvement than a less aggressive strategy as in groups 1 and 2. Low disease activity (defined by $DAS_{44} \leq 2.4$) was reached by 53%, 64%, 71% and 74% of patients in group 1, 2, 3 and 4, respectively (p=0.0004 for group 1 vs. 3, p=0.001 for group 1 vs. 4). After 2 years, patients in all four treatment groups had approximately the same improvement in disease activity and functional status irrespective of initial treatment, probably because of tight control and frequent treatment adjustments. However, the more aggressively treated patients had less radiological progression of joint damage, and during the second year more of them could be treated successfully with monotherapy, suggesting that the initial aggressive therapy did result in some long-term gains.

6. When to stop biologic agents

A significant number of patients who receive biological treatment achieve low disease activity or remission. It is often difficult to define these terms, and there are today several definitions of both low disease activity and remission. According to the 2011 ACR (American College of Rheumatology) / EULAR (EUropean League Against Rheumatism) criteria, remission of rheumatoid arthritis is defined as tender joint count ≤ 1 AND swollen joint count ≤ 1 AND C-reactive protein ≤ 1 mg/dl AND patient global assessment ≤ 1 (on a 0-10 scale) (boolean-based definition) or a Simplified Disease Activity Index score of ≤ 3.3 (Index-based definition)[28]. Other definitions of low disease activity and remission are also frequently used, as for example DAS28 score ≤ 3.2 (low disease activity) and DAS28 ≤ 2.6 (remission).

When a patient is in state of low disease activity or remission for a sufficiently long period of time (usually at least 6 months) the next step is to assess the feasibility of discontinuation of the biologic agent with the aim of maintaining the good clinical response. This is a

† Definition of EULAR responses:

DAS28 at endpoint	Improvement in DAS28 from baseline ≥1.2	>0.6 and <1.2	≤0.6
≤3.2	GOOD	MODERATE	NO
>3,2 and ≤5.1	MODERATE	MODERATE	NO
>5.1	MODERATE	NO	NO

DAS28=Disease Activity Score (based on 28 joint status)

$$DAS28= 0.56^* \sqrt{\mathbf{TJC28}} + 0.28^* \sqrt{\mathbf{SJC28}} + 0.70^*\ln(\mathbf{ESR}) + 0.014^* (\mathbf{General\ Health})$$

question of importance for reasons of safety and health economics. In various settings, the possibility has been investigated of discontinuing the biologic agent while maintaining the patient in remission on a conventional DMARD.

In the ATTRACT study 17 patients in a single centre in the UK received infliximab and all 17 experienced flare-ups after discontinuation of the biologic therapy after 2 years, with a mean time of 13.5–15.0 weeks after the end of therapy[29]. Of importance, re-introduction of infliximab after disease flare was associated with comparable responses without any safety issues. In another study Quinn et al. addressed the same question in a randomized, double-blind, placebo-controlled trial in a population of patients with early RA, with symptom duration of <12 months[2]. Induction of remission with infliximab plus MTX in early, poor prognosis RA provided not only significant reduction in synovitis and erosions at 1 year (shown by magnetic resonance imaging), but also sustained functional and quality-of-life benefits for 70% of the patients at 2 years despite infliximab withdrawal. These two studies tested the same question in different populations of RA patients; the former one in patients with longstanding disease (mean disease duration, 11 years), and the latter in patients with early RA. More recently, Tanaka et al. determined the possibility of discontinuing infliximab after attaining DAS-guided low disease activity in patients with RA in the remission induction by Remicade in RA (RRR) study[30]. Of 102 patients, 56 (55%) maintained $DAS28<3.2$ and 44 (43%) reached remission ($DAS28<2.6$) 1 year after the discontinuation of infliximab. The mean disease duration in this study was 5.9 years which suggests that discontinuation of infliximab would be possible not only in patients with early RA but also in patients with more established disease. In a post hoc analysis from the BeSt study, it was shown that significantly more patients who received initial combination therapy with infliximab and MTX achieved sustained $DAS_{44} \leq 2.4$ and were able to discontinue infliximab, compared with those with delayed introduction of the biologic agent (56% vs. 29%, $p=0.008$)[31,32]. It was also shown in the BeSt study that the shorter the symptom duration, the higher the likelihood of a biologic-free, and even a drug-free, remission. A systematic review and meta-analysis showed that patients with established RA who stopped treatment with traditional DMARDs had a significantly higher risk of disease flare or deterioration than those who continued treatment[33]. In this analysis, however, patients had RA of more than 2 years duration. Larger randomized, controlled, double-blind trials are needed in order to better approach this important issue.

Several conclusions can be drawn from the information that exists today about discontinuation of biologic DMARDs:

- Discontinuation of biologic treatment and sustained remission or low disease activity is the long-term therapeutic goal, important for matters of long-term safety and health economics.
- Biologic-free remission may be possible after achieving remission or low disease activity in a considerable proportion of patients.
- The duration of disease until the introduction of the biologic treatment may be negatively associated with the risk of deterioration after discontinuation of treatment, thus suggesting that earlier initiation of biologic treatment leads not only to better results, but also increases the possibility of withdrawal of biologic agents with maintenance of remission.

- More data about the feasibility of dose reduction or discontinuation of biological DMARDs are needed.

7. Principles for use of biologic treatment in rheumatoid arthritis

The rapid progress and advances in the field of biologic treatment in RA, combined with the high cost of these drugs and the potential long-term safety issues, makes it necessary to define clear rules that will guide the use of these agents in clinical practice.

The rheumatologist should always keep in mind that the goal of RA treatment today is remission or low disease activity, if remission cannot be achieved. Treatment efficacy should be assessed in tight time intervals and changes in treatment should be considered if the goal has not been reached[34].

As soon as the diagnosis of RA is established a synthetic DMARD (most often Methotrexate) is started with or without concomitant corticosteroids. If the goal of treatment is not achieved after 3 months, an additional DMARD can be added or a biologic agent can be introduced. As it was analyzed above, data have shown superiority of the latter choice. Especially for patients with multiple negative prognostic factors, such as seropositivity, radiographic progression and high disease activity, early aggressive treatment is strongly indicated. In the absence of these unfavorable factors one could consider testing switching of synthetic DMARD or combination of synthetic DMARD +/- corticosteroids before biologics. In patients with active RA who have not yet been treated with DMARDs there is strong evidence that biologics provide better results at the group level, but not widely used in practice based on various considerations (safety, high cost, possibility of very good effect of methotrexate).

The first biologic agent is most often a TNF inhibitor, unless contraindicated. If possible, TNF inhibitors should be combined with MTX; the clinical efficacy particularly the radiological efficacy of the combination is clearly superior to TNF inhibitor monotherapy. In case of a contraindication to TNF inhibitor therapy, a biologic agent with a different mechanism of action (rituximab, abatacept or tocilizumab) can be chosen.

About one third of patients will discontinue the first TNF inhibitor for reasons of either intolerance or inefficacy (lack of efficacy or loss of efficacy). Since the goal is still remission, even patients with moderate responses ('partial responders') should eventually be candidates for an alternative treatment.

After the failure of one biologic agent for the reasons described above, and after having perhaps tried to modify the dose of the concomitant DMARDs and/or corticosteroids with no effect, three main treatment options are available: a) optimize the dose of biologic drug; b) switch between TNF inhibitors; or c) switch to a biologic agent with a different mechanism of action.

7.1. Optimize dose of biologic

As it is shown in table 1, the TNF inhibitors have different dose intervals, ranging from once weekly (etanercept) to once every 8 weeks (infliximab). Concerning optimization of the infliximab dose, controversial data are available. In the ATTRACT trial, four different treatment regimens of infliximab were studied: infliximab 3 mg kg^{-1} every 4 and 8 weeks and 10 mg kg^{-1} every 4 and 8 weeks. At 24 weeks similar American College of Rheumatology (ACR) responses were observed. At 48 weeks, however, there was a tendency for the lowest dosage of infliximab to be less effective than the higher ones, but this difference was only significant with respect to the ACR50 responses[29].

An important question is whether dose increase or change of treatment interval can yield better results in patients with secondary loss of efficacy to infliximab. Results from uncontrolled observational studies have suggested that this might be true[35]. On the other hand, in a double-blind randomized trial, Pavelka *et al.* showed no significant difference in efficacy of two dosages of infliximab (3 and 5 mg/kg) after initial failure of the lower dosage to lead to remission[36]. Moreover, the higher dosage had a poorer safety profile. In an observational study conducted in our centre, patients in whom the dose of infliximab was increased in clinical practice appeared to have a benefit, as defined by reduction in the disease activity score (DAS28)[37]. However, patients in the control groups (i.e. patients with no change in infliximab dose and those receiving a stable dose of etanercept) also showed an improvement in DAS28. This observation suggests that the improvements were most probably attributable to regression to the mean and that no important benefit is gained from dose increases of infliximab. Finally, van den Bemt *et al.* found that 17 of 18 patients who were in clinical practice treated with infliximab at dosages higher than 3 mg/kg showed no deterioration of their RA if the dosage was reduced to 3 mg/kg[38]. In conclusion, the evidence suggests that increasing the dose of infliximab might result in loss of time, higher cost and potentially more side effects with no significant efficacy gain in most patients. Therefore, it would clearly be useful to be able to identify, using relevant biomarkers, a smaller subset of patients who might truly benefit from dose increases. Studies to investigate this possibility are currently underway.

7.2. Switching to an alternative TNF inhibitor

As it is shown in table 1, there are substantial differences between the five TNF inhibitors available today (in molecular structure, immunological actions and in pharmacokinetics). This is the reason why switching from one TNF inhibitor to another does make sense and is often used in the clinical practice, although these agents target the same cytokine. Observational studies support this argument, as a significant proportion of patients benefit from this switching. In the randomized double-blinded GO-AFTER study, patients who received golimumab after failure of a prior TNF inhibitor, showed significantly greater responses than those who received placebo[39]. However, cohort study data have shown a gradual loss of efficacy after a greater number of switches[40-44]. Thus, a first switch might provide significant improvement, whereas the effect is much less profound at the second or third switch.

7.3. Switch to a biologic with different mechanism of action

It might sound more reasonable, after the failure of TNF inhibition the next step to be change of mechanism, rather than switching between agents of the same drug class. There is strong evidence about the efficacy of rituximab, abatacept and tocilizumab after TNF treatment (figure 2). However, there is no randomized clinical trial comparing head to head these two treatment options, but there are some observational studies from national registries. In the Swiss Clinical Quality Management program for RA (SCQM-RA) registry, patients with inadequate response to TNF inhibitor treatment achieved greater reductions in DAS28 when switching to rituximab than to an alternative TNF blocker[45]. This was especially obvious when the reason for discontinuation of the previous TNF inhibitor was secondary inefficacy[46]. A small observational study by Venkatachalam *et al.* provided similar results, whilst a study reported by Buch *et al.* also demonstrated comparable results of rituximab and alternative TNF inhibitors[47,48]. Our data have shown slightly better overall results for patients who had failed TNF inhibitor therapy when treated with rituximab than with another TNF blocker, but both options provided clinical benefits[49].

In figure 3 an algorithm of biologic treatment in RA is presented[50].

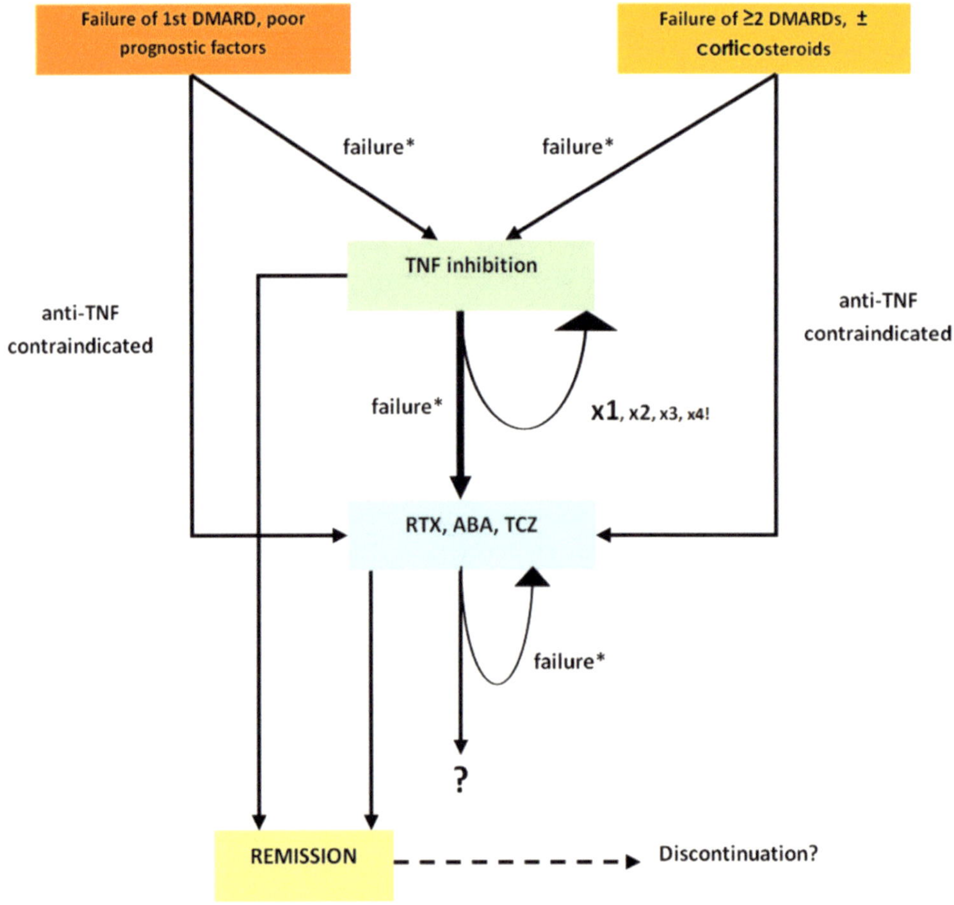

Failure*: primary or secondary loss of efficacy, intolerance or a partial, inadequate response. (After optimizing DMARD dose and/or trying combination of DMARDs).

Figure 3. Algorithm of biologic treatment in RA.

8. Conclusions

The field of RA treatment has changed dramatically after the introduction of biologic DMARDs. Despite the advances though, several issues remain to be further studied and clarified. On the one hand treatment algorithms are needed of the choice and time of introduction of biologics. On the other hand a more individualized treatment might be possible in the future. Such an approach is crucial, taking into consideration the increasing number of biologic agents, their high cost and the importance of choosing the right treatment from the beginning. These are some of the important challenges of clinical, epidemiological and basic rheumatologic research.

Author details

Katerina Chatzidionysiou
Unit for Clinical Therapy Research, Inflammatory Diseases, Karolinska Institute, Stockholm, Sweden

9. References

[1] Feldmann M, et al. *Role of cytokines in rheumatoid arthritis.* Annu Rev Immunol. 1996;14:397-440.

[2] Quinn, M.A., et al., *Very early treatment with infliximab in addition to methotrexate in early, poor-prognosis rheumatoid arthritis reduces magnetic resonance imaging evidence of synovitis and damage, with sustained benefit after infliximab withdrawal: results from a twelve-month randomized, double-blind, placebo-controlled trial.* Arthritis Rheum, 2005. 52(1): p. 27-35.

[3] St Clair, E.W., et al., *Combination of infliximab and methotrexate therapy for early rheumatoid arthritis: a randomized, controlled trial.* Arthritis Rheum, 2004. 50(11): p. 3432-43.

[4] Emery, P., et al., *Comparison of methotrexate monotherapy with a combination of methotrexate and etanercept in active, early, moderate to severe rheumatoid arthritis (COMET): a randomised, double-blind, parallel treatment trial.* Lancet, 2008. 372(9636): p. 375-82.

[5] Emery, P., et al., *Golimumab, a human anti-tumor necrosis factor alpha monoclonal antibody, injected subcutaneously every four weeks in methotrexate-naive patients with active rheumatoid arthritis: twenty-four-week results of a phase III, multicenter, randomized, double-blind, placebo-controlled study of golimumab before methotrexate as first-line therapy for early-onset rheumatoid arthritis.* Arthritis Rheum, 2009. 60(8): p. 2272-83.

[6] Breedveld, F.C., et al., *The PREMIER study: A multicenter, randomized, double-blind clinical trial of combination therapy with adalimumab plus methotrexate versus methotrexate alone or adalimumab alone in patients with early, aggressive rheumatoid arthritis who had not had previous methotrexate treatment.* Arthritis Rheum, 2006. 54(1): p. 26-37.

[7] Westhovens, R., et al., *Clinical efficacy and safety of abatacept in methotrexate-naive patients with early rheumatoid arthritis and poor prognostic factors.* Ann Rheum Dis, 2009. 68(12): p. 1870-7.

[8] Smolen, J.S., et al., *Effect of interleukin-6 receptor inhibition with tocilizumab in patients with rheumatoid arthritis (OPTION study): a double-blind, placebo-controlled, randomised trial.* Lancet, 2008. 371(9617): p. 987-97.

[9] Emery, P., et al., *Efficacy and safety of different doses and retreatment of rituximab: a randomised, placebo-controlled trial in patients who are biological naive with active rheumatoid arthritis and an inadequate response to methotrexate (Study Evaluating Rituximab's Efficacy in MTX iNadequate rEsponders (SERENE)).* Ann Rheum Dis.

[10] Tak PP, et al. *Inhibition of joint damage and improved clinical outcomes with rituximab plus methotrexate in early active rheumatoid arthritis: the IMAGE trial.* Ann Rheum Dis. 2011 Jan;70(1):39-46. Epub 2010 Oct 11.

[11] Kremer, J.M., et al., *Effects of abatacept in patients with methotrexate-resistant active rheumatoid arthritis: a randomized trial.* Ann Intern Med, 2006. 144(12): p. 865-76.

[12] Cohen, S.B., et al., *A multicentre, double blind, randomised, placebo controlled trial of anakinra (Kineret), a recombinant interleukin 1 receptor antagonist, in patients with rheumatoid arthritis treated with background methotrexate.* Ann Rheum Dis, 2004. 63(9): p. 1062-8.

[13] Maini, R., et al., *Infliximab (chimeric anti-tumour necrosis factor alpha monoclonal antibody) versus placebo in rheumatoid arthritis patients receiving concomitant methotrexate: a randomised phase III trial. ATTRACT Study Group.* Lancet, 1999. 354(9194): p. 1932-9.

[14] Weinblatt, M.E., et al., *Adalimumab, a fully human anti-tumor necrosis factor alpha monoclonal antibody, for the treatment of rheumatoid arthritis in patients taking concomitant methotrexate: the ARMADA trial.* Arthritis Rheum, 2003. 48(1): p. 35-45.

[15] Weinblatt, M.E., et al., *A trial of etanercept, a recombinant tumor necrosis factor receptor:Fc fusion protein, in patients with rheumatoid arthritis receiving methotrexate.* N Engl J Med, 1999. 340(4): p. 253-9.

[16] Keystone, E., et al., *Golimumab in patients with active rheumatoid arthritis despite methotrexate therapy: 52-week results of the GO-FORWARD study.* Ann Rheum Dis. 69(6): p. 1129-35.

[17] Genovese MC, et al. *Interleukin-6 receptor inhibition with tocilizumab reduces disease activity in rheumatoid arthritis with inadequate response to disease-modifying antirheumatic drugs: the tocilizumab in combination with traditional disease-modifying antirheumatic drug therapy study.* Arthritis Rheum. 2008 Oct;58(10):2968-80.

[18] Smolen, J., et al., *Efficacy and safety of certolizumab pegol plus methotrexate in active rheumatoid arthritis: the RAPID 2 study. A randomised controlled trial.* Ann Rheum Dis, 2009. 68(6): p. 797-804.

[19] Askling, J. et al. *Time-dependent increase in risk of hospitalisation with infection among Swedish RA patients treated with TNF antagonists.* Ann. Rheum. Dis. 66, 1339-1344 (2007).

[20] Galloway, J. B. et al. *Anti-TNF therapy is associated with an increased risk of serious infections in patients with rheumatoid arthritis especially in the first 6 months of treatment: updated results from the British Society for Rheumatology Biologics Register with special emphasis on risks in the elderly.* Rheumatology (Oxford) 50, 124-131 (2011).

[21] Greenberg, J. D. et al. *Association of methotrexate and tumour necrosis factor antagonists with risk of infectious outcomes including opportunistic infections in the CORRONA registry.* Ann. Rheum. Dis. 69, 380-386 (2010).

[22] Mariette, X. et al. *Malignancies associated with tumour necrosis factor inhibitors in registries and prospective observational studies: a systematic review and meta-analysis.* Ann Rheum Dis 2011;70:1895-1904 doi

[23] Woodrick R. S. and Ruderman E. M. *Safety of biologic therapy in rheumatoid arthritis. Nature Reviews Rheumatology* 7: p. 639-652

[24] van Vollenhoven, R.F., et al., *Addition of infliximab compared with addition of sulfasalazine and hydroxychloroquine to methotrexate in patients with early rheumatoid arthritis (Swefot trial): 1-year results of a randomised trial.* Lancet, 2009. 374(9688): p. 459-66.

[25] van Vollenhoven RF, et al. *Conventional combination treatment versus biological treatment in methotrexate-refractory early rheumatoid arthritis: 2 year follow-up of the randomised, non-blinded, parallel-group Swefot trial.* Lancet. 2012 Mar 28. [Epub ahead of print]

[26] Goekoop-Ruiterman, Y.P., et al., *Comparison of treatment strategies in early rheumatoid arthritis: a randomized trial.* Ann Intern Med, 2007. 146(6): p. 406-15.

[27] Goekoop-Ruiterman, Y.P., et al., *Clinical and radiographic outcomes of four different treatment strategies in patients with early rheumatoid arthritis (the BeSt study): a randomized, controlled trial.* Arthritis Rheum, 2005. 52(11): p. 3381-90.

[28] Felson D., et al., *American College of Rheumatology/European League Against Rheumatism provisional definition of remission in rheumatoid arthritis for clinical trials.* Arthritis & Rheumatism, 63: 573–586.

[29] Lipsky, P.E., et al., *Infliximab and methotrexate in the treatment of rheumatoid arthritis. Anti-Tumor Necrosis Factor Trial in Rheumatoid Arthritis with Concomitant Therapy Study Group.* N Engl J Med, 2000. 343(22): p. 1594-602.

[30] Tanaka, Y., et al., *Discontinuation of infliximab after attaining low disease activity in patients with rheumatoid arthritis: RRR (remission induction by Remicade in RA) study.* Ann Rheum Dis. 69(7): p. 1286-91.

[31] van der Kooij, S.M., et al., *Clinical and radiological efficacy of initial vs delayed treatment with infliximab plus methotrexate in patients with early rheumatoid arthritis.* Ann Rheum Dis, 2009. 68(7): p. 1153-8.

[32] van der Kooij, S.M., et al., *Drug-free remission, functioning and radiographic damage after 4 years of response-driven treatment in patients with recent-onset rheumatoid arthritis.* Ann Rheum Dis, 2009. 68(6): p. 914-21.

[33] O'Mahony, R., et al., *Withdrawal of DMARDs in patients with Rheumatoid Arthritis: a systematic review and meta-analysis.* Ann Rheum Dis, 2009.

[34] Smolen, J.S., et al., *EULAR recommendations for the management of rheumatoid arthritis with synthetic and biological disease-modifying antirheumatic drugs.* Ann Rheum Dis. 69(6): p. 964-75.

[35] Durez, P., et al., *A dose adjustment in patients with rheumatoid arthritis not optimally responding to a standard dose of infliximab of 3 mg/kg every 8 weeks can be effective: a Belgian prospective study.* Rheumatology (Oxford), 2005. 44(4): p. 465-8.

[36] Pavelka, K., et al., *Increasing the infliximab dose in rheumatoid arthritis patients: a randomised, double blind study failed to confirm its efficacy.* Ann Rheum Dis, 2009. 68(8): p. 1285-9.

[37] van Vollenhoven, R.F., S. Brannemark, and L. Klareskog, *Dose escalation of infliximab in clinical practice: improvements seen may be explained by a regression-like effect.* Ann Rheum Dis, 2004. 63(4): p. 426-30.

[38] van den Bemt, B.J., et al., *Sustained effect after lowering high-dose infliximab in patients with rheumatoid arthritis: a prospective dose titration study.* Ann Rheum Dis, 2008. 67(12): p. 1697-701.

[39] Smolen, J.S., et al., *Golimumab in patients with active rheumatoid arthritis after treatment with tumour necrosis factor alpha inhibitors (GO-AFTER study): a multicentre, randomised, double-blind, placebo-controlled, phase III trial.* Lancet, 2009. 374(9685): p. 210-21.

[40] Haraoui, B., et al., *Clinical outcomes of patients with rheumatoid arthritis after switching from infliximab to etanercept.* J Rheumatol, 2004. 31(12): p. 2356-9.

[41] Bingham, C.O., 3rd, et al., *Effectiveness and safety of etanercept in subjects with RA who have failed infliximab therapy: 16-week, open-label, observational study.* Curr Med Res Opin, 2009. 25(5): p. 1131-42.

[42] Buch, M.H., et al., *Therapy of patients with rheumatoid arthritis: outcome of infliximab failures switched to etanercept.* Arthritis Rheum, 2007. 57(3): p. 448-53.

[43] Furst, D.E., et al., *Open-label, pilot protocol of patients with rheumatoid arthritis who switch to infliximab after an incomplete response to etanercept: the opposite study.* Ann Rheum Dis, 2007. 66(7): p. 893-9.

[44] Bombardieri, S., et al., *Effectiveness of adalimumab for rheumatoid arthritis in patients with a history of TNF-antagonist therapy in clinical practice.* Rheumatology (Oxford), 2007. 46(7): p. 1191-9.

[45] Finckh, A., et al., *B cell depletion may be more effective than switching to an alternative anti-tumor necrosis factor agent in rheumatoid arthritis patients with inadequate response to anti-tumor necrosis factor agents.* Arthritis Rheum, 2007. 56(5): p. 1417-23.

[46] Finckh, A., et al., *Which subgroup of patients with rheumatoid arthritis benefits from switching to rituximab versus alternative anti-tumour necrosis factor (TNF) agents after previous failure of an anti-TNF agent?* Ann Rheum Dis. 69(2): p. 387-93.

[47] Venkatachalam, S., et al., *Rituximab may be more effective than switching to an alternative TNF inhibitor in rheumatoid arthritis patients who have failed other tnf inhibitors.* Rheumatology, 2008. 47: p. Ii31-Ii31.

[48] Buch, M.H., et al., *Does tumour necrosis factor (TNF)-alpha blockade differentially reduce synovial TNF-alpha expression in patients with rheumatoid arthritis?* Arthritis and Rheumatism, 2003. 48(9): p. S146-S146.

[49] Chatzidionysiou K., et al. *Rituximab vs. Anti-TNF after Failure of Anti-TNF: An Observational Study* [abstract]. Arthritis Rheum 2010;62 Suppl 10 :410

[50] Chatzidionysiou K. et al. When to initiate and discontinue biologic treatments for rheumatoid arthritis? J Intern Med. 2011 Jun;269(6):614-25.

Chapter 15

Biologic Therapy in Patients with Juvenile Idiopathic Arthritis – A Unique Single Centre Experience at the Scientific-Research Pediatric Centre in the Russian Federation

A.A. Baranov, E.I. Alexeeva, L.S. Namazova-Baranova,
T.M. Bzarova, S.I. Valiyeva, R.V. Denisova, K.B. Isayeva,
A.M. Chomakhidze, E.G. Chistyakova, T.V. Sleptsova,
E.V. Mitenko, E.I. Zelikovich, G.V. Kurilenko, E.L. Semikina,
A.V. Anikin, A.M. Stepanchenko, N.I. Taybulatov, A.V. Starikova,
I.V. Dvoryakovskiy and M.V. Ryazanov

Additional information is available at the end of the chapter

http://dx.doi.org/10.5772/48761

1. Introduction

In 10-20% of children with JIA, a wide range of extra-articular manifestations such as spiking febrile fever, carditis, pneumonitis and serositis were noted [1]. Despite the advances in modern medicine, treatment of the systemic JIA variant with glucocorticoids and immunosuppressants has not always proved effective [1,2,3]. In 50% of patients, progressively destructive changes in the joints, with recurring extra-articular manifestations, have been steadily increasing the disability level. Most children with systemic JIA take oral, intravenous or intra-articular corticosteroids. However, glucocorticoids do not control the disease, prevent the progression of cartilage bone destruction or reduce disability in patients, and their prolonged use leads to severe irreversible effects, particularly, short stature, delayed puberty, adrenal insufficiency, osteoporosis and corticosteroid dependence [1,2, 3].

Interleukin 6 (IL-6), one of the central cytokines, has been discovered to play a leading role in development of systemic JIA. When excess IL-6 is produced, extra-articular manifestations such as fever and thrombocytosis are noted [4,5]. IL-6 stimulates the production of inflammatory proteins by hepatocytes (CRP, amyloid A, haptoglobin, fibrinogen), and competitively inhibits synthesis of albumin and transferrin [6]. Anemia is one of extra-articular manifestations of systemic JIA. It develops during IL-6 stimulated secretion of hepcidin by the hepatocytes [7-10]. In normal concentrations, IL-6 enhances the synthesis of the adrenocorticotropic hormone and cortisol, as well as the production of the growth hormone and procalcitonin [10,11]. However, at higher concentrations, IL-6 blocks the production of these hormones, which leads to fatigue, sleepiness, depression, cognitive disorders and retarded growth in children with systemic JIA [10,11,12], as the activity of IL-6 is also connected with the development of amyloidosis associated JIA. Thus, inhibition of IL-6 is very important in treatment of systemic JIA. Tocilizumab was synthesized for this purpose. Tocilizumab is a humanized monoclonal antibody to IL-6 receptor [13]. Based on the positive results of clinical studies on the efficacy and safety of Tocilizumab therapy, the drug has been registered for treatment of systemic JIA [16-23].

The purpose of this study is to evaluate the efficacy and safety of Tocilizumab treatment in children with the severe refractory systemic JIA.

2. Patients and methods

In a retrospective observational study, patients with the systemic JIA, treated with Tocilizumab between June 2009 and October 2011 in the Rheumatology Department, Science Center for Children's Health of RAMS were followed. The use of Tocilizumab in all the cases was approved by the local ethics committee. Prior to treatment, written consent was taken from the parents of the children, children aged 14 and older gave written informed consent themselves.

The results of treatment of 60 children (30 girls and 30 boys) aged 6.5 (4.5; 9) years (Me (25, 75)) were given in this analysis. The mean disease duration before beginning Tocilizumab therapy was 4.5 (2.2; 6.5) years. Diagnosis of systemic JIA was made based on diagnostic ILAR criteria (International League of Associations for Rheumatology). All patients underwent standard clinical and laboratory examination. Control of hemoglobin level, the number of erythrocytes, platelets, leukocytes, ESR, serum concentration of urea, creatinine, uric acid, bilirubin, transaminases, and clinical urinalysis was performed once every two weeks. Blood pressure (BP) was checked on a daily basis.

Number of systemic manifestations, swollen, painful joints, joints with limitation of function, serum CRP level were determined on a monthly basis. Therapy efficacy was evaluated according to the ACR pedi criteria ACR30, ACR50, ACR70. The criteria included a parent's assessment of pain, parent's global evaluation, physician's global assessment of disease status using VAS, the functional ability by CHAQ, number of joints with active arthritis, number of joints with limitation of function and ESR.

The main target of therapy was status of inactive disease and remission. Inactive phase of disease was established in the absence of active synovitis, systemic manifestations, normal ESR and serum CRP level, as well as absence of disease activity on the physician's global assessment (on VAS). At the time of therapy initiation most children had active polyarthritis (Table 1). All patients revealed extra-articular manifestations of disease: spiking fever in 90% (54), carditis in 3% (2), lymphadenopathy in 86% (36), maculopapular rash in 35% (21), spleno- and hepatomegaly in 45% (27) of the patients. The number of systemic manifestations per patient was 2.5 (Table 1, Fig. 1). High clinical disease activity was accompanied by a general inflammatory reaction: hypochromic anemia in 90% (54), leukocytosis in 75% (45) and thrombocytosis in 80% (48) of patients. The median ESR was more than twice the normal value and serum CRP level increased up to 10 times (Table 1).

Index	**Value (Me (25; 75)**
number of active joints	8 (4;14)
number of joints with limitation of function	9(3;14)
number of systemic manifestations per patient	2.5 (1.5; 3.5)
ESR, mm/h	28 (18; 55)
platelets, x109/	490 (480; 640)
hemoglobin, g/L	92 (86; 98)
CRP, mg%	14 (7; 26)

Table 1. Clinical characteristic of patients with the systemic JIA included in the study.

Thus, at the beginning of therapy all patients with systemic JIA had active arthritis, severe systemic manifestations and high laboratory parameters of the disease activity with increasing disability.

Previous therapy: Prior to the Tocilizumab treatment all patients were treated with antirheumatic drugs, in various modes. In the initial stages of the disease (based on the place of residence in the territorial health care facility) 60% (36) children were prescribed oral prednisolone at a dose of 10 to 30 mg / day. All children received methylprednisolone pulse therapy at a dose of 10-30 mg / kg initially, 47 (78%) - local glucocorticoid therapy from 1 to 10 times a year, 10 (17%) were treated with TNF-blockers and 22 (37%) with anti-B cell therapy with rituximab. All children were treated with antiinflammatory drugs (NSAIDs).

Background therapy: Tocilizumab was administered in patients receiving immunosuppressive drugs (Table 2). Doses of antirheumatic drugs were stable within 3 months before Tocilizumab therapy.

Drug	Dose (Me (25; 75))	Number of children
methotrexate, mg/m^2/week	18 (15; 25)	60
cyclosporine, mg/kg/day	4 (4; 4)	46
prednisolone, mg/day	10.5 (7; 12)	36
NSAIDs	-	60

Table 2. Background therapy in patients with the systemic JIA included in the study.

Tocilizumab treatment: Tocilizumab was administered intravenously, once every two or four weeks at a dose of 8-10 mg / kg per infusion. All the children within one or two months of receiving the drug every two weeks had the interval increased to four weeks between doses. Infusions were performed for one hour, at the rate of 10 ml / h for the first 15 minutes, and then increased to 130 ml / hour.

Analysis of the efficacy was done after one month. The results indicated improvement in 52 children by 1 month, in 50 children by 3 months, in 40 children by 6 months, in 32 children by 9 months and in 24 children by the end of a year.

Statistical data processing was performed using the program STATISTICA 6.0 (StatSoft Inc., USA). Quantitative characters are shown as median (25, 75 percentiles). Changes in the quantitative traits during the treatment were evaluated using the Wilcoxon test conjugate pairs. Statistically significant differences were considered at $p < 0.05$.

2.1. Results

Tocilizumab treatment ensured reliability and marked improvement of the systemic manifestations, as well as clinical and laboratory parameters of disease activity.

Within one month after initiation of therapy, patients showed a significant decrease in number of systemic manifestations (Fig. 1). Carditis one of the serious extra-articular manifestations of systemic JIA, disappeared in all the patients. Frequency of skin rash also significantly reduced, from 21 (35%) to 13 (25%) of the cases. After the first infusion of Tocilizumab, no spikers of fever were observed in all patients (Fig. 1).

After observation of 24 patients over a year, lymphadenopathy persisted in 3 patients, rash in 2 cases and hepato / splenomegaly in 1 patient. At the end of one year of observation, the number of systemic manifestations per patient was 0.25 (Figs. 1).

In the fourth week of treatment the number of active joints significantly decreased from 8 (4, 14) to 4 (1, 14), $p < 0.01$. By the 12th month the rate was 0 ((0, 3), $p < 0.001$) (Fig. 2).

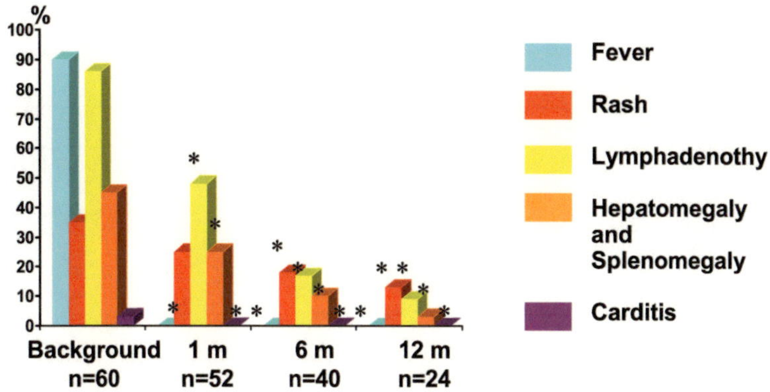

	Background	1 m	6 m	12 m
Number of systemic features per patient	**2.5**	**0.9**	**0.4**	**0.25**

Figure 1. Dynamics of Systemic Features in children with systemic JIA treated with Tocilizumab. Hereinafter: * p<0.001 – statistically significant difference compared to baseline

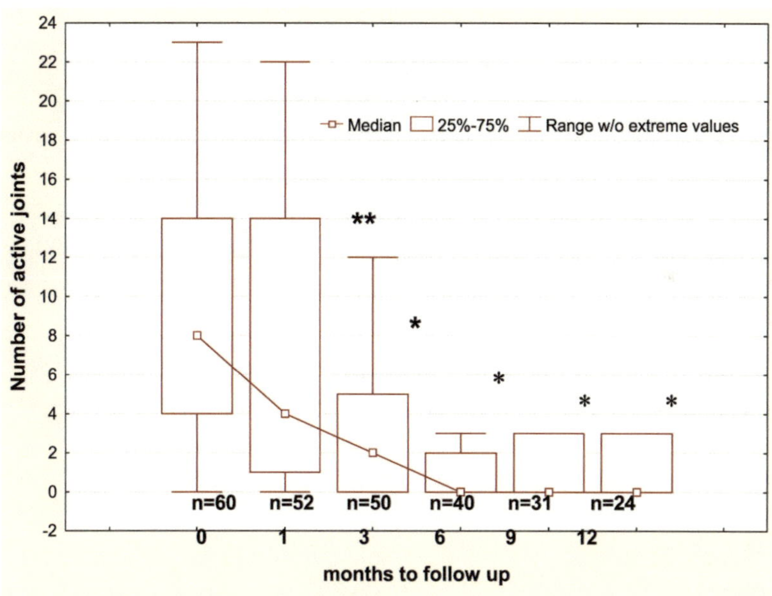

Figure 2. Dynamics in number of active joints in children with systemic JIA treated with Tocilizumab. Hereinafter: * p<0.001, ** p<0.01 – statistically significant difference compared to baseline

The same trend was observed in the joints with limitation of function. That parameter too significantly dropped after four weeks of treatment (Fig. 3). By the end of one year's observation the median number of joints with limitation of function decreased 9 times (p <0.001).

Along with the decrease in the number of joints with active arthritis, as well as joints with limitation of function, a significant improvement in functional ability of the affected joints was noted (Fig. 4). After four weeks of Tocilizumab treatment the index of functional disability by CHAQ questionnaire decreased significantly from 2.0 (1.35, 2.7) to 1,3 (0.9; 1.3), p <0.001).

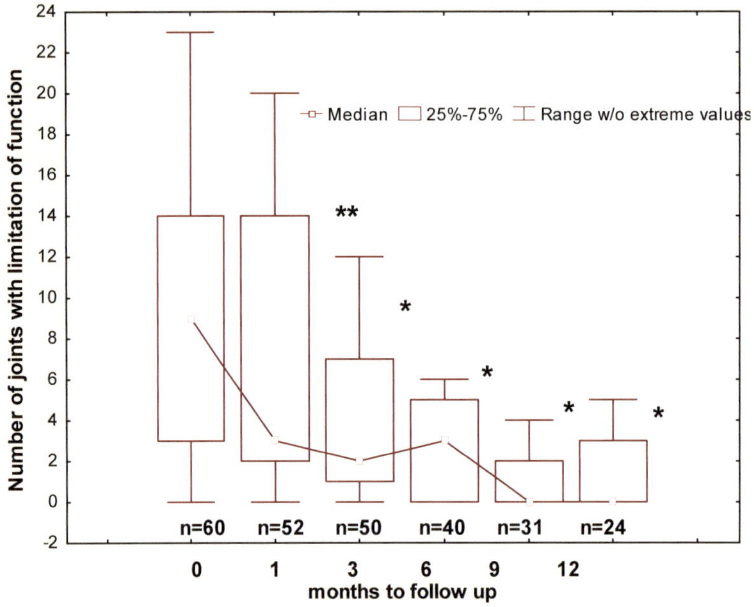

Figure 3. Dynamics in number of joints with limitation of function in children with systemic JIA treated with Tocilizumab.
Hereinafter: * p<0.001, ** p<0.01 – statistically significant difference compared to baseline

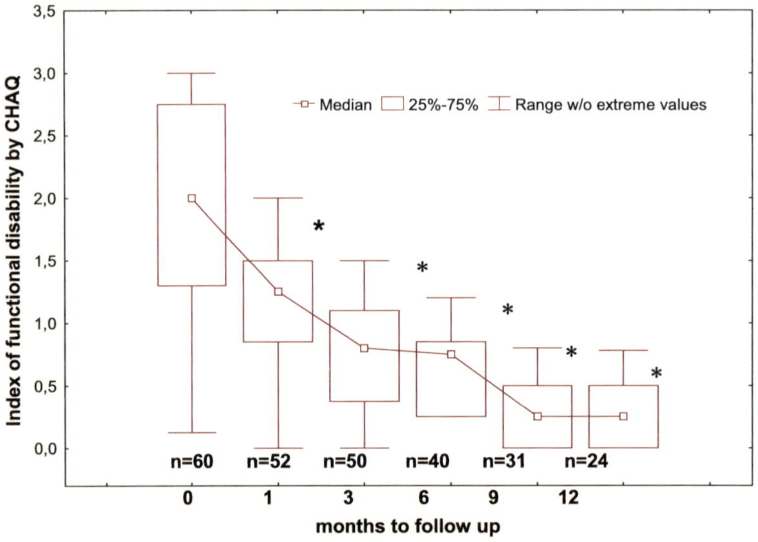

Figure 4. Dynamics in index of functional disability in children with systemic JIA treated with Tocilizumab.
Hereinafter: * p<0.001 – statistically significant difference compared to baseline

Tocilizumab therapy also influenced the laboratory parameters of the disease activity, showing significant increase in hemoglobin level (Fig. 5), decrease platelet counts, ESR, serum CRP level and normalization of these parameters by the first month of treatment (Fig. 6, 7, 8).

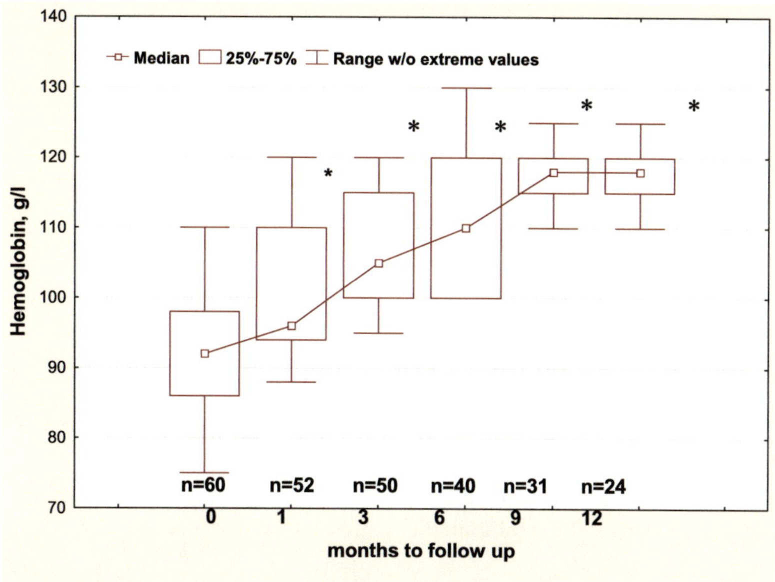

Figure 5. Dynamics in hemoglobin level in children with systemic JIA treated with Tocilizumab. Hereinafter: * p<0.001 – statistically significant difference compared to baseline

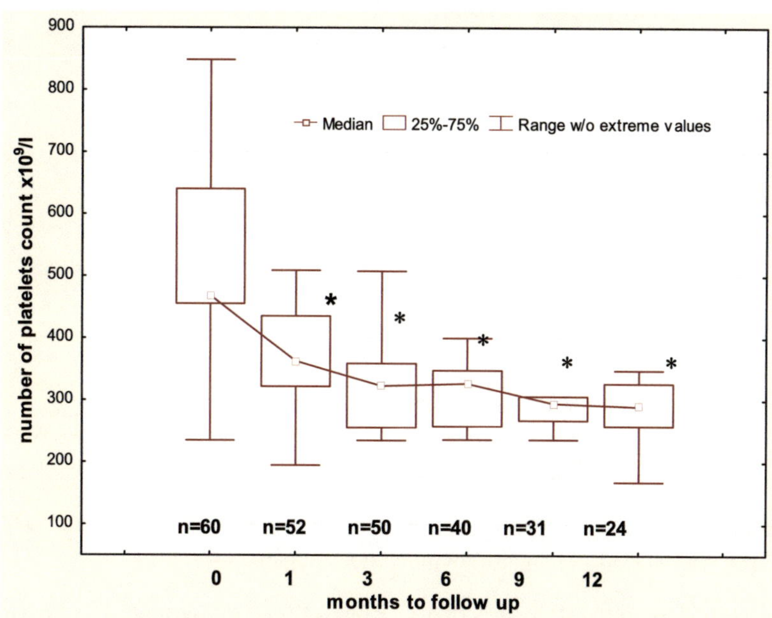

Figure 6. Dynamics in the platelets count in children with systemic JIA treated with Tocilizumab. Hereinafter: * p<0.001 – statistically significant difference compared to baseline

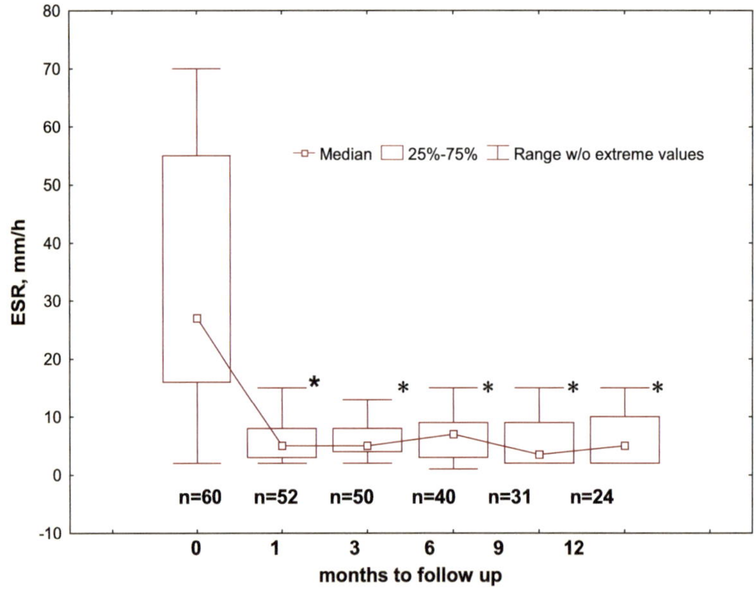

Figure 7. Dynamics in the ESR in children with systemic JIA treated with Tocilizumab. Hereinafter: * p<0.001 – statistically significant difference compared to baseline

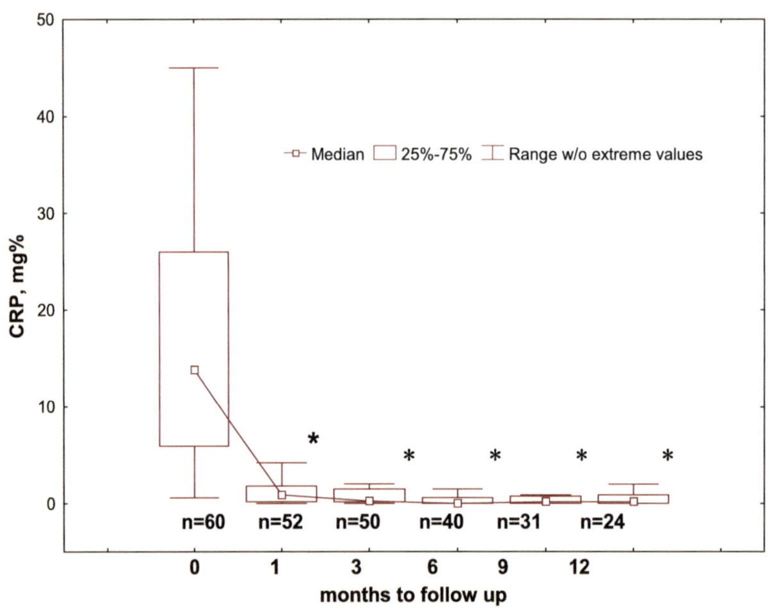

Figure 8. Dynamics in the serum CRP level in children with systemic JIA treated with Tocilizumab. Hereinafter: * p<0.001 – statistically significant difference compared to baseline

Assessment of efficacy of Tocilizumab therapy according ACRpedi criteria by one month of Tocilizumab therapy showed 30% improvement in 82% of the patients, 50% improvement in 47% of cases and 70% improvement in 29% of patients. After six months of treatment, all the children maintained improvement criteria ACR30 while 65% recorded a rate of ACR70. After a year of therapy, 50% and 70% improvement, respectively, was observed in 100% and 75% of patients (Fig. 9). In general, the efficacy of Tocilizumab after more than six months of treatment was characterized by the achievement of inactive disease status in 43% (17 of 40) patients after one year in 45% (11 of 24) patients and remission in 43 % (10 of 24).

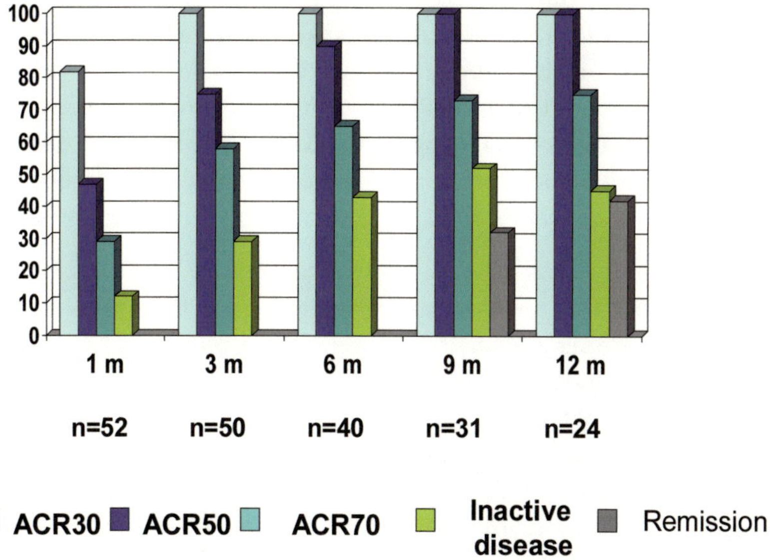

Figure 9. Response according to ACR pedi criteria in children with systemic JIA treated with Tocilizumab.

Safety assessment of Tocilizumab treatment was performed by registered adverse events (AE), laboratory parameters, based on the results of the physical examination (BP, HR), and EKG. AE were evaluated in all the patients enrolled in the study, who received at least one infusion. Tocilizumab treatment was well tolerated and most AE were mild or moderate, reversible, not limiting the course of the treatment. Infusion reactions were noted. Registered AE were differentiated into two groups, namely infectious disorders and laboratory parameters (Table 3).

Adverse events	Patients n (%)
Laboratory parameters:	
Neutropenia	25 (41%)
Thrombocytopenia	1 (2%)
Increase in alkaline phosphatase	1 (2%)
Infectious disorders:	
Cellulitis	3 (5%)
Herpes infection	4 (8%)
Acute focal pneumonia	2 (3%)

Table 3. Adverse events in patients on Tocilizumab therapy

Among the infectious AE reported, cellulitis was seen in 3 patients, exacerbation of herpes infection in 4 cases and acute focal pneumonia in 2 patients. Antibiotic therapy provided complete relief of cellulitis and pneumonia without complications. Aggravation of herpetic infection (4 cases) was not considered serious AE. Among the AE with the laboratory parameters, neutropenia was most frequently observed in the first few days after administration of the Tocilizumab, in 41% (25) of the patients. In 15 patients, the absolute neutrophil count decreased <1.000 in 1 μL, whereas in 2 patients it was 500 per 1μL. On identifying neutropenia, daily monitoring was conducted until neutrophil recovery occurred within weeks after the infusion. By reducing the number of neutrophils <1.0 x109 /L patients received the colony-stimulating factor (G-CSF) filgrastim, at a dose of 5 mg / kg, with a positive effect. All cases of neutropenia were associated with Tocilizumab infusion. None of them were accompanied by infection and it was not a cause of treatment discontinuation.

Mild thrombocytopenia was observed in one patient after 11 months of therapy. Two weeks after the regular drug administration, the platelet count decreased to 156 x109 /L. Concomitant therapy included glucocorticoids, cyclosporine, methotrexate, and NSAIDs. Thrombocytopenia was not considered serious AE, and unlikely to be the result of Tocilizumab therapy. Platelet count returned to normal within a week, without reducing the dose or interrupting the treatment. One patient reported a one-time increase in alkaline phosphatase activity to 6200 IU / L after the first injection of Tocilizumab while concomitant therapy included methotrexate and methylprednisolone. This rate returned to normal after eight days without changing the Tocilizumab treatment regimen. The AE were considered to be of no significance, and unlikely to be the result of Tocilizumab therapy.

While observing clinically significant changes in the vital functions namely, BP and HR, the EKG parameters were also observed. Treatment was discontinued in 9 patients (table 4).

Index	Patients n
Remission of disease	1
Inefficacy	1
Relapse of disease	6
Parents' refusal	1

Table 4. Causes of discontinuation of Tocilizumab treatment.

Normally, the safety profile of Tocilizumab in children is quite similar to the safety profile described earlier in adults with rheumatoid arthritis. It was within the expected range for a population of patients receiving immunosuppressive drugs. AE were manifested as mild to moderately severe infections, as well as changes in the laboratory parameters. Deaths did not occur during the period of Tocilizumab treatment. No case of discontinuation of therapy was registered due to AE development.

3. Clinical case

Patient's data: female. Age: 9 years old (born in 2002)

Diagnosis: Systemic JIA

3.1. Medical history

The girl has been sick since 2007 when she was 5 years old. Febrile fever, lymphadenopathy, inflammatory changes in the knees and ankles, high laboratory parameters of activity (ESR – 52 mm/h) were observed during the onset. The following diagnosis was set at the local in-patient facility: systemic-onset juvenile arthritis. Treatment with antibiotics, NSAIDs, oral methylprednisolone at a dose of 16 mg/day (1 mg/kg of body weight) was conducted. Fever subsided and inflammatory changes in joints resolved with treatment. Gradual reduction of methylprednisolone dose was initiated. In 6 months the dose was 4 mg per day. However, disease exacerbated again after the insolation, which manifested in febrile fever, high laboratory parameters of disease activity (ESR – 45 mm/h), swelling and pain in the elbows, metacarpophalangeal, interphalangeal joints of hands, knees and ankles. Methylprednisolone pulse therapy at a dose of 500 mg per administration was conducted 3 times at the local in-patient facility; methotrexate at a dose of 10 mg/m^2 of standard body surface area per week and NSAIDs were prescribed. Condition improved, the dose of methyprednisolone was decreased to 2 mg per day. In 6 months condition worsened again: febrile fever, exudative changes in the wrists, knees and ankles appeared. Due to persisting disease activity in 1.5 years from the disease onset, the girl was referred to the rheumatology department of Scientific Center for Children Health, RAMS. On admission to the department the child's condition was assessed as severe. The girl experienced daily febrile fevers; the joint syndrome was polyarticular, affecting wrists, knees, ankles; motions were limited and painful. The child was bothered by morning stiffness for up to 60 minutes. On admission to the department pale skin, "shadows" under the eyes, generalized lymphadenopathy also came under notice. Leukocytosis, thrombocytosis, ESR elevation, hypochromic anemia, increased serum CRP concentration (Table 5) were observed in hematology during examination. Periarticular osteoporosis and single erosions of articular surfaces were revealed according to X-ray examination of the knees. Diagnosis systemic JIA was undoubtful.

Methotrexate dose was increased up to 25 mg/m^2 of standard body surface area per week intramuscularly. 2 injections were conducted with positive effect: fever subsided, intensity of pain syndrome and exudative changes in joints reduced. The child was discharged with recommendations to continue methotrexate treatment at the place of residence. For 6 months the girl's condition remained stable.

In 6 months of methotrexate treatment at a dose of 25 mg/m^2 of standard body surface area per week, the girl started experiencing febrile fever again, duration of morning stiffness increased up to 120 minutes, exudative changes in the wrists, elbows and ankles increased (Figure 10a-d). The child fell behind in physical development, height and weight scores were below the 10th percentile (Table 5). According to hematology and immunologic blood test, activity of rheumatoid process persisted (Table 5). Based on the signs of aggressive disease course (polyarthritis, high immunologic activity, ineffectiveness of methotrexate therapy at a high dose, hormonal dependency, falling behind in physical development), the patient was prescribed treatment with genetically engineered biologic agent – Tocilizumab.

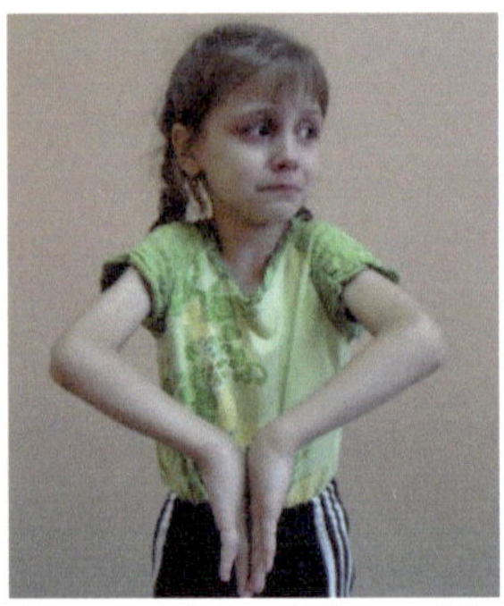

a. Functional capabilities of the wrist joints prior to Tocilizumab therapy.

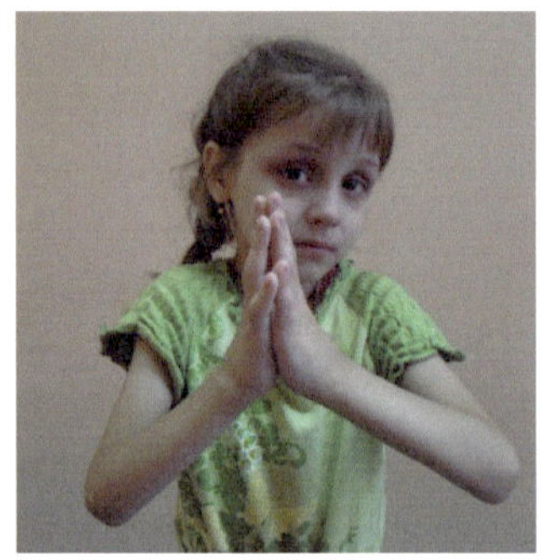

b. Functional capabilities of the wrist joints prior to Tocilizumab therapy

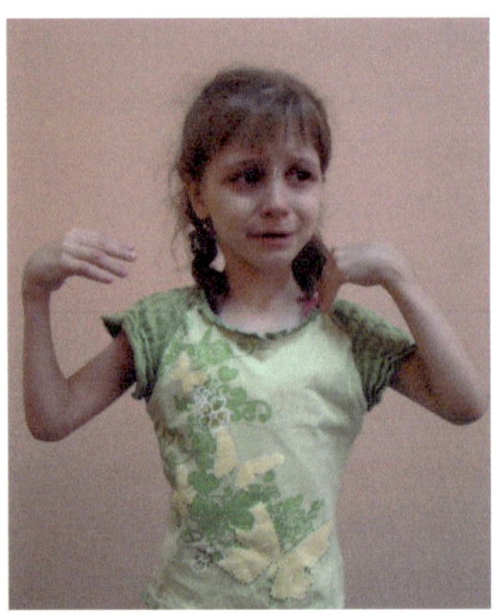

c. Functional capabilities of the elbow joints prior to Tocilizumab therapy

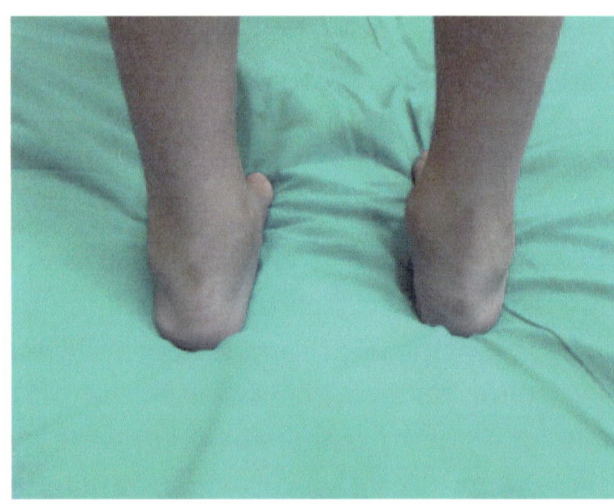

d. The swelling ankle joints prior to Tocilizumab therapy.

Figure 10.

3.2. Treatment with Tocilizumab

The drug was administered intravenously at a dose of 8 mg/kg of body weight once in 4 weeks. Drug prescription was approved by the Academic Board, Local Ethics Committee and Formulary Committees of Scientific Center for Children Health, RAMS. Child's parents have signed an informed consent for drug use.

3.3. Results of treatment

Analysis of development rate of Tocilizumab therapeutic effect has revealed that right after the first administration the fever subsided, the girl became more active, after 2 week of treatment the morning stiffness resolved (Table 5); exudative changes in the affected joints had completely resolved by the 8th week, the range of motions restored (Figure 11 a-e); laboratory parameters of disease activity normalized in 4 weeks (Table 5). Tocilizumab treatment also positively affected patient's quality of life, improved physical activity and emotional condition (Figure 11 a-e). Inactive disease status was observed in the patient in 2 months of treatment, and in 8 months the patient entered systemic JIA remission, which has been maintained for 2 years of Tocilizumab treatment.

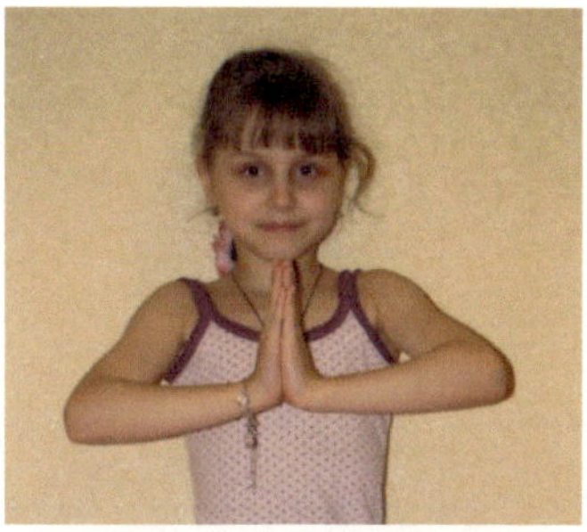

a. Functional capabilities of the wrist joints with Tocilizumab therapy at week 104.

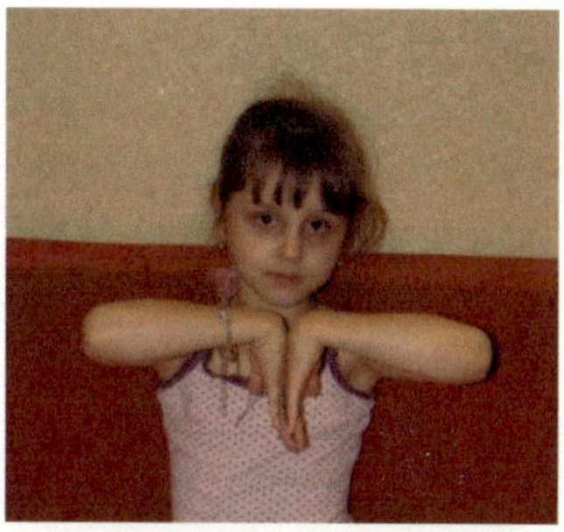

b. Functional capabilities of the wrist joints with Tocilizumab therapy at week 104

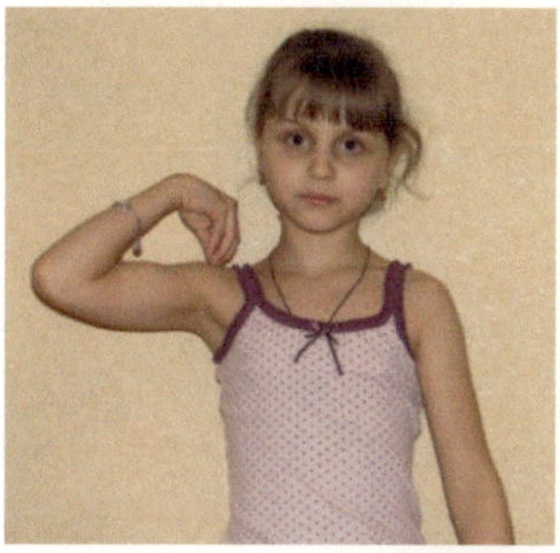

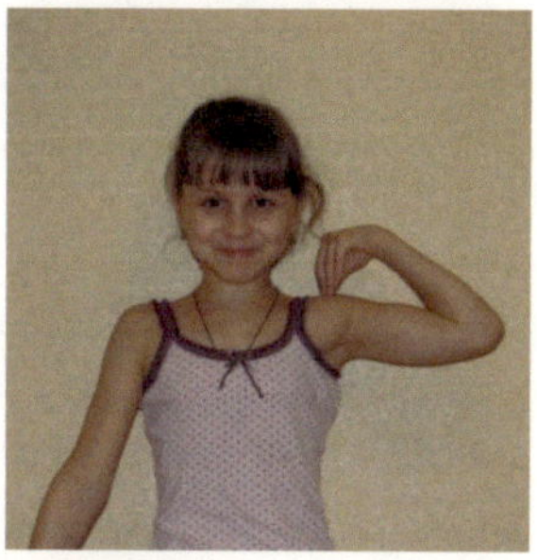

c and d. Functional capabilities of the elbow joints **with** Tocilizumab therapy at

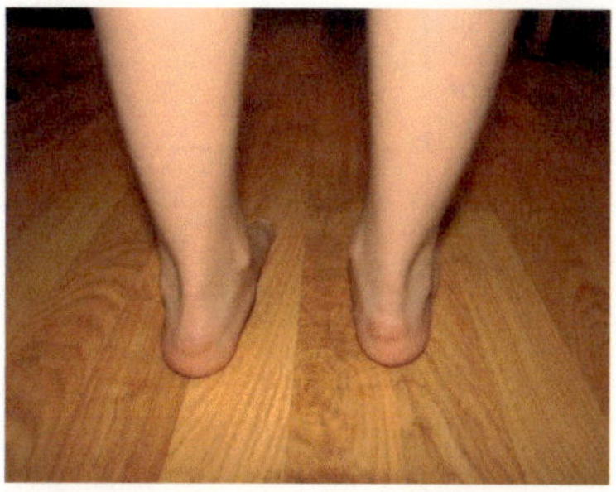

e. The absence of swelling in the ankle joints **with** Tocilizumab therapy at week

Figure 11.

The girl continues receiving intravenous Tocilizumab infusions at a dose of 8 mg/kg of body weight once in 4 weeks in combination with methotrexate (due to height and weight increase, a dose is 18 mg/m^2 of body surface area per week) and methylprednisolone at a dose of 2 mg/day. Child's physical development parameters significantly improved with Tocilizumab therapy: in 2 years the girl has grown by1 cm and weight gain was 6 kg, height and weight were in the 10th – 25th percentile range.

3.4. Adverse events

No serious adverse events were observed during the follow-up.

Parameters	Prior to the increase of methotrexate dose	Duration of Tocilizumab therapy					
		Background	Day 1	4 weeks	26 weeks	52 weeks	104 weeks
Temperature, °C	38.5	39.0	36.7	36.6	36.6	36.6	36.6
Duration of morning stiffness, minutes	60	120	no	no	no	no	no
The number of active joints	6	6	6	2	0	0	0
CHAQ index of functional disability, score	1.7	1.9	1.7	0.5	0	0	0
ESR (mm/h)	25	70	45	2	7	2	4
Hemoglobin (g/L)	88	110	110	118	120	125	128
Erythrocytes (x10^{12}/L)	3.8	4.7	4.8	5.2	5.25	5.4	5.5
Platelets (x10^9/L)	840	654	622	328	335	270	290
Leukocytes (x10^9/L)	17	22.7	17.8	7.96	6.7	8?4	7.8
CRP (mg%), normal level up to 0.8	3.85	26	16	<0.8	<0.8	<0.8	<0.8
IgG (g/L), normal range (5.72-14.74)	12.1	17.8	9.0	7.35	6.66	8.67	7.5
Height, cm	112	114	114	115	116	119	125
Weight, kg	16.5	17.5	17.5	18.0	19	20	23.5
Percentage of improvement according to $ACR_{pediatric}$ criteria	-	-	-	50%	90% Inactive disease	Disease remission	Disease remission

Table 5. Clinical and laboratory parameters of systemic JIA activity with Tocilizumab treatment in patient, 9 years old girl, over time.

4. Efficacy and safety of monoclonal human antibodies to TNFα in children with juvenile idiopathic arthritis and uveitis

4.1. Introduction

Juvenile idiopathic arthritis is a severe disabling disease associated with development of destructive arthritis and uveitis – in some patients.

Treatment with methotrexate (15 mg/m^2 of standard body surface area) provided disease control in many patients with juvenile idiopathic arthritis [26]. However, standard anti-rheumatic treatment is unlikely to provide stable remission in some patients [27-30]. Due to insufficient efficacy of methotrexate, the progression of the disease continues. Treatment of uveitis is the most complicated, because its activity is usually independent on the activity of arthritis.

Biologic drugs produced by the methods of gene engineering provide a good perspective for patients with methotrexate inefficacy. Adalimumab is one of these drugs.

Adalimumab is the recombinant IgG1 human monoclonal antibodies consisting of 1330 amino acids. The drug is manufactured by recombinant DNA technology. It binds to p55 and p75 receptors of soluble and membrane – associated TNFα. Adalimumab can activate the complement system that results in lysis of cells with superficially located TNFα. The drug has no ability to bind to or inhibit the lymphotoxin (TNFβ); it alters the levels of adhesion molecules that contribute to leukocytes migration (ELAM-1, VSAM-1, and ICAM-1). Adalimumab is administered subcutaneously once per 2 weeks; the elimination half-life of the drug is 2 weeks [31-34].

The results of controlled clinical trials and open studies demonstrated that subcutaneous administration every two weeks of the drug is safe and effective in adult patients with rheumatoid and psoriatic arthritis [34-48], as well as in children with juvenile idiopathic arthritis and uveitis [49-59].

The purpose of this study was to evaluate safety and efficacy of Adalimumab treatment in children with severe refractory juvenile idiopathic arthritis and uveitis.

4.2. Patients and methods

Enrolled: 104 patients (74 girls and 30 boys) age 10 (3; 17) years (Median (25; 75)) with oligoarticular, polyarticular, enthesitic, sistemic arthritis without active systemic manifestation no less within 1 year enthesitic types of juvenile idiopathic arthritis; in 48 patients arthritis was associated with uveitis (Table 6). Mean disease duration prior to Adalimumab administration – was 6 (2; 16) years. The diagnosis of JIA based on ILAR (International League of Associations for Rheumatology) criteria [60].

At baseline, all patients had active arthritis (Table 7). Mean number of joints with active arthritis - 5 (2; 8), mean number of joints with limitation of function – 5 (1; 7.5). High level of clinical activity of the disease was associated with general inflammation reaction. Median

ESR level was 3-fold higher compared to normal; C-reactive protein serum level was 9-fold higher compared to normal (Table 7).

Parameter	Number of patients (n=104)
Boys/girls	74/30
Age, years	10 (3; 17)
Age group 3-13 years	80(73%)
Age group 14-18 years	30(27%)
Duration of the disease, years	5.8 (2; 16)

Table 6. Demographic characteristics of patients with JIA and uveitis, included in the study

Parameter – CHAQ and number of patients – 2.0(1.3; 2.75)	Number of patients
Juvenile idiopathic arthritis Oligoarticular Polyarticular (RF-) Polyarticular (RF+) Enthesitic Systemic, without active systemic manifestations	104 41 (39%) 40 (38.5%) 7 (6.7%) 11 (11%) 5 (4.8%)
Number of joints with active joints Median (25%;75%)	5(2;8)
Number of joints with limitation of function Me (25%;75%)	5(1;7.5)
Duration of the anti-rheumatic treatment, years	2,7 (1.1;2.9)
Number of children with uveitis Bilateral uveitis Unilateral uveitis	48(46%) 32(67%) 16(33%)
Number of affected eyes	80
ESR mm/hour	30 (23; 55)
C-reactive protein, mg/l	9.5 (5; 23)

Table 7. Clinical characteristics of patients with JIA included in the study.

Uveitis was reported in 48 (44%) of patients, bilateral – in 32 (67%); unilateral uveitis – in 16 (33%) patients (Table 8).

Previous therapy. Prior to Adalimumab treatment all patients received various regimens of anti-rheumatic treatment. Due to active arthritis and uveitis development at the onset of the disease, 66 (58%) of patients had a history of prednisolone treatment (10-20 mg/day); all patients received pulse-therapy with methylprednisolone (10-20 mg/kg per administration); 86 (83%) – intra-articular (1-10 times per year), 46 (44%) – cyclosporine, 49 patients were treated with TNFα blockers: 47 (45%) with Infliximab, 2 (1.9%) with Etanercept; 5 (4.8%) children received antiB-cells therapy with Rituximab, 1 (1%) patient inhibitor of T-cells co-stimulation Abatacept. All patients were treated with non-steroid anti-inflammation drugs (NSAIDs); 48 (46%) patients with uveitis received local treatment with eye drops containing NSAIDs and glucocorticosteroids, 32(31%) - para-bulbar glucocorticoid injection (1-5 times per year)

Despite treatment, all patients experienced disease progression. At the time of enrollment they had active arthritis, elevated laboratory parameters and progressing disability. Continuous recurrent uveitis was diagnosed in 48 children.

Inclusion criteria: Ineffective treatment with methotrexate (15-25 mg/m^2 of standard body surface area, once per week, intramuscular injections; within 3 month and more) and with other immunosuppressive drugs (leflunomide, sulfasalazine, cyclosporine), progression of arthritis, vision acuity decrease, continuous recurrence of uveitis, high laboratory parameters (ESR, CRP level), and increasing functional disability.

Normal serum levels of urea, creatinine, bilirubin, ALT, AST; no significant acute or chronic infections. Patients with infections were treated with antibiotics. Prior to Adalimumab treatment all patients were examined for presence of tuberculosis – including tuberculin test (PPD test) and the chest CT. Treatment with TNFα antagonists has been recognized as a risk for active tuberculosis; some cases of latent tuberculosis could reactivate soon after treatment initiation. For this reason, worldwide health authorities recommend screening patients for latent tuberculosis and treating them before initiating anti-TNFα treatment [61]. Patients with positive or controversial PPD test (hyperemia, papule size ≥5 mm) were consulted by the phthisiatrician; and the test with tuberculin dilution was conducted (0.1, 0.1, 0.01 TU). If the tuberculosis infection was excluded, the patients received Adalimumab treatment.

The control of hemogram and serum levels of urea, creatinine, bilirubin, ALT, AST, as well as urinalysis were conducted each 2 weeks.

The following parameters were evaluated during the study: number of Active joints, number of joints with limited function, ESR and serum level of C-reactive protein; the activity of uveitis was evaluated according to criteria developed by M.J. Hogan [36]. Physician's Global Assessment of disease activity (using the 100 mm VAS scale), Parent's global evaluation of well being (using the VAS scale); evaluation of functional abilities using the CHAQ questionnaire. The effect of Adalimumab treatment was evaluated after 4, 12, 24, 36 and 52 weeks of treatment. The efficacy was evaluated according to American College of Rheumatology pediatric criteria (ACRpedi) [62].

The main target of therapy was status of inactive disease and remission [63].

Evaluation of Adalimumab treatment safety was based on the registration of adverse events and regular control of serum levels of urea, creatinine, bilirubin, ALT, AST and hemogram.

All cases of Adalimumab treatment were approved by Local Ethics Committee of the Scientific Center of children's of RAMS. Prior to treatment, children older than 14 years and children's parents were providing the written informed consent.

Background therapy. Adalimumab was administered subcutaneously once per 2 weeks; dose – 40 mg per administration; in combination with background immunosuppressive therapy (Table 8). The dose of immunosuppressive drugs remained stable for at least 3 months.

Drug	**Dose Me (25;75)**	**Number of patients n=104**
Methotrexate mg/m^2/week	20 (15; 25)	64
Cyclosporine, mg/kg/day + Methotrexate mg/m2/week	4 (4; 4)	38
Prednisolone, mg/day	10 (5; 12)	54
NSAIDs	-	104
Para-bulbar glucocorticoid injections - 32	-	48
Local treatment of uveitis with drops	-	48

Table 8. Background therapy in patients with JIA and uveitis included in the study.

The analysis of treatment efficacy was conducted after 4, 12, 24, 36, 52 weeks of treatment – in 104 of patients, accordingly.

Statistical processing of data was conducted using the STATISTICA 6.0 (StatSoft Inc., USA) program. The quantification parameters were presented as medians (25; 75 percentiles); in some cases data were presented as means ± SD. Wilcoxon's criterion was used for paired comparison. Statistically significant difference was considered to be $p<0,05$.

4.3. Results

By week 12 of treatment the statistically significant decrease in number of active joints was reported (5 (2; 8); 3 (0; 4) prior to treatment and after 12 weeks of treatment, respectively; $p< 0.05$), by week 52 there were no joints active (Figure 12).

Similar changes were reported for joints with limitation of function – statistically significant decrease in their number was observed by week 12 (5 (1; 7.5); 3 (1; 5) prior to treatment and after 12 weeks of treatment, respectively; $p< 0.05$), by week 52 the 9-fold decrease of the median parameter was reported ($p<0.05$) (Figure 13).

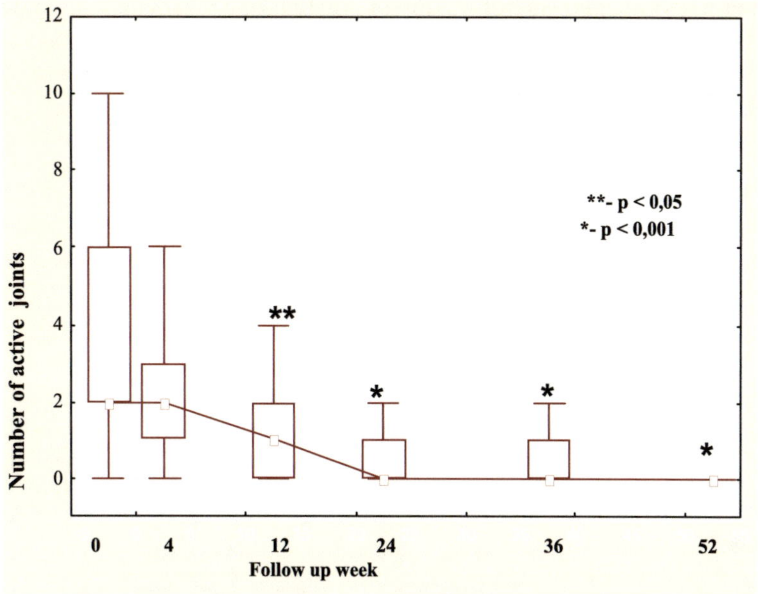

Figure 12. Dynamics in number of active joints in children with JIA treated with Adalimumab (n=104)
Hereinafter:
p<0.001, ** p<0.05 – statistically significant difference compared to baseline
by week 52 there were no joints with active arthritis

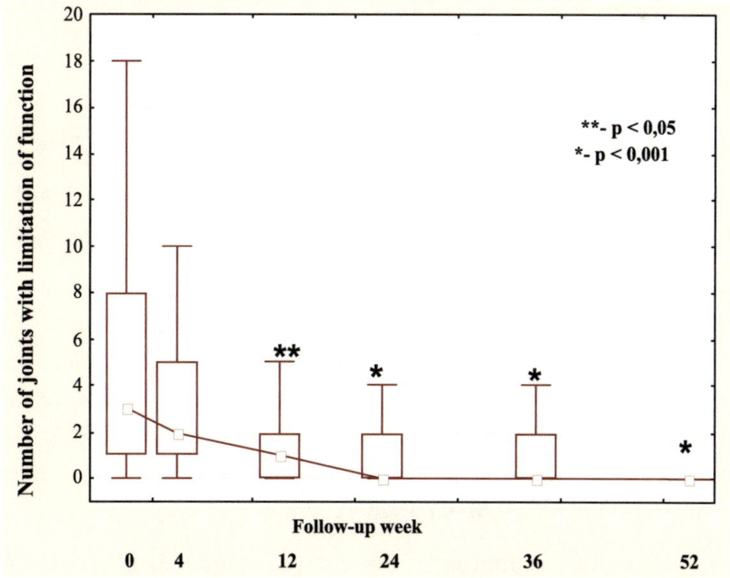

Figure 13. Dynamics in number of joints with limitation of function in children with JIA treated with Adalimumab (n=104)

The improvement of functional activity of joints after 4 weeks of Adalimumab treatment was associated with improvement of quality of life; that improvement was confirmed by the decrease in index of functional disability evaluated by CHAQ questionnaire - from 2.0 (1.3; 2.75) to 1.0 (0.6; 1.4), p<0,001.

Treatment with Adalimumab affected the laboratory parameters of disease activity.

After 4 weeks of treatment the trend to decrease in ESR was reported. By week 12 the median significantly decreased; by week 52 the median was normal in the most of patients (Figure 14).

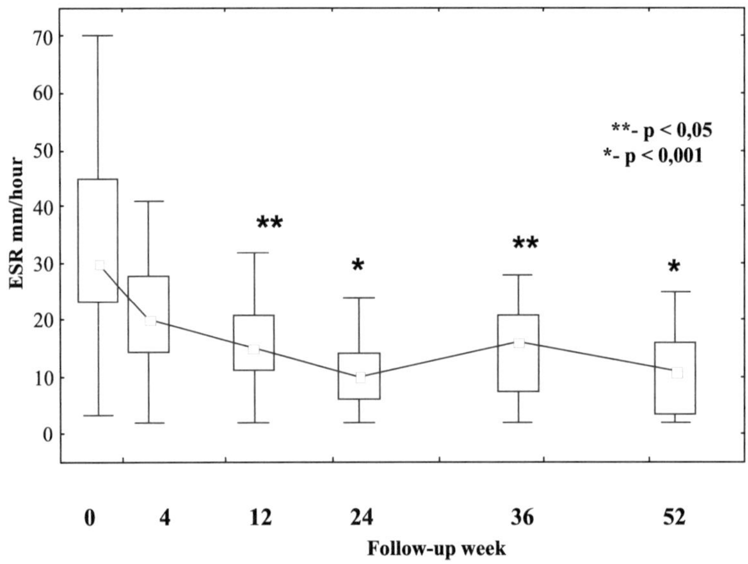

Figure 14. Dynamics in ESR in children with JIA treated with Adalimumab (n=104)

Significant decrease in the serum C-reactive protein level in all patients was observed after 8 weeks of treatment; the median parameter normalized after 12 weeks of treatment (Figure 15).

Assessment of Adalimumab efficacy according ACRpedi demonstrated that after 4 weeks of treatment the 30% improvement was achieved in 100% of patients, 50% improvement – in 80% (83), 70% improvement – in 55%(57) of patients. After 24 weeks 30% improvement was reported in 100% (104) of patients, 50% improvement – in 91% (95), 70% - in 74% (77) of patients; inactive disease was diagnosed in 55 % (58) of children. Within a year, JIA remission was diagnosed in 55% (58) of patients (Figure 16).

Prior to administration of Adalimumab, injection of conjunctiva, edema of iris, corneal precipitations, areas of inflammation in lens and optical nerve disk edema were found in all children with uveitis (Table 9).

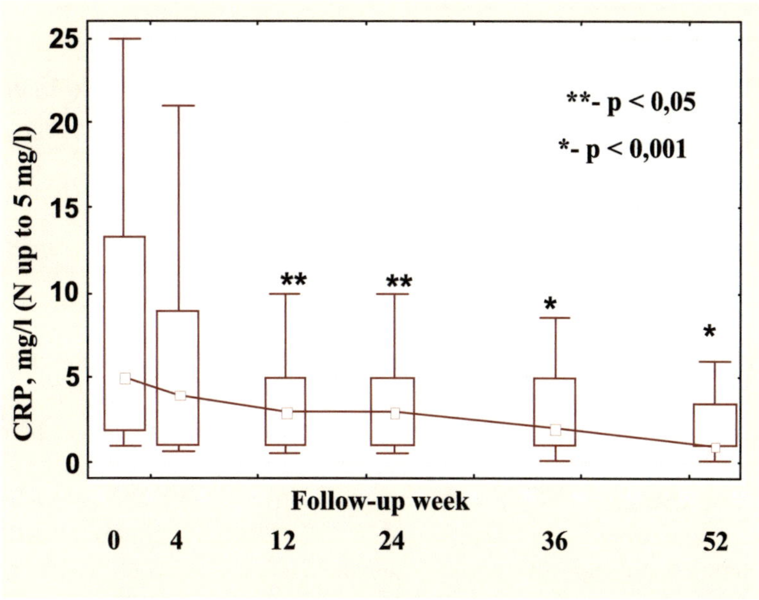

Figure 15. Dynamics in the serum CRP level in children with JIA treated with Adalimumab (n=104)

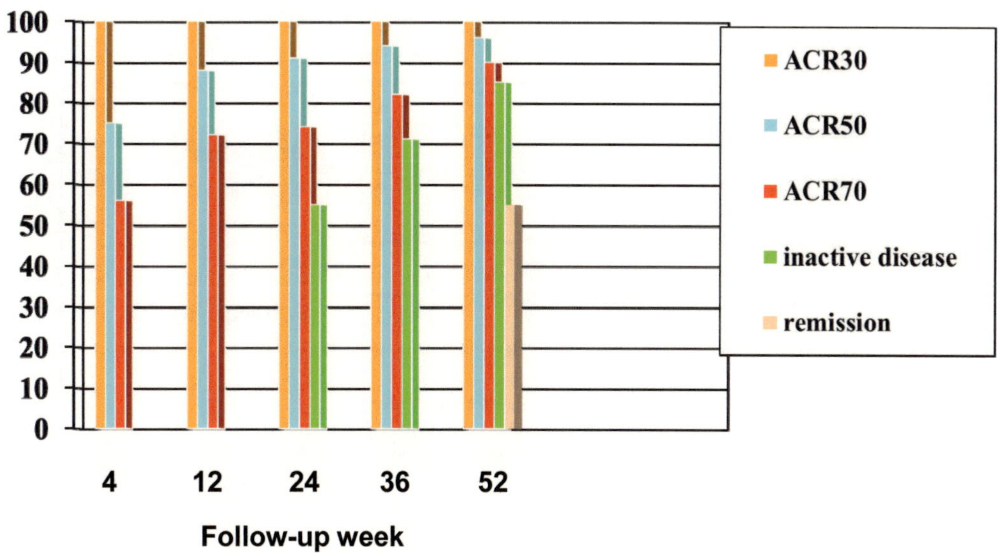

Figure 16. Response according to ACR pedi criteria in children with JIA treated with Adalimumab (n=104)

Parameter	Number of the affected eyes (n=80)
Injections of conjunctiva	85% (68/80)
Edema of iris	46% (37/80)
Corneal precipitations	40% (32/80)
Areas of inflammation in lens	21% (17/80)
Optical nerve disk edema	30% (24/80)

Table 9. Clinical manifestations of uveitis in patients with JIA included into the study

After 8 weeks of treatment complete management of conjunctiva injection, iris edema and optical nerve disk edema were reported in 55% (44/80) of the affected eyes - corneal precipitations disappeared in 45% (36/80); inflammation-associated changes of lens – in 18% (14/80) of eyes. Treatment-associated improvement of vision was found in 63 of 80 of the affected eyes; no changes of vision acuity were reported in 33 (41%) of the affected eyes. Dexamethazone eye drops were discontinued in 45% (22/48) of patients, NSAIDs eye drops – in 49% (24/48) of children; the dose of dexamethazone eye drops was reduced in 86% (41/48) of patients. The exacerbation of uveitis was persisting in 10% (8/80) of the affected eyes, subacute uveitis – in 25% (20/80); remission was found in 65% (52/80) of the affected eyes. After 24 weeks of treatment the cases of uveitis were not reported; subacute disease was observed in 22% (18/80) of eyes; remission was diagnosed in 78% (62/80) of the affected eyes. After 52 weeks of treatment remission was diagnosed in 83% of the affected eyes (66/80) (Figure 17).

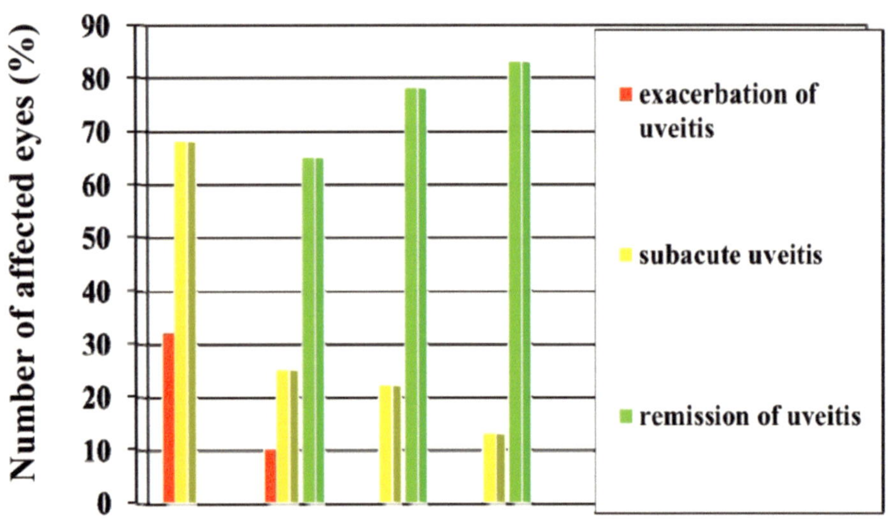

Figure 17. Efficacy of Adalimumab treatment in rheumatoid uveitis
(n=48, number of affected eyes = 80)

4.4. Adverse events related to immunosuppressive therapy

Safety evaluation was based on reported adverse events, laboratory parameters, and physical examination (evaluation of vital functions – BP, HR), and the ECG.

Adverse events were evaluated in all enrolled patients that received at least one injection of the study drug.

In general Adalimumab treatment was well-tolerated; most AE's were mild, reversible and would not result in treatment limitations. Injection reactions (occurring during the drug administration or during 24 hours after) included pain at the injection site – in 72.1 % (75) of patients; hyperemia at the injection site was reported in 48 % (50) of patients.

No cases of AE's associated with laboratory values alterations were reported.

No changes of vital functions (diastolic and systolic blood pressure, heart rate) or ECG changes were reported during the treatment course. Cases of Adalimumab discontinuation due to poor therapeutic response were not reported.

Therefore, safety profile of Adalimumab in study patients was satisfactory. Adverse events included local skin reactions at the injection sites. Adalimumab treatment was not associated with any fatal outcomes or cases of drug withdrawal due to adverse events.

One case of treatment discontinuation due to adverse events was reported in patient with suspected regional pulmonary tuberculosis. The patient was admitted to specialized hospital for further examination and development of treatment strategy. However, the diagnosis was not confirmed; the changes in lungs CT were considered to be the post-infection changes. Treatment with Adalimumab was restarted.

5. Clinical case

Patient's data: female. Age: 15 years old

Diagnosis: polyarticular JIA associated uveitis

5.1. Case history

Acute respiratory infections 3-4 times per year, rubella. Parents – practically healthy. Family history: no rheumatoid diseases reported.

Disease onset – February 1997 (age 1.5 years); swelling of the left ankle joint, walk disorders, pain associated with movements in left knee and ankle joints. The local surgeon excluded the diagnosis of acute surgical disease. Local treatment of the affected joints (ointments containing NSAIDs) was prescribed. April 1997, consultation of rheumatologist: diagnosis – juvenile rheumatoid arthritis, oligoarticular type; diclofenac-based treatment was prescribed. Treatment did not result in any decrease in swelling and pain.

Since May 1997, the patient was followed at the Rheumatology Department of one of clinics in Moscow. Disease severity was considered to be moderate. Swelling of knee and ankle joints with pain and limited mobility was reported. Blood analysis: leukocytosis (17×10^9/l), ESR increase (up to 62 mm/hour). Blood immunology analysis: positive C-reactive protein test and positive anti-nuclear factor test. Treatment: diclofenac sodium, intra-articular administration of glucocorticoids. Since January 1998 the patient was treated with methotrexate (dose 7.5 mg/m^2 of body surface/week). Methotrexate treatment was associated with mild improvements; the exacerbations of arthritis became less frequent. The intra-articular administration of glucocorticoids was conducted once per 1-2 months.

2001, spring: rheumatoid uveitis was diagnosed. Local treatment (dexamethasone eye drops, diclofenac eye drops) resulted in management of its manifestations.

Since October 2001, limited mobility of cervical part of the spine was reported; swelling of knee and ankle joints became more severe. The patient started complaining on severe morning stiffness. Only intra-articular administration of glucocorticoids resulted in certain improvements. Methotrexate dose was increased up to 10 mg/m^2 of body surface per week. July 2004: exposure to sunlight resulted in exacerbation of uveitis; combined immunosuppressive treatment (methotrexate plus cyclosporine, 3 mg/kg/day) was initiated. Combined treatment resulted in management of clinical manifestations of uveitis. Urine analysis: permanent macrohematuria was detected; therefore the immunosuppressive drugs were discontinued. Throughout a year the girl was receiving NSAIDs, with monthly intra-articular administrations of glucocorticosteroids. The treatment was ineffective. By November 2005, the number of joints affected by active arthritis increased; the polyarticular syndrome developed – elbow and radio-metacarpal joints, as well as knee and ankle joints and small joints of palms were involved. The disability was progressing. Oral prednisolone (5 mg/day) with leflunomide (10 mg/day, with gradual dose increase up to 20 mg/day) were prescribed. Despite the intra-articular administration of glucocorticoids into knee and ankle joints, complete management of the arthritis was not achieved. February 2007: prednisolone was discontinued.

Ineffective treatment with leflunomide, NSAIDs and monthly intra-articular injections of glucocorticoids were the basis for the prescription (January 2008) of anti-cytokine treatment with chimeric monoclonal antibodies to tumor necrosis factor (TNF) α (Infliximab, dose – 4.5 mg/kg). The first three infusions of Infliximab resulted in improvement; swelling of joints decreased, the duration of morning stiffness was shorter; the laboratory parameters reflecting the disease activity were decreasing. March 2008: metabolic nephropathy was diagnosed. Development of renal calculi was considered the side effect of leflunomide treatment; therefore, the drug was discontinued. March 2008: methotrexate (7.5 mg/m^2 of body surface area per week) was restarted. However, after the 4-th administration of Infliximab (same dose) resulted in exacerbation of swelling in the affected joints. The dose of Infliximab was increased up to 6.6 mg/kg. This dose of Infliximab was administered 5 times (total number of infliximab infusions – 9). Despite the dose increase, the therapy was not effective; the activity of arthritis was not changed. Therefore, intra-articular betamethasone injections (once per 1-1.5 months) were continued.

In order to develop the treatment strategy, the patient was admitted to the Rheumatology Department of the Scientific Center of Children's Health of RAMS (March 2009). It was 11 years after the onset of the disease. Disease was considered to be severe. Polyarthritis with affection of cervical spine, right shoulder joint, right elbow joint, femoral joints, knee joints, ankle joints, small joints of palms was diagnosed. The patient was unable to perform the full flexion of fingers; the movements in affected joints were limited and associated with pain. The patient complained on morning stiffness lasting up to 120 minutes. Paleness, blackness under the eyes, manifestations of hyper-corticism, associated with continuous intra-articular administration of exogenous glucocorticoids were found. The girl was in emotional depression. Blood analysis: elevated ESR (up to 57 mm/hour); serum level of C-reactive protein (up to 7.6%; normal level – up to 0.8 mg%, see Table). Computer tomography of knee joints: peri-articular osteoporosis, single erosions of bone tissue. Ophthalmologist's consultation: slowly progressing binocular rheumatoid uveitis was diagnosed.

The effect of intra-articular administration of glucocorticoids, associated with complications, and uncontrolled hormone dependency resulted in the decision to discontinue the hormone-based therapy. Analysis of health status demonstrated secondary inefficacy of the treatment with chimeric monoclonal antibodies to TNFα in combination with methotrexate. Infliximab was discontinued due to development of resistance. Despite the severe swelling of joints, glucocorticoids were not administered due to hormone dependency and growth retardation (height of the 13-years old adolescent girl was 146 cm – as of the 11-years old child).

According to the protocol of severe juvenile arthritis treatment, developed by the Scientific Center of Children's Health of RAMS, the girl was treated with pulse-therapy with methotrexate (50 mg/m^2 of body surface area) in combination with cyclosporine (4.4 mg/kg/day) .

The patient received 7 doses of methotrexate intravenously. The treatment resulted in certain improvement: the morning stiffness duration became shorter, and the girl became more active. However, the swelling of knee and ankle joints (Figure 18), limited mobility of the right shoulder joint (Figure 19), right elbow joint (Figure 20), knee joints (Figure 21), femoral joints (Figure 22) and ankle joints remained. Control blood analysis: the laboratory values reflecting the disease activity remained high (Table 10). Repeated ophthalmologic examination: manifestations of slowly progressing uveitis were found. The girl poorly tolerated methotrexate – severe headache and nausea were reported during 3 days after the drug administration. Within 1 month after the last intra-articular administration of betamethasone the withdrawal syndrome developed. It was manifested by myalgia, arthralgia, nausea, vomiting, and depression. Despite the development of the withdrawal syndrome, glucocorticoids were not restarted; active anti-rheumatic treatment was continued. The withdrawal syndrome resolved within 3 weeks.

The inefficacy of combined treatment with methotrexate (50 mg/m^2 of body surface area per week) and cyclosporine (4.4 mg/kg/day) as well as the good initial response to chimeric monoclonal antibodies to TNFα were the basis to prescribe the human antibodies to TNFα – Adalimumab.

5.2. Treatment with Adalimumab

Taking into considerations the facts mentioned above, it was decided to prescribe Adalimumab (dose – 40 mg once per 2 weeks) to patient A. The prescription was approved by the Scientific Council and the Ethics and Formulary Committees of Scientific Center for Children Health, RAMS. The parents signed the informed consent form, permitting the administration of drug. In order to exclude the diagnosis of tuberculosis prior to administration of Adalimumab, chest CT and dia-skin test (intra-cutaneous diagnostic test based on intra-cutaneous administration of 2 recombinant proteins of Mycobacterium tuberculosis) were conducted. No regional or infiltration changes were found during CT.

5.3. Results of treatment

After the exclusion of tuberculosis, Adalimumab treatment was initiated. The girl's activity improved after the first administration of the drug. Morning stiffness resolved within 2 weeks of treatment (Table 10). By the 4-th treatment week, swelling of the affected joints was completely managed; the volume of mobility has improved significantly. Within 6 weeks of Adalimumab treatment, laboratory values reflecting the disease activity returned to normal (Table 10). Control ophthalmological examination: remission of the slowly progressing uveitis was found. The girl continues receiving cyclosporine (total daily dose 4 mg/kg) and methotrexate (25 mg/m^2/week). At present, the girl has already received 10 doses of Adalimumab (40 mg); treatment was not associated with any adverse events. Treatment is associated with remission of the disease, as evaluated by clinical and laboratory values (Figure 18-22)

Therefore, this clinical report demonstrates a case of long-term juvenile idiopathic arthritis with continuous recurrence, characterized by rapid development of disability, high index of functional failure, poor quality of life, resistant to anti-rheumatic therapy, and secondary inefficacy of the chimeric monoclonal antibodies to TNFα. The Adalimumab treatment managed to overcome the resistance to chimeric antibodies and induced remission of arthritis, restoration of function of the affected joints, normalization of the laboratory values reflecting the activity of the disease. Positive effect of Adalimumab enabled the patient to overcome the severe corticosteroid dependency; the ability to decline the proposed oral prednisolone treatment strategy was achieved. Treatment results demonstrate that Adalimumab is highly effective in children with long-term polyarthritis and uveitis, resistant to various dosage regimens of methotrexate and in combination with cyclosporine, as well as with secondary resistance to chimeric antibodies to TNFα.

5.4. Adverse events

No serious adverse events were observed during the follow-up.

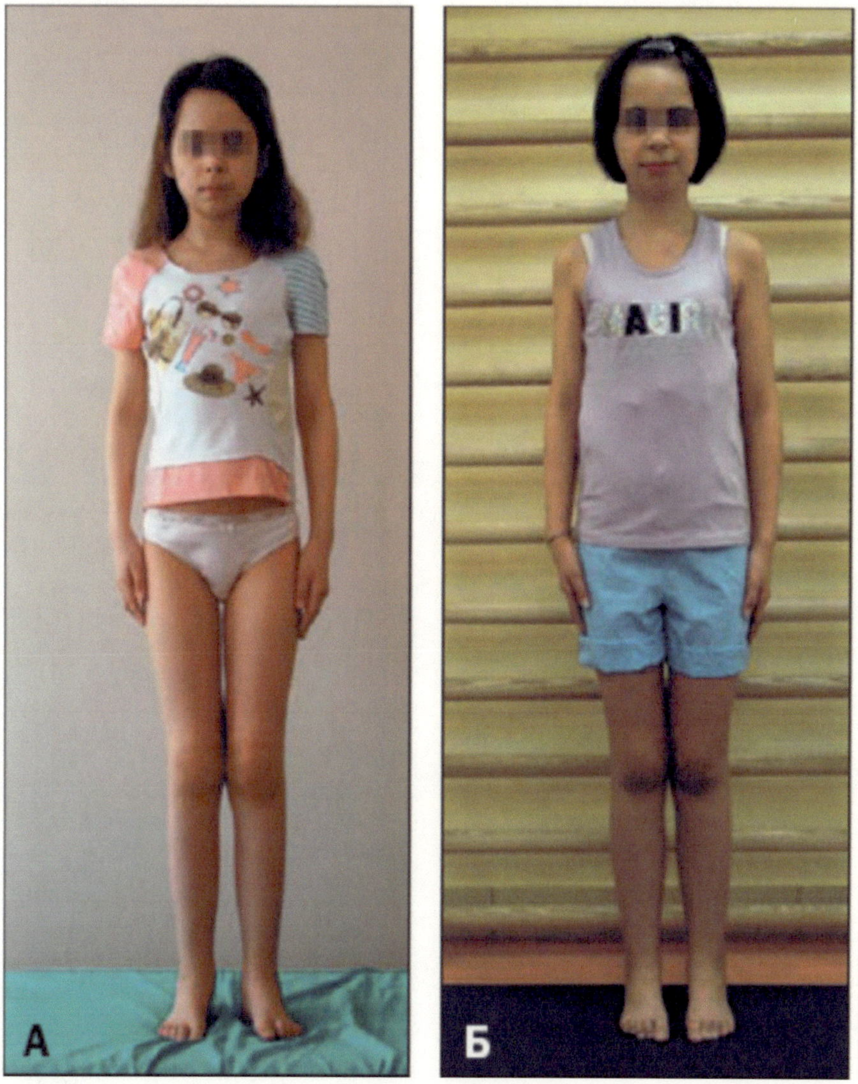

Figure 18. Patient A prior (A) and after (B) Adalimumab treatment

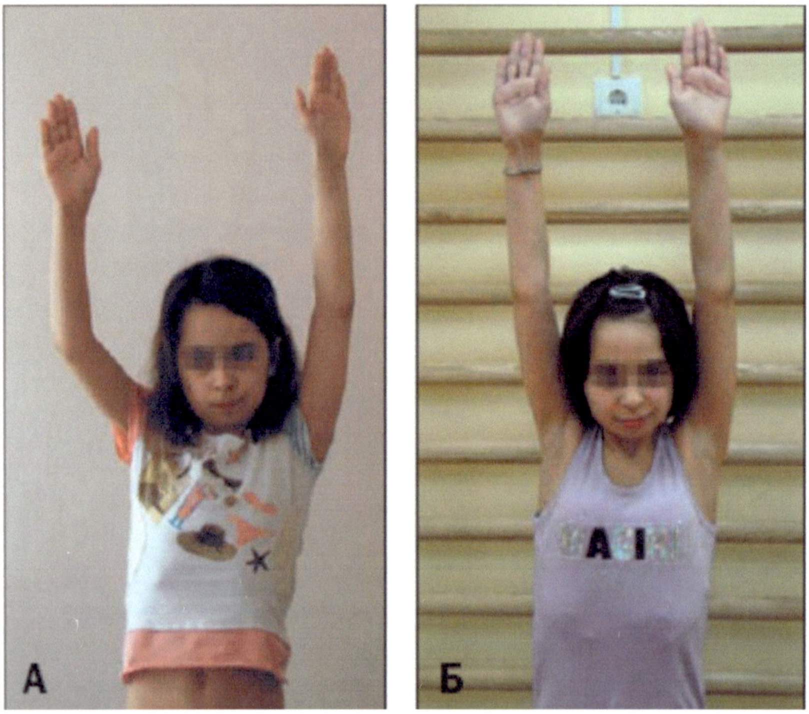

Figure 19. Functional ability of shoulder joints prior (A) and during (B) the Adalimumab treatment course

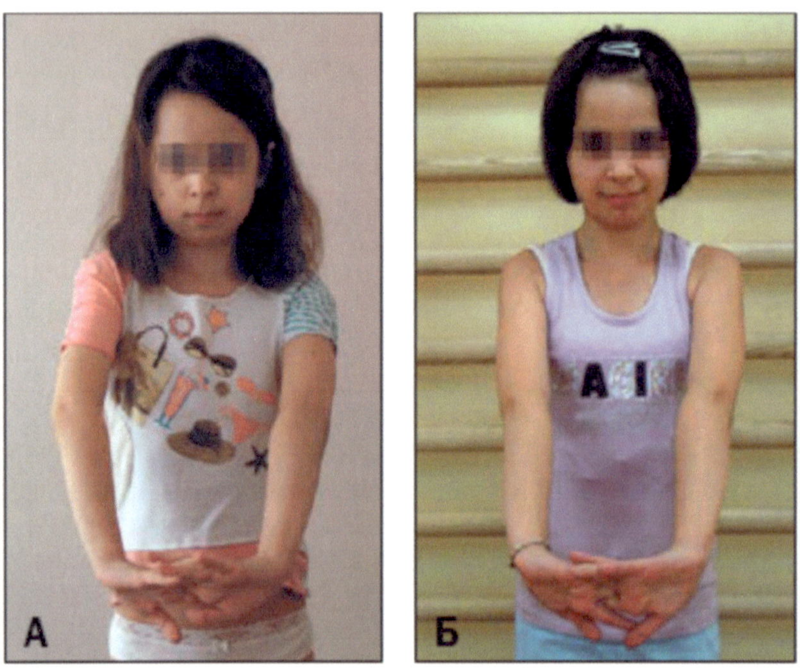

Figure 20. Functional ability of elbow joints prior (A) and during (B) Adalimumab treatment course

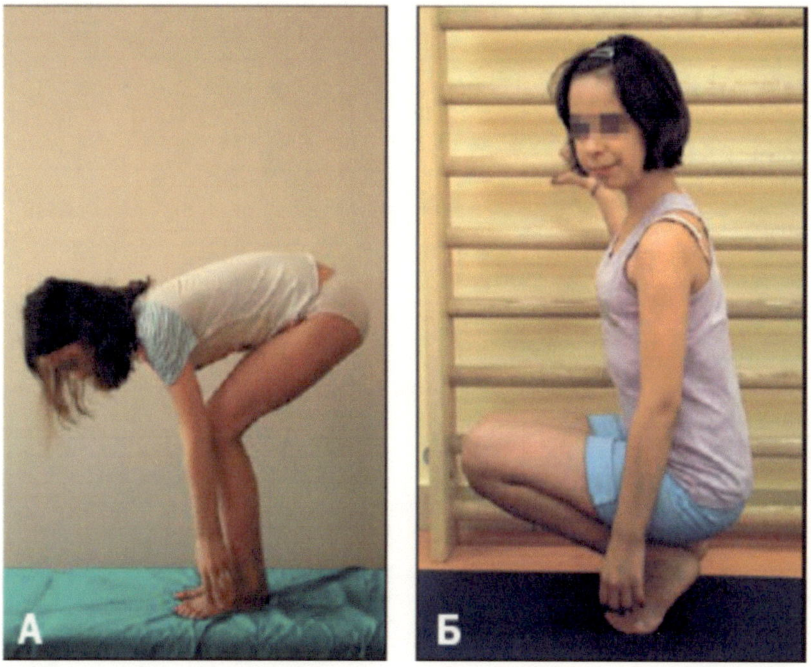

Figure 21. Functional ability of knee joints prior (A) and during (B) Adalimumab treatment course

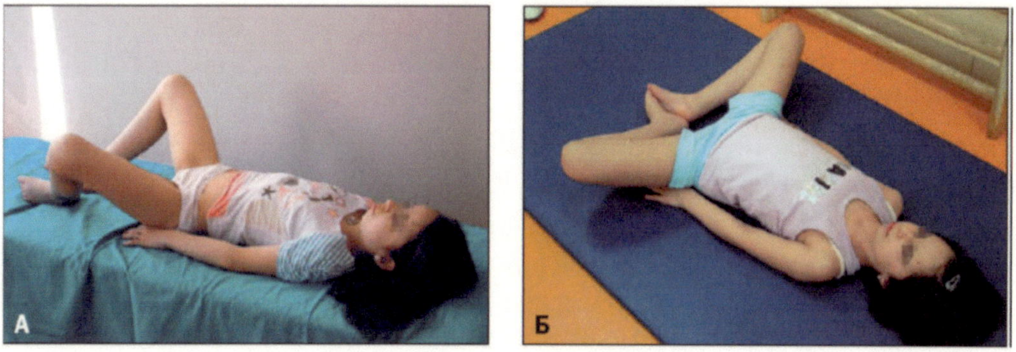

Figure 22. Functional ability of femoral joints prior (A) and during Adalimumab treatment course

Parameters	Prior to pulse-therapy with methotrexate and cyclosporine	Duration of Adalimumab therapy				
		Background	4 weeks	6 weeks	12 weeks	18 weeks
Duration of morning stiffness, min	120	100	0	0	0	0
Number of active joints	19	16	8	6	0	0
Number of joints with limitation of motion	19	15	7	4	0	0
CHAQ index of functional disability, score	1.6	1.7	1.1	0.6	0.5	0.5
Red blood cells $\times 10^{12}/l$	3.98	3.67	4.01	4.33	4.70	4.67
Hemoglobin, g/l	114	102	112	129	140	130
Leukocytes ($\times 10^9/l$)	8.	7.4	6.4	5.6	6.4	4.8
Platelets ($\times 10^9/l$)	308	426	378	313	359	287
ESR, (mm/h)	57	38	25	3	5	4
C-reactive protein, mg%	7.6	7.25	2.4	0.17	0.1	0.12
Height, cm	146	146	147	148	149	149

Table 10. Changes of clinical and laboratory parameters reflecting the activity of disease in association with Adalimumab treatment in patient a

6. Conclusion

Thus, the results of 1-year retrospective, observational trials showed high efficacy of Tocilizumab and Adalimumab in children with JIA.

Tocilizumab is effective in patients with the most severe form of juvenile idiopathic arthritis refractory to treatment with glucocorticoids, methotrexate, cyclosporine, combined immunosuppressive therapy and to TNF-α antagonists treatment. The drug induced remission of extra-articular manifestations, arthritis and normalized laboratory parameters of the disease activity without treatment with oral prednisolone, thus avoiding severe irreversible complications of glucocorticoid therapy. Tocilizumab induced disease remission in 43% of patients.

Adalimumab is effective in patients with polyarthritis associated with uveitis. The drug induced disease remission and improved functional activity and quality of life in 55% of patients. Reduction in uveitis activity and remission were reported in 83% of affected eyes. The high efficacy of Adalimumab allowed to avoid oral prednisolone and discontinue topical glucocorticoid therapy in patients with uveitis.

Both agents were well tolerated by patients; no severe serious adverse events were reported throughout the period of observation.

Author details

T.M. Bzarova, S.I. Valiyeva, R.V. Denisova, K.B. Isayeva,
A.M. Chomakhidze, T.V. Sleptsova, E.V. Mitenko, I.V. Dvoryakovskiy and M.V. Ryazanov
Scientific Center of Children's Health of RAMS, Moscow, Russia

A.A. Baranov, E.I. Alexeeva, L.S. Namazova-Baranova, E.G. Chistyakova and E.L. Semikina
Scientific Center of Children's Health of RAMS, Moscow, Russia
The First Moscow State Medical University I.M. Sechenov, Moscow, Russia

A.V. Starikova
The Helmholtz Moscow Research Institute of Eye Diseases, Moscow, Russia

7. References

[1] Cassidy J.T., Petty R.E. Juvenile idiopathic arthritis. In Cassidy JT, Petty RE, eds. Textbook of pediatric rheumatology, 6th edn. Philadelphia: WB Saunders. 2011.
[2] E.I. Alexeeva, S.I. Valeva et al. Efficacy and safety of repeat courses of rituximab treatment in patients with severe refractory juvenile idiopathic arthritis. Clinical Rheumatology 2011;(30)9:1163-1172
[3] Veldhuis G.J., Willemse PH.B., Sleijfer D.T., et al. Toxicity and efficacy of escalating dosages of recombinant human interleukin-6 after chemotherapy in patients with breast cancer or non-small-cell lung cancer // J. Clin. Oncol. 1995; 13:2585–2593.
[4] Rothwell N.J., Busbridge N.J., Lefeuvre R.A., Hardwick A.J. Interleukin-6 is a centrally acting endogenous pyrogen in the rat // Can. J. Physiol. Pharmacol. 1991; 69: 1465–1469.
[5] Castell J.V., Gomez-Lechon M.J., David M., et al. Recombinant human interleukin-6 (IL-6/BSF-2/HSF) regulates the synthesis of acute phase proteins in human hepatocytes // FEBS Lett. 1988; 232: 347–350.
[6] Nemeth E., Rivera S., Gabayan V., et al. IL-6 mediates hypoferremia of inflammation by inducing the synthesis of the iron regulatory hormone hepcidin // J. Clin. Invest. 2004; 113: P.1271–1276.
[7] Ikebuchi K., Wong G.G., Clark S.C., Ihle J.N., Hirai Y., Ogawa M. Interleukin-6 enhancement of interleukin-3-dependent proliferation of multipotential hemopoietic progenitors // Proc. Natl. Acad. Sci. USA. 1987; 84: 9035–9039.

[8] Kimura H., Ishibashi T., Uchida T., Maruyama Y., Friese P., Burstein S.A. Interleukin 6 is a differentiation factor for human megakaryocytes in vitro // Eur. J. Immunol. 1990; 20: 1927–1931.

[9] Tsigos C., Papankolaou D.A., Defensor R., Mitsiadis C.S., Kyrou I., Chrousos G.P. Dose-effects of recombinant human interleukin-6 on pituitary hormone secretion and energy expenditure // Neuroendocrinology. 1997; 66: 54–62.

[10] Heliovaara M.K., Teppo A.M., Karonen S.L., Tuominen J.A., Ebeling P. Plasma IL-6 concentration is inversely related to insulin sensitivity, and acute phase proteins associate with glucose and lipid metabolism in healthy subjects // Diabetes Obes. Metab. 2005; 7: 729–736.

[11] Cutolo M., Straub R.H. Circadian rhythms in arthritis: hormonal effects on the immune/inflammatory reaction // Autoimmun. Rev. 2008; 7: P.223–228.

[12] Nishimoto N. Kishimoto T. Humanized antihuman IL-6 receptor antibody, tocilizumab // Handb. Exp. Pharmacol. 2008; 181: 151-160.

[13] European Medicines Agency. RoActemra (tocilizumab): summary of product characteristics [online]. Available from URL: http://www.emea.europa.eu/humandoes/PDFs/EPAR/RoActemra/H-955-PI-en.pdf [accessed 2009 Mar 23].

[14] Chugai Pharmactutical Co. Actemra, a humanized antihuman IL-6 receptor monoclonal antibody obtained approval for indications of rheumatoid arthritis, polyarticular-course juvenile idiopathic arthritis and systemic-onset juvenile idiopathic arthritis [media release]. Available from URL: http://www.chugai-pharm.co.jp [accessed 2008 Sep 24].

[15] Imagawa T., Ozawa R., Miyamae T., et al. Efficacy and safety in 48-week treatment of tocilizumab in children with polyaticular course JIA with polyarticlar or olygoarticular onset // Ann. Rheum. Dis. 2007; 66(Suppl. II): 550.

[16] Yokota S., Imagawa T., Miyamae T. Safety and efficacy of up to three years of continuous tocilizumab therapy in children with systemic-onset juvenile idiopathic arthritis [SAT0536] // Ann. Rheum. Dis. 2009; 68 (Suppl. 3):715.

[17] Inaba Y., Aoki C., Ozawa R. Radiologic evaluation of large joints during tocilizumab treatment in children with systemic juvenile idiopathic arthritis [SAT0555] // Ann. Rheum. Dis. 2009; 68(Suppl. 3):720.

[18] Yokota S., Imagawa T., Mori M., et al. Efficacy and safety of tocilizumab in patients with systemic-onset juvenile idiopathic arthritis: a randomized, double-blind, placebo-controlled, withdrawal phase III trial // Lancet. 2008; 371: 998-1006.

[19] Yokota S., Miyamae T., Imagawa T., et al.: Therapeutic efficacy of humanized recombinant anti-interleukin-6 receptor antibody in children with systemic-onset juvenile idiopathic arthritis // Arthritis Rheum. 2005; 52: 818-825.

[20] Aoki C., Inaba Y., Ozawa R. Effects of tocilizumab on radiological findings in polyarticular juvenile idiopathic arthritis [OP-0145] // Ann. Rheum. Dis. 2009; 68(Suppl. 3):118.

[21] Quartier P., Maire D., Souabni L. Efficacy and safety of tocilizumab in systemic onset juvenile idiopathic arthritis in french centers [FRI0462] // Ann. Rheum. Dis. 2009; 68(Suppl. 3): 506.

[22] Kaneko U., Imagawa T., Kishi T. Discrepancy between progression of joint damage and improvement of systemic inflammation in patients with systemic-onset juvenile idiopathic arthritis treated with tocilizumab [SAT0548] // Ann. Rheum. Dis. 2009; 68(Suppl.3): 719.

[23] Yokota S., Imagawa T., Miyamae T. Safety and efficacy of up to three years of continuous tocilizumab therapy in children with systemic-onset juvenile idiopathic arthritis [SAT0536] // Ann. Rheum. Dis. 2009:.68 (Suppl. 3.): 715.

[24] De Benedetti F., Brunner H., Ruperto N.et al. Efficacy and Safety of Tocilizumab (TCZ) in Patients with Systemic Juvenile Idiopathic Arthritis (sJIA): TENDER 52-Week Data [OP0006] // Ann. Rheum. Dis. 2011;70 (Suppl 3):67

[25] Furst DE, Schiff MH, Fleischmann RM, Strand V, Birbara CA, Compagnone D, et al. Adalimumab, a fully human anti tumor necrosis factor *a* monoclonal antibody, and concomitant standard antirheumatic therapy for the treatment of rheumatoid arthritis results of STAR (Safety Trial of Adalimumab in Rheumatoid Arthritis). // J Rheumatol – 2003. – 30. – P. 2563-2571

[26] Weinblatt ME, Keystone EC, Furst DE, Moreland LW, Weisman MH, Birbara CA, et al Adalimumab, a fully human anti-tumor necrosis factor *a* monoclonal antibody, for the treatment of rheumatoid arthritis in patients taking concomitant methotrexate the ARMADA trial [published erratum appears in Arthritis Rheum 2003,48 855]. Arthritis Rheum - 2003 - 48 – P. 35-45

[27] Keystone EC, Kavanaugh AF, Sharp JT, Tannenbaum H, Hua Y, Teoh LS, et al Radiographic, clinical, and functional outcomes of treatment with adalimumab (a human anti-tumor necrosis factor monoclonal antibody) in patients with active rheumatoid arthritis receiving concomitant methotrexate therapy a randomized, placebo-controlled, 52-week trial. // Arthritis Rheum - 2004 – 50 – P. 1400-1411

[28] Van de Putte LB, Atkins C, Malaise M, Sany J, Russell AS, van Riel PL, et al Efficacy and safety of adalimumab as monotherapy in patients with rheumatoid arthritis for whom previous disease modifying antirheumatic drug treatment has failed. // Ann Rheum Dis. – 2004. – 63. – P. 508-516

[29] Mease PJ, Gladman DD, Ritchhn CT, Ruderman EM, Steinfeld SD, Choy EH, et al, for the ADEPT Study Group Adalimumab for the treatment of patients with moderately to severely active psoratic arthritis results of a double-blind, randomized, placebo-controlled trial. // Arthritis Rheum. - 2005. – 52. – P. 3279-3289.

[30] Lipsky P.E., van der Heijde D.M.F.M, St Clair E.W. et al. Infliximab and methotrexate in the treatment of rheumatoid arthritis. // N Engl J Med. – 2000. – 343. – P.1594-1602

[31] Feldman M., Brennan P., Maini R. Role of cytokines in rheumatoid arthritis. Annu. Rev. Immunol., 1996, 14, 397-440

[32] Beutler B. The rote of tumor necrosis factor in health and disease. J. Rheumatol., 1999. 26 (Suppl. 57), 16-21

[33] Aikawa NE, De Carvalho JF, Silva CA et al Immunogenicity of anti-TNFα agents in autoimmune diseases. Clinic Rev Allerg Immunol, 2010. 38(2–3):82–89

[34] Moreland LW, Cohen SB, Baumgartner SW, Tindall EA, Bulpitt K, Martin R, et al Long-term safety and efficacy of etanercept in patients with rheumatoid arthritis. // J Rheumatol - 2001. – 28. – P. 1238-44

[35] Breedveld FC, Weisman MH, Kavanaugh AF, Cohen SB, Pavelka K, van Vollenhoven R, for the PREMIER investigators, et al. The PREMIER study a multicenter, randomized, double blind clinical trial of combination therapy with adalimumab plus methotrexate versus methotrexate alone or adalimumab alone in patients with early, aggressive rheumatoid arthritis who had not had previous methotrexate treatment. // Arthritis Rheum 2006. - 54. - P: 26-37

[36] Burmester GR, Manette X Montecucco CM et al. Adalimumab alone and in combination with disease-modifying antirheumatic drugs for the treatment of rheumatoid arthritis in clinical practice the Research in Active Rheumatoid Arthritis (ReAct) trial. // Ann Rheum Dis. Published Online First 20 March 2007 doi:10.1136/ard. – 2006 066761

[37] Bombardieri S., Ruiz A.A., Fardellone P., Geusens P.. McKenna F., Unnebrink K., Oezer U., Kary S., Kupper H., Burmester G.R. on behalf of ReAct Stusy Group. Effectiveness of adalimumab for rheumatoid arthritis in patients with a history of TNF-antagonist therapy in clinical practice. // Rheumatology Advance Access published May 15, 2007 doi:10.1093/rheumatology/kem091

[38] Nicas SN, Voulgan PV, Alamanos Y *et al.* Efficacy and safety of switching from Infliximab to adalimumab a comparative controlled study. // Ann Rheum Dis. - 2006. - 65. - P: 257-60

[39] Bennett AN, Peterson P, Zain A, Grumley J, Panayi G, Kirkham B Adalimumab in clinical practice Outcome in 70 rheumatoid arthritis patients, including comparison of patients with and without previous anti-TNF exposure. // Rheumatology. - 2005. - 44. - P. 1026-31

[40] Bijl AE, Breedveld FC, Antoni CE *et. al.* Adalimumab (HUMIRA») is effective in treating patients with rheumatoid arthritis who previously failed infliximab [abstract SAT0062]. // Ann Rheum Dis/ - 2005. - 64 (Suppl III) 428

[41] Wick MC, Ernestam S, Lmdblad S, Bratt J, Klareskog L, van Vollenhoven RF Adalimumab (Humira) restores clinical response in patients with secondary loss of efficacy from infliximab (Remicade) or etanercept (Enbrel) results from the STURE registry at Karohnska University Hospital Scand. // J Rheumatol. - 2005 - 34. – P. 353-8

[42] Brocq O, Albert C, Roux C, Gerard D, Breuil V, Ziegler LE Adalimumab in rheumatoid arthritis after failed infliximab and/or etanercept therapy experience with 18 patients. // Joint Bone Spine. - 2004. – 71. P. 601-3

[43] Haibel H, Rudwaleit M, Listing J et al. Efficacy of adalimumab in the treatment of axial spondylarthritis without radiographically defined sacroiliitis: results of a twelve-week randomized, double-blind, placebo-controlled trial followed by an open-label extension up to week fifty-two. Arthritis Rheum. 2008 Jul;58(7):1981-91

[44] Wijbrandts CA, Klaasen R, Dijkgraaf MG et al. Bone mineral density in rheumatoid arthritis patients 1 year after adalimumab therapy: arrest of bone loss? Ann Rheum Dis., ARD Online First, published on April 13, 2008 as 10.1136/ard.2008.091611

[45] Kimel M, Cifaldi M, Chen N, Revicki D. Adalimumab plus methotrexate improved SF-36 scores and reduced the effect of rheumatoid arthritis (RA) on work activity for patients with early RA. J Rheumatol. 2008 Feb;35(2):206-15

[46] Лучихина Е.Л., Каратеев Д.Е.,Насонов Е.Л. Первый опыт применения адалимумаба в России: предварительные результаты 24 недельного открытого исследования. Научно-практическая ревматология. 2008, №5 стр. 59-63

[47] Lovell D.; Ruperto N.; Reiff A.; Jung Lawrence K.; Higgins G; Koné-Paut I; Jones Olcay Y.; McIlraith Melissa J.; Andhivarothai N.; Kupper H.; Giannini Edward H.; Peterson T; Martini A. Long-Term Efficacy and Safety of Adalimumab for up to 6 Years in Patients with Juvenile Idiopathic Arthritis. Abstract presented at: 75th Annual scientific meeting of the American College of Rheumatology (ACR) and the 46th Annual meeting of the Association of Rheumatology Health Professionals (ARHP); 11/5/2011 Chicago, IL; USA. Abstract MIS (7190791).

[48] Lovell Daniel J. et al. OLE DE 038 : Long-Term Efficacy and Safety of ADA for up to 6 years in Patients with JIA. ACR11 – arthritis & rheumatism volume 63, number10 (supplement) october 2011 abstract 265

[49] Luciana Breda, Marianna Del Torto, Sara De Sanctis, Francesco Chiarelli Biologics in children's autoimmune disorders: efficacy and safety. Eur J Pediatr (2011) 170:157–167

[50] Dana MR, Merayo-Lloves J, Schaumberg DA, Forster CS. Visual outcomes prognosticators in juvenile rheumatoid arthritis-associated uveitis. //Ophthalmology. - 1997. – 104. - P.236-44.

[51] Foster CS. Diagnosis and treatment of juvenile idiopathic arthritis associated uveitis. // Current Opin Ophthalmol. - 2003. – 14. – P. 395-8.

[52] BenEzra D, Cohen E, Maftzir G. Uveitis in children and adolescents. // Br J Ophthalmol. - 2006. – 89. – P. 444-8.

[53] Tynjala P., Kotaniemi K., Lindahl P., Latva K., Aalto K., Honkanen V., Lahdenne P. Adalimumab in the treatment of Juvenile Idiopathic Arthritis associated Uveitis – A Pilot Study. Abstract presented at: 8th Annual European League Against Rheumatism (EULAR 2007); June 13-16, 2007; Barcelona, Spain. Abstract THU0483.

[54] G. Schett, L C Coates, Zoe R Ash, S Finzel, P G Conaghan Structural damage in rheumatoid arthritis, psoriatic arthritis, and ankylosing spondylitis: traditional views, novel insights gained from TNF blockade, and concepts for the future. Arthritis Research & Therapy 2011, 13(Suppl 1):S4

[55] Liza B. Vazquez-cobian, MD, Thomas Flynn, MD, and Thomas J. A. Lehman, MD Adalimumab therapy for childhood uveitis. // J Pediatr. - 2006. -149.- P.572-575.

[56] Tynjälä P, Kotaniemi K, Lindahl P et. al. Adalimumab in juvenile idiopathic arthritis-associated chronic anterior uveitis. Rheumatology (Oxford). 2008 Mar;47(3):339-44. Epub 2008 Jan 31

[57] Biester S, Deuter C, Michels H et al. Adalimumab in the therapy of uveitis in childhood. Br J Ophthalmol. 2007 Mar; 91(3):274-6

[58] Heiligenhaus A, Horneff G, Greiner K et al. Inhibitors of tumour necrosis factor-alpha for the treatment of arthritis and uveitis in childhood. Klin Monatsbl Augenheilkd. 2007 Jun;224(6):526-31

[59] Foeldvari I, Nielsen S, Kümmerle-Deschner J et al. Tumor necrosis factor-alpha blocker in treatment of juvenile idiopathic arthritis-associated uveitis refractory to second-line agents: results of a multinational survey. Nat Clin Pract Rheumatol. 2007 Nov;3(11):608-9.

[60] Cassidy JT, Petty RE., Laxer R.M., Lindsley C.B. Textbook of pediatric rheumatology. 6th ed. Philadelphia: Saunders Elsevier; 2010; 794 p.

[61] Dixon W.G., Watson K., Lunt M. et al. (2006) British Society for Rheumatology Biologics Register. Rates of serious infection, including site-specific and bacterial intracellular infection, in rheumatoid arthritis patients receiving anti-tumor necrosis factor therapy^ results from the British Society for Rheumatology Biologic register. Arthritis Rheum 54(8);2368-2376.

[62] Hogan MJ., Rimura SJ., Thygeson P.. Signs and symptoms of uveitis: I. Anterior uveitis. Am. J. Ophthalmol.–1959.–Vol. 47.–P. 155–170.

[63] C.A., Ruperto N., Gannini E. et al. Preliminary criteria for clinical remission for select categories of juvenile idiopathic arthritis // J.Rheumatol. – 2004. – V.31, № 11. – P.2290-2294.